Acute Medicine

D1331038

WITHDRAWN FROM
LIBRARY
BRITISH MEDICAL ASSOCIATION

1002775

Acute Medicine

A practical guide to the management of medical emergencies

Edited by

David Sprigings

Consultant Physician 1993–2016,
Northampton General Hospital, Northampton, UK

John B. Chambers

Professor of Clinical Cardiology and Consultant Cardiologist
Guy's and St Thomas' Hospitals, London, UK

FIFTH EDITION

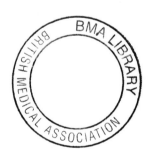

BMA LIBRARY
BRITISH MEDICAL ASSOCIATION

WILEY Blackwell

This edition first published 2018
© 2018 John Wiley & Sons Ltd

Edition History
© *2008 David Sprigings and John B. Chambers* © *1990, 1995, 2001 Blackwell Science Ltd*

All rights reserved. No part of this publication may be reproduced, stored in a retrieval system, or transmitted, in any form or by any means, electronic, mechanical, photocopying, recording or otherwise, except as permitted by law. Advice on how to obtain permission to reuse material from this title is available at http://www.wiley.com/go/permissions.

The right of David Sprigings and John B. Chambers to be identified as editors of this work has been asserted in accordance with law.

Registered Offices
John Wiley & Sons, Inc., 111 River Street, Hoboken, NJ 07030, USA
John Wiley & Sons Ltd, The Atrium, Southern Gate, Chichester, West Sussex, PO19 8SQ, UK

Editorial Office
9600 Garsington Road, Oxford, OX4 2DQ, UK

For details of our global editorial offices, customer services, and more information about Wiley products visit us at www.wiley.com.

Wiley also publishes its books in a variety of electronic formats and by print-on-demand. Some content that appears in standard print versions of this book may not be available in other formats.

Limit of Liability/Disclaimer of Warranty
The contents of this work are intended to further general scientific research, understanding, and discussion only and are not intended and should not be relied upon as recommending or promoting scientific method, diagnosis, or treatment by physicians for any particular patient. The publisher and the authors make no representations or warranties with respect to the accuracy and completeness of the contents of this work and specifically disclaim all warranties, including without limitation any implied warranties of fitness for a particular purpose. In view of ongoing research, equipment modifications, changes in governmental regulations, and the constant flow of information relating to the use of medicines, equipment, and devices, the reader is urged to review and evaluate the information provided in the package insert or instructions for each medicine, equipment, or device for, among other things, any changes in the instructions or indication of usage and for added warnings and precautions. Readers should consult with a specialist where appropriate. The fact that an organization or website is referred to in this work as a citation and/or potential source of further information does not mean that the author or the publisher endorses the information the organization or website may provide or recommendations it may make. Further, readers should be aware that websites listed in this work may have changed or disappeared between when this work was written and when it is read. No warranty may be created or extended by any promotional statements for this work. Neither the publisher nor the author shall be liable for any damages arising herefrom.

Library of Congress Cataloging-in-Publication Data

Names: Sprigings, David, editor. | Chambers, John (John Boyd), editor. |
    Preceded by (work): Sprigings, David. Acute medicine.
Title: Acute medicine : a practical guide to the management of medical
    emergencies / edited by David Sprigings, John Chambers.
Other titles: Acute medicine (Sprigings)
Description: Fifth edition. | Chichester, UK ; Hoboken, NJ : John Wiley &
Sons, Inc., 2018. |
    Preceded by Acute medicine / David Sprigings, John Chambers. 4th ed. 2008.
    | Includes bibliographical references and index.
Identifiers: LCCN 2016057155 (print) | LCCN 2016059907 (ebook) | ISBN
    9781118644287 (paperback) | ISBN 9781118644263 (pdf) | ISBN 9781118644270
    (epub)
Subjects: | MESH: Emergencies | Emergency Treatment--methods | Handbooks
Classification: LCC RC86.8 (print) | LCC RC86.8 (ebook) | NLM WB 39 | DDC
    616.02/5--dc23
LC record available at https://lccn.loc.gov/2016057155

Cover Design: Wiley
Cover Image: © Chad Baker/Jason Reed/Ryan McVay/Gettyimages

Set in 8/12 pt FrutigerLTStd-Light by Thomson Digital, Noida, India
Printed and bound in Malaysia by Vivar Printing Sdn Bhd

10 9 8 7 6 5 4 3 2 1

For Natasha and Helen

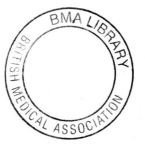

Contents

Neurological, 402

Abdominal, 446

Metabolic, 487

Skin and Musculoskeletal, 543

Haematology and Miscellaneous, 568

Section 3: Techniques and Procedures in Acute Medicine, 639

Contributors

Simon Anderson
Consultant Physician and Gastroenterologist, Guy's and St Thomas' NHS Foundation Trust, UK
Honorary Lecturer, King's College, London
Chapters 20, 21, 22, 73

Mike Beadsworth
Clinical Director, Tropical and Infectious Disease Unit, Royal Liverpool University Hospital,
Liverpool, UK
Honorary Senior Lecturer in Infectious Diseases, Department of Molecular and Clinical
Pharmacology, University of Liverpool, Liverpool, UK
Chapter 33

Nick Beeching
Senior Lecturer (Clinical) in Infectious Diseases, Department of Clinical Sciences, Liverpool
School of Tropical Medicine, Liverpool, UK
Honorary Consultant in Infectious Diseases, Tropical and Infectious Disease Unit, Royal
Liverpool University Hospital, Liverpool, UK
Chapters 33, 34

Ajay Bhalla
Consultant Stroke Physician and Honorary Senior Lecturer, Department of Ageing and Health,
Guy's and St Thomas' NHS Foundation Trust, UK
Chapters 65, 66

Michael Canty
Specialty Registrar in Neurosurgery, Institute of Neurological Sciences, Queen Elizabeth University Hospital,
Glasgow, UK
Chapters 29, 67, 70, 72

Vito Carone
Partnerships in Care, Meadow View Hospital, Glenworth, UK
Chapters 81, 82, 83, 84

Paul Carroll
Consultant Endocrinologist, Guy's and St Thomas' NHS Foundation Trust, UK
Chapters 85, 90, 91, 92, 93, 94

John B. Chambers
Consultant Cardiologist and Professor of Clinical Cardiology at Guy's and St Thomas' Hospitals, London
Chapters 6, 7, 10, 39, 45, 46, 47, 48, 49, 50, 51, 52, 53, 54, 55, 105, 114

Mas Chaponda
Consultant in Infectious Diseases, HIV Services, Royal Liverpool University Hospital, Liverpool, UK
Honorary Senior Lecturer in Clinical Pharmacology, Department of Molecular and Clinical
Pharmacology, University of Liverpool, Liverpool, UK
Chapter 34

Vincent Connolly
Regional Medical Director, North, NHS Improvement & Consultant Physician, James Cook University Hospital,
Middlesbrough, UK
Introduction

Simon Conroy
Honorary Professor of Geriatric Medicine, Department of Health Sciences, College of Medicine,
Biological Sciences and Psychology, University of Leicester, Centre for Medicine, UK
Chapters 5, 31

Michael Cooklin
Consultant Cardiologist, Guy's and St Thomas' Hospitals, London
Chapters 40, 41, 42, 43, 44, 58

John Corcoran
Clinical Research Fellow and Honorary Specialty Registrar
Oxford Centre for Respiratory Medicine, Churchill Hospital, Oxford, UK
Chapter 122

James Crane
Clinical Research Fellow in Diabetes and Endocrinology
Guy's and St Thomas' NHS Foundation Trust, UK
Chapters 85, 90, 91, 92, 93, 94

Alexandra Croom
Consultant Allergist, Spire Leicester Hospital, Leicester UK
Chapters 27, 38

Martin Crook
Consultant in Clinical Biochemistry and Metabolic Medicine, Guy's, St Thomas' and Lewisham and
Greenwich NHS Trusts, UK
Visiting Professor, University of Greenwich and Trinity College Dublin, UK
Chapters 85, 86, 87, 88, 89

Nemesha Desai
Consultant Dermatologist, St John's Institute of Dermatology, Guy's and St Thomas' NHS Foundation Trust, UK
Chapters 26, 96

Andrew Dixon
Consultant Gastroenterologist, Kettering General Hospital NHS Trust, UK
Chapters 74, 75, 76

Louise Free
Consultant in Palliative Medicine, St Wilfrid's Hospice and East Sussex Healthcare NHS Trust,
Eastbourne, UK
Chapter 110

Charlotte Frise
Consultant in Obstetric Medicine and General Medicine, Oxford University Hospitals NHS Foundation Trust, UK
Honorary Senior Clinical Lecturer in Obstetric Medicine, Nuffield Department of Obstetrics and Gynaecology,
University of Oxford, UK
Chapter 32

Matthew Frise
Specialty Registrar in General Internal Medicine and Intensive Care Medicine
Oxford Deanery, UK
Chapters 59, 112

Luna Gargani
Institute of Clinical Physiology, National Research Council, Pisa, Italy
Chapter 114

Francesca Garnham
Consultant in Emergency Medicine, Guys and St Thomas' NHS Foundation Trust, UK
Chapters 108, 109

David Garry
Consultant in Intensive Care Medicine & Anaesthetics, Oxford University Hospitals NHS Foundation Trust, UK
Chapter 117

Guy Glover
Consultant in Critical Care, Guy's and St Thomas' NHS Foundation Trust, King's College London, UK
Chapter 35

Rob Hallifax
Clinical Research Fellow, Oxford University Hospitals NHS Foundation Trust, UK
Chapter 64

Claire Harrison
Consultant Haematologist, Guy's and St Thomas' NHS Foundation Trust, UK
Chapters 100, 102

Deborah Hay
Honorary Consultant Haematologist and Clinical Tutor for Pathology, Nuffield Division of Clinical Laboratory
Sciences, Radcliffe Department of Medicine, University of Oxford, UK
Chapter 101

Carolyn Hemsley
Infectious Diseases and Microbiology Consultant, Department of Infectious Diseases,
Guy's and St Thomas' NHS Foundation Trust, UK
Chapter 80

Catherine Hildyard
Specialist Registrar in Haematology, Oxford University Hospitals NHS Foundation Trust, UK
Chapter 103

Sandeep Hothi
Specialty Registrar in Cardiology and General Internal Medicine, Glenfield Hospital, Leicester, UK
Chapters 8, 9, 116, 119, 120, 121

Jo Howard
Consultant Haematologist, Sickle Cell Service, Guy's and St Thomas' NHS Foundation Trust, UK
Chapter 104

Manohara Kenchaiah
Consultant Physician and Endocrinologist
Northampton General Hospital NHS Trust, UK
Chapters 81, 82, 83, 84

John L. Klein
Consultant Microbiologist, Department of Infectious Diseases, Guy's and St Thomas' NHS Foundation Trust, UK
Chapters 52, 68, 95, 98

Ruth Lamb
Consultant Dermatologist, St George's University Hospital NHS Foundation Trust & Consultant
Dermatologist, Hidradenitis Suppurativa Clinic, Guy's and St Thomas' NHS Foundation Trust, UK
Chapter 26

Nigel Langford
Honorary Senior Lecturer to University of Leicester, Consultant in Acute Medicine and Clinical Pharmacology,
University Hospitals of Leicester, Leicester Royal Infirmary, UK
Chapter 36

Tom Lloyd
Former Senior Medicolegal Advisor, Medical Protection Society, London, UK
Chapter 111

Raashid Luqmani
Professor of Rheumatology, Nuffield Department of Orthopaedics, Rheumatology and Musculoskeletal Science,
University of Oxford, UK
Chapter 99

Bridget MacDonald
Consultant Neurologist, Croydon University and St George's Hospitals, UK
Chapter 16

Lucy Mackillop
Consultant Obstetric Physician, Oxford University Hospitals NHS Foundation Trust
Honorary Senior Clinical Lecturer, Nuffield Department of Obstetrics and Gynaecology, University of Oxford, UK
Chapter 32

Seshi Manam
Consultant Dermatologist, Guy's and St Thomas' NHS Foundation Trust, UK
Chapter 96

Swapna Mandal
Consultant Respiratory Physician, Royal Free NHS Foundation Trust, UK
Chapter 60

Janine Mansi
Consultant Medical Oncologist, Guy's and St Thomas' NHS Foundation Trust and Biomedical Research Centre, King's College, London, UK
Chapter 105

Charlotte Masterton-Smith
Specialty Registrar in Acute Medicine, Kingston Hospital, UK
Chapter 56

Angelique Mastihi
Medical Protection Society, Edinburgh, UK
Chapter 111

Tristan McMullan
Consultant Ophthalmologist, Northampton General Hospital NHS Trust, UK
Chapter 19

Roshan Navin
Consultant Physician in Acute Internal Medicine, Guy's and St Thomas' NHS Foundation Trust, UK
Chapter 57

Jim Newton
Consultant Cardiologist, Oxford University Hospitals NHS Foundation Trust, UK
Chapters 45, 46

Claire van Nispen tot Pannerden
Consultant in Infectious Diseases, Guy's and St Thomas' NHS Foundation Trust, UK
Chapter 80

Kannan Nithi
Consultant Neurologist & Neurophysiologist, Northampton General Hospital NHS Trust, UK
Chapter 123

Kevin O'Kane
Consultant in Acute Internal Medicine, Guy's & St Thomas' NHS Foundations Trust, UK
Senior Lecturer in Medicine, King's College, London, UK
Chapters 56, 57

Marlies Ostermann
Consultant in Critical Care & Nephrology at Guy's & St Thomas' Foundation Trust, London, UK
Chapters 1, 2, 25

Ojaswini Pathak
Consultant Geriatrician, University Hospitals of Leicester, UK
Chapters 5, 31

Nayia Petousi
Clinical Lecturer in Respiratory Medicine, Nuffield Department of Medicine, University of Oxford, UK
Chapter 11

Ioannis Psallidas
Honorary Consultant Respiratory Physician, Junior Lecturer, University College, RESPIRE2 ERS Fellow,
Oxford Centre for Respiratory Medicine, Respiratory Trials Unit,
Oxford University Hospitals NHS Foundation Trust, UK
Chapter 12

Simon Rinaldi
Senior Clinical Researcher, University of Oxford, UK
Chapters 3, 14, 15, 17, 18, 71

Tony Rudd
Professor of Stroke Medicine King's College London, UK
Consultant Stroke Physician, Guy's & St Thomas' NHS Foundation Trust, UK
National Clinical Director Stroke NHS England
Chapters 65, 66

Sophia Savva
Specialist Registrar in Gastroenterology, Digestive Diseases Centre, University Hospitals Leicester
Chapters 74, 75, 76

Manu Shankar-Hari
Consultant, Intensive Care Medicine, Guy's and St Thomas' NHS Foundation Trust, London, UK.
Clinician Scientist, National Institute for Health Research (2017–2022)
Chapter 35

Udi Shmueli
Consultant Gastroenterologist, Northampton General Hospital NHS Trust, UK
Chapter 73

Nadia Short
Consultant Physician in Acute Internal Medicine, Honorary Senior Lecturer in Medicine, Guy's and St Thomas' NHS Foundation Trust, UK.
Chapter 114

David Sprigings
Consultant Physician (1993-2016), Northampton General Hospital NHS Trust, UK
Chapters 1, 2, 4, 6, 7, 8, 9, 10, 19, 25, 30, 36, 39, 40, 41, 42, 43, 44, 47, 48, 49, 53, 54, 55, 58, 68, 69, 95, 106, 107, 109, 116, 118, 119, 120, 121

Eui-Sik Suh
Consultant Respiratory Physician, Darent Valley Hospital, Dartford and Gravesham NHS Trust, UK
Chapter 61

Kehinde Sunmboye
Consultant Rheumatologist, University Hospitals of Leicester, UK
Chapters 28, 97, 98, 124

Nick Talbot
NIHR Academic Clinical Lecturer in Respiratory Medicine, Nuffield Department of Medicine, University of Oxford, UK
Chapter 37

Ambika Talwar
Clinical Research Fellow and Respiratory Registrar Oxford University Hospitals NHS Foundation Trust, UK
Chapter 115

Christopher Turnbull
Clinical Research Fellow, Oxford Centre for Respiratory Medicine, Oxford, UK
Chapter 113

Vimal Venugopal
Specialist Registrar in Diabetes & Endocrinology, University Hospitals of Leicester NHS Trust, UK
Chapters 81, 82, 83, 84

Ben Warner
Specialist Registrar in Gastroenterology & Hepatology
Research Fellow, Guy's and St Thomas' NHS Foundation Trust, UK
Chapters 23, 24, 77, 78, 79, 125

Mark Wilkinson
Consultant Hepatologist, Guy's and St Thomas' NHS Foundation Trust, UK
Chapters 23, 24, 77, 78, 79, 125

Ahmed Yousuf
Respiratory Registrar, Department of Respiratory Medicine, Churchill Hospital, Oxford, UK
Chapters 13, 62, 63

Preface

For the medical patient presenting with an undifferentiated emergency, the best outcome is achieved when initial assessment is by an experienced generalist, and subsequent care, if needed, by the appropriate specialist.

This book is written for the generalist: it aims to guide the trainee and provide an aide-memoire for the more experienced physician, to diagnose and manage the broad range of problems and diseases encountered in the emergency department, ambulatory care centre, acute medical unit or on the wards.

For this edition, we have enlisted experts to write or revise chapters; as previously, our intention has been to produce a step-by-step practical guide to the management of medical emergencies, grounded in national and international guidelines. The emphasis is on care of the patient in the first 24 hours, but guidance beyond this is also provided, as well as instructions on how to perform practical procedures. Clear advice on when to call for specialist help is given. Bed-side ultrasonography is beginning to transform acute medicine, and a new chapter summarizes its uses.

David Sprigings
John B. Chambers

Evolution of acute medicine: the development of ambulatory emergency care

VINCENT CONNOLLY

Acute medicine as a specialty

The specialty of acute medicine was developed to streamline the assessment and care of patients with acute illness or exacerbations of long-term conditions. Patients accepted on an acute medical unit (AMU) are assessed on arrival by a senior doctor and assigned to one of four streams of care:

- Ambulatory emergency care, for same-day treatment and discharge without using a hospital bed
- Short-stay (<72 hours) inpatient care
- Organ-specific disease requiring inpatient care from a specialist team
- Frail older patients, for whom comprehensive geriatric assessment (Chapter 31) is needed.

An acute physician requires the clinical skills to manage patients with a broad range of clinical problems, and in each of the care streams described above. This chapter focuses on ambulatory emergency care (Box 1).

Ambulatory emergency care (AEC)

- This is usually run by specialists in acute medicine, but can also be part of emergency medicine, surgery or paediatrics. Delivery requires rapid assessment by a senior physician, usually a consultant.
- Referrals are accepted from (Figure 1):
  - The emergency department
  - General practitioners and community nurses
  - Inpatient wards as part of a step-down approach to discharge
  - Other hospitals and clinics

Box 1 Ambulatory emergency care (AEC)

An effective AEC service can improve patient care and system efficiency.
  The essentials for a highly functioning service are:
- Senior clinician presence throughout the opening hours
- Clear patient-selection criteria
- Agreed pathways for high-volume clinical presentations
- Access to a multi-disciplinary team to support care plans for older people
- Appropriate infrastructure to meet the demand, particularly staffing

---

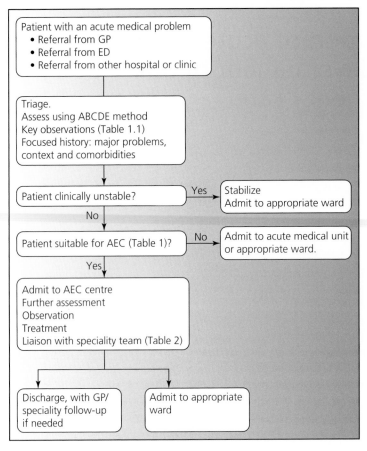

Figure 1 Ambulatory emergency care (AEC) in acute medicine.

- If suitable for AEC, the patient and relatives or carers must be informed that the plan is for same-day care then discharge, since the initial expectation after referral is often that an inpatient admission will be needed.
- The initial assessment must establish suitability for AEC.

Is the clinical condition suitable for AEC?

Is the patient actually well enough for early outpatient review? Alternatively, is the patient sick enough to require inpatient admission? National Early Warning Score (NEWS) can help (Table 1.2), but must be interpreted individually in the clinical context and working diagnosis. For example, a patient on long-term domiciliary oxygen may have a high NEWS but be clinically stable and suitable for AEC; a young person with low oxygen saturation levels may not trigger concern, even with a sub-massive PE.

The Amb score (Table 1) is also useful. A composite score of 5 or more suggests that the patient is suitable for AEC. The Amb score can be a particularly useful tool when less experienced staff are responsible for streaming, to help build confidence in the process.

Can the AEC unit deliver the required care?

Is there access to required back-up services: diagnostics; support by a community heart failure team; and ability to give parenteral antibiotics seven days a week.

Are staffing levels adequate in the face of current patient load and concerns like sickness and annual leave?

Table 1 The Amb Score.

Factor	Score
	1 if applicable, 0 if not applicable
Female sex	
Age <80 years	
Has access to personal/public transport	
IV treatment not anticipated	
Not acutely confused	
National Early Warning Score = 0	
Not discharged from hospital within previous 30 days	
Total Amb score	0–7
	A score of 5 or more suggests the patient is suitable for AEC

Can the AEC unit cope with the patient's personal needs?

These include feeding, toileting and behaviour. It is possible to manage frail older people with confusion or delirium in the AEC unit if the appropriate support is available.

Patient presentations to AEC

The clinical scenarios suitable for management in the AEC unit are in four main categories.

Diagnostic exclusion

Examples include:

- Chest pain with no acute ECG changes and low coronary risk. The patients can await troponin assays on AEC.
- Sudden onset severe headache in the absence of other neurological symptoms or signs. Exclusion of subarachnoid haemorrhage or other potentially serious diagnoses, with a CT of the brain and possibly a lumbar puncture, can be delivered in AEC.
- Suspected pulmonary embolism if haemodynamically stable. A CTPA (see Chapter 57) according to clinical scores can be performed.
- Non-specific abdominal pain.

Management of specific conditions

Patients may present with an easily recognizable diagnosis, for example DVT, cellulitis, atrial fibrillation, for which the patient requires a clinical management plan. There is often a need for confirmatory diagnostic tests, which should be readily available, or in the case of cellulitis, an outpatient parenteral intravenous antibiotic service. The patient may need to return to the AEC service for ongoing management or referral to another service for follow-up.

Management after risk-stratification

This group of clinical scenarios uses validated risk stratification tools to identify suitable patients for AEC. Examples include the Glasgow-Blatchford score for acute upper gastrointestinal bleeding, the Hestia score for suspected pulmonary embolism and the CURB-65 score for pneumonia. These scoring systems stratify patients as to their suitability for an AEC management pathway. This supports clinical decision making but is not a substitute for it. The stratification tools should be readily available for use, with the result recorded in the healthcare records.

Procedures

Some important clinical procedures can be performed, for example drainage of pleural effusions, knee aspiration and paracentesis. These may not be true emergencies, but are needed quickly for therapeutic or diagnostic purposes. Referrals in the evening can be seen the next day for the procedure, with follow-up investigations and referral as individually appropriate.

The procedures should always be carried out or directly supervised by a competent senior clinician. Another benefit of this model is that it is a training opportunity for junior medical staff.

The frail older patient

Frail older people are often admitted to hospital beds, although the clinical presentation with significant functional decline does not suggest serious illness. The involvement of a multi-disciplinary team within AEC can support the patient's needs. For example, an elderly patient who has fallen and fractured the inferior pubic ramus requires analgesia, walking and toileting aids at home and regular home visits until their functional status has returned to normal. This can all be initiated in an AEC service without hospital admission.

Many AEC services do not care for confusion or delirium, but some tailor their resources to support management at home.

AEC infrastructure and processes

Location

Many of the lessons concerning the development of AEC mirror those learned in the development of day surgery.

The unit consists of offices and trolleys and placing it close to the emergency department or acute medicine unit increases referrals.

Staffing

Adequate staffing capacity to match the demand for services. Typically a consultant should be available for 12 hours per day with support from junior medical staff. There will be a mix of nurse practitioners, staff nurses and healthcare assistants. Some units combine medical and surgical AEC by sharing the facilities and nursing staff.

Diagnostic support

Diagnostic support for the AEC service is needed, for example designated slots for Doppler ultrasound for DVT, CT pulmonary angiograms for suspected pulmonary embolism or an agreement to provide imaging within specified time scales, such as CT head scans within one hour of request. The time scales for diagnostics need to reflect the overall timescales for effective operation of the AEC unit; this should include the reporting of any imaging.

Pathways and checklists

Local pathways for common clinical scenarios reduce variability of care and increase speed and efficiency. Exclusion criteria should be minimized.

A safety checklist incorporated into the healthcare records helps to ensure that vital checks are carried out, for example:
- NEWS check
- Pain management
- Cannula check
- Radiology results
- Medication advice

Follow-up arrangements should be agreed.

Table 2 Clinical teams in the ambulatory emergency care network.

- Chronic obstructive pulmonary disease outreach team
- Rapid access chest pain clinic
- Transient ischaemic attack/stroke clinic
- Pleural diseases clinic
- Pain management team
- Falls clinic
- Multi-disciplinary functional assessment team
- Rapid response team
- Diabetes nurse specialist
- Palliative care team
- Heart failure team

Patient information

Patients should be provided with a simple information booklet explaining the AEC service, the working diagnosis, treatment plan and follow-up arrangements. The booklet should include what to do in the event of symptom recurrence or treatment complications, with a contact telephone number for in hours and out of hours. This provides a safety net for the patient and feedback for the team.

Networking

The back-up network of services (Table 2) should be made aware of the AEC service, in particular where it is and how it operates. The option of being able to make direct patient referrals especially out of hours and at weekends can significantly improve the quality of patient care. These services contribute to educating the patient about their chronic conditions.

Audit

Audit data should be collected to monitor the AEC unit's safety and effectiveness:
- Outcome metrics:
  - Mortality rate in acute medicine
  - Proportion of patients returning directly to their own home
- Process metrics:
  - Percentage of patients assessed within 15 min of arrival
  - Percentage of patients that have a medical assessment within 60 min
- Balancing metric:
  - Percentage of patients re-attending or re-admitted within seven days

Further reading

Ambulatory Emergency Care website: http://www.ambulatoryemergencycare.org.uk/.
Connolly V, Thompson D (2014) *Acute care toolkit 10: Ambulatory emergency care*. London: RCP. https://www.rcplondon.ac.uk/guidelines-policy/acute-care-toolkit-10-ambulatory-emergency-care.

SECTION 1
Presentations in Acute Medicine

General

CHAPTER 1

The critically ill patient

MARLIES OSTERMANN AND DAVID SPRIGINGS

Key features of the critically ill patient are severe respiratory, cardiovascular or neurological derangement, often in combination, reflected in abnormal physiological observations (Tables 1.1 and 1.2). Principles of management are summarised in Box 1.1 and Figure 1.1.

Priorities

Make a rapid but systematic assessment using the ABCDE approach.

While doing this, collect information about the patient, the current problem, the context and comorbidities. Attach monitoring (ECG and oxygen saturation) and secure venous access.

Box 1.1 The critically ill patient: principles of management (Resuscitation Council (UK))

Use the Airway, Breathing, Circulation, Disability, Exposure (ABCDE) approach to assess and treat the patient.

Do a complete initial assessment and re-assess regularly.

Treat life-threatening problems before moving to the next part of assessment.

Assess the effects of treatment.

Recognize when you will need extra help. Call for appropriate help early.

Use all members of the team. This enables interventions (e.g. assessment, attaching monitors, intravenous access), to be undertaken simultaneously.

Communicate effectively – plan approach.

The aim of the initial treatment is to keep the patient alive, and achieve some clinical improvement. This will buy time for further treatment and making a diagnosis.

Remember: it can take a few minutes for treatments to work, so wait a short while before reassessing the patient after an intervention.

Acute Medicine: A Practical Guide to the Management of Medical Emergencies, Fifth Edition. Edited by David Sprigings and John B. Chambers.
© 2018 John Wiley & Sons Ltd. Published 2018 by John Wiley & Sons Ltd.

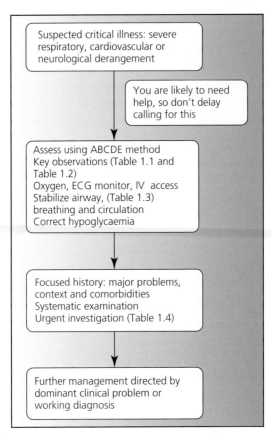

Figure 1.1 Approach to the patient with suspected critical illness.

Airway and breathing

- Ensure the airway is clear. If the patient is unconscious, remove dentures if loose and aspirate the pharynx, larynx and trachea with a suction catheter. See Chapter 112 for detailed advice on airway management.
- If there is no reflex response (gagging or coughing) to the suction catheter or the respiratory rate is <8/min, a cuffed endotracheal tube should be inserted, preferably by an anaesthetist. Before this is done, ventilate the patient using a bag-mask system with 100% oxygen.
- What is the respiratory rate? Rates <8 or >30/min signify potential critical illness. Is there respiratory distress, shown by dyspnoea, tachypnoea, ability to speak only in short sentences or single words, agitation and sweating? Is arterial oxygen saturation <90% despite breathing 40% oxygen? This indicates severe impairment of gas exchange. See Chapter 11 for management of respiratory failure.

Circulation

- Remember that a 'normal' blood pressure may be maintained by vasoconstriction and does not mean that organ perfusion is adequate. Signs of low cardiac output include confusion and agitation, cold extremities, sweating, oliguria and metabolic acidosis.
- Heart rates <40 or >130/min with signs of low cardiac output require urgent correction: see Chapters 39–44 for management of arrhythmias.
- If systolic BP is <80 mmHg, or has fallen by more than 40 mmHg and there are signs of low cardiac output, urgent correction is needed. Look carefully at the JVP, which may provide an important clue to the diagnosis.

Table 1.1 Nine key observations in suspected critical illness.

Observation	Signs of critical illness	Action
Airway	Evidence of upper airway obstruction (Table 1.3)	See Table 1.3 and Chapter 112 for management of the airway
Respiratory rate	Respiratory rate <8 or >30/min	Give oxygen (initially 60–100%) Connect a pulse oximeter Check arterial oxygen saturation and blood gases See Chapter 11 for management of respiratory failure
Arterial oxygen saturation	SaO_2 <90%	Give oxygen (initially 60–100% if there are other signs of critical illness) Check arterial blood gases (Chapter 118)
Heart rate	Heart rate <40 or >130/min with signs of impaired organ perfusion	Give oxygen 60–100% Connect an ECG monitor and obtain IV access See Chapters 39–44 for management of cardiac arrhythmias
Blood pressure	Systolic BP <90 mmHg or fall in systolic BP by more than 40 mmHg, with signs of impaired organ perfusion	Give oxygen 60–100% Connect an ECG monitor and obtain IV access See Chapter 2 for management of hypotension/shock
Perfusion	Signs of impaired organ perfusion: cool/ mottled skin with capillary refill time >2 s; agitation/reduced conscious level; oliguria	Give oxygen 60–100% Connect an ECG monitor and obtain IV access See Chapter 2 for management of hypotension/shock
Conscious level	Reduced conscious level (unresponsive to voice)	Stabilize airway, breathing and circulation Endotracheal intubation if GCS 8 or less Exclude/correct hypoglycaemia Give naloxone if opioid poisoning is possible See Chapter 3 for further management of the patient with reduced conscious level
Temperature	Core temperature <36 or >38 °C, with hypotension, hypoxaemia, oliguria or agitation/reduced conscious level	See Chapter 35 for further management of sepsis syndrome
Blood glucose	Blood glucose <4 mmol/L with signs of hypoglycaemia (sweating, abnormal behaviour, reduced conscious level, seizures)	Give 100 mL of 20% glucose or 200 mL of 10% glucose over 15–30 min IV, or glucagon 1 mg IV/IM/SC See Chapter 81

GCS, Glasgow Coma Scale score
AVPU scale: alert = GCS 14 or 15; voice responsive = GCS 12; pain responsive = GCS 8; unresponsive = GCS 3.

If there are no signs of pulmonary oedema, give IV fluid (500 mL crystalloid over 15 min). If hypovolaemia or vasodilatation is likely (suspect vasodilatation if the pulses are bounding), lay the patient flat and elevate the foot of the bed. See Chapter 2 for further management of hypotension and shock.

Neurological status ('disability' – 'da brain')

- What is the conscious level (assessed using the Glasgow coma scale score (GCS) (p. 20))? If the GCS is <9, contact an anaesthetist immediately, as the patient may need urgent endotracheal intubation.
- If the conscious level is reduced, you must exclude hypoglycaemia by immediate stick test. If blood glucose is <4.0 mmol/L, give 100 mL of 20% glucose or 200 mL of 10% glucose over 15–30 min IV, or glucagon 1 mg IV/IM/SC. Recheck blood glucose after 10 min, if still below 4.0 mmol/L, repeat the above IV

Table 1.2 National Early Warning Score (NEWS).

National Early Warning Score (NEWS)*

PHYSIOLOGICAL PARAMETERS	3	2	1	0	1	2	3
Respiratory Rate	≤8		9 - 11	12 - 20		21 - 24	≥25
Oxygen Saturations	≤91	91 - 93	94-95	≥96			
Any Supplemental Oxygen		Yes		No			
Temperature	≤35.0		35.1 - 36.0	36.1 - 38.0	38.1 - 39.0	≥39.1	
Systolic BP	≤90	91 - 100	101 - 110	111 - 219			≥220
Heart Rate	≤40		41 - 50	51 - 90	91 - 110	111 - 130	≥131
Level of Consciousness				A			V, P, or U

*The NEWS initiative flowed from the Royal College of Physicians' NEWS Development Implementation Groups NEWSDIG, and was jointly developed and funded in collaboration with the Royal College of Physicians, Royal College of Nursing, National Outreach Forum and NHS Training for innovation.
Source: Royal College of Physicians. National Early Warning Score (NEWS): Standardising the assessment of acute illness severity in the NHS. Report of a working party. London: RCP, 2012.

Level of Consciousness: A, Alert; V, responds to Voice; P, responds to Pain; U, Unresponsive.

The NEWS scoring system

In some settings, patients will have a impaired level of consciousness as a consequence of sedation, eg following surgical procedures. Thus, the assessment of consciousness level and necesslty to escalate care should be considered in the time-limited context of the appropriateness of the consciousness level in relation to recent sedation.

For patients with known hypercapnoeic respiratory failure due to chronic obstructive pulmonary disease (COPD), recommended British Thoracic Society target saturations of 88–92% should be used. These patients will still 'score' if their oxygen saturations are below 92 unless the score is 'reset' by a competent clinical decision-maker and patient-specific target oxygen saturations are prescribed and documented on chart and in the clinical notes.

All supplemental oxygen when administered, must be prescribed.

The National Early Warning Score (NEWS) thresholds and triggers

NEWS	Clinical risk
0	Low
Aggregate 1 – 4	
RED score* (Individual parameter scoring 3)	Medium
Aggregate 5 – 6	
Aggregate 7 or more	High

glucose treatment. In patients with malnourishment or alcohol use disorder, there is a remote risk of precipitating Wernicke encephalopathy by a glucose load: prevent this by giving thiamine 100 mg IV before or shortly after glucose administration. See Chapter 81 for further management of hypoglycaemia.

- If the respiratory rate is <12/min or the pupils are pinpoint, or there is other reason to suspect opioid poisoning, give naloxone. Give up to 4 doses of 800 µgm IV every 2–3 min until the respiratory rate is around 15/min. Further doses may be needed (see p. 233).
- If you suspect benzodiazepine overdose may be the cause, give flumazenil, 200 µgm IV over 15 s; if needed, further doses of 100 µgm can be given at 1-min intervals up to a total dose of 2 mg.
- If there are recurrent or prolonged major seizures, treat with diazepam 10–20 mg IV or lorazepam 2–4 mg IV: see Chapter 16 for management of seizures.
- Examine the eyes and pupils, and check for neck stiffness.
- Make a rapid assessment of limb tone and power: is there lateralized weakness?

Exposure (entire examination)

- Check for abdominal tenderness and guarding. If the patient has severe abdominal pain or generalized abdominal tenderness, and is shocked (systolic BP <90 mmHg with cold skin), the likely diagnosis is generalized peritonitis, mesenteric infarction, severe pancreatitis or ruptured abdominal aortic aneurysm (Table 21.1).
- Examine the limbs, spine and perineum for evidence of ischaemia or a septic focus.

Further management

Investigation of the critically ill patient is given in Table 1.4. Further management is directed by the dominant clinical problem or working diagnosis.

Table 1.3 Assessment and stabilization of the airway.

	Signs of acute upper airway obstruction	Causes of acute upper airway obstruction	Action if you suspect upper airway obstruction
Conscious patient	Respiratory distress* Inspiratory stridor Suprasternal retraction Abnormal voice Coughing/choking	Foreign body Anaphylaxis (Chapter 38) Angioedema (Chapter 27)	Sit the patient up Give high-flow oxygen Call for urgent help from an anaesthetist and ENT surgeon Specific management of cause of obstruction
Unconscious patient	Respiratory arrest Inspiratory stridor Gurgling Grunting/snoring	Above causes Tongue and soft tissues of oropharynx Inhalation of foreign body, secretions, blood, vomitus	Head-tilt/chin-lift manoeuvre Remove dentures if loose and aspirate the pharynx, larynx and trachea with a suction catheter Call for urgent help from an anaesthetist See Chapter 112 for management of the airway Specific management of cause of obstruction

* Respiratory distress is shown by dyspnoea, tachypnoea, ability to speak only in short sentences or single words, agitation and sweating.

Table 1.4 Investigation of the critically ill patient.

Immediate

Arterial blood gases, pH and lactate

ECG

Blood glucose

Plasma sodium, potassium, urea and creatinine

Full blood count

Urgent

Chest X-ray

Echocardiography if hypotension/shock

Cranial CT if reduced conscious level or focal signs

Coagulation screen if low platelet count, suspected coagulation disorder, jaundice or purpura

Biochemical profile

Amylase if abdominal pain or tenderness

C-reactive protein

Blood culture if suspected sepsis

Urine stick test

Toxicology screen (serum 10 mL and urine 50 mL) if suspected poisoning

Further reading

Capana M, Ivya J, Rohlederb T, Hickman J, Huddleston JM. (2015) Individualizing and optimizing the use of early warning scores in acute medical care for deteriorating hospitalized patients. *Resuscitation* 93, 107–112.

Royal College of Physicians (2012) *National Early Warning Score (NEWS): Standardising the assessment of acute illness severity in the NHS*. Report of a working party. London: RCP. https://www.rcplondon.ac.uk/projects/outputs/national-early-warning-score-news.

CHAPTER 2

Hypotension and shock

MARLIES OSTERMANN AND DAVID SPRIGINGS

- Shock is acute circulatory failure associated with inadequate oxygen utilization by the cells, resulting in organ dysfunction and lactic acidosis (>2 mmol/L).
- Compensatory mechanisms may initially maintain the blood pressure, but hypotension is usually present:
  - Systolic blood pressure (SBP) <90 mmHg or mean arterial pressure (MAP) <65 mmHg
  - Fall in systolic BP >40 mmHg
- Causes of shock are given in Table 2.1. Up to one-third of patients admitted to ICU have shock predominantly caused by sepsis.
- Monitor vital signs in patients at risk (e.g. acute coronary syndrome, pneumonia) to detect the first signs of developing shock and take prompt action to reverse this.

Priorities

Initial management is summarized in Figure 2.1.

1 If hypovolaemia or vasodilatation is likely, lay the patient flat and elevate the foot of the bed.

2 Give oxygen. Place an IV cannula. Attach an ECG monitor. Check oxygen saturation. Make a rapid clinical assessment (Table 2.2). Look carefully at the JVP, and assess skin temperature and perfusion. Investigations needed urgently are given in Table 2.3.

   Questions to ask yourself include:
- Is there obvious haemorrhage from the gastrointestinal tract or other site (e.g. abdominal aortic aneurysm) (Chapters 73 and 74)?
- Is there a major arrhythmia (Chapter 39)?
- Is there ECG evidence of an acute coronary syndrome (ST segment elevation or depression, new left bundle branch block) (Chapters 45 and 46)?
- Is there associated pulmonary oedema, indicating cardiogenic shock (Chapter 49)?
- Is there fever, or other features pointing to sepsis (Chapter 35)?
- Is pulmonary embolism possible (Chapter 57)? Hypotension and hypoxaemia without pulmonary oedema suggest pulmonary embolism or sepsis; in this setting, a raised JVP would favour pulmonary embolism and a low JVP sepsis.
- Is tension pneumothorax a possibility (e.g. recent central vein cannulation) (Chapter 64)?
- Could this be anaphylaxis (Chapter 38)? If the patient has recently been exposed to a potential allergen, and has urticaria, erythema, angio-oedema or wheeze, treat as anaphylaxis and give adrenaline 0.5–1 mg IM (0.5–1 mL of 1 in 1000 solution). Further management is detailed in Chapter 38.

3 If hypotension does not respond promptly, put in a bladder catheter so that urine output can be monitored. The urine output is a rough guide to renal blood flow and cardiac output; the target is >0.5 mL/kg/h.

Acute Medicine: A Practical Guide to the Management of Medical Emergencies, Fifth Edition. Edited by David Sprigings and John B. Chambers.
© 2018 John Wiley & Sons Ltd. Published 2018 by John Wiley & Sons Ltd.

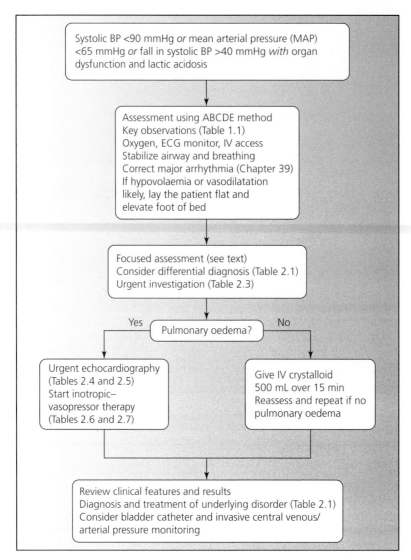

Figure 2.1 Management of hypotension and shock.

If there is obvious haemorrhage:

- Get help from a gastroenterologist (if you are dealing with suspected upper gastrointestinal haemorrhage) or a surgeon (see Chapters 73 and 74).
- Place a second large-bore IV cannula (e.g. grey Venflon).
- Rapidly transfuse crystalloid until the systolic BP is around 100 mmHg. Start transfusing blood as soon as it is available. If systolic BP is still <90 mmHg despite 1 L of crystalloid, and cross-matched blood is not yet available, use grouped but not cross-matched blood and save a sample of the transfused blood for a retrospective cross-match.
- Aim for a haemoglobin concentration of 80 g/L.

Table 2.1 Differential diagnosis of hypotension and shock.

Hypovolaemia
Haemorrhage
Urinary loss
Gastrointestinal fluid loss
Cutaneous loss (e.g. burns)
Third-space sequestration (e.g. acute pancreatitis)

Cardiac obstruction
Pulmonary embolism (Chapter 57)
Cardiac tamponade (Chapter 54)
Tension pneumothorax (Chapter 64)

Cardiac pump failure (see Chapter 49)
Acute myocardial infarction (usually associated with pulmonary oedema, except when due to right ventricular infarction)
Acute myocardial ischaemia (usually associated with pulmonary oedema)
Arrhythmia (especially when associated with valve disorder, e.g. severe aortic stenosis, or impaired left ventricular function, in which case usually associated with pulmonary oedema)
Acute aortic or mitral regurgitation (due to endocarditis, aortic dissection, papillary muscle or chordal rupture) (always associated with pulmonary oedema)
Ventricular septal rupture complicating myocardial infarction (often associated with pulmonary oedema)

Vasodilatation
Sepsis
Drugs and toxins
Anaphylaxis
Acute adrenal insufficiency (Addisonian crisis)

Table 2.2 Clinical signs pointing to the cause of hypotension.

Cause of hypotension	Pulse volume	Skin temperature	Jugular venous pressure
Hypovolaemia	Low	Cool	Low
Cardiac obstruction or pump failure	Low	Cool	Normal or raised
Vasodilatation	Normal or increased	Warm	Low

Table 2.3 Urgent investigation in hypotension.

ECG
Chest X-ray
Echocardiography if indicated (see Tables 2.4, 2.5)
Arterial blood gases, pH and lactate; in refractory cases, central venous oxygen saturation and veno-arterial partial pressure of CO_2
Blood glucose
Plasma sodium, potassium, urea and creatinine
Full blood count
Group and screen (cross-match six units if acute haemorrhage suspected)
Coagulation screen if low platelet count, suspected coagulation disorder, jaundice or purpura
Blood culture
Urine stick test

Table 2.4 Indications for urgent echocardiography in the hypotensive patient.

Suspected cardiac tamponade
- Hypotension and breathlessness following placement of central venous cannula or pacing lead, or in a patient with known cancer
- Raised jugular venous pressure
- Pulsus paradoxus >10 mmHg

Suspected acute major pulmonary embolism
- Risk factors for venous thromboembolism
- Raised jugular venous pressure
- Hypoxaemia

Hypotension with pulmonary edema

Unexplained severe hypotension

- Correct clotting abnormalities. If the prothrombin time is >1.5 x control, give vitamin K 10 mg IV and 2 units of fresh frozen plasma. If the platelet count is <75 × 10^{12}/L, give platelet concentrate. Recheck the platelet count if >4 units of blood have been transfused. If fibrinogen is <1.5 g/L, give cryoprecipitate.
- Consider tranexamic acid.

If there is cardiogenic shock (hypotension with pulmonary oedema):
- Correct major arrhythmias (Chapters 39–44).
- If there is ECG evidence of ST-segment-elevation acute coronary syndrome, consider primary angioplasty if feasible (Chapter 45).
- Arrange urgent echocardiography to assess right and left ventricular function and to exclude ventricular septal rupture, pericardial tamponade and acute aortic or mitral regurgitation (Table 2.5).
- Increase the inspired oxygen, aiming for an oxygen saturation of >90%/arterial PO$_2$ >8 kPa. If these targets are not met despite an inspired oxygen concentration of 60%, use a continuous positive airway pressure system

Table 2.5 Echocardiographic findings in hypotension.

Cause of hypotension	IVC	LV size	LV contraction	RV size	RV contraction
Hypovolaemia	Flat	Small	Increased	Small	Increased
Sepsis	Flat	Normal or large	Normal, reduced or increased	Normal or large	Normal or reduced
LV dysfunction due to ischaemia	Normal or dilated	Large	Reduced regionally or globally	Normal	Normal (unless associated RV infarction)
Acute major pulmonary embolism	Dilated	Normal or small	Normal or increased	Large	Reduced
Cardiac tamponade	Dilated	Normal or small	Normal or increased	Normal or small	Diastolic free wall collapse
RV infarction	Dilated	Normal or large if associated LV inferior infarction	Normal or reduced if associated inferior infarction	Large	Reduced

IVC, inferior vena cava; LV, left ventricular; RV, right ventricular.

Table 2.6 Choice of inotropic/vasopressor therapy.

Cause of hypotension	Choice of therapy
Left ventricular failure	Dobutamine or phosphodiesterase inhibitor if systolic BP is >90 mmHg
	Levosimendan or phosphodiesterase inhibitor
Right ventricular infarction	Dobutamine if systolic BP is 80–90 mmHg
Pulmonary embolism	Noradrenaline if systolic BP is <80 mmHg
Cardiac tamponade while awaiting pericardiocentesis	Noradrenaline
Septic shock	Noradrenaline
	Dobutamine should be added if cardiac output is low
Anaphylactic shock	Adrenaline

Table 2.7 Inotropic/vasopressor therapy: dosages.

Drug	Dosage (µg/kg/min)	Effect
Adrenaline	0.05	Beta-1 inotropism and beta-2 vasodilatation
	0.05–5	Beta-1 inotropism and alpha-1 vasoconstriction
Dobutamine	5–40	Beta-1 inotropism and beta-2 vasodilatation
Dopamine	5–10	Beta-1 inotropism
	10–40	Alpha-1 vasoconstriction
Noradrenaline	0.05–5	Alpha-1 vasoconstriction and beta-1 inotropism
Milrinone	0.375–0.75	Phosphodiesterase inhibitor; inotropy and vasodilatation
Levosimendan	0.1	Calcium-sensitizing agent; inotropy and vasodilatation

(Chapter 113). Intubation and mechanical ventilation may be appropriate in some patients: discuss this with an intensivist and cardiologist.

- Start inotropic/vasopressor therapy (Tables 2.6 and 2.7).
  Diuretics are relatively ineffective in patients with cardiogenic shock, but can be used in case of fluid overload once the cardiac output has increased (as shown by improvement in the patient's mental state and skin perfusion): if renal function is normal, give Furosemide 40 mg IV.
- Providing the systolic BP has increased to at least 100 mmHg, start a nitrate infusion, initially at low dose (e.g. isosorbide dinitrate 2 mg/h).
- If the patient is not improving, consider haemodynamic monitoring using pulse contour or thermodilution techniques to allow more accurate titration of therapy. Adjust the doses of inotrope/vasopressor +/– nitrate, aiming for normalization of tissue perfusion parameters (serum lactate, urine output, skin perfusion).
- Discuss management with a cardiologist if you suspect a surgically correctable cause (e.g. papillary muscle rupture) or there is evidence of acute myocardial ischaemia without infarction (Chapter 46).

Further management

The key points in the management of hypotension/shock are to:
- Make a diagnosis and give specific treatment (e.g. pericardiocentesis for tamponade, PCI for ACS, cardiac surgery for ruptured papillary muscle). Seek help from an intensivist and, in the case of cardiogenic shock, a cardiologist.

- Correct cardiac arrhythmias.
- Correct hypovolaemia while avoiding fluid overload.
- Correct hypoxia and biochemical abnormalities.
- Use inotropic/vasopressor therapy if there is refractory hypotension.

1 Make a diagnosis and give specific treatment:
- Consider the causes in Table 2.1.
- Echocardiography is indicated if the diagnosis remains unclear.
- Give hydrocortisone 200 mg IV if the patient has been on previous long-term steroid treatment (prednisolone >7.5 mg daily) or you suspect acute adrenal insufficiency (Chapter 90).

2 Correct cardiac arrhythmias:
- Ventricular tachycardia or supraventricular tachycardia with a ventricular rate >150 min should be treated with DC cardioversion (Chapter 121).
- Acute atrial fibrillation: consider DC cardioversion if the ventricular rate is >140 min, after correction of hypoxia and electrolyte disorders. Otherwise, give amiodarone IV (via a central line; 300 mg in glucose 5% over 60 min, followed by 900 mg over 24 h). Most drugs used to control the ventricular rate in atrial fibrillation are contraindicated in hypotension. Digoxin is largely ineffective when sympathetic drive is high.
- If there is severe bradycardia (heart rate <40 min), give atropine 0.6–1.2 mg IV, with further doses at 5-min intervals up to a total dose of 3 mg if the heart rate remains below 60 min. If there is little response to atropine, use an external transcutaneous pacing system or put in temporary pacing wire (Chapter 119).

3 Correct hypovolaemia:
- If there is obvious hypovolaemia (appropriate clinical setting; low JVP with flat neck veins), give IV fluid (blood, colloid or crystalloid as appropriate to the cause). There is no role for a central line unless the patient needs inotropic medication.
- If the evidence for hypovolaemia is less certain, but there are no clinical signs of fluid overload, give a fluid challenge, especially if the JVP is difficult to assess.
- If systolic BP remains <90 mmHg despite correction or exclusion of hypovolaemia, search for and treat other causes of hypotension, of which sepsis is the most likely. In patients with acute bleeding, relative hypotension can be accepted until the bleeding is stopped surgically. In sepsis with prior systemic hypertension, a MAP >65 mmHg may be needed to prevent acute kidney injury.
- There is no single value of LV filling pressure or CVP that should guide fluid replacement; instead, multiple methods should be used, including dynamic measures (e.g. pulse-pressure variability on the arterial line or the change in IVC diameter on leg raising).
- Even in fluid-responsive patients, titrate fluid carefully to avoid hypervolaemia
- If BP remains low, inotropic–vasopressor therapy will be needed.

4 Correct hypoxia and biochemical abnormalities:
- Maintain PaO_2 >8 kPa (60 mmHg), arterial saturation >90%.
- Severe metabolic acidosis may contribute to hypotension. It is crucial to identify the cause of metabolic acidosis so that the correct treatment can be initiated. Causes of metabolic acidosis are given on p. 249. If arterial pH is <7.1 and falling, consider giving 50 mL of 8.4% sodium bicarbonate whilst waiting for a response to treatment of the underlying disease. Recheck arterial pH after 30 min.

5 Use inotropic/vasopressor therapy if there is refractory hypotension:
- If systolic BP remains <90 mmHg (MAP <65 mmHg) with signs of hypoperfusion (associated with low central venous oxygen saturation) despite correction of hypovolaemia, start inotropic/vasopressor therapy whilst searching for the underlying cause.
- Inotropes are not indicated for a low LV ejection fraction on echocardiography without signs of low cardiac output.

- Invasive central venous and arterial pressure monitoring is recommended.
- Choice of therapy and dosages are summarized in Tables 2.6 and 2.7.
- Discuss with a cardiologist whether intra-aortic balloon counterpulsation (balloon pump) or left ventricular assist device is indicated as a bridge to definitive treatment (e.g. surgery for a ruptured papillary muscle).

Further reading

Francis GS, Bartos JA, Adatya S (2014) Inotropes. *J Am Coll Cardiol* 63, 2069–2078.

Mackenzie DC, Noble VE (2014) Assessing volume status and fluid responsiveness in the emergency department. *Clin Exp Emerg Med* 1, 67–77. http://dx.doi.org/10.15441/ceem.14.040.

Roshdy A, Francisco N, Rendon A, Gillon S, Walker D (2014) Critical Care Echo Rounds: Haemodynamic instability. *Echo Research and Practice*, September. DOI: 10.1530/ERP-14-0008.

Task force of the European Society of Intensive Care Medicine (2014) Consensus on circulatory shock and hemodynamic monitoring. *Intensive Care Med* 40, 1795–1815. DOI: 10.1007/s00134-014-3525-z.

CHAPTER 3

Reduced conscious level

SIMON RINALDI

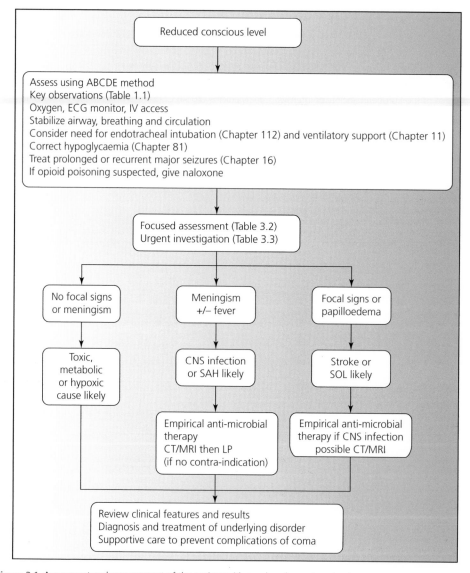

Figure 3.1 Assessment and management of the patient with a reduced conscious level.

Acute Medicine: A Practical Guide to the Management of Medical Emergencies, Fifth Edition. Edited by David Sprigings and John B. Chambers.
© 2018 John Wiley & Sons Ltd. Published 2018 by John Wiley & Sons Ltd.

A reduced conscious level is characterized by impaired awareness and decreased responsiveness to external stimuli. Akinetic mutism, functional unresponsiveness, severe neuromuscular impairment and the locked-in syndrome can sometimes be mistaken for a reduced conscious level.

In patients aged <40, poisoning is the commonest cause of a reduced conscious level not due to trauma, and in those >60, stroke. However, the differential diagnosis is broad (Table 3.1). Stabilization of the patient, with rapid identification and treatment of reversible causes, is required to achieve a good outcome. Management is summarized in Figure 3.1.

Priorities

1 Stabilize the airway, breathing and circulation

For detailed guidance, see Chapters 1, 59, 112 (airway management), 11 and 113 (management of respiratory failure) and 2 (management of hypotension and shock).

Table 3.1 Causes of a reduced conscious level.

Without localizing signs or meningism	With meningism (+/ − localizing signs)	With localizing signs
Toxic Alcohol, drugs, carbon monoxide		
Metabolic/endocrine Hypoxia, hypercapnia, hypoglycaemia, hyperglycaemic ketoacidosis/hyperosmolar states, hypo/hypernatraemia, uraemia, hepatic encephalopathy, hypercalcaemia, Addisonian crisis, dysthyroidism, hypo/ hyperthermia, Wernicke's	Pituitary apoplexy	Wernicke's encephalopathy, hypo/ hyperglycaemia, sodium shifts
Vascular Shock, hypertensive encephalopathy, eclampsia, venous sinus thrombosis	Subarachnoid haemorrhage	Brainstem infarction, cerebral infarction with mass effect, venous sinus thrombosis, cerebral/pontine/cerebellar haemorrhage
Infective Severe systemic infection	Bacterial meningitis, viral meningo-encephalitis, cerebral malaria	Herpes simplex encephalitis, subdural empyema, abscess, septic emboli
Inflammatory Paraneoplastic or autoimmune encephalitis (limbic encephalitis (with or without VGKC, GABA$_B$R, or AMPAR antibodies)), NMDAR encephalitis, Hashimoto's encephalopathy		Bickerstaff's brainstem encephalitis, acute disseminated encephalo-myelitis (ADEM), autoimmune encephalitis
Seizure Post-ictal state, status epilepticus		Post-ictal, status epilepticus
Tumour Paraneoplastic, acute hydrocephalus	Carcinomatous meningitis	Brain tumour
Trauma Concussion		SDH, EDH, other traumatic brain injury

Table 3.2 Focused assessment of the patient with reduced conscious level.

History

History will usually need to be obtained from third party sources such as family and friends, paramedics, GPs and existing medical records. It is important to establish:

Tempo and pattern of onset (abrupt, gradual, fluctuating)

Any prodromal symptoms? (fever, headache, vomiting, anorexia, altered behaviour, seizure, focal neurological deficits)

History of trauma (head injury, neck manipulation)

Past history (systemic, neurological, psychiatric)

Possibility of alcohol/drug intoxication

Current medications/immunosuppression/anti-coagulants

History of exposure or foreign travel

Examination

Vital signs (respiratory rate, pulse, blood pressure, temperature, oxygen saturation)

Conscious level (using Glasgow Coma Scale score (Figure 3.2))

Meningism?

Signs of trauma?

Skin colour, rash?

Eye signs (Figure 3.3)

Pupillary size and light reflex, corneal reflex?

Papilloedema? (indicates raised ICP of >12 h duration or malignant hypertension) Spontaneous venous pulsations? (absence more sensitive, but less specific, for raised ICP)

Eye movements (tracking, spontaneous, oculocephalic response (OCR) to passive head turn, conjugate or dysconjugate gaze deviation?)

Focal signs (asymmetry of tone, movement, deep tendon reflexes, extensor plantar)

Breath odour (uraemic, hepatic, ketotic)

General examination (murmur, bruit, pulmonary disease, evidence of liver disease, pertitonism, urinary retention)

2 Exclude and correct hypoglycaemia
- If blood glucose is <4.0 mmol/L, give 100 mL of 20% glucose or 200 mL of 10% glucose over 15–30 min IV, or glucagon 1 mg IV/IM/SC.
- Recheck blood glucose after 10 min, if still below 4.0 mmol/L, repeat the above IV glucose treatment.
- In patients with malnourishment or alcohol-use disorder, there is a remote risk of precipitating Wernicke's encephalopathy by a glucose load: prevent this by giving thiamine 100 mg IV before or shortly after glucose administration. See Chapter 81 for further management of hypoglycaemia.

3 Treat prolonged or recurrent major seizures
- Take into account prehospital treatment. Give lorazepam (which is less likely to cause respiratory suppression) 0.1 mg/kg (typically 4–8 mg) IV over 5–10 min (Table 16.2), midazolam 10 mg buccally (NICE-recommended, but only licensed in patients <18 years), or diazepam 10–20 mg IV at a rate of <2.5 mg/min (faster injection rates carry the risk of sudden apnoea).
- If the seizure does not terminate, give a second dose, to a maximum total dose of lorazepam 8 mg or diazepam 40 mg.
- See Chapter 16 for further management of seizures/status epilepticus.

4 Give naloxone, if opioid poisoning is possible or must be excluded
- If the respiratory rate is <12/min, or the pupils are pinpoint, or there is other reason to suspect opioid poisoning, give naloxone 800 µgm IV every 2–3 min up to a total dose of 3200 µgm or until the respiratory rate is >15/min.
- If there is a response to bolus naloxone, start an IV infusion: add naloxone 2000 µgm to 500 mL glucose 5% or normal saline (4 µgm/mL) and titrate against the respiratory rate and conscious level. The plasma half-life of naloxone is 1 h, shorter than that of most opioids.

Table 3.3 Investigation of the patient with reduced conscious level.

All patients

Blood glucose

Plasma sodium, potassium, urea and creatinine

Liver function tests, albumin and calcium

Full blood count

C-reactive protein

Blood culture if temperature <36 °C or >38 °C

Arterial blood gases and pH

Chest X-ray

ECG

With focal neurological signs

CT head (with CT angiography if basilar artery occlusion possible)

With meningism

CT head, then LP if no cause identified

If cause remains unidentified, consider

CT/LP (if not yet done)

Plasma osmolality (see Table 11.3)

Toxicology screen (send serum (10 mL) and urine (50 mL)).

Prothrombin time

Arterial ammonia level

Cortisol

Thiamine/red cell transketolase

Blood film

Autoantibody screen (VGKC, NMDAR, GABA$_B$R, AMPAR, TPO, paraneoplastic, GQ1b)

MRI brain

EEG

- In patients who have taken partial opioid agonists such as buprenorphine, methadone and tramadol, repeated large (1200 μgm) doses of naloxone may be required to achieve a satisfactory response.
- If there is no response to naloxone, opioid poisoning is excluded.

5 **Give flumazenil, if coma is a complication of the therapeutic use of benzodiazepine in hospital**

Give flumazenil 200 μgm IV over 15 s; if needed, further doses of 100 μgm can be given at 1-min intervals up to a total dose of 2 mg.

6 **Once the patient is stabilized, make a full clinical assessment (Table 3.2) and arrange urgent investigation (Table 3.3)**

- Document the level of consciousness in objective terms, using the Glasgow Coma Scale (see Figure 3.2).
- Examine for signs of head injury (e.g. scalp laceration, bruising, bleeding from an external auditory meatus or from the nose). If there are signs of head injury, assume additional cervical spine injury until proved otherwise: the neck must be immobilized in a collar and X-rayed before you check for neck stiffness and the oculocephalic response.
- Check for neck stiffness.
- Record the size of pupils and their response to bright light (Figure 3.3). Examine the fundi.
- Check the oculocephalic response. This is a simple but important test of an intact brainstem. Rotate the head to left and right. In an unconscious patient with an intact brainstem, both eyes rotate in the opposite direction from movement of the head.

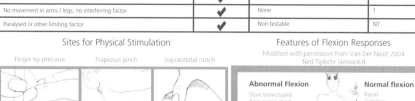

GLASGOW COMA SCALE : Do it this way

GCS at 40 | EYES VERBAL MOTOR

Institute of Neurological Sciences NHS Greater Glasgow and Clyde

CHECK
For factors Interfering with communication, ability to respond and other injuries

OBSERVE
Eye opening , content of speech and movements of right and left sides

STIMULATE
Sound: spoken or shouted request
Physical: Pressure on finger tip, trapezius or supraorbital notch

RATE
Assign according to highest response observed

Eye opening

Criterion	Observed	Rating	Score
Open before stimulus	✔	Spontaneous	4
After spoken or shouted request	✔	To sound	3
After finger tip stimulus	✔	To pressure	2
No opening at any time, no interferring factor	✔	None	1
Closed by local factor	✔	Non testable	NT

Verbal response

Criterion	Observed	Rating	Score
Correctly gives name, place and date	✔	Orientated	5
Not orientated but communication coherently	✔	Confused	4
Intelligible single words	✔	Words	3
Only moans / groans	✔	Sounds	2
No audible response, no interferring factor	✔	None	1
Factor interferring with communication	✔	Non testable	NT

Best motor response

Criterion	Observed	Rating	Score
Obey 2-part request	✔	Obeys commands	6
Brings hand above clavicle to stimulus on head neck	✔	Localising	5
Bends arm at elbow rapidly but features not predominantly abnormal	✔	Normal flexion	4
Bends arm at elbow, features clearly predominantly abnormal	✔	Abnormal flexion	3
Extends arm at elbow	✔	Extension	2
No movement in arms / legs, no interferring factor	✔	None	1
Paralysed or other limiting factor	✔	Non testable	NT

Sites for Physical Stimulation

Finger tip pressure   Trapezius pinch   Supraorbital notch

Features of Flexion Responses

Modified with permission from Van Der Naalt 2004 Ned Tijdschr Geneeskd

Abnormal Flexion
Slow stereotyped
Arm across chest
Forearm rotates
Thumb clenched
Leg extends

Normal flexion
Rapid
Variable
Arm away from body

For further information and video demonstration visit www.glasgowcomascale.org

Graphic design by Margaret Frej based on layout and illustrations from Medical Illustration M I • 268093

Figure 3.2 Glasgow Coma Scale. Source: http://www.glasgowcomascale.org/. Accessed August 2016. Reproduced with permission of Sir Graham Teasdale.

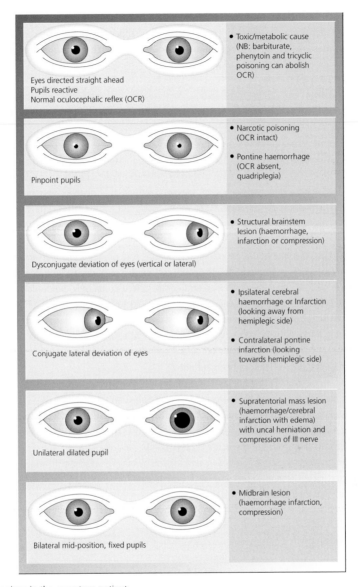

Figure 3.3 Eye signs in the comatose patient.

• Examine the limbs: tone, response to a painful stimulus (nailbed pressure), tendon reflexes and plantar responses.

7 Make a diagnosis

The differential diagnosis for reduced consciousness can be split into three groups on the basis of the presence or absence of focal signs and meningism (Table 3.1).

• **If bacterial meningitis or viral meningo-encephalitis are possible** (because of fever and meningism), empirical anti-microbial therapy (with cefotaxime (plus ampicillin in patients over 55 or at increased risk of listeria infection) and aciclovir) should be started immediately, after taking blood for culture. See Chapters 68 and 69.

- **If acute adrenal insufficiency is possible (Chapter 90)** give hydrocortisone 200 mg IV. Fludrocortisone is not required in addition as this dose of hydrocortisone has sufficient mineralocorticoid action.
- **If CT shows a mass lesion or hydrocephalus, seek urgent advice from a neurosurgeon.**

Further management

- Further management is directed by the working diagnosis, based on the clinical signs, CT findings and laboratory results (Table 3.1).
- Patients with a reduced conscious level should be nursed in a high-dependency or intensive-care unit.
- In all patients, regular reassessment of the depth of coma, eye signs and neurology is required to establish any progression or resolution. Complications arising from coma, such as pressure injury of skin and muscle, deep vein thrombosis, respiratory infection/aspiration and contractures need to be considered and pre-empted where possible. Some patients, for example those with a malignant MCA territory infarct, may require close monitoring and repeat neuroimaging if neurosurgical intervention/decompressive craniectomy is being considered.
- Induced hypothermia can improve the neurological prognosis for coma after cardiac arrest.
- In some patients no cause is apparent for their reduced conscious level. Early in the presentation, it is reasonable to give glucose, thiamine, naloxone and corticosteroid empirically, before laboratory results are available, if hypoglycaemia, Wernicke's encephalopathy, opioid toxicity or acute adrenal insufficiency are possible.
- For those remaining in cryptogenic coma there are a number of considerations:
  - Could this be a coma mimic, such as functional unresponsiveness?
  - Has non-convulsive status epilepticus been excluded?
  - Could this be an autoimmune/paraneoplastic encephalopathy (for which serological diagnostic support may be delayed or inconclusive)? Should empirical immunosuppression be trialled?
  - Has existing brain pathology (or extreme age) resulted in more prolonged or deeper coma than otherwise expected – for example following a brief seizure or lesser degrees of metabolic derangement – or produced misleading localizing signs despite the acute process being non-focal?
- It is also important to remember that the history and toxicology may not disclose the ingestion of all relevant drugs, that hepatic encephalopathy can occur with normal liver function tests, and that CSF PCR does not detect all cases of viral encephalitis.

Further reading

Edlow JA, Rabinstein A, Traub SJ, Wijdicks EF. (2014) Diagnosis of reversible causes of coma. *Lancet* 384, 2064–2076.

Royal College of Physicians (2013) Prolonged disorders of consciousness: National clinical guidelines. London, RCP, https://www.rcplondon.ac.uk/guidelines-policy/prolonged-disorders-consciousness-national-clinical-guidelines.

Traub SJ, Wijdicks EF. (2016) Initial diagnosis and management of coma. *Emerg Med Clin North Am* 34, 777–793.

CHAPTER 4

Delirium

DAVID SPRIGINGS

Consider delirium (Box 4.1) in patients with:

- Abnormal cognitive function (confusion, impaired concentration, slow responses to questions – the patient described as a 'poor historian').
- Abnormal mood ('depression' developing in hospital).
- Abnormal perception (visual or auditory hallucinations).
- Abnormal behaviour (restlessness, agitation or reluctance to mobilize; unwillingness to eat or drink; abnormal sleep-wake cycle).
- Abnormal social behaviour (withdrawal from social contact; unwillingness to cooperate with care – the patient described as 'uncooperative' or 'difficult').

Several neuropsychiatric disorders may give rise to abnormal consciousness, language, memory or behaviour, and should be considered in the differential diagnosis of delirium (Table 4.1).

Causes of delirium are given in Appendix 4.1, and diagnoses to consider in specific patient groups in Table 4.2. Assessment of the patient with delirium is summarized in Figure 4.1.

Box 4.1 Delirium

Delirium is a functional brain disorder, characterized by disturbances of consciousness, attention and cognition. The term 'acute confusional state' is often used synonymously with delirium, although delirium is preferred, as confusion (uncertainty about what is happening, intended, or required) is not specific to delirium and its medical definition is imprecise.

It can reflect a primary neurological disorder, substance intoxication or withdrawal, an adverse effect of drugs (especially those with an anticholinergic effect), or a systemic disorder such as sepsis (Appendix 4.1).

In sepsis, delirium may be caused by cytokines which enter the brain and activate microglia. Microglia then release molecules which cause neuronal dysfunction and thus delirium. Failure of cholinergic inhibition of microglia (due to neurodegenerative disease, or drugs with an anticholinergic effect) may amplify the microglial response to inflammatory cytokines.

It is distinguished from dementia (with which it may coexist, as dementia is a major risk factor for delirium) by its speed of onset (over hours or days) and reversibility with correction of the underlying cause.

Delirium is clinical diagnosis; criteria are given in Table 4.1.

Acute Medicine: A Practical Guide to the Management of Medical Emergencies, Fifth Edition. Edited by David Sprigings and John B. Chambers.
© 2018 John Wiley & Sons Ltd. Published 2018 by John Wiley & Sons Ltd.

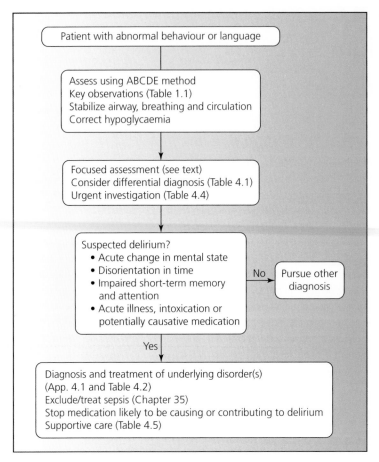

Figure 4.1 Assessment of the patient with delirium.

Priorities

1 Make a rapid assessment to ensure that airway, breathing and circulation are not compromised. Check blood glucose and correct hypoglycaemia (Chapter 81).

2 Assess the mental state. This can be done using the ten-item abbreviated mental test score (Table 4.3) or equivalent.
   - The diagnosis of delirium is based on the criteria shown in Table 4.1. Delirium is characterized by a change in the mental state (occurring over hours or days, often fluctuating over the course of the day), associated with a causative acute medical or toxic illness (Appendix 4.1).
   - The duration of the patient's abnormal mental state, as assessed by a reliable witness, often helps distinguish delirium from dementia (which may of course coexist).

3 What is causing delirium?
   - Establish current symptoms, context and past history by talking to family members, carers or hospital staff, and reviewing relevant medical records.
   - Check the drug chart. Many drugs may cause delirium, notably benzodiazepines, tricyclics, analgesics (including NSAIDs), lithium, corticosteroids, and medications for parkinsonism.

Table 4.1 Differential diagnosis of acutely disturbed behaviour or language.

Diagnosis	Comment
Delirium	Diagnostic criteria:* • There is a disturbance of consciousness, that is, reduced clarity of awareness of the environment, with reduced ability to focus, sustain or shift attention. • There is a change in cognition, such as memory deficit, disorientation, language disturbance, or the development of a perceptual disturbance that is not better accounted for by a pre-existing dementia. • The disturbance has developed over a short period of time (usually hours to days) and tends to fluctuate during the course of the day. • There is evidence from the history, examination or laboratory findings that the disturbance is caused either by the direct physiological consequences of a general medical condition, or by substance intoxication/withdrawal, or by medication.
Acute psychosis (manic or schizophrenic)	Typical features of acute psychosis include: • Hallucinations • Delusions • Confused and disturbed thoughts • Lack of insight and self-awareness Assume a diagnosis of delirium rather than acute psychosis if: • The patient is older than 40 with no previous psychiatric history • There is a history of alcohol or substance-use disorder • There are major medical comorbidities • There is disorientation, clouding of consciousness or decreased alertness, or • Physiological observations are abnormal
Other psychiatric disorders	Agitated depression, anxiety disorder, borderline and anti-social personality disorders may result in acutely disturbed behaviour.
Non-convulsive status epilepticus (NCSE)	In NCSE, there are often mild clonic movements of the eyelids, face or hands, or simple automatisms. The EEG is abnormal.
Transient global amnesia	Abrupt onset of antegrade amnesia without clouding of consciousness or loss of personal identity. Cognitive impairment is limited to amnesia, and there are no focal neurological or epileptic signs. Symptoms resolve within 24 h.
Fluent dysphasia	Speech is fluent but with meaningless words, unnecessary phrases and nonsensical grammar. There is no clouding of consciousness.

* Source: American Psychiatric Association (2000) *Diagnostic and Statistical Manual*, 4th edition.

- If the patient was admitted with delirium, find out exactly what drugs were being taken prior to admission: if necessary, contact the patient's general practitioner to check which drugs were prescribed, and ask relatives to collect all medications in the home.
- Review the physiological observations and make a systematic examination. Check for focal chest signs, abdominal tenderness or guarding, urinary retention, faecal impaction, pressure ulceration and cellulitis. Are there abnormal neurological signs? As a minimum, examine for neck stiffness and lateralized weakness, and check the plantar responses.
- Consider non-convulsive status epilepticus if there are mild clonic movements of the eyelids, face or hands, or simple automatisms. Diazepam (10 mg IV, at a rate of <2.5 mg/min) may terminate the status with improvement in conscious level. Seek advice from a neurologist.

Table 4.2 Causes of delirium to consider in specific patient groups.

Patient group	Common causes
Older patient in emergency dept	Acute infection
	Adverse effect of medication
	Electrolyte disorder
	Stroke
	Subdural haematoma
Younger patient in emergency dept	Alcohol intoxication
	Poisoning with cocaine, amphetamine and other psychoactive drugs
	Primary neurological disorder (e.g. encephalitis)
Older patient with delirium after surgery	Acute infection
	Adverse effect of medication
	Urinary retention
	Faecal impaction
Patient from psychiatric hospital	Neuroleptic malignant syndrome
	Primary neurological disorder (e.g. encephalitis, brain tumour)
Patient with alcohol use disorder	Alcohol intoxication or withdrawal
	Wernicke encephalopathy
	Decompensated chronic liver disease
	Acute infection (e.g. pneumonia, spontaneous bacterial peritonitis)
Patient with cancer	Adverse effect of medication (e.g. opioid toxicity)
	Brain or meningeal metastases
	Electrolyte disorder (e.g. hyponatraemia, hypercalcaemia)
	Paraneoplastic effect

Reference: Oxford Clinical Diagnosis and Treatment eds Davey & Sprigings, OUP 2018. Reproduced with permission.

Table 4.3 Abbreviated mental test score.

- Age
- Time (to nearest hour)
- Address for recall at end of test – this should be repeated by the patient to ensure it has been heard correctly: 42 West Street
- Year
- Name of hospital
- Recognition of two people (e.g. doctor, nurse)
- Date of birth (day and month sufficient)
- Year of 2nd World War
- Name of present monarch
- Count backwards 20–1

Each correct answer scores one mark. The healthy elderly score 8–10.

Source: Qureshi KN, Hodkinson HM (1974) Evaluation of a ten-question mental test in the institutionalized elderly. *Age and Ageing* 3, 152–157. Reproduced with permission of Oxford University Press.

Table 4.4 Urgent investigation in delirium.

Blood glucose
Plasma sodium, potassium, urea and creatinine
Liver function tests, albumin and calcium
Full blood count
Prothrombin time or international normalized ratio (INR) if suspected liver disease
C-reactive protein
Blood culture if temperature <36 or >38 °C
Urine stick test; microscopy and culture if stick test abnormal or evidence of sepsis
ECG
Chest X-ray
Arterial blood gases if arterial oxygen saturation <92% or new chest signs
Neuroimaging, if indicated: see text (point 4)
Lumbar puncture, if indicated: see text (point 5)
EEG, if indicated: see text

- Are there signs suggesting liver failure (jaundice, asterixis, ascites, signs of chronic liver disease)? See Chapter 77 for further management of acute liver failure and decompensated chronic liver disease.
- In patients with delirium in the context of alcohol-use disorder, check for other signs of Wernicke's encephalopathy: nystagmus, VI nerve palsy (unable to abduct the eye) and ataxia (wide-based gait; may be unable to stand or walk). See Chapter 106 for management.
- Test a urine specimen if available for white cells, blood and protein. If there is fever or low temperature, new focal chest signs or oxygen saturation is <94% breathing air, arrange a chest X-ray. Other investigations needed are given in Table 4.4.

4 **Neuroimaging** (by CT or MRI) is indicated if:
  - Delirium followed a fall or head injury.
  - A primary neurological disorder (e.g. encephalitis) is suspected.
  - There are new focal neurological signs.
  - There is papilloedema or other evidence of raised intracranial pressure.
  - The patient has cancer, HIV-AIDS or other cause of immunosuppression.
  - The patient's behaviour prevents adequate neurological examination.
  - No systemic cause for the delirium is apparent.

5 **Lumbar puncture** with examination of the cerebrospinal fluid should be done (assuming no contraindication to lumbar puncture) if:
  - Meningitis (Chapter 68) or encephalitis (Chapter 69) is suspected.
  - The patient is febrile and no systemic focus of infection is found.
  - The cause of delirium remains unclear.

6 **Electroencephalography (EEG)** is indicated if:
  - Non-convulsive status epilepticus or encephalitis is suspected.
  - It is unclear if the diagnosis is delirium or psychosis.
  - No cause for delirium is apparent, despite investigation.

Further management

- Identify and treat the underlying cause (Appendix 4.1; Table 4.2).
- Ensure comprehensive supportive care (Table 4.5), with avoidance of physical restraint, and anticipation and prevention of complications of delirium (e.g. dehydration, constipation, pressure ulceration).

Table 4.5 Supportive care of the patient with delirium.

Exclude/treat sepsis
Stop medications likely to be causing or contributing to delirium
Prevent dehydration: ensure adequate fluid intake
Exclude/relieve urinary retention
Exclude/prevent constipation
Exclude/prevent pressure ulceration
Assess for/relieve pain
Prevent DVT: give thromboprophylaxis if indicated
Prevent sleep disturbance
Ensure spectacles and hearing aid are worn if needed
Reality orientation: give the patient information about time, place and person, repeated at regular intervals

- Review the drug chart. Avoid unnecessary medications, especially those with an anticholinergic effect.
- If needed, to relieve severe distress or prevent injury, give short-term therapy (one week or less) with haloperidol (in a dose of <3 mg daily) or olanzapine (the latter is contraindicated in patients with dementia).

Appendix 4.1 Causes of delirium.

Category of disorder	Examples/comment
Primary neurological disorders	Head injury
	Post-ictal state
	Non-dominant parietal lobe stroke
	Subdural haematoma
	Subarachnoid haemorrhage
	Non-convulsive status epilepticus
	Meningitis
	Encephalitis
	Raised intracranial pressure
Substance intoxication or withdrawal	Alcohol intoxication or withdrawal
	Wernicke's encephalopathy
	Intoxication with amphetamine and amphetamine-type drugs, benzodiazepines, cannabis, cocaine, opioids and other psychoactive substances
	Withdrawal of opioids
Adverse effect of drugs	Benzodiazepines, tricyclics, analgesics (including NSAIDs), lithium, high-dose corticosteroids, and drugs for parkinsonism
	Neuroleptic malignant syndrome (Appendix 69.2)
Sepsis	Urinary or respiratory tract infections are the commonest causes.
	Bacterial meningitis (Chapter 68), infective endocarditis (Chapter 52) and intra-abdominal sepsis (e.g. cholangitis (Chapter 35) should also be considered in the patient with delirium and signs of sepsis.
	Exclude malaria if there has been recent travel to an endemic region (Chapter 33).
Other systemic disorders	Hypoglycaemia
	Hyperglycaemic states
	Any organ failure
	Severe electrolyte disorders
	Severe endocrine disorders
	Other metabolic disorders
	Hypothermia

Further reading

Fong TG, Davis D, Growdon ME, Albuqerque A, Inouye SK. (2015) The interface between delirium and dementia in elderly adults. *Lancet Neurol* 14, 823–832.

Inouye SK, Westendorp RGJ, Saczynski JS. (2013) Delirium in elderly people. *Lancet* 383, 911–922.

National Institute for Health and Care Excellence (2010) Delirium: prevention, diagnosis and management. Clinical guideline (CG103) Reviewed January 2015. https://www.nice.org.uk/guidance/cg103?unlid=9628712972016102061852

Woodford HJ, George J, Jackson M. (2015) Non-convulsive status epilepticus: a practical approach to diagnosis in confused older people. *Postgrad Med J* 91, 655–661.

CHAPTER 5

Falls in older people

SIMON CONROY AND OJA PATHAK

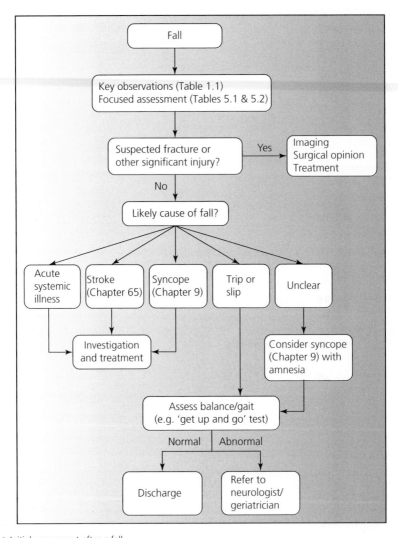

Figure 5.1 Initial assessment after a fall.

Acute Medicine: A Practical Guide to the Management of Medical Emergencies, Fifth Edition. Edited by David Sprigings and John B. Chambers.
© 2018 John Wiley & Sons Ltd. Published 2018 by John Wiley & Sons Ltd.

Priorities

1 Assess the patient for acute illness and injury (Tables 5.1 and 5.2).

If there is a suspected fracture or other significant injury, arrange appropriate imaging and request a surgical opinion.

2 Could the fall be due to syncope?

See Chapter 9 for the assessment of syncope.

3 If there is no evidence pointing to syncope as the cause of the fall, you will need to consider other factors that may have challenged balance. 'Mechanical fall' is often used to imply that a severe cause has been excluded, but it is better to decide why a fall has occurred, so that steps can be taken to prevent a recurrence. A fall is not a diagnosis but a symptom with multiple possible causes. Falls can result from deficits in one or more of:

- Sensory inputs: vision, proprioception and vestibular function (impairments may be due to stroke, diabetic retinopathy, cataracts)
- Central processing of sensory information
- Effector mechanisms: muscle strength and balance
- Postural blood pressure control, with orthostatic hypotension exacerbating poor balance
- Environmental factors, such as loose rugs

Further management

Testing your theories

Having put together a formulation for the reasons behind the fall, encompassing a range of sensory and motor issues, you can then proceed to test your theories by physical examination.

- You will need a Snellen chart, tuning fork and the ability to examine the neuromuscular system. It is not usual to test vestibular function in the acute setting unless you suspect benign positional paroxysmal vertigo (BPPV), in which case a Hallpike test can usually be carried out at the bedside.
- A useful test of function is the 'get up and go' test. Check the patient is able to stand (if they can straight-leg-raise in bed, they should be able to stand) and walk. Usual footwear should be worn, and usual walking aid used. Ask the patient to stand up from a standard chair, and walk a distance of at least 3 m, then turn and get back to the chair. There is no need to time the test. People who cannot 'get up and go' unaided are at increased risk of future falls.
- You will usually work with therapy colleagues to confirm the reasons behind the fall.
- You may need to do some focused investigations but be sure you know why you are doing them and how you will interpret the results

Box 5.1 Falls

A fall is commonly defined as 'unintentionally coming to rest on the ground, floor or other lower level'. This excludes coming to rest against furniture, wall, or other structure, and also excludes syncope.

One-third of community-dwelling older people fall each year, as do 50% of those aged 85 and over.

Although most falls do not result in serious harm, they are potentially serious, and may result in injury, fear of falling and social isolation.

Falls have a major impact on hospital services, and are an important cause of carer strain and admission to long-term care.

Multifactorial interventions delivered to fallers are effective in reducing falls rates by 25%.

Table 5.1 Focused assessment after a fall.

History
Circumstances of fall (e.g. place, time of day, witnessed)
Symptoms before fall (e.g. presyncope/syncope, palpitations, acute illness)
Injuries sustained (facial injury following fall suggests syncope with failure of protective reflexes)
Contributory factors (e.g. dementia, previous stroke, parkinsonism, lower limb joint disorders, foot disorders)
Previous falls (how many in past year?)
Previous syncope
Usual effort tolerance (e.g. able to climb stairs; able to walk on flat; able to manage activities of daily living)
Walking aids used
If fall at home, are there environmental hazards (ask family/carer), for example loose rugs, poor lighting?
Current medications (e.g. sedatives, hypnotics, antidepressants, antihypertensives, multiple drugs)
Alcohol history
Social history: living at home or residential/nursing home resident?
Examination
Physiological observations including BP sitting and standing
Systematic examination (focal neurological abnormalities, severe aortic stenosis)
Injuries sustained (check for head injury, fracture, joint dislocation, soft tissue bruising and laceration)
Assess mental state (e.g. abbreviated mental test score, see Table 4.3)
If the patient does not have evidence of acute illness or injury, screen for neurological and musculoskeletal disorders with
the 'get up and go' test: ask the patient to stand up from a chair, walk 3 m and return: can this be done without
difficulty or unsteadiness (see text)?

Table 5.2 Investigation after a fall.

ECG
Blood glucose
Plasma sodium, potassium, urea and creatinine
Full blood count
Urinalysis – only if symptoms of UTI, not routine
Further investigation directed by clinical features

Preventing falls

Once you have a set of reasons as to why the patient fell, you will need to put in place management plans for each
of the issues.

- This may involve further diagnostics (e.g. testing for reversible causes of peripheral neuropathy), referral to
  therapeutic interventions (e.g. falls service for outpatient strength and balance training, or referral for a more
  detailed visual assessment).
- Depending on the context, you may need a rapid response for people going home, in the form of community
  rehabilitation services.
- The environment is important. If going home, a home hazards assessment should be undertaken (e.g. by the
  community therapy teams). If being admitted, inform the ward team if the patient is at high risk of falls (e.g.
  those that fail the 'get up and go' test) and therefore requires careful surveillance.

Medication is an important cause of falls. Consider using a structured approach to medication review, such as
the STOPP/START criteria. Key medications for risk-benefit balance include:

- Diuretics (are they really needed? What is the patient's state of hydration?)
- Anti-hypertensives (look for labile blood pressure dropping beyond the range of cerebral autoregulation)
- Psychoactive medication (SSRIs increase falls risk, sedatives impair balance)
- Neuroleptics may provoke Parkinsonism

Warfarin or other anticoagulants are sometimes stopped because of falls. Unless someone is falling weekly or more often, do not stop warfarin unless there are other considerations, since the benefits usually outweigh the risks.

Dementia is a major consideration. Ensure you check cognition, as the presence of dementia increases falls risk, and often makes interventions more difficult to implement. You will need to involve the full MDT in people with falls and dementia, as well as carers.

Despite addressing all of the above and implementing a multifactorial management plan, you will usually only reduce the rate of falls by 25% per year. So you will need to ensure that you have mitigated the consequences of future falls by ensuring that:

- The patient has access to help if they do fall.
- The patient knows how to fall safely and get back up (the falls programme will often address this).
- The potential consequences of a fall are addressed, such as fracture risk http://www.shef.ac.uk/FRAX/tool.jsp?locationValue=9). Consider adding bone protection. Vitamin D can reduce the rate of falls by about 20%, so it is usually worth adding it to the prescription.

Further reading

Rimland JM, Abraha I, Dell'Aquila G, *et al.* (2016) Effectiveness of non-pharmacological interventions to prevent falls in older people: a systematic overview. *PLOS ONE*. DOI: 10.1371/journal.pone.0161579. 25 August.

Cardiorespiratory

CHAPTER 6

Cardiac arrest in hospital

DAVID SPRIGINGS AND JOHN B. CHAMBERS

- This chapter summarizes the management of cardiac arrest in hospital (Box 6.1), following the 2015 Guidelines of the UK Resuscitation Council (https://www.resus.org.uk/resuscitation-guidelines/in-hospital-resuscitation/).
- All hospital medical staff should know how to respond to cardiac arrest, and should regularly rehearse cardiopulmonary resuscitation (CPR).
- It is also important to recognize when attempts at CPR would not be justified, so that patients are not subjected to an inappropriate intervention at the end of their lives (see Appendix 6.1).

Initial management

Figure 6.1 shows the algorithm for the initial management of in-hospital cardiac arrest or peri-arrest.

If the patient has a monitored and witnessed cardiac arrest, and a manual defibrillator is rapidly available:

- Confirm cardiac arrest and shout for help.
- If the initial rhythm is VF/pVT, give up to three quick successive (stacked) shocks.
- Rapidly check for a rhythm change and, if appropriate, check for a pulse and other signs of a return of spontaneous circulation (ROSC) after each defibrillation attempt.
- Start chest compressions and continue CPR for two minutes if the third shock is unsuccessful. These initial three stacked shocks are considered as giving the first shock in the ALS algorithm (Figure 6.2).

Box 6.1 In-hospital cardiac arrest

In-hospital cardiac arrest (IHCA) occurs in two groups of patients that differ in pathophysiology and underlying cardiac rhythm (Table 6.1):
- Ventricular fibrillation/pulseless ventricular tachycardia (VF/pVT) (~25% total). This is typically due to myocardial ischaemia or primary cardiac disease.
- Pulseless electrical activity (PEA) (~50% total) or asystole (~25% total), usually as the result of prolonged hypoxia, hypotension or other severe metabolic derangement from non-cardiac disease. For this second group of patients, better outcomes may be achieved by earlier recognition, diagnosis and treatment of critical illness (Chapter 1), so that progression to cardiac arrest is forestalled.

Acute Medicine: A Practical Guide to the Management of Medical Emergencies, Fifth Edition. Edited by David Sprigings and John B. Chambers.
© 2018 John Wiley & Sons Ltd. Published 2018 by John Wiley & Sons Ltd.

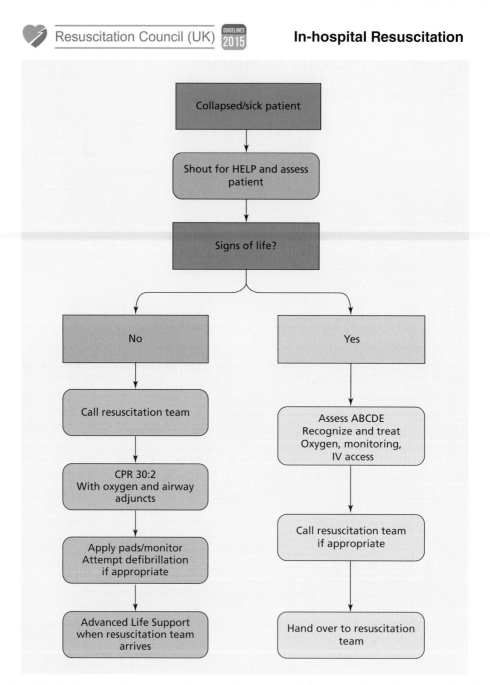

Figure 6.1 Algorithm for initial management of In-hospital cardiac arrest or peri-arrest. Source: Resuscitation Council. Reproduced with permission of the Resuscitation Council (UK).

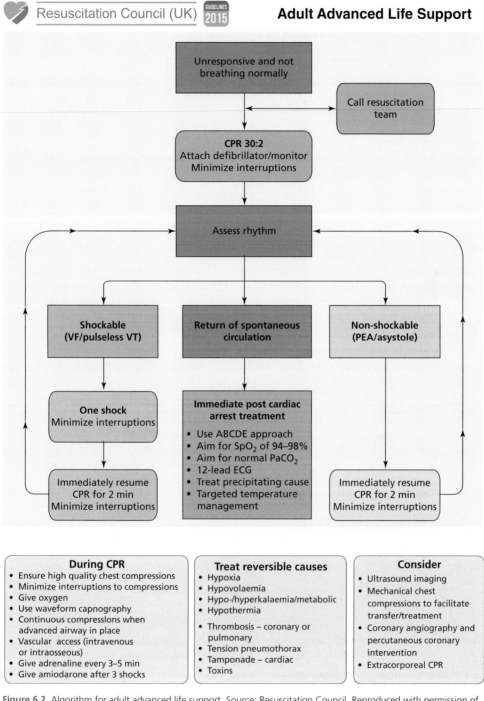

Figure 6.2 Algorithm for adult advanced life support. Source: Resuscitation Council. Reproduced with permission of the Resuscitation Council (UK).

Further management

Figure 6.2 shows the algorithm for advanced life support in adults.
- Each cycle consists of 2 min of CPR followed by assessment of the rhythm and, if the rhythm is compatible with a spontaneous output, check the pulse.
- Adrenaline 1 mg is given every 3–5 min (i.e. every other cycle of CPR) until ROSC is achieved.

1 Airway maintenance and ventilation
Airway
See Chapters 59 and 112.
- Use head tilt and chin lift or jaw thrust to open the airway. Use suction to clear the airway if needed. Place an oropharyngeal or nasopharyngeal device to maintain an open airway.
- Endotracheal intubation or placement of a supraglottic airway can be done by an experienced operator.

Ventilation
See Chapter 112.
- Use a bag-valve device, which allows ventilation with 100% oxygen. Aim for a tidal volume of 400–600 mL. This is adequate for oxygenation, and less likely to cause gastric insufflation (which increases the risk of vomiting and aspiration) than larger volumes. Over-ventilation may also cause barotrauma, pneumothorax and cardiovascular compromise.
- The ratio of chest compressions to ventilations should be 30:2. However, if an endotracheal tube or supraglottic airway has been placed, give 8–10 ventilations/min, not synchronized with chest compressions.
- Waveform capnography enables end-tidal CO_2 ($E_T CO_2$) to be monitored during CPR. Measurement of $E_T CO_2$ can confirm appropriate placement of an endotracheal tube, assess the adequacy of CPR and indicate ROSC (when $E_T CO_2$ increases) during CPR.

2 Chest compression
- Chest compressions should be performed at a rate of 100–120/min.
- Compress the chest by 5–6 cm, allowing the chest to recoil completely after each compression.
- Minimize interruptions to chest compression. To maintain high-quality chest compression, ideally change the person doing chest compressions after each cycle of CPR.

3 Defibrillation for ventricular fibrillation/pulseless ventricular tachycardia (VF/pVT)
- Place the sternal electrode to the right of the sternum, below the clavicle. Place the apical electrode in the mid-axillary line, clear of any breast tissue.
- Continue chest compressions during defibrillator charging. Remove any oxygen mask or nasal cannulae and place them at least 1 m away from the patient's chest during defibrillation.
- Deliver defibrillation with an interruption in chest compressions of no more than 5 seconds. Immediately resume chest compressions following defibrillation. Only check the pulse between shocks if the ECG waveform changes to one compatible with a spontaneous output. Deliver the first shock with an energy of at least 150 J. If this is unsuccessful, deliver the second and subsequent shocks with a higher energy level if the defibrillator is capable of this. If VF/pVT recurs during a cardiac arrest (refibrillation), give subsequent shocks with a higher energy level if the defibrillator is capable of this.

4 Pulseless electrical activity (PEA)/asystole
- Check electrode positions and contacts before concluding the rhythm is not VF/pVT.
- Consider the potentially reversible causes of cardiac arrest with PEA/asystole and address these (Table 6.1).

Table 6.1 Causes of cardiac arrest.

With ventricular fibrillation (VF)/pulseless ventricular tachycardia (pVT)
Acute coronary syndrome
Ischaemic heart disease with previous myocardial infarction
Other structural heart disease (e.g. dilated or hypertrophic cardiomyopathy)
Wolff-Parkinson-White syndrome
Channelopathies (e.g. long QT syndrome, Brugada syndrome)

With pulseless electrical activity (PEA) or asystole
Hypovolaemia
Hypoxaemia
Hypokalaemia/hyperkalaemia/hypocalcaemia
Hypothermia

Toxins (poisoning)
Tamponade: cardiac
Tension pneumothorax
Thromboembolism: pulmonary

---

5 Specific drug therapy and drug delivery
- If a central venous line is not already in place, put a wide-bore cannula in a large peripheral vein. Use a flush of 20 mL of normal saline and elevation of the limb after drug administration to facilitate delivery to the central circulation.
- If IV access is not possible, the intraosseous route can be used.

Adrenaline
- Give adrenaline 1 mg IV every 3–5 min (i.e. every other cycle of CPR) until ROSC is achieved.

Amiodarone
- Give amiodarone 300 mg IV if VF/pVT persists after a total of three shocks.

Sodium bicarbonate
- Sodium bicarbonate (50 mL of 8.4% solution (50 mmol)) should only be given for cardiac arrest due to severe hyperkalaemia or tricyclic poisoning.

Fibrinolytic therapy
- Fibrinolytic therapy should be considered for cardiac arrest in the setting of proven or suspected pulmonary embolism: see Chapter 57. In this circumstance, CPR may need to be continued for 60–90 minutes.

6 Focused echocardiography/ultrasonography during CPR
See Chapter 114.
- Focused echocardiography/ultrasonography by an experienced operator may help identify a potentially reversible cause of cardiac arrest (e.g. cardiac tamponade, pulmonary embolism, hypovolaemia).
- If the probe is placed just before chest compressions are paused for a planned rhythm assessment, views can be obtained within 10 seconds.

7 Management of tachycardia and bradycardia after ROSC
- See Figures 6.3 and 6.4.
- Further information about the management of arrhythmias is given in Chapters 39–44.

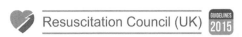

Resuscitation Council (UK)

Tachycardia Algorithm (with pulse)

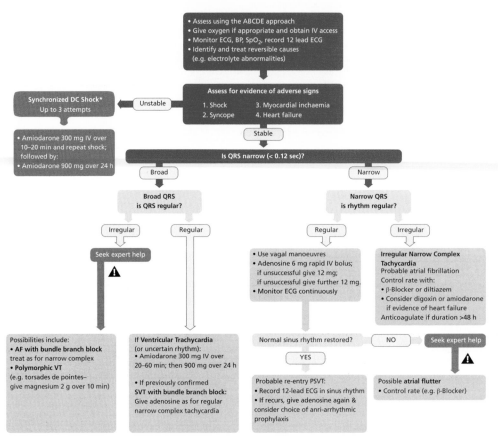

Figure 6.3 Tachycardia with pulse. Source: Resuscitation Council. Reproduced with permission of the Resuscitation Council (UK).

8 When to stop resuscitation

- Resuscitation should be stopped if a: 'Do not attempt cardiopulmonary resuscitation' (DNACPR) order (Appendix 6.1) has been written, or the circumstances of the patient indicate that one should have been.
- Resuscitation should be stopped if there is refractory asystole for more than 20 min (except when cardiac arrest is due to hypothermia). Resuscitation should not be stopped while the rhythm is ventricular fibrillation.
- Absence of cardiac motion on echocardiography during CPR is highly predictive of death, but should not be the sole basis for the decision to stop CPR.

9 After successful resuscitation

- Protect the airway until the patient is fully conscious. Adjust inspired oxygen to achieve arterial oxygen saturation 94–98%. Mechanical ventilation should be continued if:
  - The patient's conscious level is reduced (Glasgow Coma Scale score 8 or below).
  - There is severe pulmonary oedema.
  - Arterial PO_2 is <9 kPa or PCO_2 is >6.5 kPa.

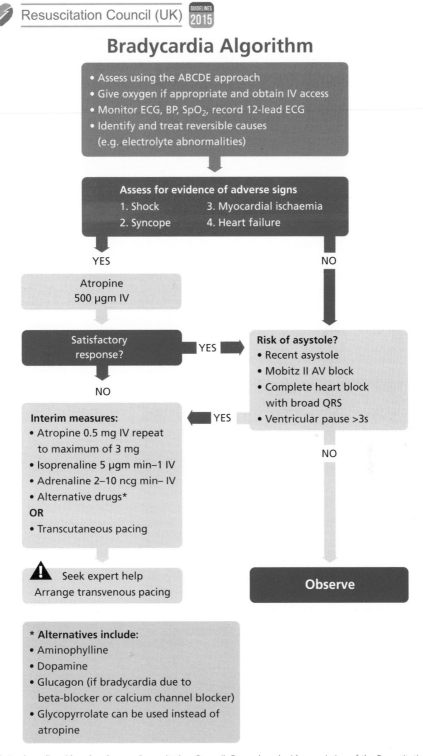

Figure 6.4 Bradycardia with pulse. Source: Resuscitation Council. Reproduced with permission of the Resuscitation Council (UK).

Table 6.2 Urgent investigation after successful resuscitation.

ECG (? acute coronary syndrome, long QT interval)
Chest X-ray (? pulmonary oedema, pneumothorax, rib fracture)
Echocardiography (? structural heart disease, right and left ventricular size and systolic function, pericardial effusion)
Arterial blood gases and pH
Plasma sodium, potassium, calcium and magnesium
Plasma urea and creatinine
Blood glucose
Plasma troponin

- Insert a nasogastric tube to decompress the stomach and prevent splinting of the diaphragm by gastric distension in patients needing mechanical ventilation.
- Check arterial blood gases and other blood tests (Table 6.2). Maintain ECG monitoring. Record a 12-lead ECG, and check the blood pressure. Arrange a chest X-ray. Perform focused echocardiography/ ultrasonography.
- Decide why the arrest occurred, and take action to deal with the underlying causes.
  - If there is evidence of ST elevation acute coronary syndrome, consider revascularization by thrombolysis or PCI (Table 25.2).
  - If cardiac arrest was due to primary brady-asystole (Chapter 44), arrange placement of a temporary pacing system (Chapter 119).
  - Correct derangements of plasma potassium, calcium and magnesium (Chapters 86–88).
  - Arrange CT brain if conscious level is reduced or a primary neurological cause for cardiac arrest is suspected.
- Transfer the patient to the appropriate ward (CCU, HDU or ITU), with ECG monitoring during transfer. Prevent sepsis: IV lines inserted without sterile technique during the resuscitation should be changed.
- Protect the brain:
  - Optimize cerebral perfusion. Correct arrhythmias that are causing haemodynamic instability (Figures 6.3 and 6.4; Chapters 39–44). Post-resuscitation myocardial dysfunction (lasting 24–48 h) may result in hypotension and low cardiac output, requiring inotropic vasopressor support (Chapter 2).
  - Control seizures (Chapter 16).
  - Control blood glucose (Chapters 81 and 82).
  - Treat hyperthermia by fanning, tepid sponging or paracetamol.
  - If there is coma, therapeutic hypothermia (32–36 °C, for 24 h) is indicated.

Appendix 6.1 Decisions about cardiopulmonary resuscitation

The management plan for all hospital inpatients should include consideration as to whether CPR should be attempted in the event of cardiac arrest.
- This decision must involve the patient, unless the patient lacks capacity for this (Chapter 111).
- When a patient lacks this capacity, the senior clinician responsible for the patient should make the decision, having consulted with those close to the patient, unless the patient has recorded their wishes in an Advance Decision to Refuse Treatment or has a representative with legal authority (e.g. Power of Attorney) to make such decisions (Chapter 111).
- All discussions and decisions about CPR must be recorded fully and clearly, preferably using a standard form (e.g. Figure 6.5), and communicated to all members of the medical and nursing team caring for the patient. The decision about CPR should be reviewed:

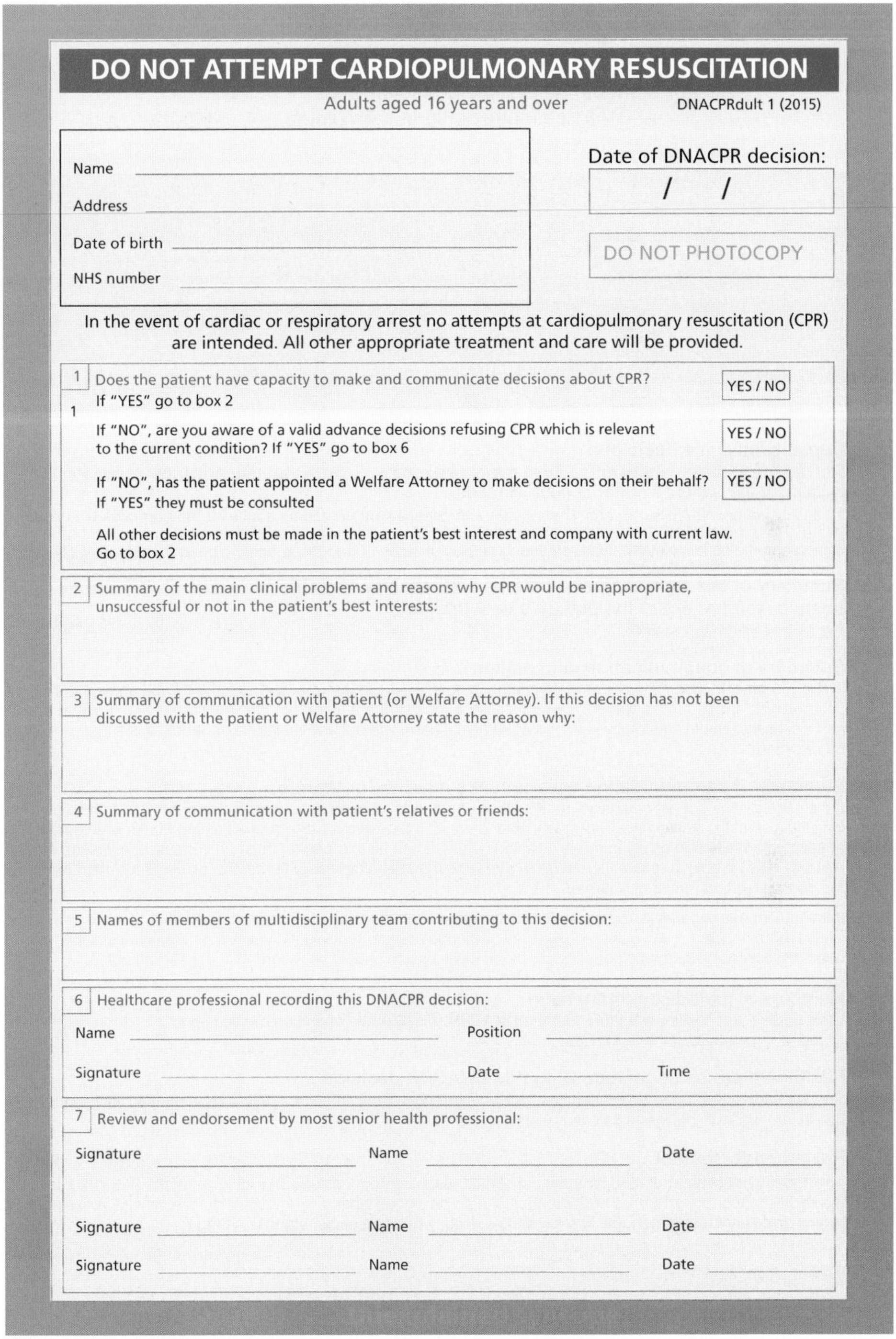

DO NOT ATTEMPT CARDIOPULMONARY RESUSCITATION

Adults aged 16 years and over   DNACPRdult 1 (2015)

Name _____

Address _____

Date of birth _____

NHS number _____

Date of DNACPR decision:

/   /

DO NOT PHOTOCOPY

In the event of cardiac or respiratory arrest no attempts at cardiopulmonary resuscitation (CPR) are intended. All other appropriate treatment and care will be provided.

1	Does the patient have capacity to make and communicate decisions about CPR?	YES / NO

1   If "YES" go to box 2

If "NO", are you aware of a valid advance decisions refusing CPR which is relevant to the current condition? If "YES" go to box 6 — YES / NO

If "NO", has the patient appointed a Welfare Attorney to make decisions on their behalf? YES / NO
If "YES" they must be consulted

All other decisions must be made in the patient's best interest and company with current law.
Go to box 2

2 Summary of the main clinical problems and reasons why CPR would be inappropriate, unsuccessful or not in the patient's best interests:

3 Summary of communication with patient (or Welfare Attorney). If this decision has not been discussed with the patient or Welfare Attorney state the reason why:

4 Summary of communication with patient's relatives or friends:

5 Names of members of multidisciplinary team contributing to this decision:

6 Healthcare professional recording this DNACPR decision:

Name _____   Position _____

Signature _____   Date _____ Time _____

7 Review and endorsement by most senior health professional:

Signature _____ Name _____ Date _____

Signature _____ Name _____ Date _____

Signature _____ Name _____ Date _____

Figure 6.5 Do Not Attempt Cardiopulmonary Resuscitation (DNACPR) form. Source: Resuscitation Council. Reproduced with permission of the Resuscitation Council (UK).

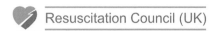 Resuscitation Council (UK)

This form should be completed legibly in black ball-point ink
All sections should be completed

- The patient's full name, date of birth and address should be written clearly.
- The date of recording the decision should be entered.
- This decision will be regarded as "INDEFINITE" unless it is clearly cancelled or a definite review date is specified.
- The decision should be reviewed whenever clinically appropriate or whenever the patient is transferred from one healthcare setting to another, admitted from home or discharged home.
- If the decision is cancelled the form should be crossed through with 2 diagonal lines in black ball-point ink and "CANCELLED" written clearly between them, signed and dated by the healthcare professional cancelling the decision.

1. **Capacity/advance decisions**
    Record the assessment of capacity in the clinical notes. Ensure that any advance decision is valid for the patient's current circumstances.
    16 and 17-year-olds: Whilst 16- and 17-year-olds with capacity are treated as adults for the purposes of consent, parental responsibility will continue until they reach age 18. Legal advice should be sought in the event of disagreements on this issue between a young person of 16 or 17 and those holding parental responsibility.

2. **Summary of the main clinical problems and reasons why CPR would be inappropriate unsuccessful or not in the patient's best interests**
    Be as specific as possible.

3. **Summary of communication with patient…**
    There is a presumption in favour of involving the patient. State clearly what was discussed and agreed. If this decision was not discussed with the patient state the reason. If a patient is in the final stages of a terminal illness and discussion would cause physical or psychological harm without any likelihood of benefit this situation should be recorded.

4. **Summary of communication with patient's relatives or friends**
    If the patient does not have capacity their relatives or friends must be consulted and may be able to help by indicating what the patient would decide if able to do so. If the patient has made a Lasting Power of Attorney, appointing a Welfare Attorney to make decisions on their behalf, that person must be consulted. A welfare Attorney may be able to refuse life-sustaining treatment on behalf of the patient if this power is included in the original Lasting Power of Attorney.

    If the patient has capacity ensure that discussion with others does not breach confidendiality.
    State the names and relationships of relatives or friends or other representatives with whom this decision has been discussed. More detailed description of such discussion should be recorded in the clinical notes.

5. **Members of multidisciplinary team…**
    State names and positions. Ensure that the DNACPR decision has been communicated to all relevant members of the healthcare team.

6. **Healthcare professional recording this DNACPR decision**
    This will vary according to circumstances and local arrangements. In general this should be the most senior healthcare professional immediately available.

7. **Review/endorsement…**
    The decision must be endorsed by the most senior healthcare professional responsible for the patient's care at the earliest opportunity. Further endorsement should be signed whenever the decision is reviewed. A fixed review date is not recommended. Review should occur whenever circumstances change.

DNACPRnotes_adult_2015

Figure 6.5 Do Not Attempt Cardiopulmonary Resuscitation (DNACPR) form. Source: Resuscitation Council. Reproduced with permission of the Resuscitation Council (UK).

- If requested by the patient, or those close to the patient.
- Whenever there is a significant change in the patient's clinical condition.
- When the patient moves from one care setting to another (including transfer between wards or teams in a hospital).

Further reading

European Resuscitation Council Guidelines (2015) https://cprguidelines.eu/.

Resuscitation Guidelines. Resuscitation Council (UK) https://www.resus.org.uk/resuscitation-guidelines/.

CHAPTER 7

Acute chest pain

JOHN B. CHAMBERS AND DAVID SPRIGINGS

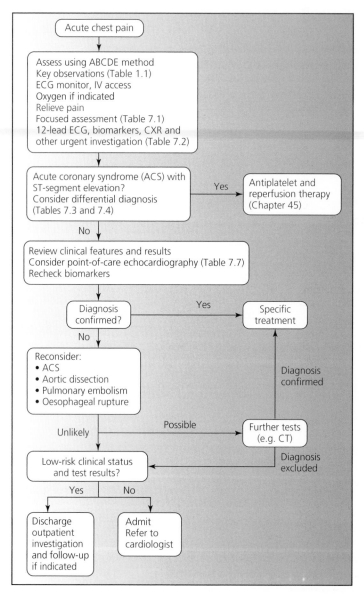

Figure 7.1 Assessment of the patient with acute chest pain.

Acute Medicine: A Practical Guide to the Management of Medical Emergencies, Fifth Edition. Edited by David Sprigings and John B. Chambers.
© 2018 John Wiley & Sons Ltd. Published 2018 by John Wiley & Sons Ltd.

Box 7.1 Causes of acute chest pain.

	Common	Less common or rare
Coronary	Acute coronary syndrome	Angina due to tachyarrhythmia
Other	Pulmonary embolism	Stress cardiomyopathy
cardiovascular	Pericarditis	Myocarditis/myopericarditis
		Aortic dissection and other aortic syndromes
Oesophageal	Gastro-oesophageal reflux	Oesophageal candidiasis (chest pain on
	Oesophageal motility disorder	swallowing)
		Other infective and inflammatory causes of
		oesophagitis
		Oesophageal rupture
Pulmonary	Pneumonia	Pneumothorax
	Other lower respiratory tract	Pneumomediastinum
	infections	Vaso-occlusive sickle crisis
	Pleurisy	
Chest wall	Benign chest wall pain	Vertebral crush fracture
	Rib contusion and fracture	Chest wall involvement by cancer
	Intercostal muscle strain	Referred pain from thoracic spine
	Costochondritis	
Intra-abdominal*		Pancreatitis
		Peptic ulcer
		Biliary tract disease
Skin		Herpes zoster

* Usually upper abdominal rather than chest pain.

Acute chest pain has a broad differential diagnosis (Box 7.1), ranging from benign to life-threatening disorders. Consider the potentially lethal causes in all patients; these include acute coronary syndrome (ACS), pulmonary embolism and aortic dissection.

The management of acute chest pain is summarized in Figure 7.1.

Priorities

1 While taking a focused history (Table 7.1), check the pulse and blood pressure, listen over the lungs and:
- Attach ECG and oxygen saturation monitors.
- Give oxygen if the patient has severe pain, is breathless, or if arterial oxygen saturation by pulse oximetry is <92%.
- Put in an IV cannula and take blood for urgent investigation including biomarkers (Table 7.2).
- Relieve severe pain with morphine 5–10 mg IV plus an antiemetic, for example prochlorperazine 12.5 mg IV.
2 Correct major arrhythmias (Chapter 39) or hypotension (Chapter 2).
3 Complete your clinical assessment, record a 12-lead ECG, and compare it with previous ECGs if available. If chest pain persists, repeat the ECG every 15 min. If you suspect ACS but the ECG is normal, include modified leads (lateral and right sided leads) as left circumflex coronary territory or right ventricular ischaemia may not appear with standard lead positions.
- The working diagnosis is ST-segment elevation acute coronary syndrome (STE-ACS) if there is:
  - ST segment elevation in two or more adjacent leads
  - Left bundle branch block, not known to be old
  - The chest pain is consistent with myocardial ischaemia and has lasted >20 min

Table 7.1 Focused assessment in acute chest pain.

History

Onset and characteristics of the pain

Instantaneous onset with pain 'migrating' to back, neck or jaw suggests aortic dissection (Chapter 50).

Radiation to the back alone is non-specific and can occur with myocardial, oesophageal and musculoskeletal pain.

Previous similar chest pain brought on by effort and relieved by rest (within 10 min), such as exertional angina?

Pleuritic (worse on inspiration and affected by posture) occurs with pericarditis, pneumonia, pulmonary embolism and chest wall pain.

After oesophageal instrumentation (suspect perforation) or insertion of a central line (suspect pneumothorax)?

After severe vomiting, suspect spontaneous oesophageal rupture.

Associated features

Neurological symptoms, even minor transient blurring of vision, suggest aortic dissection.

Haemoptysis suggests pulmonary embolism.

Purulent sputum.

Past history

Known coronary disease? Other known pathology potentially causing chest pain, e.g. gastroesophageal reflux.

Has there been a previous myocardial infarction with similar pain?

Risk factors

For ischaemic heart disease (cigarette smoking, hypertension, hyperlipidaemia, diabetes, family history of early coronary disease).

For venous thromboembolism (page 355 Table 56.1).

For aortic dissection (hypertension, Marfan syndrome, pregnancy).

Examination

Blood pressure in both arms (>15 mmHg difference in systolic pressure is abnormal), and the presence and symmetry of major pulses (if abnormal, consider aortic dissection).

Jugular venous pressure (if raised, consider pulmonary embolism or pericardial effusion with tamponade).

Murmur (if you hear the early diastolic murmur of aortic regurgitation, aortic dissection must be excluded).

Pericardial or pleural rub.

Signs of pneumothorax, consolidation or pleural effusion.

Localized chest wall or spinal tenderness (significant only if pressure exactly reproduces the spontaneous pain).

Subcutaneous emphysema around the neck (which may occur with oesophageal rupture and pneumothorax).

Are there any gross neurological abnormalities (suggesting dissection or vertebral crush fracture)?

- If the diagnosis is STE-ACS, arrange coronary angiography with a view to primary PCI. If primary PCI is not available, give thrombolysis without delay unless contraindicated (Table 45.2).
- If the history is not typical of myocardial ischaemia, consider the differential diagnosis (Tables 7.3 and 7.4), and seek urgent advice from a cardiologist before giving thrombolysis.

Table 7.2 Urgent investigation in acute chest pain.

ECG immediately on admission, repeated every 15 min if chest pain persists (if acute coronary syndrome suspected but ECG is normal, include modified leads (lateral and right sided leads) as left circumflex coronary territory or right ventricular ischaemia may not appear with standard lead positions)

Chest X-ray

Biomarkers

Point-of-care echocardiography (Table 7.7)

Full blood count

Blood glucose

Plasma sodium, potassium and creatinine

Table 7.3 Causes of ST-segment elevation other than acute coronary syndrome.

Cause	Clinical features
Acute pericarditis	Pain positional and worse on inspiration, pericardial rub, may not have coronary risk factors, may have viral prodrome (ECG see Table 7.4). Echocardiography shows no wall motion abnormality and may show pericardial fluid.
Stress cardiomyopathy (Takotsubo syndrome)	Usually follows emotional shock in a >65-year-old female (Table 45.5). Characteristic appearances on echocardiography, but angiography usually required to exclude coronary disease.
Early repolarization	A non-cardiac cause of pain associated with early repolarization can be confusing, but there will be no evolution of ECG changes (see Table 7.2) and no troponin release.
Aortic dissection	Dissection down the right coronary artery occurs in around 3% of acute type A dissections so this is rare. Consider if the chest pain is of immediate onset, radiates to the neck or back and is associated with neurological symptoms or signs. See Chapter 50.
Acute pancreatitis	Rare cause of ST segment changes. The history is atypical of a cardiac origin. See Chapter 79.

4 At this point, you need to review systematically the information you have from clinical assessment, ECG, chest X-ray and biomarkers. Points to note on the chest X-ray are summarized in Table 7.5.

5 Biomarker results (Table 7.6) must be interpreted in the clinical context. Troponin levels should be checked on admission then at three hours after the onset of chest pain (high-sensitivity cardiac troponin T; hs-cTpT) or after 12 hours (cardiac troponin T; cTpT).

- Normal levels at three hours after admission of myoglobin, hs-cTpT (12 hours for cTpT) and D-dimer rule out acute coronary syndrome (provided the ECG is normal), pulmonary embolism (in patients at low clinical risk) and aortic dissection (within 24 h of onset of symptoms).

Table 7.4 Comparison of ECG features of ST segment elevation acute myocardial infarction, early repolarization and acute pericarditis.

ECG feature	Myocardial infarction	Early repolarization	Acute pericarditis
ST segment morphology	Convex upwards	Convex upwards	Concave upwards
Typical magnitude of ST elevation	1–10 mm	1–2 mm	1–5 mm
Distribution of ST elevation	Inferior, anterior and lateral patterns	Commonly septal, rarely limb leads	Both limb and chest leads
ST depression in V1	In posterior infarction	Rare	Common
ST elevation in V6	In infero- or anterolateral infarction	Uncommon	Common
ST/T wave evolution	Uniform in all involved leads	Does not occur	Various stages occur concurrently
Pathological Q waves	Commonly develop	Never develop	Never develop
PR segment depression	Not seen	Not seen	May be seen
Rhythm disturbances	May occur	Do not occur	Supraventricular tachyarrhythmias may occur

Table 7.5 Chest X-ray abnormalities possible in pulmonary embolism, aortic dissection and oesophageal rupture.

Diagnosis	Possible abnormalities (on PA and lateral films)
Pulmonary embolism	Focal infiltrate
	Segmental collapse
	Raised hemidiaphragm
	Pleural effusion
Aortic dissection	Widening or double lumen to aortic knuckle
	Irregular aortic contour
	Discrepancy in diameter of ascending and descending thoracic aorta
	Pleural effusion
	Mediastinal widening
	Displacement of calcified intima
Oesophageal rupture	Mediastinal and subcutaneous emphysema
	Paraspinal mass
	Pleural effusion

Table 7.6 Plasma markers of myocardial necrosis.

Marker	Rises after:	Peaks at:	Returns to normal:
Myoglobin	1–4 h	6–7 h	24 h
Troponin T* (high-sensitivity assay)	1 h	3–4 h	10–14 days (3–4 after unstable angina)
Troponin I or T (standard assay)	3–12 h	24 h	5–10 days
Myocardial B-fraction of creatine kinase (CK-MB)	4–8 h	12–20 h	2–3 days

*See Table 46.3 for causes of raised plasma troponin other than acute coronary syndrome.

6 Consider a point-of-care echocardiogram (Table 7.7). This is not widely available and must only be performed by an operator who is trained in echocardiography and subject to the processes of the main echocardiography department (including quality control, continuing education, second opinion):

- Normal wall motion in the presence of chest pain reduces the likelihood of an ACS. In the presence of ST segment elevation this helps differentiate acute pericarditis from ACS.
- A dissection flap is visible in up to 90% cases of proximal (Type A) aortic dissection.
- A pericardial effusion associated with chest pain suggests acute pericarditis or dissection.
- In clinically suspected pulmonary embolism associated with shock, a dilated RV with raised TR V max is sufficient evidence to give thrombolysis.

Further management

If the diagnosis is still not obvious, consider other causes (Box 7.7) and ask yourself how closely the clinical picture matches the profile of any of the potentially lethal causes.

Table 7.7 Point-of-care echocardiography in acute chest pain.

Clinically suspected diagnosis	Echocardiographic finding
Acute coronary syndrome	Regional wall motion abnormality
	Generalized LV systolic dysfunction if established coronary disease
Acute pericarditis	Pericardial effusion
	Normal LV/RV wall motion (unless there is associated myocarditis, with elevated troponin)
Pulmonary embolism	Dilated, hypokinetic RV (see Table 57.5)
Aortic dissection	**Type A (involving ascending aorta)**
	Dilated ascending aorta
	Dissection flap (seen in 90%)
	Aortic regurgitation
	Pericardial effusion (if there has been retrograde dissection into the pericardial space)
	Type B (involving only the descending thoracic aorta)
	A flap in the descending thoracic or abdominal aorta (50–70% cases)

Could you be missing an acute coronary syndrome (Chapters 45 and 46)?

- Remember that the pain of myocardial ischaemia and oesophageal pain (due to acid reflux or spasm) may be indistinguishable. Both may radiate to the back or arms, and both may be burning or gripping in quality. Both may be relieved transiently by belching. Angina may occur after meals, but usually during exercise after meals.
- The presence of ST segment depression or T wave inversion strongly favours an acute coronary syndrome rather than oesophageal pain. A normal ECG does not exclude unstable angina. The differential diagnosis of ST segment changes is given in Table 7.1.
- The first sign of acute myocardial infarction may be hyperacute peaking of the T wave, which is often overlooked. If present, give aspirin and nitrate, and repeat the ECG in 20–30 min.
- If the history is compatible with myocardial ischaemia, or the patient is at moderate or high risk of ischaemic heart disease, admit for observation. Repeat the ECG initially after 1 h and await cTpT levels.
- A normal hs-cTpT on admission and after three hours excludes an ACS, provided the ECG is normal. If there are cardiac risk factors and there is no alternative cause for the pain, a cardiology referral should be made for consideration of secondary prophylaxis and further outpatient investigation. A coronary CT scan can be considered for patients with a low QRisk (<20%). Stress echocardiography or a myocardial perfusion scan are indicated for those with an intermediate risk (20–65%)

Could you be missing pulmonary embolism (Chapter 56)?

- One or more risk factors for venous thromboembolism (Table 56.1) are found in 80–90% of patients with pulmonary embolism. In the absence of these, pleuritic chest pain is more likely to be caused by pneumonia or pleurisy.
- In patients at low clinical risk, pulmonary embolism is excluded by a normal D-dimer level.

Could you be missing aortic dissection (Chapter 50)?

- Aortic dissection must be excluded by contrast CT if:
  - The chest pain was instantaneous in onset.

- There are associated neurological abnormalities.
- The patient has Marfan syndrome, known dilated aortic root or bicuspid aortic valve, or is pregnant.
- Remember that the pulses and chest X-ray are normal in at least 50% of patients with aortic dissection. If you suspect aortic dissection, seek urgent advice on further management from a cardiologist.
- An acute dissection is very unlikely with a normal D-dimer level (within 24 h of onset of symptoms).

Could you be missing oesophageal rupture (Chapter 75)?

Spontaneous oesophageal rupture is very rare. Typically the pain follows vomiting (while, in acute myocardial infarction, vomiting follows pain).

- Check the chest X-ray for mediastinal gas (a crescentic radiolucent zone, which may be retrocardiac or along the right cardiac border), a pleural effusion or a widened mediastinum.
- If you suspect oesophageal rupture, put the patient nil by mouth and start antibiotic therapy with coamoxiclav and metronidazole. Discuss further management with a gastroenterologist or surgeon.

Could you be missing a pneumothorax (Chapter 64)?

This usually causes breathlessness rather than chest pain resembling myocardial ischaemia. Look again at the chest X-ray. It is easy to miss a small apical pneumothorax.

Further reading

Chambers JB, Marks EM, Hunter MS (2015) The head says yes but the heart says no: what is non-cardiac chest pain and how is it managed? *Heart* 101, 1240–1249. DOI: 10.1136/heartjnl-2014-306277.

Pollak P, Brady W (2012) Electrocardiographic patterns mimicking ST Segment elevation myocardial infarction. *Cardiol Clin* 30, 601–615. http://dx.doi.org/10.1016/j.ccl.2012.07.012.

Rybicki FJ, Udelson JE, Peacock WF, *et al.* (2016) Appropriate utilization of cardiovascular imaging in emergency department patients with chest pain: a joint report of the American College of Radiology Appropriateness Criteria Committee and the American College of Cardiology Appropriate Use Criteria Task Force. *J Am Coll Cardiol* 67, 853–879.

Vafaie M, Biener M, Mueller M, *et al.* (2014) Analytically false or true positive elevations of high sensitivity cardiac troponin: a systematic approach. *Heart* 100, 508–514.

CHAPTER 8

Palpitations

SANDEEP HOTHI AND DAVID SPRIGINGS

When assessing the patient with palpitation who presents to the emergency department, you need to address four questions:
- What is the haemodynamic status of the patient?
- What is the cardiac rhythm?
- Is there evidence of underlying structural or coronary heart disease, pre-excitation or channelopathy?
- What systemic factors may have triggered or exacerbated the patient's symptoms?

Priorities

While taking a focused history (Tables 8.1–8.2), check the pulse and blood pressure, auscultate the lungs and:
- Attach ECG and oxygen saturation monitors.
- Give oxygen if the patient is breathless, or if arterial oxygen saturation by pulse oximetry is <92 %.
- If there is evidence of haemodynamic instability, put in an IV cannula and take blood for urgent investigation including relevant biomarkers (Table 8.3).

If there is imminent cardiac arrest, call the arrest team and manage along standard lines (see Chapter 6).

If there is a reduced level of consciousness, severe pulmonary oedema, chest pain or systolic BP is <90 mmHg:
- Record a 12-lead ECG (if possible) for later analysis (Table 8.4).
- If the heart rate is >150/min: call an anaesthetist in preparation for DC cardioversion starting at 200 J (Chapter 121).
- If the heart rate is <50/min: give atropine 0.6–1.2 mg IV, with further doses at 5-min intervals up to a total dose of 3 mg if the heart rate remains below 60/min. If the bradycardia is unresponsive or recurs, use an external cardiac pacing system or insert a temporary transvenous pacemaker (Chapter 119).
- Seek advice on further management from a cardiologist.

If the patient is haemodynamically stable, there is time to make a working diagnosis and plan management.
- Complete your clinical assessment (Tables 8.1–8.2), record a 12-lead electrocardiogram and a long rhythm strip, arrange a chest X-ray, and consider other investigations (Table 8.3).
- Carefully assess the ECG (Table 8.4).
- Are there any systemic factors which may have triggered or exacerbated the patient's symptoms (Table 8.5)? The patient can now be placed in one of two groups:

Acute Medicine: A Practical Guide to the Management of Medical Emergencies, Fifth Edition. Edited by David Sprigings and John B. Chambers.
© 2018 John Wiley & Sons Ltd. Published 2018 by John Wiley & Sons Ltd.

Table 8.1 Assessment of the patient with palpitation.

Description	See Table 8.2.
Positional factors	Extrasystoles may be felt on lying down in the left lateral decubitus or supine positions. AV nodal re-entrant tachycardia may be precipitated by bending over and then standing up and may terminate on lying down.
Syncope	Syncope during palpitation is a sign of haemodynamic compromise, either from ventricular tachycardia (VT) or occasionally SVT. VT must be excluded.
Relation to exercise	Exercise can trigger right ventricular outflow tract ventricular tachycardia, catecholaminergic polymorphic ventricular tachycardia (CPVT) and some forms of congenital long QT syndrome (LQTS). Atrial fibrillation (AF) can also be triggered by the onset or offset of exercise. Inappropriate sinus tachycardia may follow physical or emotional stress.
Emotional stress	Most likely to induce sinus tachycardia, but can occasionally trigger SVT or VT.
Anxiety	A quick screening question is: 'Have you experienced brief periods, for seconds or minutes, of an overwhelming panic or terror that was accompanied by racing heartbeats, shortness of breath, or dizziness?' Other causes should be considered before attributing to anxiety.
Drug history	Caffeine, illicit drugs (e.g. cocaine, amphetamines, 'ecstasy') and alcohol can trigger arrhythmias.
Prescribed drugs	Arrhythmias can be caused by anti-arrhythmics, thyroxine, theophyllines, beta-adrenoreceptor agonists, antidepressants and antipsychotics.*
Cardiac history	Symptoms or signs of cardiac disease may suggest specific arrhythmias. Ischaemic heart disease and cardiomyopathies raise the possibility of ventricular arrhythmias. Mitral valve disease predisposes to atrial fibrillation.
Medical history	Thyrotoxicosis, anaemia and phaeochromocytoma may result in palpitations and arrhythmias. Pregnancy may also result in palpitations and arrhythmias.
Family history	Ischaemic heart disease, early-onset atrial fibrillation, channelopathies and cardiomyopathies have a genetic component.

*For a full list see: http://www.sads.org.uk/drugs-to-avoid/

1 Persistent arrhythmia

Further management is determined by the type of arrhythmia and the context: see Chapters 39–44. Consider if there are any systemic factors which may have triggered the arrhythmia (Table 8.5). Consider discharge for patients with atrial fibrillation or flutter, provided that:

- They are haemodynamically stable (no or only mild symptoms, heart rate <100/min, systolic BP >110 mmHg).
- No systemic trigger requiring specific treatment is apparent (e.g. sepsis).
- Stroke/thromboembolic prophylaxis has been addressed (see Chapters 43 and 103).
- Rate-control (rather than cardioversion) is appropriate, at least in the short term.
- A plan of management has been agreed and follow-up arranged.

2 ECG shows sinus rhythm/sinus tachycardia

Possibilities are a paroxysmal arrhythmia (resolved before the ECG was recorded) or palpitation due to awareness of sinus rhythm/sinus tachycardia.

Table 8.2 Pointers in the description of palpitation.

Type of palpitation	Subjective description	Heartbeat	Onset and termination	Trigger situations	Possible associated symptoms
Extrasystolic	'Skipping/ missing a beat', 'sinking of the heart'	Irregular, interspersed with periods of normal heartbeat	Sudden	Rest	—
Tachycardiac	'Beating wings' in the chest	Regular or irregular, markedly accelerated	Sudden	Physical effort, cooling down	Syncope, dyspnoea, fatigue, chest pain
Anxiety-related	Anxiety, agitation	Regular, slightly accelerated	Gradual	Stress, Anxiety attacks	Tingling in the hands and face, Lump in the throat, atypical chest pain, sighing dyspnoea
Pulsation	Heart pounding	Regular, normal frequency	Gradual	Physical effort	Asthenia

Type of arrhythmia	Heartbeat	Trigger situations	Associated symptoms	Vagal manoeuvres
AVRT, AVNRT	Sudden onset regular with periods of elevated heart rate	Physical effort, changes in posture	Polyuria, neck pulsation	Sudden interruption
Atrial fibrillation	Irregular with variable heart rate	Physical effort, cooling down, post meal, alcohol intake	Polyuria	Transitory reduction in heart rate
Atrial tachycardia and atrial flutter	Regular (irregular if A-V conduction is variable) with elevated heart rate			Transitory reduction in heart rate
Ventricular tachycardias	Regular with elevated heart rate	Physical effort	Signs/symptoms of haemodynamic impairment	No effect

Source: Raviele A, Giada F, Bergfeldt L, *et al.* (2011) Management of patients with palpitations: a position paper from the European Heart Rhythm Association. *Europace* 13, 920–934. Reproduced with permission of Oxford University Press.

Paroxysmal arrhythmia

Patients with 'red-flag' features should be considered for inpatient investigation: seek advice from a cardiologist. Red-flag features include:

- Associated syncope or
- Palpitation triggered during exercise or
- Evidence of structural heart disease, accessory pathway or channelopathy (murmur, signs of heart failure, abnormal 12-lead ECG) or
- Family history of sudden death or cardiomyopathy

Other features for which admission may be indicated are summarized in Table 8.6. In the absence of such features, the patient can be discharged: arrange ambulatory ECG monitoring, to establish cardiac rhythm at the time of symptoms, and follow-up with the GP or a cardiologist.

Table 8.3 Urgent investigation of the patient with palpitation.

ECG
Blood glucose
Plasma sodium, potassium, calcium and magnesium
Plasma creatinine
Plasma TSH
Plasma troponin if acute coronary syndrome suspected
Plasma BNP or NT-pro-BNP if heart failure suspected
Urine drug screen if illicit drug use considered
Chest X-ray
Echocardiogram if there is clinical evidence of an underlying structural abnormality or there is a proven sustained or non-sustained arrhythmia
ECG monitoring:
- 24-hour ECG if frequent ventricular extrasystoles seen on 12-lead ECG, or if palpitation occurs at least daily
- 7-day ECG monitoring if palpitation occurs approximately weekly
- ECG event recorder (smartphone-based systems now available)
- Implantable ECG loop recorder (for selected high-risk patients)
Exercise ECG, in selected patients
Electrophysiological study, in selected patients with cardiology advice

Table 8.4 ECG in the patient with suspected paroxysmal arrhythmia (i.e. recorded after palpitation has resolved).

ECG feature	Comment
Supraventricular extrasystoles	Occur in healthy people as well as those with heart disease. In the absence of associated cardiac disease, have a benign prognosis. If palpitation due to awareness of supraventricular extrasystoles is suspected, arrange: • 24-h ECG monitoring to establish relation to symptoms, quantify frequency and assess for paroxysmal atrial fibrillation. • Echocardiography to assess cardiac structure and function.
Ventricular extrasystoles	May occur in healthy people, but are more strongly associated with heart disease than supraventricular extrasystoles. If palpitation due to awareness of ventricular extrasystoles is suspected, arrange: • 24-h ECG monitoring to establish relation to symptoms, quantify frequency, and determine if monomorphic or polymorphic. • Echocardiography to assess cardiac structure and function. • Exercise ECG to establish effort tolerance, assess response of ventricular extrasystoles to exercise and whether ventricular tachycardia can be induced, and screen for ischaemic heart disease.
Sinus bradycardia (rate <50/min) or sinus pauses	May reflect sinoatrial disorder with associated paroxysmal atrial fibrillation.
Short PR interval (<120 ms)	Look for other features of Wolff-Parkinson-White (WPW) syndrome: delta wave, widened QRS complex. If WPW present, discuss management with a cardiologist before discharge.

Table 8.4 (*Continued*)

ECG feature	Comment
Right-axis deviation (QRS predominantly negative in lead I and positive in lead II)	Consider pulmonary hypertension or pulmonary embolism.
Left-axis deviation (QRS predominantly positive in lead I and negative in lead II)	As an isolated abnormality, usually of no significance.
Right bundle branch block (RBBB)	Consider pulmonary hypertension or pulmonary embolism. Consider Brugada syndrome (ECG shows RBBB pattern with coved or saddle back ST-elevation in leads V1-V3).
Left bundle branch block (LBBB)	May reflect structural heart disease or conducting system disease. Arrange echocardiography.
Left ventricular hypertrophy	May be seen in: • Severe hypertension • Aortic valve disease • Hypertrophic cardiomyopathy
Pathological Q waves	Usually reflect previous myocardial infarction (with associated risk of ventricular tachycardia (Chapter 40)). May also be seen in hypertrophic cardiomyopathy or WPW syndrome (pseudoinfarct pattern).
Dominant R wave in V1	May be seen in: • Right ventricular hypertrophy • RBBB • WPW syndrome • Posterior myocardial infarction • Duchenne muscular dystrophy with cardiomyopathy • Normal variant
Long QT interval	Long QT interval may reflect congenital channelopathy (long QT syndrome) or acquired disorder (due to drugs (see http://www.sads.org.uk/drugs-to-avoid/), or metabolic disorder (e.g. hypokalaemia or hypocalcaemia)), or a combination of these factors. QT interval >500 ms is associated with high risk of polymorphic ventricular tachycardia (torsade de pointes) (Chapter 41).
Short QT interval	Short QT interval may reflect congenital channelopathy (short QT syndrome) or acquired disorder (e.g. due to acidosis, hyperkalaemia or hypercalcaemia), or a combination of these factors. Short QT syndrome is associated with atrial and ventricular arrhythmias.
T wave inversion	May be seen in: • Structural heart disease (e.g. severe aortic stenosis) • Cardiomyopathies • Acute coronary syndrome • Myopericarditis • Subarachnoid haemorrhage • Stress cardiomyopathy

Table 8.5 Systemic factors which may trigger or exacerbate palpitation.

Psychological factors (e.g. generalized anxiety disorder, panic disorder)
Sepsis
Hypovolaemia with postural hypotension
Postural orthostatic tachycardia syndrome
Anaemia
Pregnancy
Pulmonary embolism
Hypoglycaemia
Thyrotoxicosis
Phaeochromocytoma
Caffeine excess
Alcohol excess/alcohol withdrawal
Prescribed drugs (e.g. inhaled salbutamol, nifedipine, drugs with anticholinergic effect; see http://www.sads.org.uk/
drugs-to-avoid/)
Recreational drugs (e.g. cannabis, cocaine, amphetamine)
Electrolyte derangement (hypo- or hyperkalaemia, hypo- or hypercalcaemia, hypomagnesaemia)

Advice on discharge:
- Avoid excess caffeine, excess alcohol, substance use.
- Return if palpitation recurs.
- Keep a symptom diary.
- Follow-up after ambulatory ECG monitoring.

Palpitation due to awareness of sinus rhythm/sinus tachycardia

Consider if there are any systemic factors which may have triggered sinus tachycardia (Table 8.5). Admit if there is evidence of acute illness requiring inpatient management.

Table 8.6 When to admit the patient with palpitation.

Diagnostic purposes
Severe structural heart disease (e.g. severe valve disease, complex congenital heart disease, cardiomyopathy, severely impaired left ventricular systolic function (ejection fraction <35%)), suspected or ascertained
Primary electrical heart disease (channelopathy), suspected or ascertained
Family history of sudden death
Need to perform electrophysiological study, invasive investigations or in-hospital telemetric monitoring

Therapeutic purposes
Bradyarrhythmias requiring implantation of pacemaker
Cardiac device malfunction not rectifiable by reprogramming
Ventricular tachyarrhythmias requiring immediate interruption and/or implantable cardoverter-defibrillator (ICD)
implantation or catheter ablation
Supraventricular tachycardias requiring interruption immediately or in a short time, or catheter ablation
Presence of heart failure or other symptoms of haemodynamic compromise
Severe structural heart diseases requiring surgery or interventional procedures
Severe systemic causes (see Table 8.5)
Severe psychotic decompensation

Source: Raviele A, Giada F, Bergfeldt L, *et al.* (2011) Management of patients with palpitations: a position paper from the European Heart Rhythm Association. *Europace* 13, 920–934. Reproduced with permission of Oxford University Press.

Discharge if there is no evidence of significant acute illness, no red-flag features (see above), a normal cardiac examination and ECG. Follow-up should be with the GP.

Further reading

Gale CP, Camm AJ (2016) Assessment of palpitations. *BMJ* 352, h5649. http://dx.doi.org/10.1136/bmj.h5649.
Raviele A, Giarda F, Bergfeldt L, *et al.* (2011) Management of patients with palpitations: a position paper from the European Heart Rhythm Association. *Europace* 13, 920–934. http://dx.doi.org/10.1093/europace/eur130.

CHAPTER 9

Transient loss of consciousness

SANDEEP HOTHI AND DAVID SPRIGINGS

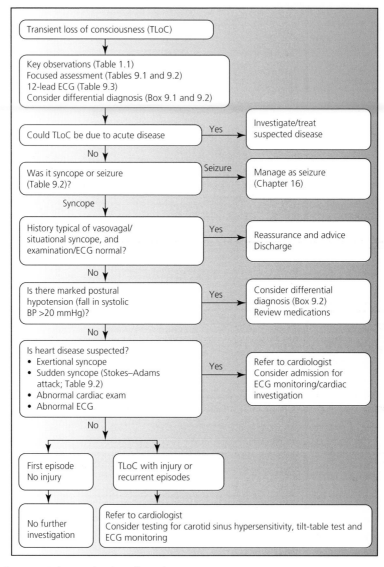

Figure 9.1 Assessment after transient loss of consciousness.

Acute Medicine: A Practical Guide to the Management of Medical Emergencies, Fifth Edition. Edited by David Sprigings and John B. Chambers.
© 2018 John Wiley & Sons Ltd. Published 2018 by John Wiley & Sons Ltd.

Box 9.1 Causes of transient loss of consciousness.

Transient global cerebral hypoperfusion: syncope (Box 9.2)
Metabolic disorders:
- Hypoglycaemia
- Severe hypoxia
- Hyperventilation with hypocapnia
Poisoning with alcohol and psychoactive drugs
Epilepsy
Migraine
Vertebrobasilar transient ischaemic attack
Subclavian steal syndrome
Subarachnoid haemorrhage

The causes of transient loss of consciousness (TLoC) (Box 9.1) can usually be differentiated by a detailed history taken from the patient and any eyewitnesses (Tables 9.1 and 9.2), supplemented by the examination findings and a careful review of the ECG (Table 9.3). Further investigation may be needed for definitive diagnosis.

- Risk-stratification is important, as patients at low risk of serious adverse events can be discharged from the emergency department.
- The assessment of the patient with transient loss of consciousness is summarized in Figure 9.1.

Priorities

1 Is transient loss of consciousness related to acute disease?

Consider those acute diseases which may be associated with TLoC:
- Major arrhythmias (Chapters 39–44)
- Acute coronary syndrome (Chapters 45 and 46)
- Pulmonary embolism (Chapter 57)
- Aortic dissection (Chapter 50)
- Subarachnoid haemorrhage (Chapter 67)
- Rapid blood loss and other cause of hypovolaemia (Chapters 73 and 74)
- Hypoglycaemia (Chapter 81)

These patients will typically have other symptoms (e.g. headache, chest pain, breathlessness) or abnormal physiological observations (e.g. hypotension). Further assessment and management of these diseases is given in the corresponding chapters.

2 Was transient loss of consciousness due to syncope or a seizure?
- A detailed history will usually allow syncope (defined as TLoC due to global cerebral hypoperfusion (Box 9.2)) to be differentiated from seizure (Tables 9.1 and 9.2).
- Involuntary movements (including tonic-clonic seizures, after 30 s of cardiac arrest) are common in syncope, and should not be interpreted as necessarily indicating epilepsy.
- Further management of the patient after a generalized seizure is given in Chapter 16.

3 Admit or discharge?

High-risk features warranting admission for inpatient management include:
- Suspicion of acute disease causing syncope (see 1. above)
- Evidence of significant structural or ischaemic heart disease, or the presence of heart failure
- Clinical (e.g. exertional syncope) or ECG features (Table 9.3) suggesting arrhythmic syncope

Table 9.1 Focused assessment after transient loss of consciousness.

History

Background
Any previous similar attacks
Previous significant head injury (i.e. with skull fracture or loss of consciousness)
Birth injury, febrile convulsions in childhood, meningitis or encephalitis
Family history of epilepsy
Cardiac disease associated with ventricular arrhythmia (previous myocardial infarction, hypertrophic or dilated cardiomyopathy, heart failure)
Medications
Alcohol or substance use
Sleep deprivation

Before the attack
Prodromal symptoms: were these cardiovascular (e.g. dizziness, palpitations, chest pain) or focal neurological symptoms (aura)?
Circumstances, for example exercising, standing, sitting or lying, asleep
Precipitants, for example coughing, micturition, head-turning

The attack
Were there any focal neurological features at the onset: sustained deviation of the head or eyes or unilateral jerking of the limbs?
Was there a cry (may occur in tonic phase of fit)?
Duration of loss of consciousness
Associated tongue biting, urinary incontinence or injury
Facial colour changes (pallor common in syncope, uncommon with a fit)
Abnormal pulse (must be assessed in relation to the reliability of the witness)

After the attack
Immediately well or delayed recovery with confusion or headache?

Examination
Conscious level and mental state (confirm the patient is fully oriented)
Pulse, blood pressure, respiratory rate, arterial oxygen saturation, temperature
Systolic BP sitting or lying, and after 2 min standing (a fall of >20 mmHg is abnormal; note if symptomatic or not)
Arterial pulses (check major pulses for asymmetry and bruits)
Jugular venous pressure (if raised, consider pulmonary embolism, pulmonary hypertension, heart failure or cardiac tamponade)
Heart murmurs (aortic stenosis and hypertrophic cardiomyopathy may cause exertional syncope; atrial myxoma may simulate mitral stenosis)
Neck mobility (does neck movement induce presyncope? Is there neck stiffness?)
Presence of focal neurological signs: as a minimum, check visual fields, limb power, tendon reflexes and plantar responses
Fundi (check for haemorrhages or papilloedema)

- Abnormal physiological observations
- Major comorbidities
4 Advice to discharged patients

Driving
- As a general rule, any patient who has had TLoC must not drive until specialist assessment has been completed and they have been advised by the specialist that they may drive.

Table 9.2 Features differentiating a generalized seizure from vasovagal syncope and cardiac syncope due to arrhythmia (Stokes-Adams attack).

	Generalized seizure	Vasovagal syncope	Cardiac syncope due to arrhythmia
Occurrence when sitting or lying	Common	Rare	Common
Occurrence during sleep	Common	Does not occur	May occur
Prodromal symptoms	May occur, with focal neurological symptoms, head turning, automatisms	Typical, with dizziness, sweating, nausea, blurring of vision, disturbance of hearing, yawning	Often none; palpitation may precede syncope in tachyarrhythmias
Focal neurological features at onset	May occur, and signify focal cerebral lesion	Never occur	Never occur
Tonic-clonic movements	Characteristic, occur within 30 s of onset	May occur after 30 s of syncope (secondary anoxic seizure)	May occur after 30 s of syncope (secondary anoxic seizure)
Facial colour	Flush or cyanosis at onset	Pallor at onset and after syncope	Pallor at onset, flush on recovery
Tongue biting	Common (lateral border)	Rare	Rare
Urinary incontinence	Common	May occur	May occur
Injury	May occur	Uncommon	May occur
After the attack	Confusion common	Nauseated and 'groggy'	Usually well

Table 9.3 The ECG after transient loss of consciousness.

ECG feature	Comment
Sinus bradycardia (rate <50/min) or sinus pauses	May reflect sinoatrial disorder. Pacing indicated for syncope with sinus bradycardia <40/min or sinus pauses >3 s.
Sinus tachycardia	Many possible causes. Consider: • Pulmonary embolism • Aortic dissection • Rapid blood loss and other cause of hypovolaemia
First-degree AV block	Raises the possibility of intermittent second- or third-degree AV block, but as an isolated abnormality is usually of no significance.
Second-degree AV block	Likely to be the cause of syncope: indication for pacing.
Third-degree (complete) AV block	Likely to be the cause of syncope: indication for pacing. Arrange echocardiography to check for associated structural heart disease and assess left ventricular function.
Atrial fibrillation	May reflect sinoatrial disorder of underlying structural heart disease. Indication for echocardiography.
Paced rhythm	Pacemaker failure is rare but should be excluded. Arrange for interrogation of device to determine rhythm at the time of TLoC.
Short PR interval (<120 ms)	Look for other features of Wolff-Parkinson-White (WPW) syndrome: delta wave, widened QRS complex. If WPW present, discuss management with a cardiologist.
Right-axis deviation (QRS predominantly negative in lead I and positive in lead II)	Consider pulmonary hypertension or pulmonary embolism.

(continued)

Table 9.3 (*Continued*)

ECG feature	Comment
Left-axis deviation (QRS predominantly positive in lead I and negative in lead II)	As an isolated abnormality, usually of no significance.
Right bundle branch block (RBBB)	Consider pulmonary hypertension or pulmonary embolism. Consider Brugada syndrome (ECG shows RBBB pattern with ST-elevation in leads V1–V3).
Left bundle branch block (LBBB)	May reflect structural heart disease or conducting system disease. Arrange echocardiography.
Bifascicular block (RBBB or LBBB with right-axis or left-axis deviation), with or without first-degree AV block	Significantly increases the likelihood that syncope was due to intermittent AV block.
Left ventricular hypertrophy	May be seen in: <ul><li>Severe hypertension</li><li>Aortic valve disease</li><li>Hypertrophic cardiomyopathy</li></ul>
Pathological Q waves	Usually reflect previous myocardial infarction (with associated risk of ventricular tachycardia (Chapter 40)). May also be seen in hypertrophic cardiomyopathy or WPW syndrome (pseudoinfarct pattern).
Dominant R wave in V1	May be seen in: <ul><li>Right ventricular hypertrophy</li><li>RBBB</li><li>WPW syndrome</li><li>Posterior myocardial infarction</li><li>Duchenne muscular dystrophy with cardiomyopathy</li><li>Normal variant</li></ul>
Short QT interval	Short QT interval may reflect congenital channelopathy (short QT syndrome) or acquired disorder (e.g. due to acidosis, hyperkalaemia or hypercalcaemia), or a combination of the two. Short QT syndrome is associated with atrial and ventricular arrhythmias.
Long QT interval	Long QT interval may reflect congenital channelopathy (long QT syndrome) or acquired disorder (due to drugs (see http://www.sads.org.uk/drugs-to-avoid/), or metabolic disorder (e.g. hypokalaemia or hypocalcaemia)), or a combination of the two. QT interval >500 ms is associated with high risk of polymorphic ventricular tachycardia (torsade de pointes) (Chapter 41).
T wave inversion	May be seen in: <ul><li>Structural heart disease (e.g. severe aortic stenosis)</li><li>Cardiomyopathies</li><li>Acute coronary syndrome</li><li>Myopericarditis</li><li>Subarachnoid haemorrhage</li><li>Stress cardiomyopathy</li></ul>

- Patients who have had typical vasovagal syncope while standing, with a reliable prodrome, may continue to drive and need not notify the DVLA.
- Consult the guidelines of the Driver and Vehicle Licensing Agency (DVLA) (available online at: www.gov.uk/dvla/fitnesstodrive).

Occupational issues

- Working patients who have had TLoC should be given advice on the implications of the episode for health and safety at work and any action they must take to ensure the safety of themselves and other people. They should inform their occupational health department.

Box 9.2 Causes of syncope.

Mechanism	Subtype	Comment
Reflex (neurally-mediated)	Vasovagal	Typically follows pain, emotional distress or prolonged standing. Diagnose when there are no features suggesting an alternative diagnosis, and the clinical features are concordant (Table 9.2).
	Situational	Diagnose when there are no features suggesting an alternative diagnosis and syncope occurred in typical circumstances (e.g. micturition while standing, or a prolonged bout of coughing).
	Carotid sinus hypersensitivity (CSH)	Diagnose in patients aged 60 and over with TLoC, when there are no features suggesting an alternative diagnosis, and testing for CSH (Table 9.4) is positive.
	Atypical form	Diagnose when there no features suggesting an alternative diagnosis, testing for CSH is negative, and tilt-table testing provokes symptoms.
Orthostatic hypotension	Primary autonomic failure	For example in multiple system atrophy, Parkinson's disease with autonomic failure.
	Secondary autonomic failure	For example in diabetes mellitus or amyloidosis.
	Drug-induced	Many drugs may cause or contribute to orthostatic hypotension, including alpha blockers, antidepressants, antihypertensive agents, drugs for Parkinson's disease and diuretics.
	Volume depletion	See Chapter 2.
Cardiovascular	Bradyarrhythmia	See Chapter 44.
	Tachyarrhythmia	See Chapters 40–43.
	Structural cardiac disease	This includes valve disease (notably severe aortic stenosis; see Chapter 51), congenital heart disease and cardiomyopathies. ECG and echocardiography typically show characteristic abnormalities.
	Acute myocardial ischaemia	See Chapters 45 and 46.
	Aortic dissection	See Chapter 50.
	Pulmonary embolism	See Chapter 57.
	Severe pulmonary hypertension	May result in exertional syncope. There may be clinical signs of right ventricular failure (e.g. elevated jugular venous pressure). ECG and echocardiography typically show characteristic abnormalities.

Table 9.4 Testing for carotid sinus hypersensitivity.

Indicated in patients aged 60 and over with unexplained syncope.

Contraindications include the presence of a carotid bruit, recent myocardial infarction, recent stroke or a history of ventricular tachycardia.

Begin with the patient lying.

Attach an ECG monitor with a printer and check the blood pressure.

The carotid sinus lies at the level of the upper border of the thyroid cartilage just below the angle of the jaw.

Perform carotid sinus massage for up to 15 s whilst recording a rhythm strip. Press posteriorly and medially over the artery (first on the right, and if this is negative on the left) with your thumb or index and middle fingers.

If the test is negative, repeat with the patient sitting.

An abnormal response is defined by a sinus pause >3 s or a drop in systolic blood pressure >50 mmHg. If these occur, discuss with a cardiologist whether pacemaker implantation is indicated.

Suspected cardiovascular cause

- Patients waiting for cardiovascular assessment should be advised to return to the emergency department in the event of a further episode. If TLoC occurred during exercise, or there is evidence of structural heart disease or an abnormal ECG, they should be advised not to exercise until the assessment has been completed, and the management plan should be discussed with a cardiologist before discharge.

Suspected epilepsy

See Chapter 16 for the advice you should give to patients after a generalized seizure.

Further management

Probable vasovagal syncope

- Give advice to the patient on avoiding action to take in the event of prodromal symptoms. Muscle clenching (leg crossing and arm tensing/hand grip) can prevent progression to syncope.
- If there have been recurrent episodes with significant impact on quality of life or with high risk of injury, arrange a tilt-table test with cardiology follow-up: pacing may be considered for patients with a pronounced cardio-inhibitory response (typically prolonged asystole).

Suspected arrhythmic syncope

The choice of ECG monitoring depends on the frequency of episodes and the presence or absence of heart disease. Patients with high-risk features (see above) should be admitted for investigation. For those without high-risk features, recommendations for ECG monitoring are:

- TLoC at least several times a week: Holter monitoring (up to 48 hours if necessary)
- TLoC every 1–2 weeks: external event recorder
- TLoC infrequently (less than once every two weeks): implantable event recorder

Unexplained syncope

- For patients with suspected carotid sinus hypersensitivity, and for those with unexplained syncope who are aged ≥60 years, carotid sinus massage should be the initial investigation (Table 9.4).
- For other patients with unexplained syncope, and those with negative testing for carotid sinus hypersensitivity, ambulatory ECG monitoring should be done (see above).

Further reading

National Institute for Health and Care Excellence (2010) Transient loss of consciousness ('blackouts') in over 16s. Clinical guideline (CG109) Last updated: September 2014. https://www.nice.org.uk/guidance/cg109.

Wieling W, van Dijk N, de Lange FJ, *et al.* (2015) History taking as a diagnostic test in patients with syncope: developing expertise in syncope. *Eur Heart J.* 36, 277–280. http://dx.doi.org/10.1093/eurheartj/ehu478.

CHAPTER 10

Acute breathlessness

DAVID SPRIGINGS AND JOHN B. CHAMBERS

Box 10.1 Acute breathlessness

Acute breathlessness is usually due to cardiorespiratory disease, but may result from a broad range of disorders including sepsis and neuromuscular disease.

Among patients presenting to the emergency department, the commonest causes are acute heart failure, exacerbation of chronic obstructive pulmonary disease or asthma, and pneumonia. More than one disorder may be present, particularly in older patients or those with long-term conditions.

Although uncommon, three immediately life-threatening conditions – upper airway obstruction, tension pneumothorax and cardiac tamponade – should be considered in the relevant context or in the presence of characteristic clinical features.

Assessment and initial management of the patient with acute breathlessness are summarized in Figure 10.1.

Priorities

1 Assess the airway, breathing and circulation (Chapter 1).
- Attach ECG and oxygen saturation monitors. Give oxygen 35% by mask. Increase the inspired oxygen concentration if arterial oxygen saturation is <90%. Secure venous access.
- Focused assessment is summarized in Table 10.1, and investigations needed urgently in Table 10.2.

2 If **upper airway obstruction** is likely, because of abnormal voice, stridor (Box 10.2) or the clinical setting, sit the patient up and give high-flow oxygen. Call the resuscitation team and an ear, nose and throat (ENT) surgeon, in case tracheostomy is needed. Further assessment and management of upper airway obstruction is described in detail in Chapter 59.

3 If there are signs of **tension pneumothorax** with impending cardiorespiratory arrest, insert a large-bore needle into the second intercostal space in the mid-clavicular line on the side with absent or reduced breath sounds. Further management of tension pneumothorax is described in Chapter 64.

4 If **cardiac tamponade** is likely (risk factor for pericardial effusion, especially cancer, with raised jugular venous pressure and pulsus paradoxus (Box 10.2) palpable over the radial artery, see Chapter 54), obtain immediate echocardiography and perform pericardiocentesis if pericardial effusion with cardiac tamponade is confirmed (see Chapter 120 for the technique of pericardiocentesis).

5 If there is **respiratory failure** (respiratory distress; respiratory rate <8 or >30 breaths/min; agitation or reduced conscious level; oxygen saturation <90% despite high-flow oxygen), call the resuscitation team and/or intensive care team. Further management of respiratory failure is described in Chapter 11.

Acute Medicine: A Practical Guide to the Management of Medical Emergencies, Fifth Edition. Edited by David Sprigings and John B. Chambers.
© 2018 John Wiley & Sons Ltd. Published 2018 by John Wiley & Sons Ltd.

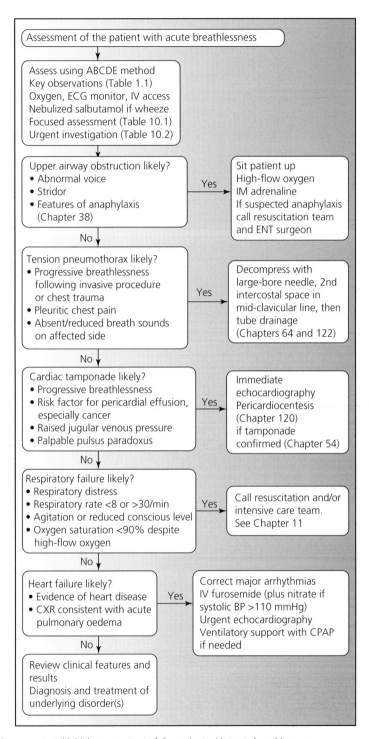

Figure 10.1 Assessment and initial management of the patient with acute breathlessness.

Table 10.1 Focused assessment of the patient with acute breathlessness.

Known cardiac or respiratory disease?
Associated chest pain (pleuritic or non-pleuritic)?)
Associated cough, with purulent sputum or haemoptysis?
Change in sputum volume or purulence if chronic productive cough?
Risk factors for venous thromboembolism (Table 56.1)?)
Usual exercise capacity and any recent change?
Temperature, heart rate, blood pressure, jugular venous pressure, respiratory rate.
Stridor or wheeze?
Signs of heart failure?
Focal lung crackles.
Peak expiratory flow rate, related to predicted normal.

Table 10.2 Urgent investigation in acute breathlessness.

Chest X-ray
Arterial blood gases, pH and lactate if oxygen saturation is <90%, sepsis is suspected or diagnosis is unclear
ECG (except in patients under 40 with pneumothorax or acute asthma)
Echocardiogram if suspected cardiac disease
Full blood count
Plasma sodium, potassium and creatinine
Blood glucose
Plasma biomarkers:
- Fibrinogen degradation products (d-dimer) if there are risk factors for venous thromboembolism (Table 56.1)
- BNP or NT-proBNP if clinical features of cardiac disease or abnormal ECG, and in patients with suspected exacerbation of COPD
- Troponin if clinical features of cardiac disease or abnormal ECG
- C-reactive protein if possible sepsis

Box 10.2 Stridor and pulsus paradoxus.

Stridor is a high-pitched sound, heard more loudly over the neck than the chest, in contrast to wheeze. Inspiratory stridor is a feature of laryngeal obstruction; expiratory stridor, of tracheobronchial obstruction; and biphasic stridor, of glottic or subglottic obstruction.

Causes of stridor include upper airway obstruction with a foreign body, angioedema, and vocal cord dysfunction.

Pulsus paradoxus is an exaggeration of the normal inspiratory fall in systolic blood pressure to >10 mmHg. When marked, it may be palpable in the radial artery, with the radial pulse disappearing on inspiration. The 'paradox' is that the pulse disappears despite cardiac contraction.

Pulsus paradoxus is a characteristic feature of cardiac tamponade (but may not always occur, e.g. if there is an atrial septal defect or severe aortic regurgitation). It may also be present in acute severe asthma and right ventricular infarction.

6 If there is **wheeze**, give nebulized salbutamol, 1 mg of nebulizer solution diluted in 2 mL of normal saline.
  • If the patient is hypoxic (oxygen saturation <90%), but does not have known chronic obstructive pulmonary disease (COPD), the nebulizer should be driven with oxygen: check the necessary flow rate on the nebulizer packaging.
  • If the patient has COPD with known or potential CO_2 retention, use air as the driving gas.
7 If there are signs of **heart failure** with pulmonary oedema (see Chapters 47 and 48):
  • Correct major arrhythmias.
  • Give furosemide 40 mg IV.
  • Provided systolic BP is >110 mmHg, give sublingual nitrate followed by IV nitrate infusion (e.g. isosorbide dinitrate 2 mg/h, increasing by 2 mg/h every 15–30 min) until breathlessness is relieved or systolic blood pressure falls below 100 mmHg or to a maximum of 10 mg/h, or buccal administration of nitrate (glyceryl trinitrate buccal tablet, 5 mg)
  • Consider non-invasive ventilation if there is respiratory distress (see Chapters 11 and 113).
  • Obtain urgent echocardiography (Table 48.2 and Chapter 114).

Further management

Review the ECG and chest X-ray arterial blood gas results. Check previous results (e.g. echocardiography, CT and pulmonary function tests).

The clinical assessment and results of first-line investigations should enable you to make a differential diagnosis and working diagnosis. Your differential diagnosis should be broad, and your working diagnosis must be repeatedly re-assessed in the light of the patient's progress.

Further management of specific disorders is given in Section 2.

Problems

Pneumonia or pulmonary oedema?
• Differentiation can sometimes be difficult. Pulmonary oedema may be localized and when severe (alveolar) may produce an air-bronchogram. The radiological signs of pulmonary oedema are modified by the presence of lung disease.
• The two diagnoses may co-exist: patients with heart failure are at increased risk of pneumonia; those with COPD are at increased risk of heart failure; and pneumonia may trigger acute atrial fibrillation and cause heart failure.
• Pulmonary oedema is unlikely if there are no clinical or ECG features to suggest significant cardiac disease and the plasma BNP level is <100 pg/mL (NT-proBNP <400 pmol/L).
• If in doubt, treat for both. If fever and a productive cough are absent, and the white cell count is <15 × 10⁹/L or C-reactive protein <10 mg/L, give diuretic alone and assess the response. Repeat the chest X-ray the following day.
• Arrange echocardiography to clarify the diagnosis if there are clinical or ECG abnormalities or the plasma BNP is >100 pg/mL (NT-proBNP >400 pmol/L).

Breathlessness with a raised jugular venous pressure
• This combination may be seen in acute major pulmonary embolism, heart failure with biventricular involvement, chronic hypoxic lung disease complicated by cor pulmonale, and cardiac tamponade.
• Obtain immediate echocardiography to clarify the diagnosis.

Table 10.3 Breathlessness with clear lungs on chest X-ray.

Disorder	Arterial PO$_2$	Arterial PCO$_2$	Arterial pH	Suggestive clinical features
Acute asthma (Chapter 60)	Normal or low	Low	High	Wheeze with reduced peak flow, diurnal variability, family history, atopy.
Exacerbation of COPD (Chapter 61)	Low	May be high	Normal or low	Fever, wheeze and productive cough; smoking history. Exacerbations in winter.
Pulmonary embolism (Chapter 57)	Normal or low	Low	High	Risk factors for thromboembolism (Table 56.1).
Acute coronary syndrome (Chapters 45 and 46)	Normal (unless pulmonary oedema)	Normal	Normal	Coronary risk factors, previous exertional breathlessness, abnormal ECG or raised troponin.
Sepsis (Chapter 35)	Normal or low	Low	Low	Low or high temperature, raised white count and C-reactive protein, raised lactate.
Metabolic acidosis (Chapter 37)	Normal or high	Low	Normal or low	Hyperventilation, diabetes, or renal failure, drug overdose.
Pre-radiological pneumonia[†]	Low	Low	High	Fever, raised white count and C-reactive protein.
Hyperventilation without organic disease	Normal or high	Low	High	Often emotional stress, resolves with rebreathing or breathing exercises.

COPD, chronic obstructive pulmonary disease.

[†] Most commonly due to viruses or *Pneumocystis jirovecii* (Table 34.4).

Breathlessness with clear lungs on chest X-ray
See Table 10.3.

Further reading

Bohadana A, Izbicki G, Kraman SS. (2014) Fundamentals of lung auscultation *N Engl J Med* 370, 744–751. DOI: 10.1056/NEJMra1302901.

Dharmarajan K, Strait KM, Tinetti ME, *et al.* (2016) Treatment for multiple acute cardiopulmonary conditions in older adults hospitalized with pneumonia, chronic obstructive pulmonary disease, or heart failure. *Journal of the American Geriatrics Society* 64, 1574–1582. DOI: 10.1111/jgs.14303.

Francis GS, Felker GM, Tang WHW. (2016) A test in context: critical evaluation of natriuretic peptide testing in heart failure. *J Am Coll Cardiol* 67, 330–337.

CHAPTER 11

Acute respiratory failure

NAYIA PETOUSI

Respiratory failure is defined as inadequate gas exchange resulting in hypoxaemia.

- Acute respiratory failure develops over a time course of minutes (hyperacute), hours or days (sub-acute), whereas chronic respiratory failure develops over weeks, months or years.
- Respiratory failure is subdivided into:
  - **Type 1**: PaO_2 <8 KPa and normal or low $PaCO_2$
  - **Type 2**: PaO_2 <8 KPa with a raised $PaCO_2$ >6 KPa
- Type 1 respiratory failure is caused primarily by ventilation/perfusion (V/Q) mismatch and usually relates to diseases within the respiratory system. Type 2 respiratory failure is caused by alveolar hypoventilation, with or without V/Q mismatch and can thus be caused by diseases both intrinsic and extrinsic to the respiratory system.
- The causes of acute respiratory failure are given in Table 11.1. Remember there may often be a combination of disease processes, for example pneumonia on a background of pulmonary fibrosis or heart failure. There may also be an acute-on-chronic presentation, for example decompensated chronic respiratory failure in a patient with an exacerbation of chronic obstructive pulmonary disease.
- In patients who develop acute respiratory failure while they are already inpatients, the commonest causes are hospital-acquired pneumonia, pulmonary embolism, pulmonary oedema and sedative drugs (e.g. opioids).

The management of the patient with suspected acute respiratory failure is summarized in Figures 11.1 and 11.2.

Priorities

1 Is urgent intubation and/or ventilation required?
Assess if there is severe upper airway obstruction (see Chapter 59: Upper airway obstruction), inability to protect airway due to decreased consciousness (see Chapter 112: Airway management), impending respiratory or cardiac arrest, severe hypoxia despite oxygen treatment or severe acidosis/hypercapnia.

2 Prevent life-threatening hypoxia
Oxygen therapy is key in preventing life-threatening hypoxia, but caution should be taken. Patients known to suffer from COPD may have chronic respiratory failure with hypercapnia; in these patients hypoxia acts as a stimulus to ventilatory drive and abolishing it completely may make respiratory failure worse. These patients need controlled oxygen therapy. Thus, try to establish early, with the means of an arterial blood gas (see Chapter 118), whether the patient has type 1 or type 2 respiratory failure and instigate appropriate oxygen therapy (Figure 11.2).

Acute Medicine: A Practical Guide to the Management of Medical Emergencies, Fifth Edition. Edited by David Sprigings and John B. Chambers.
© 2018 John Wiley & Sons Ltd. Published 2018 by John Wiley & Sons Ltd.

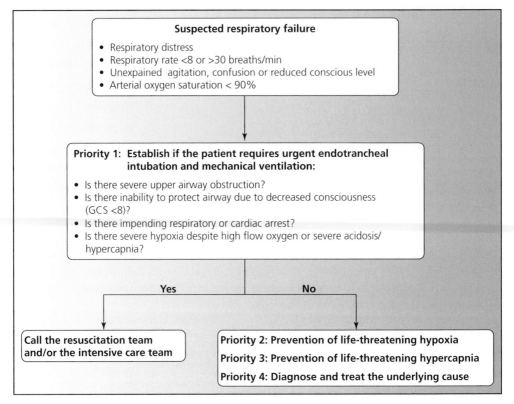

Figure 11.1 Management of the patient with suspected acute respiratory failure: priorities.

3 Prevent life-threatening hypercapnia

Patients in type 2 respiratory failure will require controlled oxygen therapy via a Venturi mask, aiming for SaO_2 of 88–92% (Figure 11.2). Monitoring with repeat ABGs is important. If high $PaCO_2$ or acidosis persists, assisted ventilation will be required.

4 Diagnose and manage the underlying cause (Tables 11.1, 11.2 and 11.3)

Careful history and examination (see Table 11.2) and appropriate investigations (see Table 11.3) are paramount. Management will largely be determined by the working diagnosis as well as the response to the initial treatment. Some treatments need to be instigated quickly. For example:

- Inhaled bronchodilator therapy (e.g. salbutamol 2.5–5 mg) and steroids (e.g. prednisolone 30–40 mg) in acute exacerbation of asthma or COPD (see Chapter 61).
- Intravenous diuretic (e.g. furosemide 40–80 mg) in acute pulmonary oedema (see Chapter 47).
- Antibiotic therapy in pneumonia (see Chapters 62 and 63).
- Anticoagulation (e.g. low-molecular-weight heparin) in pulmonary embolism (see Chapter 57).
- Chest physiotherapy in the presence of copious respiratory secretions which impair adequate gas exchange.
- Drainage of a large pleural effusion or pneumothorax (see Chapters 12 and 64).
- Non-invasive ventilation in acidotic hypercapnic respiratory failure in acute exacerbation of COPD that fails to respond to initial treatment and controlled oxygen therapy (see Table 11.4 and Chapters 61 and 113).

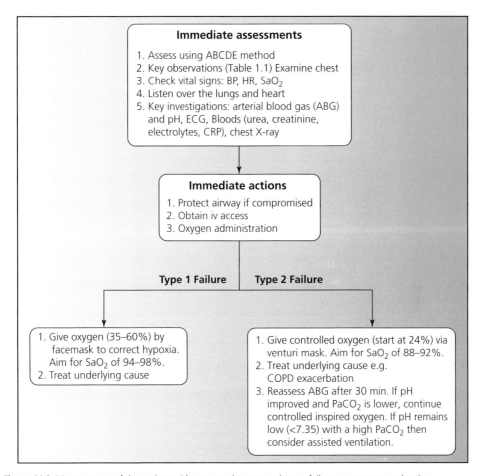

Figure 11.2 Management of the patient with suspected acute respiratory failure: assessment and action.

Table 11.1 Causes of acute respiratory failure.

Type 1 Respiratory Failure	Type 2 Respiratory Failure
Pneumonia	**Reduced central respiratory drive**
Pulmonary embolism	Sedative drugs, for example opiates/opioids, benzodiazepines, alcohol
Acute exacerbation of COPD	Head trauma
Acute exacerbation of asthma	Space-occupying CNS lesion
Pulmonary fibrotic lung disease	Cerebrovascular accident
Pulmonary oedema (heart failure)	**Neuromuscular and thoracic wall disease**
Acute Respiratory Distress Syndrome (ARDS)	Cervical cord lesion
Pneumothorax	Guillain-Barré syndrome
	Myasthenia gravis
	Poliomyelitis
	Diaphragmatic paralysis

(*continued*)

Table 11.1 (*Continued*)

Type 1 Respiratory Failure	Type 2 Respiratory Failure
	Flail chest
	Chest wall deformity (acute on chronic)
	Respiratory disease
	Acute upper airway obstruction (foreign body or reduced conscious level)
	Acute exacerbation of COPD
	Severe life-threatening asthma
	Pneumothorax
	Factors that can worsen respiratory failure of any cause
	Sedative drugs: benzodiazepines, opioids
	Aspiration of secretions or gastric contents
	Respiratory muscle fatigue
	Low cardiac output
	Severe obesity
	Chest wall abnormality, for example kyphoscoliosis
	Large pleural effusion
	Pneumothorax

Table 11.2 Clinical assessment in acute respiratory failure.

History

Is the patient known to suffer from an underlying cardiopulmonary disease, for example asthma, COPD, heart disease?
Are there features to suggest infection, for example fever, cough, purulent sputum or increase in sputum volume?
Is there chest pain (pleuritic or non-pleuritic)?
What is the rate of onset of the presentation? Is it acute, sub-acute or chronic?
Background
Usual functional status
Careful drug history, for example opiates, benzodiazepines, respiratory or cardiac medications
Social history: occupation, smoking, alcohol excess
Examination
Drowsiness (GCS)
Tachypnoea
Cyanosis
Tachycardia or bradycardia
Blood pressure
Tremor, bounding pulse, flap/asterixis
Raised JVP, peripheral oedema
Chest wall abnormalities (kyphoscoliosis, flail chest post trauma)
Paradoxical movement of the diaphragm
Chest examination:
   Wheeze (consider: asthma, COPD, heart failure)
   Fine inspiratory crackles (consider: heart failure, fibrosis)
   Coarse crackles (consider: bronchiectasis, pneumonia)
   Bronchial breathing (consider: pneumonia)
   Dull percussion note, reduced air entry (consider: pleural effusion)
   Hyper-resonant percussion note, reduced air entry (consider: pneumothorax)
   Peak expiratory flow (if patient is able to perform)
Neurological examination: are there features of a chronic neurological disease? Are there focal neurological features?

Table 11.3 Investigation in acute respiratory failure.

Chest X-ray
Arterial blood gases, pH and lactate
ECG
Full blood count
C-reactive protein
Blood glucose
Creatinine and electrolytes
Plasma BNP or NT-proBNP
Blood culture
Sputum microscopy and culture

Also consider:
Thoracic ultrasonography if chest X-ray abnormal
Echocardiography if suspected cardiac disease
Neurological investigation if suspected CNS or neuromuscular disease (see Chapter 17).

- Reversal of the effects of narcotic drugs (e.g. naloxone in opiate overdose, flumazenil in benzodiazepine overdose) (see Chapter 36).

5 Institute assisted ventilation if indicated (Tables 11.4 and 11.5)

If, following treatment of the underlying problem, oxygen requirements remain high (e.g. >60%) or there is persistent acidosis with hypercapnia, assisted ventilation (invasive or non-invasive) should be considered, if appropriate given the clinical situation. See Tables 11.4 and 11.5, and Chapter 113.

Table 11.4 Non-invasive ventilation in acute respiratory failure.

Mode of ventilation	Indications	Contraindications	Disadvantages and complications
Continuous positive airway pressure (CPAP)	Cardiogenic pulmonary oedema	Recent facial, upper airway, or upper gastrointestinal surgery Vomiting or bowel obstruction Unconscious or uncooperative patient Copious secretions (relative) Haemodynamic instability Undrained pneumothorax	Patient must be conscious and cooperative Discomfort from tightly fitting facemask Bloating due to aerophagia May fail
Bilevel positive airway pressure (BiPAP)	Acidotic type 2 respiratory failure in acute exacerbation of COPD Acidotic type 2 respiratory failure in patient with chest wall deformity		

Remember:
Before commencing non-invasive ventilation, an action plan needs to be in place in the event of failure, that is, whether this is ceiling of treatment or whether invasive ventilation should follow.

Table 11.5 Invasive ventilation in acute respiratory failure.

Mode of ventilation	Indications	Contraindications	Disadvantages and complications
Endotracheal intubation and mechanical ventilation	Upper airway obstruction	Patient has expressed wish not to be ventilated	Need for sedation and paralysis
	Impending respiratory arrest	Chronic respiratory disease with severely impaired functional capacity and/or severe comorbidity	Pharyngeal, laryngeal and tracheal injury
	Airway at risk because of reduced conscious level (GCS <8)	Irreversible extensive neurological damage	Ventilator-associated pneumonia
	Oxygenation failure: PaO_2 <7.5–8 kPa, despite supplemental oxygen/NIV Ventilatory failure: respiratory acidosis with pH <7.25		Ventilator-induced lung injury (e.g. barotrauma) Weaning may pose ethical difficulties

Further reading

Goligher EC, Ferguson ND, Brochard LJ. (2016) Clinical challenges in mechanical ventilation. *Lancet* 387, 1856–1866.

Davidson AC, Banham S, Elliott M, *et al*. (2016) British Thoracic Society/Intensive Care Society Acute Hypercapnic Respiratory Failure Guideline Development Group. BTS/ICS Guidelines for the ventilatory management of acute hypercapnic respiratory failure in adults. *Thorax* 71, ii1–ii35. https://www.brit-thoracic.org.uk/document-library/clinical-information/acute-hypercapnic-respiratory-failure/bts-guidelines-for-ventilatory-management-of-ahrf/.

Pepin JL, Timsit JF, Tamisier R, Borel JC, Levy P, Jaber S. (2016) Prevention and care of respiratory failure in obese patients. *Lancet Respir Med* 4, 407–418.

O'Driscoll R, Howard L, Earis J, Mak V, on behalf of the BTS Emergency Oxygen Guideline Group (2015) BTS Guidelines for oxygen use in adults in healthcare and emergency settings (https://www.brit-thoracic.org.uk/document-library/clinical-information/oxygen/emergency-oxygen-guideline-2015/bts-full-guideline-for-oxygen-use-in-adults-in-healthcare-and-emergency-settings-2015/).

Stephen Chapman, Grace Robinson, John Stradling, Sophie West, and John Wrightson (2014) Oxford Handbook of Respiratory Medicine (3 ed.), OUP.

CHAPTER 12

Pleural effusion

IOANNIS PSALLIDAS

Pleural effusion is a feature of a wide range of diseases. Transudative and exudative effusions (Tables 12.1 and 12.2) are caused by distinctive pathogenic mechanisms, and Light's criteria should be used for their differentiation.

Evaluation requires clinical assessment, imaging (by chest X-ray and thoracic ultrasonography) and examination of pleural fluid. Assessment and management of pleural effusion is summarized in Figure 12.1.

Priorities

Clinical assessment and imaging

The clinical assessment is summarized in Table 12.3.

- Review the history, with a focus on occupational exposures, drugs, risk factors for pulmonary embolism or tuberculosis, extrapleural sources (e.g. ascites) and comorbid conditions.
- Review the chest X-ray. Pleural effusion results in basal shadowing obscuring the hemidiaphragm with a concave upper border. Massive effusion demonstrates a complete 'white-out' of the hemithorax with mediastinal displacement away from the effusion. If mediastinal shift is not present, consider the possibility of a co-existing bronchial obstruction with the effusion (e.g. lung cancer).
- Thoracic ultrasonography is more sensitive than chest radiography in detecting pleural effusion and also provides additional diagnostic information as to the cause of the effusion (exudative, empyema, malignant pleural effusion).

Thoracentesis

- There is no need for thoracentesis if the patient has an obvious reason for pleural effusion (e.g. small bilateral pleural effusions and a history of heart failure).
- It may be diagnostic (50–60 mL of fluid) and/or therapeutic (target: symptomatic relief).
- Pleural fluid examination should be analysed carefully. Vital diagnostic clues may lie in simple inspection or smell. Tests needed are summarized in Table 12.4.
  - If pleural infection is suspected send fluid in blood culture bottles in addition to a plain tube.
  - Cytology (approximately 40–50 mL should be sent for malignant cell identification and for cell differential diagnosis). The sensitivity of the technique for detecting malignant pleural effusion is around 60% (i.e. false-negative rate 40%) and the additional yield from sending more than two specimens of pleural fluid taken on different occasions is low.
  - If pleural fluid pH is needed, use ABG analyser (but do not analyse a purulent sample, as this is unnecessary and may damage the machine).
  - Additional tests may be indicated, depending on clinical scenario (e.g. chylomicrons, cholesterol, triglycerides, adenosine deaminase, amylase).

Acute Medicine: A Practical Guide to the Management of Medical Emergencies, Fifth Edition. Edited by David Sprigings and John B. Chambers.
© 2018 John Wiley & Sons Ltd. Published 2018 by John Wiley & Sons Ltd.

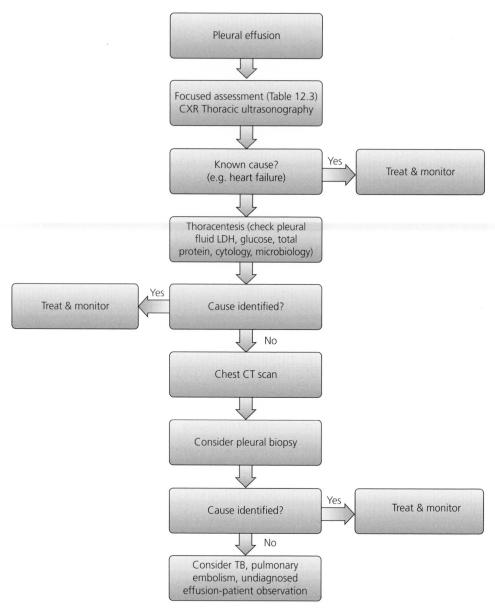

Figure 12.1 Investigation of pleural effusion.

Categorizing an effusion as a transudate or an exudate

To answer this important question, Light's criteria should be employed. The effusion is an exudate if it meets one of the following criteria:

- Pleural fluid protein/serum protein ratio >0.5
- Pleural fluid LDH/serum LDH ratio >0.6
- Pleural fluid LDH greater than two-thirds of the upper limit of normal serum LDH

Table 12.1 Causes of transudative pleural effusion.

Cause	Comment
Heart failure	Increased interstitial fluid, which crosses the visceral pleura and enters the pleural space. Investigate further if atypical features are present (unilateral effusion, fever, chest pain).
Nephrotic syndrome	Usually bilateral effusions, decreased oncotic pressure causing transudate effusion.
Cirrhosis with ascites	Predominantly right-sided pleural effusion and often ascites is present. Ascitic fluid migration to the pleural space through diaphragmatic defects.
Hypoalbuminaemia (serum albumin <25 g/L)	Associated with oedema.
Hypothyroidism	May be transudate or exudate, commonly in combination with ascites, pericardial effusion and cardiac failure.
Meigs' syndrome	In women with ovarian or other pelvic tumours (either bilateral or unilateral).
Urinothorax	Due to urine obstruction that causes retroperitoneal urine leak. pH usually low, pleural fluid smells of urine and pleural fluid creatinine > serum creatinine is diagnostic.
Constrictive pericarditis	Increases IV hydrostatic pressure, associated with oedema.

Light's criteria correctly identify almost all exudates, but mis-classifies about 20% of transudates as exudates. If a transudative effusion is suspected (e.g. due to heart failure or cirrhosis) and none of the biochemical measurements is >15% above the cutoff levels for Light's criteria, the difference between serum and the pleural fluid protein is measured. If the difference is >31 g/L, the effusion is probably a transudate.

Table 12.2 Causes of exudative pleural effusion.

Cause	Comment
Pleural infection (parapneumonic effusion and empyema)	Most common cause in young patients; empyema is defined as pus in the pleural cavity.
Malignancy	Most common cause in older patients and a frequent cause of massive effusions.
Tuberculosis	Delayed hypersensitivity reaction to mycobacteria released into the pleural space. AFB and pleural fluid culture often negative.
Chylothorax	Often milky effusions, diagnosis with presence of chylomicrons or pleural fluid triglyceride level >1.24 mmol/L.
Oesophangeal rupture	pH <7.20, increased levels of salivary amylase.
Pulmonary embolism	Almost always exudative; bloody in <50%; it should be suspected when dyspnoea is disproportionate to size of effusion, or when patient is hypoxic.
After coronary artery bypass surgery (CABG)	Commonly left sided pleural effusions and most resolve spontaneously. If <30 days of surgery, blood stained due to post-operative bleeding. If >30 days of surgery: clear fluid due to immune reaction.
Acute pancreatitis	Pleural fluid pancreatic amylase may be raised.
Rheumatoid arthritis	Typical low pleural fluid glucose (<1.6 mmol/L).
Yellow nail syndrome	Triad of nail discolouration, lymphoedema and pleural effusion.

Table 12.3 Focused assessment of the patient with pleural effusion.

History

Dyspnoea

Pleuritic chest pain, chest discomfort or 'heaviness', pain referred to the shoulder or abdomen

Dry cough

Symptoms of malignancy: loss of appetite, energy, weight

Symptoms of infection: fever, sputum, night sweats

May also be asymptomatic

Examination

Reduced chest expansion

Reduced tactile vocal fremitus

Dull percussion

Reduced breath sounds

Pleural friction rub may be heard in patient with pleural inflammation

Table 12.4 Pleural fluid analysis: (1) In all patients; (2) Additional tests for exudative effusions.

Pleural fluid analysis (1): In all patients	
Test	**Comment**
Visual inspection	Blood-stained effusion (pleural fluid haematocrit 1–20% of peripheral haematocrit) is likely to be due to malignancy, pulmonary embolism or trauma. Purulent fluid signifies empyema.
Protein and lactate dehydrogenase (LDH)	These are the only tests needed if the effusion is likely to be a transudate. Pleural fluid LDH correlates with the degree of pleural inflammation. Exudative pleural effusions have a protein concentration >30 g/L. If the pleural fluid protein is around 30 g/L, Light's criteria are helpful in distinguishing between a transudate and exudate. An exudate is identified by one or more of the following: • Pleural fluid protein to serum protein ratio >0.5 • Pleural fluid LDH to serum LDH ratio >0.6 • Pleural fluid LDH more than two-thirds the upper limit of normal for serum LDH

Pleural fluid analysis (2): Additional tests for exudative pleural effusion	
Test	**Comment**
Pleural fluid pH and glucose (check these if parapneumonic or malignant pleural effusion is suspected. Send sample in heparinized syringe for measurement of pH in blood gas analyser).	Low pH (<7.3)/low glucose (<3.3 mmol/L) pleural fluid may be seen in: • Complicated parapneumonic effusion and empyema • Malignancy • Rheumatoid or lupus pleuritis • Tuberculosis • Oesophageal rupture
Cytology (total and differential cell count; malignant cells).	Neutrophilia (>50% cells) indicate acute pleural disease. Lymphocytosis is seen in malignancy, tuberculous pleuritis and in pleural effusions after CABG. The yield of cytology is influenced by the histological type of malignancy: >70% positive in adenocarcinoma, 25–50% in lymphoma, 10% in mesothelioma.
Microbiology (Gram stain culture; markers of tuberculosis (TB)).	Send fluid for markers of TB if TB is suspected or there is a pleural fluid lymphocytosis.

Table 12.4 (*Continued*)

Pleural fluid analysis (2): Additional tests for exudative pleural effusion

Test	Comment
Other tests depending on clinical setting (e.g. amylase, triglyceride).	Elevated pleural fluid amylase is seen in the acute pancreatitis and oesophageal rupture. Check triglyceride level if chylothorax is suspected (opaque white effusion); chylothorax (triglyceride >1.1 g/L) is due to disruption of the thoracic duct by trauma or lymphoma.

CABG, coronary artery bypass graft.

Further management

Treatment of symptoms and underlying disorder

- The effusion itself generally does not require treatment if the patient is asymptomatic.
- Many effusions resorb spontaneously when the underlying disorder is treated, especially effusions due to heart failure, pulmonary embolism or after CABG.
- Pleuritic pain can usually be managed with NSAIDs or other oral analgesics.

Drainage of a symptomatic effusion

- Therapeutic aspiration is a sufficient treatment for many symptomatic effusions and can be repeated for effusions that re-accumulate. Seek advice from a chest physician.
- In most cases, 1–1.5 L of pleural fluid can be aspirated with careful attention to the development of chest symptoms; re-expansion pulmonary oedema is a recognized but rare consequence of large-volume aspiration. Pleural aspiration should be stopped if the patient develops chest tightness, chest pain or severe coughing
- Effusions that are chronic, recurrent and causing symptoms, can be treated with pleurodesis or by intermittent drainage with an indwelling catheter.

Specific management for parapneumonic effusions and empyema

- Seek advice from a chest physician. For indications for chest drain insertion see Table 12.5.
- All patient with pleural infection should be treated with antibiotics (refer to local hospital prescribing guidelines) and treatment options ought to be rationalized with culture and sensitivity results of the pleural fluid or blood cultures (note that anaerobes are frequently difficult to culture and may coexist with other organisms).
- Refer to a thoracic surgeon if there is persistent sepsis after 5–7 days of maximum therapy with antibiotics and pleural fluid drainage.

Table 12.5 Indications for chest tube insertion for parapneumonic effusions/empyema.[*]

Pleural fluid pH <7.20 or pleural fluid glucose <3.3 mmol/L
Purulent pleural fluid
Pleural fluid positive culture or Gram stain

[*] The ideal chest drain size is subject to debate but small (<14 F) drains may be as effective as larger ones (>14 F) in the management of empyema, and cause less pain and discomfort. Regular flushes with normal saline (0.9%) are needed (20 mL four times per day).

Specific management for malignant pleural effusions

- Seek advice from a chest physician.
- Asymptomatic effusions and those causing dyspnoea unrelieved by thoracentesis do not require additional procedures.
- If dyspnoea caused by malignant pleural effusion is relieved by thoracentesis but fluid and dyspnea re-develop, definitive treatment is required (talc pleurodesis or placement of an indwelling pleural catheter).
- Pleurodesis is performed by instilling a sclerosing agent into the pleural space in order to seal the visceral and parietal pleura and eliminate the space. The most effective and commonly used sclerosing agent is talc. Talc pleurodesis can be performed either by the insertion of a small chest tube (10–14 F) as a slurry or by medical thoracoscopy as a poudrage.
- Indwelling pleural catheter (IPC) drainage is the preferred approach for ambulatory patients because hospitalization is not necessary for catheter insertion and the pleural fluid can be drained intermittently into vacuum bottles. IPC is the preferred option for patients with significant trapped lung (when tumour encases the visceral pleura and prevents lung re-expansion).
- Chest CT scan with pleural phase contrast (late venous phase) is useful in distinguishing nodular, mediastinal or circumferential pleural thickening (features present in around 80% of cases of malignant pleural disease).
- Pleural tissue biopsy for histological or microbiological examination may be indicated. Pleural biopsy can be performed using image-guided (CT or US guidance) techniques or via medical thoracoscopy. Both techniques have significantly better results compared to closed pleural biopsies. Thoracoscopy also offers diagnostic and therapeutic approaches to patients with pleural effusion (e.g. talc poudrage pleurodesis).
- Bronchoscopy has no role in investigating pleural effusions, and is only used if the chest CT scan is suggestive of parenchymal abnormities that require further investigation, or if main bronchial obstruction is suspected.
- Even after extensive investigations, 25% of pleural effusions remain undiagnosed. These are often due to occult pulmonary embolism, TB, viral infection or cancer.

Further reading

Corcoran JP, Wrightson JM, Belcher E, DeCamp MM, Feller-Kopman D, Rahman NM (2015) Pleural infection: past, present, and future directions. *Lancet Respir Med* 3, 563–577.

Light RW (2013) The Light criteria: the beginning and why they are useful 40 years later. *Clin Chest Med* 34, 21–26. http://dx.doi.org/10.1016/j.ccm.2012.11.006.

Psallidas I, Kalomenidis I, Porcel JM, Robinson BW, Stathopoulos GT (2016) Malignant pleural effusion: from bench to bedside. *European Respiratory Review* 25, 189–198. DOI: 10.1183/16000617.0019-2016.

CHAPTER 13

Cough and haemoptysis

AHMED YOUSUF

Cough

Cough is defined as a forced expulsive manoeuvre, usually against a closed glottis, and is associated with a characteristic sound. It is a very common and usually self-limiting symptom (Box 13.1). Occasionally, it is the presenting symptom of a serious underlying condition such as lung cancer or pulmonary tuberculosis (Table 13.1). Management of the patient with cough is summarized in Figure 13.1.

Management

Management is directed by the working diagnosis.

Clinical assessment (Tables 13.2 and 13.3), a chest X-ray and other investigations (Table 13.4) will identify the cause and guide management.

- If gastro-oesophageal reflux disease is considered as the cause of cough, a therapeutic trial of treatment with a proton pump inhibitor for minimum of two months should be considered (e.g. omeprazole 20 mg 12-hourly or lansoprazole 15 mg 12-hourly).
- Patients with pulmonary tuberculosis who are smear-positive (i.e. Acid-fast bacilli seen on sputum microscopy) are potentially infectious. If they are admitted, ensure that they are isolated and local infection control procedures are followed. Contact your microbiology or respiratory department immediately for advice. If they are in the community, inform the TB nurse, microbiology consultant and Public Health England (Health Protection Scotland in Scotland).

Box 13.1 Definitions.

Acute cough: Cough lasting less than three weeks. It is most commonly due to upper respiratory tract infection, with a benign course. Clinical signs indicating a serious cause that warrants inpatient admission are given in Table 13.3.

Chronic cough: Cough lasting more than eight weeks. In the absence of worrying clinical features (Table 13.3), the patient can be discharged and investigated in general respiratory or specialist cough clinic.

Acute Medicine: A Practical Guide to the Management of Medical Emergencies, Fifth Edition. Edited by David Sprigings and John B. Chambers.
© 2018 John Wiley & Sons Ltd. Published 2018 by John Wiley & Sons Ltd.

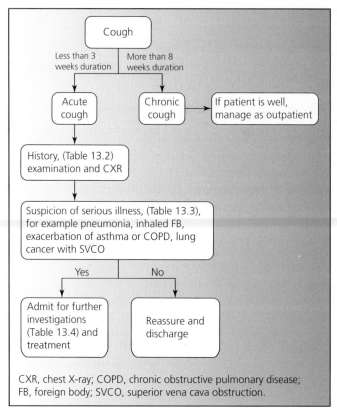

Figure 13.1 Management of cough.

Table 13.1 Causes of cough.

Upper respiratory tract infection (accounts for 90% of acute cough)[*]

Lower respiratory tract infection[*] (Chapter 62)

Pulmonary tuberculosis[*†]

Airways disease[†] (chronic obstructive pulmonary disease, asthma)

Bronchiectasis[†]

Lung cancer[*†]

Gastro-oesophageal reflux disease[†]

Upper airway cough syndrome[†] (previously known as post-nasal drip syndrome)

Angiotensin-converting-enzyme (ACE) inhibitor therapy[†]

[*] Common cause of acute cough.
[†] Common cause of chronic cough.

Table 13.2 Cough history.

Duration of cough

Associated symptoms: fever, night sweats, weight loss, haemoptysis, breathlessness, chest pain

History of tuberculosis or contact with tuberculosis

History of other respiratory disease

Foreign travel

Symptoms of gastro-oesophageal reflux disease (heart burn, acid reflux, pain on swallowing)

Post-nasal drip syndrome (feeling of excess mucus accumulating in the back of the throat, feeling of mucus dripping from the nose into back of the throat)

Triggers to cough (e.g. dust, wind, smoke)

Drug history (enquire specifically about angiotensin-converting-enzyme (ACE) inhibitors)

Smoking history

Occupational history

History of asbestos exposure

Table 13.3 Clinical signs warranting inpatient admission of the patient with cough.

Respiratory rate >30 breaths/min

Oxygen saturation <92%, (if no history of chronic hypoxia)

Use of accessory muscles of respiration

Tachycardia >130/min

Systolic blood pressure <90 mmHg or diastolic blood pressure <60 mmHg

Haemoptysis

Fever

Chest pain

Suspicion of inhaled foreign body

Table 13.4 Investigations.

Full blood count – raised eosinophil level may direct you to consider eosinophilic airways disease as the cause of cough. CRP – raised CRP could be due to respiratory tract infection.

CXR – everyone with history of cough should have a baseline CXR. Approximately 30% of chest radiographs requested for investigating the cause of cough are abnormal.

CT chest: if the CXR is abnormal (e.g. suspicious of lung cancer, interstitial lung disease).

Sputum for acid-fast bacilli (AFB) staining, microscopy and culture – if the patient is in high-risk group for TB (e.g. homeless, alcohol dependent, immunosuppressed, Asian or Afro-Caribbean background, previous history of pulmonary TB).

Bronchoscopy, if there is suspicion of inhaled FB (usually in children and elderly).

Investigations in outpatient setting

Three early morning sputum samples for TB culture.

Spirometry: reversibility test (for obstructive airways disease), airway provocation test with mannitol or methacholine for cough variant asthma.

Bronchoscopy: patients presenting with small haemoptysis, suspected TB with non-productive cough or suspected lung cancer can be referred to respiratory physicians for outpatient bronchoscopy.

Fibreoptic laryngoscopy: in patients with suspected upper airways pathology as the cause of cough, laryngoscopy may show changes associated with laryngeal inflammation and oedema.

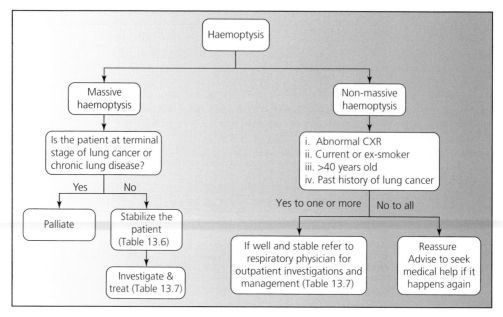

Figure 13.2 Management of haemoptysis.

Haemoptysis

Haemoptysis is coughing up blood, either mixed with sputum or on its own, from the respiratory tract (Table 13.5).

- Management is summarized in Figure 13.2. Haemoptysis can be distinguished from haematemesis by its colour and pH: haemoptysis is bright red and alkaline, haematemesis is brown ('coffee ground') and acidic. Bleeding from the nasopharynx may be mistaken for haemoptysis: if in doubt, ask the advice of ENT surgeon.
- In the majority of cases, haemoptysis originates from the bronchial circulation. Bronchial arteries usually arise directly from the aorta and carry blood at systemic blood pressure. Therefore, bleeding that originates from bronchial circulation causes massive haemoptysis; if left untreated it has a mortality rate of up to 80%. Management of massive haemoptysis is summarized in Table 13.6.
- Haemoptysis can be classified as small or massive, based on the volume of blood expectorated in 24 hours. A pragmatic definition of massive haemoptysis is 200 mL of blood loss in 24 hours, or haemoptysis significant enough to impair gas exchange and cause haemodynamic compromise, regardless of the duration of haemoptysis.
- Investigation of haemoptysis is given in Table 13.7.

Management of massive haemoptysis

The priority is to stabilize the patient, identify the bleeding site and stop the bleeding (Table 13.6). Active intervention is not appropriate for all patients and in some cases (e.g. end-stage lung cancer, end-stage chronic pulmonary or cardiac disease) a palliative approach might be the best option.

Table 13.5 Causes of haemoptysis.

Cause	Comment
Lung cancer[*]	Frank haemoptysis or blood stained sputum, weight loss, cough
Tuberculosis[*]	Cough, fever, night sweat, weight loss
Bronchiectasis[*]	Chronic cough with purulent sputum, previous episodes of haemoptysis
Pneumonia[*]	'Rusty' sputum, fever, cough, signs of consolidation
Lung abscess[*]	Purulent sputum, fever, chest pain
Pulmonary embolism[*]	Pleuritic chest pain, breathlessness
Pulmonary oedema[*]	Frothy 'pink' sputum, breathlessness, ↑JVP
Vasculitides[†]	Granulomatosis with polyangiitis (formerly known as Wegner's), Goodpasture's syndrome, SLE
Mycetoma[†]	Fungal ball on CXR, previous TB
Arteriovenous malformation[†]	Recurrent haemoptysis, Osler-Weber-Rendu syndrome (telangiectasia)
Iatrogenic[†]	Post-lung biopsy or bronchoscopy

[*] Common,
[†] Rare

Table 13.6 Management of massive haemoptysis.

1. Airway protection and ventilation: this could be achieved by sitting up the patient, or lying the patient on the bleeding side (if known) to avoid spillage of blood to the unaffected lung. Give oxygen to maintain oxygen saturation of above 94%.
2. Cardiovascular support:
   - Insert two large bore (at least 16 gauge) cannulas
   - Send blood for FBC/cross match/clotting screen
   - Fluid resuscitation
   - Blood transfusion (if Hb <80)
   - Arterial +/− CVP line (preferably in HDU/ICU)
3. Assess patient's GCS, if <8 or unable to protect airway, ask for anaesthetist's help to protect the airway
4. Correct clotting as per hospital protocol
5. Give IV tranexamic acid (1 g TDS, avoid if known renal failure)
6. Give nebulized adrenaline (1 mL of 1:1000 with 4 mL of NaCl 0.9%)
7. Give IV terlipressin (2 mg IV stat, then 1 mg IV every 4–6 h)

Once patient is stabilized arrange:
1. Bronchoscopy (flexible or rigid): for diagnostic and therapeutic (injecting cold saline or 1:20,000 adrenaline, cryocautery, diathermy) purposes.
2. Endovascular embolization: most effective and minimally invasive procedure in managing massive haemoptysis.
3. Surgery: resection of the bleeding lobe (if all other measures have failed).

Table 13.7 Investigation of haemoptysis.

Full blood count
Clotting screen
Creatinine and electrolytes
ECG
Auto-antibodies (ANA, ANCA, anti-GBM), urine dip and microscopy for red cells casts, if vasculitides are suspected
Arterial blood gases if O_2 saturations <92% or pleuritic chest pain, or breathless.
CXR can help with lateralizing bleeding and may reveal a focal or diffuse lung involvement. It has 35–50% positive diagnostic yield. A quarter of patients presenting with hemoptysis due to malignancy will have normal CXR.
Sputum Ziehl-Neelsen stains and culture.
CTPA to exclude PE and identify bleeding site. It will also help to identify other causes of haemoptysis (e.g. lung cancer). Performing CT scan before bronchoscopy will improve diagnostic yield.
Bronchoscopy (flexible or rigid): it helps to visualize the airways and localize the site of bleeding. Diagnostic (biopsy, bronchial wash) and therapeutic interventions (e.g. injecting cold saline or adrenaline cryocautery and diathermy) can be undertaken.

Further reading

Larici AR, Franchi P, Occhipinti M. (2014) Diagnosis and management of hemoptysis. *Diagn Interv Radiol* 20, 299–309.

National Institute for Care and Health Excellence. Clinical Knowledge Summaries. Cough. Last revised June 2015. http://cks.nice.org.uk/cough.

Smith JA, Woodcock A. Chronic cough (2016) *N Engl J Med* 375, 1544–1551.

Thomas A, Lynch G. (2011) Management of massive haemoptysis. http://www.frca.co.uk/Documents/225% 20Massive%20Haemoptysis.pdf.

http://cks.nice.org.uk/cough.

http://www.issc.info/cough.pdf.

Neurological

CHAPTER 14

Neurological diagnosis in acute medicine

Simon Rinaldi

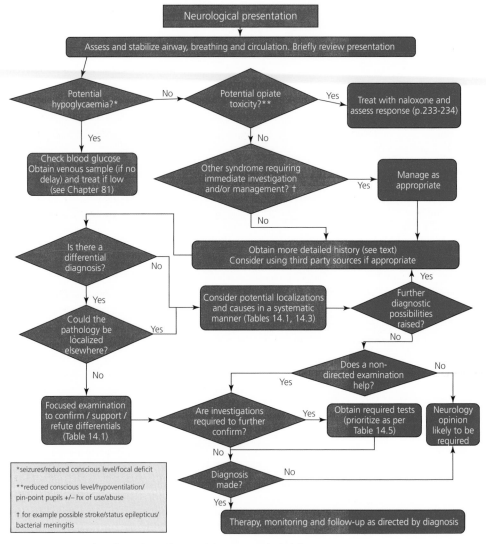

Figure 14.1 Approach to the patient with potential acute neurological disease.

Acute Medicine: A Practical Guide to the Management of Medical Emergencies, Fifth Edition. Edited by David Sprigings and John B. Chambers.
© 2018 John Wiley & Sons Ltd. Published 2018 by John Wiley & Sons Ltd.

Box 14.1 Neurological diagnosis in acute medicine.

- About 10–20% of patients on an acute medical ward have a neurological problem such as stroke, headache, seizure and disorders of consciousness.
- Differential diagnosis in neurology involves identifying where the lesion is (from the history and neurological examination) and what it is (often primarily from the time course of the illness). This guides investigation and further management.

Priorities

- Identify or exclude an immediately life-threatening disorder (see Figure 14.1, Table 14.1) such as stroke, cord compression, or meningo-encephalitis.
- The history (Table 14.2) is usually the critical step in establishing a differential diagnosis:
  - Pattern recognition may suggest some diagnoses, for example an acute onset, right sided hemiparesis with dysphasia and homonymous hemianopia in a hypertensive smoker is recognized as a left cerebral hemisphere anterior circulation stroke.
  - In more difficult cases, a logical system for working through potential diagnoses can be based on the localization (Table 14.3) or temporal evolution of symptoms (Table 14.4).
- A systematic 'full' or 'screening' neurological examination is not usually indicated. It may be better to target the examination to test the differential diagnostic hypotheses generated during history taking (Table 14.5).
  - Asymptomatic areas should still be examined. For example, demonstrating normal arm function in suspected spinal cord compression is helpful in placing the lesion below the level of the cervical cord.
  - Remember that performance in the different domains is not independent. For example a patient with limb weakness may appear uncoordinated despite normal proprioceptive and cerebellar function.
- The distinction between upper and lower motor neuron pathology and the implication of certain patterns of weakness is discussed in further detail in Chapter 17. Specific patterns of visual loss also have clear value in localization (Chapter 19).
- Table 14.6 summarizes the indications and limitations of the tests most often needed.

Further management

- Some presentations may allow discharge and deferred outpatient investigations following initial assessment, with or without a short period of observation, for example gradual-onset resolving headache without red flag features or signs (Chapter 15) or a fully resolved solitary seizure without systemic upset (Chapter 16).
- Transient symptoms may not be benign:
  - Transient loss of consciousness suggestive of intermittent raised ICP/CSF outflow obstruction will require urgent neurosurgical management (Chapter 72).
  - Suspected cardiac syncope will require cardiac workup (Chapter 9).
  - Transient ischaemic attacks (TIAs) require urgent assessment even if all symptoms have resolved; clinical scoring schemes provide an indication regarding how quickly subsequent investigations should be performed (Chapter 66).

Table 14.1 Priority differential diagnoses to consider based on presentation.

Presentation	Always consider
Coma	Hypoglycaemia, drug toxicity, intracranial haemorrhage/SOL with brainstem herniation, non-convulsive status, functional unresponsiveness*
Acute ataxia/vertigo	Cerebellar stroke (haemorrhage/infarction)
Hemiparesis	Stroke[†]
Paraparesis	Spinal cord compression/stroke[‡]
Quadriparesis	Spinal cord compression/stroke, brainstem infarction[‡]
Acute severe headache	Subarachnoid haemorrhage, venous sinus thrombosis
Transient loss of consciousness	Cardiac syncope, transient CSF outflow obstruction, seizure
Status epilepticus	Non-epileptic attack disorder,* underlying cause for status?
Seizure, fever, dysphasia	(Herpes simplex) encephalitis
Meningism +/− rash, fever	Bacterial meningitis
Saddle anaesthesia, sphincter disturbance, back pain	Cauda equina compression
Monocular visual loss	Giant cell arteritis, optic neuritis, 'ophthalmological causes'
Homonymous hemianopia	Stroke[†]
New onset Horner's	Carotid dissection, apical lung tumour
IIIrd nerve palsy	Uncal herniation, aneurysm (typically PCoM)
VIth nerve palsy	SOL/raised ICP
Postural/morning headache	SOL/raised ICP

* Functional presentations are included here not because they are intrinsically dangerous but because of the risk of iatrogenic harm from unnecessary drug treatment and/or intubation.
[†] If acute.
[‡] Brainstem and spinal cord stroke more frequently has a stuttering onset so must still be considered in sub-acute presentations.

For patients requiring admission, there should be a clear plan for monitoring:
- What is to be monitored?
- How often should observations be performed?
- What are the thresholds for action?
    These should be clearly documented and communicated to the relevant staff.
- The patients requiring closest monitoring are typically those in whom potentially life-threatening complications may occur, especially when these may be subtle and when interventions are available to modify the disease course, for example:
  - Neuromuscular respiratory failure. Symptoms can be minimal even with profound hypoventilation, emphasizing the need for regular vital capacity measurement.
  - Patients with or at risk of coma and rising ICP. This may range from regular assessment of conscious level and/or pupillary and other reflexes, to serial imaging studies and invasive ICP monitoring.

Table 14.2 Focused history-taking in acute neurological disease.

Weakness? Numbness? Pain/headache? Unsteadiness? Dizziness? Altered consciousness? Visual disturbance?
Cognitive/higher mental dysfunction? Speech and language disturbance?
Swallowing difficulty? Sphincter disturbance?
Chronology of different symptoms? Previous episodes? Distribution? Speed of onset? Aggravating/relieving factors?
Progression (in time and space)? Fluctuating?
Trigger/prodromal illness?
Functional consequences?
Systemic upset? Rash? Weight loss? Appetite? Diet?
Drugs and medications? Missed/extra doses? Newly prescribed/taken?
Past history? Family history? Smoking? Alcohol? Recreational drugs?
Occupation? Toxin exposure? Handedness?

Table 14.3 Anatomical localization in neurological diagnosis.

Anatomical structure	Associated clinical features
Meninges	Headache, neck stiffness, photophobia
Cerebrum	
• **Cortical**	Seizure, dysphasia, hemianopia, neglect, apraxia, dyscalculia, other disturbances of higher cortical function
• **Subcortical**	Bradyphrenia, executive dysfunction, personality change
• **Pyramidal**	Pyramidal distribution weakness, hyper-reflexia, spasticity, extensor plantar
• **Extrapyramidal**	Tremor, rigidity, bradykinesia, hemiballismus, chorea
• **Diffuse**	Reduced conscious level, impaired attention
Cerebellum	Nystagmus, dysarthria, dysmetria, ataxia, dysdiadokokinesis
Brainstem	'Crossed' (e.g. ipislateral facial and contralateral limb weakness with a pontine lesion), other cranial nerve deficits +/- long tract signs, 'locked-in', quadriparesis
Spinal cord	Paraparesis or quadriparesis, sensory level (may be suspended, crossed and/or dissociated), extensor plantars, sphincter and autonomic dysfunction
Motor neurons/anterior horn	Mixed upper and lower motor neuron signs, fasciculations
Nerve roots	Radicular pain (deep within limb or radiating 'electric shock'), weakness in a group of muscles, localized areflexia
Dorsal root ganglia	Ataxia, pseudoathetosis, areflexia
Plexus	Pain then weakness > sensory disturbance, involves multiple root and nerve territories
Peripheral nerve	
• **Mononeuropathy**	Characteristic pattern of selective muscle weakness and sensory loss in a single limb
• **Axonal**	Weakness proportional to wasting (distal > proximal), glove and stocking sensory loss
• **Demyelinating**	Proximal and distal weakness out of proportion to wasting, global areflexia
• **Small fibre**	Pain, selective loss of pin-prick and temperature sensation, autonomic dysfunction, preserved power and reflexes
Neuromuscular junction	Fatigable diplopia, ptosis, dysarthria, facial and proximal limb weakness, no sensory loss
Muscle	Characteristic distribution of weakness (often proximal), wasting, myalgia, no sensory loss

Table 14.4 Temporal evolution: what is the lesion?

Temporal evolution	Likely cause
Instantaneous maximum deficit	Vascular/stroke, acute compression/trauma
Over seconds	Seizure (especially if stereotyped and recurrent)
Over minutes	Migraine, 'amyloid spell'
Over hours to days	Inflammatory (MS, GBS), infective
Over weeks to months	Neoplastic, chronic compression
Over months to years	Degenerative

Table 14.5 Focused examination in acute neurological disease.

Domain	Tests
Conscious level	Glasgow Coma Scale score/AVPU scale
Higher mental function	Orientation? Registration? Attention/concentration? Recall/memory? Language? Object recognition (visual/tactile)? Verbal fluency? Executive function? Follows (increasingly complex) commands? Visuospatial function? Calculation?
Meninges	Neck stiffness? Kernig's? Photophobia? Rash? Temperature?
Extrapyramidal	Tremor? Rigidity? Bradykinesia? Gait? Postural instability? Chorea? Hemiballismus?
Cerebellum	Nystagmus? Dysarthria? Dysmetria? Intention tremor? Dysdiadokokinesis? Ataxia?
Cranial nerves	II – acuity, fields, fundi, pupils
	III/IV/VI – eye movements, ptosis, fatigability?
	V/VII – facial sensation and movements, including jaw
	VIII – hearing, vestibular function
	IX/X – palatal elevation/cough/speech/swallow
	XI – shoulder elevation/head turn
	XII – tongue inspection/protrusion/strength
Limbs	Inspection – wasting? Fasciculations? Dyskinesia? Drift? Rash?
	Tone – hypotonic/hypertonic? Spastic? Rigid?
	Power – proximal versus distal? Symmetric? MRC grade? Fatigable? Functional/collapsible weakness?
	Deep tendon reflexes – asymmetric? Absent? Present with reinforcement? Reduced? Normal? Brisk?
	Plantar response – flexor? Extensor? Mute?
	Gait – ataxic/wide based? Foot drop? Spastic? Parkinsonian?
	Coordination – finger nose, heel shin, dysdiadokokinesis?
	Sensation – distribution affected? Modality affected (pin-prick, temperature, vibration, light touch, proprioception)?

Table 14.6 Diagnostic testing in acute neurological disease.

Test	Comment
Lumbar puncture	Critical part of the investigation of CNS infection and subarachnoid haemorrhage. May provide supportive role in diagnosis of CNS and PNS inflammatory disorders. Contraindications, technique and interpretation are further discussed in Chapter 123.
CT brain	Invaluable in the workup of suspected haemorrhagic/vascular pathology (SAH, EDH/SDH, stroke, venous sinus thrombosis) and where raised ICP or a mass lesion are acute concerns. Benefits from availability, rapidity, and sensitivity in detecting acute haemorrhage. Spatial resolution of contrast CT-A exceeds that of MR-A. CT-V may also provide more diagnostic clarity than MR-V in suspected venous sinus thrombosis.

Table 14.6 (*Continued*)

Test	Comment
MRI brain	Provides improved visualization of posterior fossa/brainstem structures and spinal cord over CT. MR images may be virtually diagnostic of CNS demyelination and even HSV encephalitis. DWI/ADC sequences can be extremely useful for clarifying diagnostically difficult stroke/TIA presentations.
EEG	Most useful acutely in the evaluation of possible non-convulsive status or for differentiating (ongoing) epileptic from non-epileptic seizures. An inter-ictal EEG lacks the sensitivity or specificity to rule in or out epileptic seizures and it is prudent to carefully consider and/or discuss such requests in advance.
EMG/nerve conduction studies	EMG can help distinguish neurogenic from myogenic causes of weakness, but it is worth noting that spontaneous activity suggestive of denervation can take up to two weeks from the point of injury to develop. Likewise, nerve conduction studies can prove entirely normal, particularly in the early stages of an acute neuropathy such as GBS. Specialist protocols (repetitive stimulation and/or single fibre EMG) are required to evaluate the neuromuscular junction (e.g. in suspected myasthenia). Again, these tests do not make or break a diagnosis of in isolation, and will often require specialist input to interpret correctly.
Vital capacity	A spirometric assessment of vital capacity is an absolute requirement in the safe management of patients at risk of neuromuscular respiratory failure (typically GBS or myasthenia gravis in the acute setting). An adult vital capacity of <1.5 L/<20 mL/kg is of immediate concern and warrants discussion with ICU as a minimum. At <1 L/15 mL/kg, or with a fall of 50% from baseline on serial testing, prompt ICU involvement is required. Peak flow or arterial blood gas measurements are inadequate substitutes.

EEG, electroencephalography; EMG, electromyography; GBS, Guillain-Barré syndrome.

Box 14.2 Neurological diagnosis – alerts.

Uncertainty about the diagnosis can sometimes be reduced by retaking the history and again following the scheme set out in Figure 14.1. Sometimes a period of time is required – for other symptoms to manifest or for a critical test result to become available – before the diagnosis is apparent.

In difficult cases, it is worth considering:

- Whether longstanding pathology might be clouding or modifying the clinical presentation
- Whether there may be multiple active pathologies
- Whether the syndrome might be attributable to a multifocal disease process

Examples of the latter include multiple sclerosis, mitochondrial disease, vasculitis and paraneoplastic disorders.

Be wary of concluding that a presentation is functional simply because it appears bizarre or difficult to explain. It is also inadvisable to make a functional diagnosis by exclusion alone. Look for supportive positive (e.g. internal inconsistency, distractability) as well as negative (e.g. no hard neurological signs) features and weigh up the other possibilities; this will reduce the chance of making an incorrect diagnosis.

Further reading

O'Brien MD (2014) Use and abuse of physical signs in neurology. *Journal of the Royal Society of Medicine* 107, 416–421. DOI: 10.1177/0141076814538785

Shibasaki H, Hallett M. (2016) *The Neurologic Examination: Scientific Basis for Clinical Diagnosis*. Oxford University Press.

Stone J, Reuber M, Carson A. (2013) Functional symptoms in neurology: mimics and chameleons. *Pract Neurol* 13, 104–113.

CHAPTER 15

Acute headache

SIMON RINALDI

Most patients presenting to the emergency department with acute headache have migraine. A minority have life-threatening disorders such as subarachnoid haemorrhage or bacterial meningitis. The clinical assessment (Table 15.1) enables you to place the patient in one of three groups, guiding differential diagnosis, investigation (Table 15.2) and further management.

1 Acute headache with any 'red-flag' features: fever, reduced conscious level, papilloedema, neck stiffness or focal neurological signs

Causes are given in Table 15.3.

- If the patient is febrile, or the index of suspicion for CNS infection is high, take blood cultures and start antibiotic/antiviral therapy to cover bacterial meningitis (Chapter 68) and herpes simplex encephalitis (Chapter 69). Next, obtain CSF to confirm the diagnosis, identify the pathogen, and direct further therapy. CT should always be performed before lumbar puncture (Chapter 123) with:
  - Focal neurological signs
  - Altered consciousness
  - Papilloedema
  - Immunosuppression, or
  - Recent seizure (within two weeks)
- Tuberculous and cryptococcal meningitis should considered in at-risk groups (see Appendices 68.1 and 68.2). Meningism may be absent or mild in these diseases.
- Infectious diseases acquired abroad (e.g. malaria, typhoid) should be considered in patients with the relevant travel history (Chapter 33).
- When subarachnoid haemorrhage is suspected (see below and Chapter 67), CT is the initial investigation of choice and LP is likely to be more useful if delayed until 12 hours after the onset of headache.

2 Headache with local signs

Causes and management are summarized in Table 15.4.

3 Acute headache with no abnormal signs

Causes are given in Table 15.5.

- Always consider subarachnoid haemorrhage (Chapter 67) and giant-cell arteritis (see below and Chapter 99).
- Formal criteria state that a headache cannot be diagnosed as migraine or tension-type headache until multiple episodes have occurred. While such criteria highlight the increased difficulty in diagnosing a single episode, it may still be appropriate to treat migraine-like headache as such if other more serious causes have been satisfactorily excluded.

Acute Medicine: A Practical Guide to the Management of Medical Emergencies, Fifth Edition. Edited by David Sprigings and John B. Chambers.
© 2018 John Wiley & Sons Ltd. Published 2018 by John Wiley & Sons Ltd.

Table 15.1 Focused assessment of the patient with acute headache.

History

How did the headache start? Instantaneous onset? How long did it take to reach maximum intensity?

Context of onset? With exertion? Orgasmic? On postural change? On waking?

Still present? How long has it lasted?

Syncope at onset?

How severe? Worst headache ever?

Distribution (unilateral, diffuse, localized)

Nausea/vomiting? Photo/phonophobia? Pulsating quality? Inability to continue routine physical activities? (All associated with but not specific for migraine)

Associated systemic, neurological or visual symptoms (e.g. syncope/presyncope, limb weakness, speech disturbance, blurring of vision, transient blindness, diplopia, scalp tenderness, jaw claudication, malaise, myalgia/stiffness, scotomata, fortification spectra). Did these precede or follow the headache?

Background

Medication history and possible exposure to toxins

Recent travel abroad?

Immunosuppressed or known malignancy?

Disorders associated with increased risk of aneurysmal subarachnoid haemorrhage: polycystic kidney disease, Ehlers-Danlos syndrome type IV, pseudoxanthoma elasticum, fibromuscular dysplasia, sickle cell disease, alfa-1 antitrypsin deficiency

Family history of migraine or subarachnoid hemorrhage?

Examination

Key observations: airway, respiratory rate, arterial oxygen saturation, heart rate, blood pressure, perfusion, consciousness level, temperature, blood glucose

Neck stiffness (in both flexion and extension)?

Focal neurological signs?

Horner syndrome (partial ptosis and constricted pupil: if present, consider carotid artery dissection)?

Visual acuity and fields

Fundi (papilloedema or retinal haemorrhage?)

Signs of dental, ENT or ophthalmic disease?

Temporal artery tenderness or loss of pulsation?

Table 15.2 Urgent investigation in acute headache.

Full blood count

Coagulation screen if suspected intracranial haemorrhage

ESR and C-reactive protein

Blood glucose

Creatinine and electrolytes

Skull X-ray if suspected sinus infection

Blood culture if suspected bacterial meningitis

CT scan if suspected stroke or meningitis/encephalitis

LP if suspected subarachnoid haemorrhage or meningitis/encephalitis, provided there are no contraindications (Chapter 123)

ESR, erythrocyte sedimentation rate; LP, lumbar puncture.

Table 15.3 Causes of acute headache with 'red-flag' features: fever, reduced conscious level, papilloedema, neck stiffness or focal neurological signs.

Cause	Chapter or reference/comment
Vascular	
Stroke	Chapter 65
Subarachnoid haemorrhage	Chapter 67
Cerebral venous sinus thrombosis	Headache usually of gradual onset but may be 'thunderclap'
Subdural haematoma	Table 65.4
Hypertensive encephalopathy	Table 55.4
Pituitary apoplexy	Chapter 93
Cerebral vasculitis	Table 65.4, Chapter 99
Infective	
Bacterial meningitis	Chapter 68
Viral encephalitis	Chapter 69
Brain abscess	Headache usually localized to side of abscess; may be of gradual or sudden onset
Subdural empyema	Complication of paranasal sinusitis, otitis media, or mastoiditis
Tuberculous meningitis	Appendix 68.1
Cryptococcal meningitis	Appendix 68.2
Toxoplasma encephalitis	Chapter 34
Systemic infection with headache/ meningism	In returning travellers, include malaria and typhoid in the differential diagnosis (Chapter 33)
Others	
Poisoning with amphetamine/cocaine	Table 36.2
Other causes of raised intracranial pressure	Chapter 72
Hyperviscosity syndrome	Due to high levels of immunoglobulin (e.g. Waldenstrom macroglobulinaemia) or cells (e.g. polycythaemia, leukaemias)
Severe hyponatraemia	Chapter 85
Malignant meningitis (carcinoma, melanoma, lymphoma, leukaemia)	CSF typically shows raised protein concentration and high lymphocyte count; diagnosis confirmed by cytology

Table 15.4 Acute headache with local signs.

Cause	Comment/management
Acute sinusitis	Suspect from associated fever, facial pain especially on bending over, mucopurulent nasal discharge, and tenderness on pressure over the affected sinus. Obtain X-rays of the sinuses, looking for mucosal thickening, a fluid level or opacification. Treatment is with coamoxiclav (or erythromycin and metronidazole if allergic to penicillin) and steam inhalations. Discuss management with an ENT surgeon.
Acute angle-closure glaucoma	Usually unilateral; eye red and injected, visual acuity reduced due to corneal clouding, pupil fixed. Refer urgently to an ophthalmologist.
Giant-cell arteritis	See text, Appendix 19.1 and Chapter 99.
Temporomandibular joint disorder	A group of disorders affecting the temporomandibular joint (TMJ) and the muscles of mastication. Signs include limitation of jaw opening, tenderness to palpation of the TMJ and palpable spasm of masseter and internal pterygoid muscles. Seek advice from an oral surgeon.
Cervicogenic headache	Headache referred from disorder of the cervical spine.
Mucormycosis	Diabetes, orbital and facial pain, periorbital and orbital cellulitis, proptosis, purulent nasal discharge, mucosal necrosis.

Table 15.5 Acute headache with no abnormal signs.

Cause	Comment
Tension-type headache	Usually described as pressure or tightness around the head.
	Does not have the associated symptoms or aura of migraine (although some patients may have both types of headache).
Migraine	See Table 15.6 for diagnostic criteria.
Medication-overuse headache	Suspect in patients who have frequent or daily headaches despite (or because of) the regular use of medications for headache.
Drug-related	Seen with nitrates, nicorandil and dihydropyridine calcium antagonists and sildenafil.
Toxin exposure	Seen with carbon monoxide poisoning (Chapter 36).
Subarachnoid haemorrhage	Around 20% of patients with subarachnoid haemorrhage have acute headache with no other signs. See text and Chapter 67.
Giant cell arteritis	See text and Chapter 99.
Cerebral venous thrombosis	Headache frequently precedes other symptoms, and can be the only symptom. Onset may be 'thunderclap', acute or progressive
Pituitary apoplexy	Usually associated with ophthalmoplegia and reduced visual acuity. See Chapter 93.
Carotid or vertebral arterial dissection	Unilateral headache, which may be accompanied by neck pain. May follow neck manipulation or minor trauma.
	Usually accompanied by other signs (ischaemic stroke, Horner syndrome or pulsatile tinnitus).
Spontaneous intracranial hypotension	Due to leak of CSF from spinal meningeal defects or dural tears.
	Headache worse on standing and relieved by lying down (like post-LP headache). May be accompanied by nausea and vomiting, dizziness, auditory changes, diplopia, visual blurring, interscapular pain and/or radicular pain in the arms or legs.
Benign (idiopathic) 'thunderclap' headache	Assumes subarachnoid haemorrhage and cerebral venous thrombosis have been excluded.

Subarachnoid haemorrhage

- If the headache was abrupt in onset, reaching maximum intensity within minutes at most, subarachnoid haemorrhage must be excluded by CT, followed by examination of the CSF if the CT is normal or equivocal.
- CT is most sensitive for detection of subarachnoid haemorrhage if done within 12 h of onset of headache. Examination of the CSF by spectrophotometry to detect bilirubin (a breakdown product of haemoglobin) is the most reliable method of confirming or excluding subarachnoid haemorrhage. Bilirubin is reliably present in CSF from 12 h to 2 weeks after haemorrhage (occasionally longer). Lumbar puncture should therefore be delayed >12 h after the onset of headache unless meningitis is a possibility.
- Further management of subarachoid haemorrhage is detailed in Chapter 67.

Giant-cell arteritis

- Consider in any patient aged 50 or over with headache, which will usually be of days or a few weeks in duration.
- Associated symptoms include malaise, weight loss, jaw claudication, scalp tenderness and visual changes (amaurosis fugax, diplopia and partial or complete loss of vision).
- If the ESR is >50 mm/h and/or C-reactive protein raised, and/or the temporal artery is thickened or tender (feel 2 cm above and 2 cm forward from the external auditory meatus), start prednisolone. For patients with visual symptoms (who should be seen by an ophthalmologist the same day), give 60 mg as a one-off dose. For those

Table 15.6 Diagnostic criteria for migraine.

Migraine without aura
- Attacks lasting 4–72 h (but in some cases may be longer than this – 'status migrainosus')
- At least two of the following characteristics:
  - Unilateral
  - Pulsating
  - Moderate to severe
  - Aggravated by movement
    (NB: migraine headache may be bilateral or vary unilateral/bilateral during a single episode; may be continuous).
- At least one associated symptom:
  - Nausea or vomiting
  - Photophobia or phonophobia

Migraine with aura
- One or more transient focal neurological aura symptom
- Gradual development of aura symptom over >4 min, or several symptoms in succession
- Aura symptoms last 4–60 min
- Headache follows or accompanies aura within 60 min

without visual symptoms, give 40–60 mg daily (minimum 0.75 mg/kg). Also give aspirin 75 mg daily, if not contraindicated, and a proton pump inhibitor for gastroprotection.
- Arrange urgent review by a rheumatologist (and ophthalmologist if ophthalmic involvement is suspected).
- See Chapter 99.

Migraine
- Diagnostic criteria are given in Table 15.6. The first migraine headache usually occurs between the ages of 10 and 30.
- Treatment of an acute attack is with an NSAID, triptan, dispersible aspirin or paracetamol and an antiemetic, for example metoclopramide 10 mg IM or domperidone (available in suppository form). Combination therapy with a triptan and NSAID/paracetamol may be more effective.

Further reading

Angus-Leppan H. (2013) Migraine: mimics, borderlands and chameleons. *Pract Neurol* 13, 308–318.
Ducros A. (2012) Reversible cerebral vasoconstriction syndrome. *Lancet Neurol* 11, 906–917.
Headache Classification Committee of the International Headache Society (IHS) (2013) The International Classification of Headache Disorders, 3rd edition (beta version). *Cephalalgia* 33, 629–808. https://www.ichd-3.org/.

CHAPTER 16

Seizures and epilepsy

BRIDGET MACDONALD

Box 16.1 Generalized tonic-clonic status epilepticus

Defined as a generalized tonic-clonic seizure (GTCS) lasting more than 30 min or repeated seizures without recovery of normal alertness in between. As 98% of GTCS self-terminate in two minutes, any seizure lasting >5 minutes should be treated as status unless that patient is known habitually to have longer seizures.

Prompt treatment is needed to reduce cerebral damage and metabolic complications (hypoglycaemia, lactic acidosis and hyperpyrexia) and prevent mortality.

Mortality in status epilepticus occurs with both under and over-treatment

Generalised tonic-clonic seizure

Priorities

Airway, breathing and circulation

- Clear the airway. Place a nasopharyngeal airway if needed to maintain a clear airway (Chapter 112).
- Put the patient in the lateral semiprone position. Attach an ECG monitor and oxygen saturation monitor.
- Give high-flow oxygen and obtain IV access.
- Take blood for urgent investigation (Table 16.1).

Exclude hypoglycaemia

Check blood glucose immediately by stick test. If blood glucose is <4.0 mmol/L:

- Give 100 mL of 20% glucose (or 200 mL of 10% glucose) over 15–30 min IV, or glucagon 1 mg IV/IM/SC.
- Recheck blood glucose after 10 min; if still <4.0 mmol/L, repeat the above IV glucose treatment.
- In patients with malnourishment or alcohol use disorder, there is a remote risk of precipitating Wernicke's encephalopathy by a glucose load; prevent this by giving thiamine 100 mg IV before or shortly after glucose administration.

See Chapter 81 for further management of hypoglycaemia.

Acute Medicine: A Practical Guide to the Management of Medical Emergencies, Fifth Edition. Edited by David Sprigings and John B. Chambers.
© 2018 John Wiley & Sons Ltd. Published 2018 by John Wiley & Sons Ltd.

Table 16.1 Investigation in status epilepticus or after a first seizure.

Immediate
Blood glucose
Sodium, potassium, calcium, magnesium and creatinine
Arterial blood gases and pH (not required after first seizure)

Later
Full blood count
Blood culture (x2) if febrile
Liver function tests
Anticonvulsant levels (if on therapy), consider toxic screen
Serum (10 mL) and urine sample (50 mL) at 4 °C for toxicology screen if poisoning suspected or cause of seizure unclear
ECG (NB A missed diagnosis of cardiac arrhythmia is more likely to lead to sudden death than a missed diagnosis of epilepsy. Look for long QT interval, conduction abnormality (e.g. left bundle branch block), Q waves indicative of previous myocardial infarction, evidence of left ventricular hypertrophy. If present, consider arrhythmia rather than seizure, arrange echocardiography and cardiology follow-up.)
Chest X-ray
Cranial CT scan*
Lumbar puncture (after CT) if suspected subarachnoid haemorrhage, meningitis or encephalitis
EEG (this test requires judgement as to when necessary: discuss with a neurologist)

---

* CT scan should be performed immediately after control of status epilepticus or after a first seizure if any of the following features is present:
- Focal neurological deficit
- Reduced conscious level
- Fever
- Recent head injury
- Persistent headache
- Known malignancy
- Warfarin or other anticoagulation
- HIV-AIDS

For patients after a first seizure who are fully recovered and have no abnormal signs, CT can be done at a later date.

Give a benzodiazepine

- Take into account pre-hospital treatment. Give **lorazepam** (which is less likely to cause respiratory suppression) 0.1 mg/kg (typically 4–8 mg) IV over 5–10 min (Table 16.2), **midazolam** 10 mg buccally (NICE-recommended, but only licensed in patients <18 years), or **diazepam** 10–20 mg IV at a rate of <2.5 mg/min (faster injection rates carry the risk of sudden apnoea).

What is the likely cause of the seizure? (Table 16.3)

Obtain the history from all available sources including emergency information or health app on mobile telephone, and make a systematic examination of the patient. Check the blood results.

- Correct severe hyponatraemia (plasma sodium <120 mmol/L) with hypertonic saline (Chapter 85).
- Correct severe hypocalcaemia (plasma total calcium <1.5 mmol/L) with calcium gluconate 1 g IV (10 mL of 10% solution) (Chapter 87).
- Correct hypomagnesaemia (Chapter 88)
- Give dexamethasone 10 mg IV if the patient is known to have a brain tumour or active vasculitis.
- If patient is known to have epilepsy, restart any antiepileptic medication stopped within the last three weeks (via a nasogastric tube if IV or rectal preparations are not available).

Table 16.2 Drug therapy for generalized convulsive status epilepticus.

Drug	Dose	Comments
First line		
Lorazepam	0.1 mg/kg, give 4–8 mg IV	Dose can be repeated once after 20 min. Ampoules contain lorazepam 4 mg in 1 mL. Dilute 1 : 1 with water for injection. Longer duration of action and less likely to cause sudden hypotension or respiratory arrest than diazepam.
or		
Midazolam	10 mg in 1 or 2 mL (depends on manufacturer) bucally	In accord with NICE adult status guidelines but only licensed for those aged <18 years).
or		
Diazepam	10–20 mg IV at a rate of <2.5/min.	Risk of sudden apnoea with faster injection. Dose should not be repeated more than twice, or to a total dose >40 mg because of the risk of respiratory depression and hypotension.
Second line		
Phenobarbital	Loading dose: 10 mg/kg to a maximum of 1000 mg, given at 100 mg/min. Maintenance dose 1–4 mg/kg/day given IV, IM or PO	Contraindicated in acute intermittent porphyria. Hypotension. Respiratory impairment due to sedation.
or		
Phenytoin	Loading dose: 20 mg/kg IV (max dose 2 g). Infusion rate should not exceed 50 mg/min. Maintenance dose of 100 mg 6–8-hourly IV, adjusted according to plasma level. Do not give more than one loading dose and do not load a patient who is taking oral phenytoin.	Monitor blood pressure and ECG (as risk of arrhythmia). Give through separate large-bore IV cannula, as alkaline and will precipitate other drugs. Valproate and levetiracetam are alternative second-line drugs
Third line		
Midazolam	0.1–0.2 mg/kg/h by IV infusion	
or		
Propofol	2 mg/kg IV bolus, then repeat bolus if necessary. Maintenance dose 5–10 mg/kg/h by IV infusion	
or		
Thiopentone	100–250 mg IV bolus, then 50 mg bolus every 3 min until burst suppression on EEG Maintenance dose 2–5 mg/kg/h by IV infusion	

Further management

If fitting continues:

- Transfer the patient to the ICU and discuss management with an anaesthetist and neurologist.
- Consider the possibility of psychogenic status epilepticus (Table 16.4), which is not uncommon. Definitive diagnosis may require EEG.
- Give either phenobarbital or phenytoin (Table 16.2) (please note the difference in time to treatment dose being given – many experts prefer phenobarbital for this reason).

If there is refractory status epilepticus

If fitting continues despite phenytoin or phenobarbital IV:

- The patient should be intubated and ventilated.
- Midazolam, propofol or thiopentone should be given (Table 16.2), preferably with EEG monitoring.

Table 16.3 Causes of tonic-clonic status epilepticus.

In a patient known to have epilepsy

Poor compliance with therapy, therapy recently reduced or stopped, or altered drug pharmacokinetics

Drug interaction causing alteration of their normal maintenance level

Intercurrent infection

Alcohol withdrawal

Alcohol or substance use

In a patient not known to have epilepsy

Stroke, especially haemorrhagic stroke

Encephalitis

Brain tumour

Brain abscess (including toxoplasmosis)

Arteriovenous malformation

Meningitis

Acute head injury

Cerebral malaria

Metabolic disorder: cerebral anoxia from cardiac arrest, acute kidney injury, hyponatraemia, hypocalcaemia, hypomagnesaemia, hepatic encephalopathy

Poisoning: alcohol, tricyclics, phenothiazines, theophylline, cocaine, amphetamines, MDMA ('ecstasy'), heroin

Cerebral vasculitis

Hypertensive encephalopathy

Pre-eclampsia/eclampsia

Once fitting has stopped

- Determine the cause (Table 16.3).
- Ask advice from a neurologist on further management; in complex patients with a past history of epilepsy, speak to their usual consultant where possible.

After a first generalized tonic–clonic seizure

Was it a seizure? (Table 9.2)

Distinguishing between a seizure and syncope requires a detailed history, taken from the patient and any eyewitnesses. Points to cover include the following:

Background

- Any previous similar attacks (including partial seizures such as déjà vu or myoclonic jerks in morning)
- Previous significant acquired brain injury (i.e. complicated or premature birth, trauma with skull fracture or loss of consciousness >1 h, meningitis or encephalitis, stroke)

Table 16.4 Characteristics of dissociative seizures (non-epileptic attack disorder).

Asynchronous bilateral movements of the limbs, asymmetrical clonic contractions, pelvic thrusting and side-to-side movements of the head, often intensified by restraint

Gaze aversion, resistance to passive limb movement or eye-opening, focus on face if mirror used and eyes held open

Avoidance of the hand falling on to the face

Incontinence, tongue biting and injury rare (but can occur)

Normal or volitional pattern chest wall movements

Normal tendon reflexes, plantar responses, blink, corneal and eyelash reflexes

Absence of metabolic complications

No post-ictal confusion (drowsiness and dysarthria may be due to benzodiazepine given to treat suspected seizure)

Features differentiating a generalized seizure from vasovagal and cardiac syncope (Stokes-Adams attack).

	Generalized seizure	Vasovagal syncope	Cardiac syncope (Stokes-Adams attack)
Occurrence when sitting or lying	Common	Rare	Common
Occurrence during sleep	Common	Does not occur	May occur
Prodromal symptoms	May occur with focal neurological symptom, automatisms or hallucinations	Typical with sweating, dizziness, nausea, blurring of vision, yawning	Often none; palpitation may occur
Focal neurological features at onset	May occur (signifies focal cerebral lesion)	Never occurs	Never occurs
Tonic-clonic movements	Characteristic; occurs within 30 s of onset	May occur after 30 s of syncope (secondary anoxic seizure)	May occur after 30 s of syncope (secondary anoxic seizure)
Facial colour	Flushing or cyanosis at onset	Pallor at onset	Pallor at onset; flushing afterwards
Tongue biting	Common	Rare	Rare
Urinary incontinence	Common	Uncommon	May occur
Injury	May occur	Uncommon	May occur
After the attack	Confusion common	Nauseated and 'groggy'	Usually well

- Febrile seizures in childhood (age six months to six years)
- Family history of epilepsy
- Cardiac disease (previous myocardial infarction, hypertrophic or dilated cardiomyopathy, long QT interval (at risk of ventricular tachycardia))
- Drug therapy
- Alcohol or substance use
- Sleep deprivation

Before the attack

- Prodromal symptoms: were these cardiovascular (e.g. dizziness, palpitation, chest pain) or focal neurological (aura)?
- Circumstances, for example exercising, standing, sitting or lying, asleep
- Precipitants, for example coughing, micturition, head-turning

The attack

- Were there any focal neurological features at the onset: sustained deviation of the head or eyes or unilateral jerking of the limbs (bilateral 'twitching' is common in syncope)?
- Was there a cry (may occur in tonic phase of seizure)?
- Duration of seizure (must be assessed in relation to the reliability of the witness).
- Associated tongue biting, urinary or faecal incontinence or injury.
- Facial colour changes (pallor common in syncope, uncommon with a seizure).
- Abnormal pulse (must be assessed in relation to the reliability of the witness).
- Eyes rolled up consistent with syncope, eyes open and staring in any direction consistent with seizure.
- Waxing and waning of long duration consistent with non-epileptic attack (dissociative seizure).

After the attack

- Immediately well or delayed recovery with confusion or headache? (fatigue common after syncope, somnolence more common after seizure).
- Was speech normal?

Is there evidence of an underlying cause of seizure?

- Are there any focal neurological signs? Like an aura preceding the seizure, these indicate a structural cause.
- Are there features of meningitis (Chapter 68), encephalitis (Chapter 69) or subarachnoid haemorrhage (Chapter 67)?
- Does the patient have a systemic disease requiring urgent treatment, for example acute liver failure, hyperosmolar hyperglycaemic state?

If the patient is well

- Discharge if fully recovered and supervision by an adult for the next 24 h can be arranged.
- Advise the patient not to drive (in writing, as memory may be impaired after a seizure).
- Give first aid advice for seizure recurrence, also bathing and kitchen safety advice (see 'epilepsy app' from Epilepsy Action or National Society for Epilepsy).
- Outpatient investigation (CT if indicated) and follow-up by a neurologist should be arranged. EEG is not routine but is likely to be needed if seizure, not syncope, suspected in a person <23 years.
- In general, anticonvulsant therapy should be started after a second seizure (not a first one) – local advice should be sought for choice of starting medication (which will be carbamazepine, lamotrigine or valproate).

After a generalized seizure in a patient with known epilepsy

- Take blood for anticonvulsant levels.
- If the current history deviates from the usual pattern of seizures, consider intercurrent infection, alcohol use or poor compliance with therapy (an 'epilepsy app' can help with compliance).
- If the patient has had a typical seizure and is fully recovered, CT is not necessary.
- Discharge (with outpatient follow-up arranged) if the patient is fully recovered and has no evidence of acute illness. Advise the patient not to drive.

Alcohol withdrawal seizures

- Alcohol withdrawal seizures consist of 1–6 tonic-clonic seizures without focal features, which begin within 48 h of stopping drinking (although may occur up to seven days after stopping drinking if the patient has been taking a benzodiazepine). They are usually brief and self-limiting.
- Patients who have had withdrawal seizures once are highly likely to have a recurrence if they withdraw again.
- Patients with alcoholic hepatitis or chronic liver disease may have coagulation abnormalities, and if so, subdural haematoma should be excluded by CT.
- Cranial CT scan is not needed after suspected withdrawal seizures if:
  - A clear history of alcohol withdrawal is obtained
  - The seizures have no focal features
  - There is no evidence of head injury
  - There are no more than six seizures
  - The seizures do not occur over a period >6 h
  - Post-ictal confusion is brief
- Management of alcohol withdrawal is described in Chapter 106.

Further reading

Betjemann JP, Lowenstein DH (2015) Status epilepticus in adults. *Lancet Neurol* 14, 615–624.

Glauser T, Shinnar S, Gloss D, *et al.* (2016) Evidence-Based Guideline: Treatment of convulsive status epilepticus in children and adults: Report of the Guideline Committee of the American Epilepsy Society. *Epilepsy Currents* 16, 48–61. http://dx.doi.org/10.5698/1535-7597-16.1.48.

CHAPTER 17

Weakness and paralysis

SIMON RINALDI

Paralysis is a complete loss of voluntary movement. Weakness is a reduction in the force of voluntary movement, and is a result of pathology affecting the motor pathway at any point from the cerebral hemisphere to the muscle fibre (Box 17.1). Weakness can be life-threatening if respiratory muscles are involved.

- Stroke (Chapter 65), multiple sclerosis and spinal cord injury (Chapter 70) are the major central nervous system pathologies causing weakness.
- Guillain-Barré syndrome (GBS) (Chapter 71) is the commonest cause of acute neuromuscular paralysis.

Pathologies at different localizations produce distinctive syndromes (Table 17.1). They are broadly divided into upper motor neuron (UMN) or lower motor neuron (LMN) syndromes with specific features (Table 17.2). Combined UMN and LMN signs raise the possibility of motor neuron disease, but can also indicate dual pathology.

Priorities

You need rapidly to identify those patients:
- With acute stroke, who may be candidates for thrombolysis (Chapter 65)
- At risk of neuromuscular respiratory failure
- Who require urgent imaging and/or neurosurgical opinion (Figure 17.1)

Box 17.1 Medical Research Council (MRC) scale for assessment of muscle power.

Grade	Description
0	No contraction
1	Flicker or trace of contraction
2	Active movement with gravity eliminated
3	Active movement against gravity
4	Active movement against gravity and resistance
	Grades 4-, 4 and 4+ may be used to indicate movement against slight, moderate and strong resistance respectively
5	Normal power

Acute Medicine: A Practical Guide to the Management of Medical Emergencies, Fifth Edition. Edited by David Sprigings and John B. Chambers.
© 2018 John Wiley & Sons Ltd. Published 2018 by John Wiley & Sons Ltd.

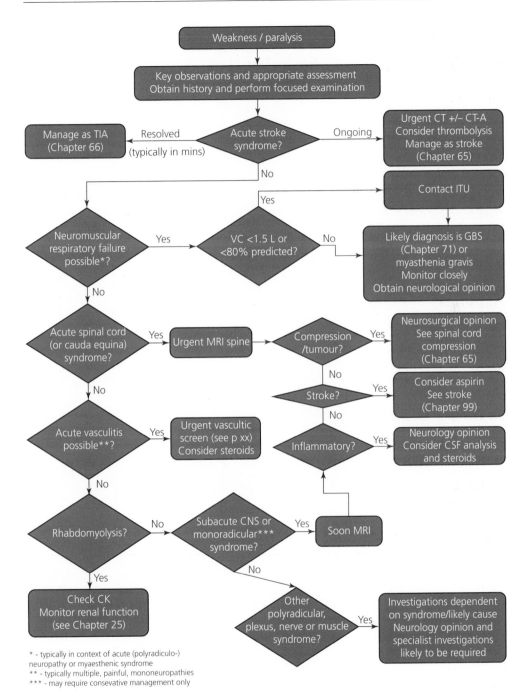

Figure 17.1 Assessment of the patient with weakness or paralysis.

Table 17.1 Localization of the cause of weakness by clinical syndrome.

Localization	Syndrome(s)	Additional features	Possible pathology
Brain	Hemiplegia	Homonymous hemianopia, ipsilateral sensory loss, dysphasia, dysphagia	Stroke, MS, tumour, migraine, post-ictal, hypoglycaemia
• **MCA territory**	• Face/arm > leg		
• **ACA territory**	• Leg > face/arm		
• **Lacunar**	• Face = arm = leg, no cortical signs		
	Isolated monoplegia	Typically part of limb only ('cortical hand'), no sensory loss	Stroke, MS, tumour, post-ictal
Brainstem			
• **Midbrain**	Weber	Ipsilateral IIIrd and contralateral hemiplegia	Stroke
• **Pons**	Quadriplegia	Bulbar palsy, horizontal gaze paralysis, delirium	Stroke, central pontine myelinolysis
	Millard-Gubler	Ipsilateral VIth/VIIth, contralateral arm and leg weakness	Stroke, MS
• **Medial medulla**	Djerine	Ipsilateral XIIth, contralateral hemiplegia and loss of proprioception/ vibration	Stroke, MS
Spinal cord	Anterior cord	Para/quadriplegia, sensory level, sphincter disturbance, proprioception/ vibration (relatively) spared	Anterior spinal artery thrombosis, cord compression, tumour, radiation
	Transverse myelitis	Para/quadriplegia, sensory level, constricting/band-like pain	MS, inflammatory, tumour, post-infectious, viral, dural AVM
	Posterior cord	Sensory ataxia, vibration sensation loss	B12/copper deficiency, HIV, syphilis, tumour, dural metastasis, MS
	Brown Séquard (hemi-cord)	Ipsilateral weakness and loss of proprioception/vibration, contralateral loss of pain and temperature	MS, penetrating injury, tumour
	Conus medullaris	Prominent sphincter involvement, saddle anaesthesia, mixed UMN/LMN signs	Disc prolapse, tumour
	Central cord	Suspended, dissociated sensory level	Syrinx, MS, acute compression, intramedullary tumour
Spinal roots	Cauda equina	Back/radicular pain, sphincter disturbance, dermatomal sensory loss	Disc prolapse, tumour, arachnoiditis, lumbar canal stenosis
	Polyradiculopathy	Proximal and distal weakness, areflexia in affected limbs, back/radicular pain, sensory symptoms > sensory signs	GBS/CIDP, leptomeningeal infiltration (e.g. lymphoma), Lyme, VZV/viral
	Monoradiculopathy	Weakness in a group of muscles in one limb, pain radiating down limb +/− sensory loss in corresponding dermatome	Degenerative, disc prolapse, tumour, VZV/viral

Plexus	Brachial or lumbar-sacral plexopathy	Pain (often in groin or shoulder) before weakness, patchy/minimal sensory loss	Diabetes, idiopathic, infiltrative (cancer/lymphoma), radiation, infective
Peripheral nerve	Demyelinating	Proximal and distal weakness without wasting, global areflexia, early vibration loss	GBS/CIDP, paraproteinaemic
	Axonal	Distal weakness and sensory loss, wasting, reflex loss in weak limbs/at ankles only	Alcohol, nutritional, diabetes, critical illness, paraneoplastic
	Mononeuropathy	Weakness in one area of one limb +/− sensory loss and wasting	Compression, trauma
	Multiple mononeuropathies (mononeuritis multiplex)	Pain, systemic features of vasculitis	Vasculitis, cancer, sarcoid, lymphoma, amyloid, HIV, multiple pressure palsies
Neuromuscular junction (myasthenic)	Generalized	Fatigable proximal weakness, dysphagia, dysarthria, neuromuscular respiratory failure, no sensory loss	Autoimmune (myasthenia gravis)
	Ocular	Fatigable diplopia/ptosis	Autoimmune, Botulism (if 'descending' weakness)
	Lambert-Eaton	Dry mouth/autonomic dysfunction, supressed reflexes which return post exercise	Paraneoplastic, non-paraneoplastic
Muscle	Proximal myopathy	Myalgia, rash	Inflammatory (dermatomyositis), steroids, statins
	Rhabdomyolysis	Myalgia, dark urine/myoglobinuria	Crush injury, malignant hyperthermia, neuroleptics
	Other	Inclusion body, limb-girdle, fascio-scapulo-humeral, distal patterns	Genetic/degenerative (rarely present acutely)

Table 17.2 Features of lower motor neuron (LMN) and upper motor neuron (UMN) weakness.

	LMN	UMN
Tone	Normal/decreased	Spastic
Deep tendon reflexes	Supressed/lost	Exaggerated
Plantar response	Flexor/mute	Extensor
Fasciculations	May be present	Absent
Atrophy	Pronounced (if axonal process)	Slight (reflecting disuse)
Distribution of weakness	Individual muscles may be affected, bilaterally innervated muscles can be involved	Groups of muscles affected, 'pyramidal' pattern;* bilaterally innervated muscles spared

* Extensors weaker than flexors in arms, flexors weaker than extensors in legs.

The clinical assessment is summarized in Table 17.3.

Diagnostic tests are directed by the clinical picture, although some tests should be considered for all patients (Table 17.4). Acute stroke and spinal cord/cauda equina syndromes require urgent neuroimaging.

Table 17.3 Focused assessment of the patient with weakness.

History

Time and speed of onset and progression (instant, seconds, hours, days, weeks; resolving, stable, fluctuating/fatigable, worsening)?

Distribution? (hemi-, quadri-, para-, monoplegia, localized, proximal, distal, axial)

Cranial nerve distribution involvement? (facial, bulbar, ocular/diplopia)

Headache?

Other associated pain? Character? Myelopathic (constricting)? Radicular (shooting/deep ache)? Localized to entrapment sites or plexus? Neuropathic (paraesthesia)? Myalgic?

Sensory loss (chapter 18)? Distribution? Saddle?

Sphincter disturbance? Dysphasia/hemianopia/other cortical symptoms?

Functional impairment? Walking? Stairs/chairs? Fine motor tasks? Breathing?

Prodromal illness/infection? Trauma? Compression? Arising from sleep?

Systemic upset? Weight loss? Diet/malnutrition? Alcohol/drug/toxin exposure?

Vascular risk factors?

Past neurological or systemic disease?

Examination

Rapid assessment of ABC/vital signs/glucose

If acute stroke, possible CT scanning +/− thrombolysis now takes priority

Assess distribution of weakness, tone and reflex pattern as per Table 3.1

Check for cranial nerve and higher mental dysfunction. Is there dysphasia?

Perform sensory testing with a hypothesis in mind:

Hemisensory loss? Sensory level? Suspended? Dissociated/crossed? (Check both spinothalamic and dorsal column modalities) Saddle? Dermatomal? Glove and stocking? In territory of single peripheral nerve? Normal? (See Chapter 18)

Test for fatigability if appropriate

Ptosis +/− diplopia developing or worsening with prolonged upgaze? Reduction in power after repetitive muscle contraction?

Check vital capacity if neuromuscular respiratory failure possible

General examination to look for cause

Bruit? AF? Rash? Cachexia? Lymphadenopathy? Organomegaly?

Table 17.4 Urgent investigation of the patient with weakness.

To consider in all patients
Glucose, FBC, U+Es, LFTs, calcium, magnesium, ESR/CRP, clotting, TFTs, ABGs, cultures, ECG, CXR
If acute stroke possible
Urgent CT head +/− CT-A, lipids, carotid Dopplers (if anterior circulation)
Spinal cord/cauda equina syndromes
MRI spine +/− LP, B_{12}/folate, copper, syphilis, HIV, CMV and VZV serology
Polyradiculopathy/acute neuropathy
NCS, LP, blood film, B_{12}/folate/thiamine, Borrelia/*C;jejuni*/CMV/EBV/HIV/*Mycoplasma* serology, anti-ganglioside and anti-paraneoplastic antibodies, serum and urine protein electrophoresis with immunofixation, urinary porphyrins
Multiple mononeuropathies/mononeuritis multiplex
ANA/ENA, ANCA, Cryoglobulins, ACE, HIV serology, paraneoplastic antibodies, blood film, NCS/EMG, Schirmer's test, LP, nerve biopsy, PMP22 genetics (of multiple pressure palsies), anti-GM1 antibodies (if pure motor)
Mononeuropathy
No tests may be required, NCS (rarely helpful acutely)
Myasthenic syndromes
NCS/EMG (with repetitive stimulation/single fibre EMG), anti-acetylcholine receptor and anti-MUSK antibodies (myasthenia gravis), anti-voltage gated calcium channel antibodies (LEMS), CT thorax (both)

Further management

Further management is directed by the working diagnosis.

- Patients with acute stroke should be admitted to a specialist stroke unit, have an assessment of their swallow performed, and be regularly monitored for deterioration and the development of complications (Chapter 65).
- Patients with GBS (Chapter 71) and myasthenia need regular vital capacity checks and involvement of ICU in the event of deterioration, but may be suitable for the general ward in the absence of respiratory compromise. The former group also requires monitoring for arrhythmia and other forms of autonomic disturbance, which are also seen with spinal cord infarction.
- In other spinal cord syndromes, admission and repeat neurological assessment is likely to be required to inform the need for and timing of surgical intervention.
- Patients with multiple mononeuropathies and rhabdomyolysis need admission for monitoring and treatment.

Box 17.2 Weakness and paralysis – alerts.

A common pitfall is to fail to distinguish true neurological weakness from its mimics. Patients with systemic illness, infections, cachexia and depression may report weakness when objective tests of strength are normal. Conversely, patients with systemic illness, pain, or functional disorders may have apparent weakness on examination without there being any neurological dysfunction. In the latter group the observation of give-way weakness, a positive Hoover sign, or inconsistency between the examination findings and functional performance may provide the diagnosis.

In acute stroke and (especially) acute spinal cord syndromes, UMN signs may be initially absent. Likewise, areflexia in GBS may not be seen in the early stages of the disease process. You should not place undue weight on one aspect of the clinical assessment, but rather consider all aspects of the history and examination together.

In difficult cases, reassessment after stabilization, following analgesia and initial investigations, and at intervals thereafter, may be required to reach the correct diagnosis.

- Those with subacute CNS syndromes may be suitable for outpatient investigation, dependent on the presence of ongoing deterioration and the severity of the deficit.
- Patients with monoradiculopathy or mononeuropathy can usually be discharged if systemically well, not progressing and if a benign cause is likely.
- In all immobile patients, pressure sores, deep vein thrombosis, respiratory infection/aspiration and contractures need to be prevented and addressed.

Further reading

Asimos AW (2015) Evaluation of the adult with acute weakness in the emergency department. UpToDate, last updated May 2015. http://www.uptodate.com/contents/evaluation-of-the-adult-with-acute-weakness-in-the-emergency-department?source=search_result&search=weakness+and+paralysis&selectedTitle=1%7E150.

Martin RA, Rosenfeld J, Bauer DW Weakness: Practical guide for family physicians. American Academy of Neurology. https://www.aan.com/uploadedfiles/website_library_assets/documents/4.cme_and_training/2.training/4.clerkship_and_course_director_resources/fm_chp4.pdf

CHAPTER 18

Acute sensory symptoms

SIMON RINALDI

- Sensory symptoms are a result of altered perception of pain, temperature, touch or proprioception. They may be positive (dysaesthesia) or negative (hypoaesthesia). They are commonly, but not invariably, associated with weakness (Chapter 17).
- Sensory symptoms can result from pathology anywhere in the nervous system, although disease processes restricted to the muscle, neuromuscular junction, or motor neuron should not produce sensory signs.
- Points to bear in mind in the interpretation of the sensory examination are summarized in Box 18.1.

Priorities

You need to rapidly identify those patients:
- With acute stroke, who may be candidates for thrombolysis (Chapter 65)
- At risk of neuromuscular respiratory failure
- Who require urgent imaging and/or neurosurgical opinion (Figure 18.1)

The clinical assessment is summarized in Table 18.1. The diagnosis is suggested by characteristics of the symptoms:

Box 18.1 Acute sensory symptoms – alerts.

The sensory examination can be difficult to perform and interpret.

Patients may over report minor qualitative differences in an attempt to 'help' the examiner, provide inconsistent responses, or fail to appreciate what is being asked of them.

Some deficits may only be apparent when specifically tested for (e.g. parietal signs or positive Romberg test).

Directed testing to confirm or refute a predefined hypothesis can help avoid these pitfalls, for example, by specifically testing for a sensory level or 'glove and stocking' loss. Even so, the distribution of sensory loss can sometimes seem baffling and inconsistent with the rest of the diagnostic formulation. Reference to dermatome and peripheral nerve field charts, or the appreciation that the sensory signs and symptoms may be due to some other coexistent pathology (e.g. chronic diabetic neuropathy), will sometimes clarify matters.

It is sometimes worth considering whether the diagnosis is made clearer when the sensory signs are disregarded. Functional sensory symptoms can also cause confusion. Typical patterns of functional loss are a complete hemisensory disturbance, which returns abruptly to normal in the midline (although this can be seen with thalamic pathology) and widespread spinothalamic and dorsal column modality loss confined to a single limb (typically abruptly 'cut off' at the groin or shoulder). In many cases, the sensory examination mantra 'do it last, trust it least' proves sage advice.

Acute Medicine: A Practical Guide to the Management of Medical Emergencies, Fifth Edition. Edited by David Sprigings and John B. Chambers.
© 2018 John Wiley & Sons Ltd. Published 2018 by John Wiley & Sons Ltd.

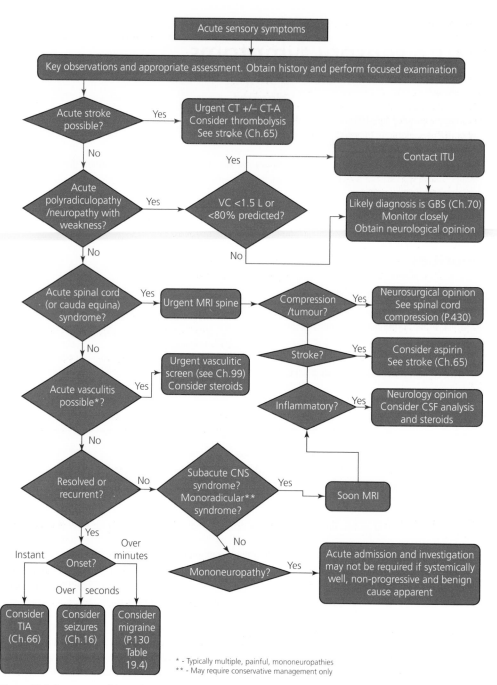

Figure 18.1 Assessment of the patient with acute sensory symptoms.

Table 18.1 Focused assessment of the patient with acute sensory symptoms.

History

Onset? Progression (Table 18.2)? Fluctuating? Intermittent? Recurrent? Aggravating/relieving factors? Triggers?
Character (Table 18.3) and distribution (Table 18.4, Figure 18.2)?
Associated weakness (Chapter 17)? Headache (Chapter 15)?
Sphincter disturbance? Dysphasia/cortical symptoms/hemianopia?
Functional impairment? Sensory ataxia (worse in dark/eyes closed)?
Prodromal illness infection? Trauma? Compression? Arising from sleep?

Background

Systemic upset? Weight loss? Diet/malnutrition? Alcohol/drug/toxin exposure?
Past neurological or systemic disease?
Diabetes? Vascular risk factors?

Examination

Even with a predominantly (or purely) sensory presentation, it is almost always advisable to leave the sensory examination until last, having already developed a clear hypothesis regarding the expected abnormality.
Rapid assessment of ABC/vital signs/glucose
If acute stroke possible CT scanning +/− thrombolysis now takes priority
Assess for any weakness, and alteration of tone, and reflexes (Chapter 17)
Assess visual function and cranial nerves
Check vital capacity if GBS possible
Perform sensory testing with a prior hypothesis/expected distribution (Table 18.4; Figure 18.2). Use unaffected region to check patient appreciates what normal sensation is and understands the response expected. Proceed from abnormal to normal areas, mapping out the borders between areas of abnormal and normal sensation.
Check spinothalamic (pain/temperature) and dorsal column (vibration/proprioception/light touch) modalities
Look for other signs if proprioceptive loss. Rombergism? Pseudoathetosis?
Look for parietal signs if appropriate. Two-point discrimination? Astereognosis? Agraphesthesia? Extinction?
Provocation tests if appropriate (Phalen's/Tinnel's/Spurling's)
General examination to look for cause: Bruit? AF? Rash? Cachexia? Lymphadenopathy? Organomegaly?

- Speed of progression (Table 18.2)
- Character (Table 18.3)
- Distribution (Table 18.3; Figure 18.2)

Diagnostic tests are directed by the clinical picture, although some tests should be considered for all patients Table 18.4).

- Acute stroke and spinal cord/cauda equina syndromes require urgent neuroimaging.
- Investigation for syndromes with the potential for both motor and sensory involvement are given in Table 17.4.
- With a single focal-onset sensory seizure, MRI is the imaging modality of choice (and can usually be performed as an outpatient) although there may be situations when immediate CT is the more pragmatic choice.

Table 18.2 Clues to the pathology from the tempo of sensory symptoms.

Speed of progression	Likely cause
Instantaneous maximum deficit	Vascular/stroke, acute compression/trauma
Seconds	Seizure (especially if stereotyped and recurrent)
Minutes	Migraine, amyloid spell/attack
Hours to days	Inflammatory (MS, GBS), infective
Weeks to months	Tumour, chronic compression
Months to years	Inherited/genetic, degenerative

Table 18.3 Localization: clues from the history.

Character	Likely localization
Complete loss (anaesthesia)	Central
'Complex' symptoms (formication, 'running water')	Central
Tight band	Myelopathy
Electric shock, shooting, ache deep within limb	Radiculopathy
Tingling/paraesthesia	Large fibre neuropathy
Burning/hot/cold	Small fibre neuropathy
Hyperaesthesia	Partial peripheral nerve damage
Asymptomatic (signs without symptoms)	Inherited/genetic, functional

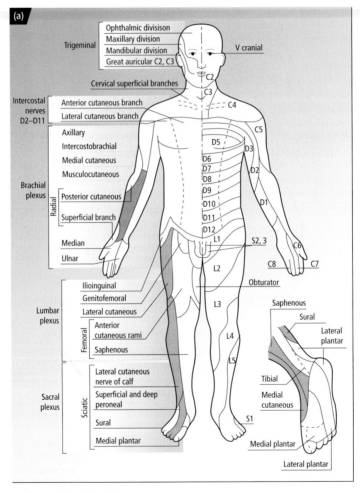

Figure 18.2 Sensory innervation of the skin.
   Cutaneous areas of distribution of spinal segments and sensory fibres of the peripheral nerves:
   (a) anterior and (b) posterior views.
   Source: Walton J. (1993). *Brain's Diseases of the Nervous System,* 10th edition. Reproduced with permission of Oxford University Press.

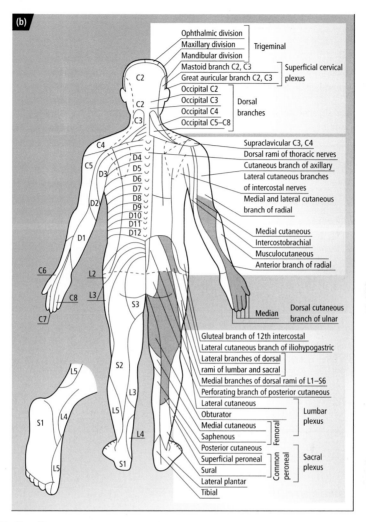

Figure 18.2 (*Continued*)

Table 18.4 Localization: clues from the examination.

Distribution	Localization
Hemisensory	Parietal, subcortical, thalamic, none (functional)
Crossed (ipsilateral face and contralateral body)	Brainstem
Sensory level	Spinal cord
Suspended, dissociated sensory level (pain and temperature only)	Central cord
Crossed sensory level (ipsilateral weakness and posterior column loss, contralateral pain and temperature loss)	Hemi-cord (Brown Séquard)
Dermatomal	Spinal nerve root(s)
Saddle	Cauda equina

(*continued*)

Table 18.4 (*Continued*)

Distribution	Localization
Patchy, single limb	Plexopathy
Glove and stocking	Generalized peripheral neuropathy
Discrete (non-dermatomal) area in single limb	Single peripheral nerve, central (usually cortical)
No sensory loss	Muscle, NMJ, motor neuron, motor cortex

Table 18.5 Urgent investigation of the patient with acute sensory symptoms.

To consider in all patients

Blood glucose level
Plasma sodium, potassium and creatinine level
Liver function tests
Thyroid function
Calcium, magnesium
Serum ACE level
B_{12}/folate levels
Haemoglobin level and white count
ESR or C-reactive protein
Antinuclear antibody titres
Paraneoplastic antibodies
HIV serology
12-lead electrocardiogram
Chest X-ray

Further management

- Further management is directed by the working diagnosis.
- Sensory symptoms may predispose to injury and falls and these risks need to be evaluated and addressed.
- Neuropathic pain is frequent, may respond poorly to standard analgesic preparation, typically requiring neuropathic pain agents such as amitriptyline, gabapentin and/or pregabalin.

Further reading

Briemberg HR, Amato AA Approach to the patient with sensory loss. UpToDate, last updated May 2015. https://www.uptodate.com/contents/approach-to-the-patient-with-sensory-loss?source=search_result&search=approach%20to%20the%20patient%20with%20sensory%20loss&selectedTitle=1~150.

CHAPTER 19

Loss of vision

Tristan McMullan and David Sprigings

The visual pathway extends from the cornea to the occipital cortex (Figure 19.1). Visual loss may indicate ocular, intracranial or systemic disease that requires prompt intervention to preserve sight. Clinical assessment (Table 19.1; Figure 19.2) will narrow the differential diagnosis and determine further management.

Giant cell arteritis should be considered in any patient over 50 with new-onset visual symptoms: it can present with transient visual loss in one eye (amaurosis fugax), persistent visual loss due to retinal or optic nerve ischaemia (may rarely affect both eyes) or diplopia.

Sudden or gradual?

Sudden loss of vision typically (but not exclusively) reflects vascular disease, and gradual loss of vision, a non-vascular disorder (Table 19.2).

One or both eyes?

Loss of vision in one eye indicates disease of that eye or optic nerve.

Bilateral visual loss occurs with systemic disease or focal disorders involving the visual pathway from the optic chiasm back to the occipital cortex.

Patients may report loss of vision in only one eye, even though both eyes are affected. With a homonymous hemianopia, the patient may only be aware of the visual loss in the eye with the temporal field defect, despite having a nasal visual field defect in the fellow eye.

Persistent or transient?

Sudden painless persistent loss of vision is usually due to ischaemia/infarction or haemorrhage at some point along the visual pathway, but is also a feature of retinal detachment (Table 19.3). Sudden transient loss of vision has a range of ocular, vascular and neurological causes (Table 19.4).

Central or peripheral visual field?

Central blurring or vision loss is typical of macular pathology (e.g. diabetic maculopathy).

Acute Medicine: A Practical Guide to the Management of Medical Emergencies, Fifth Edition. Edited by David Sprigings and John B. Chambers.
© 2018 John Wiley & Sons Ltd. Published 2018 by John Wiley & Sons Ltd.

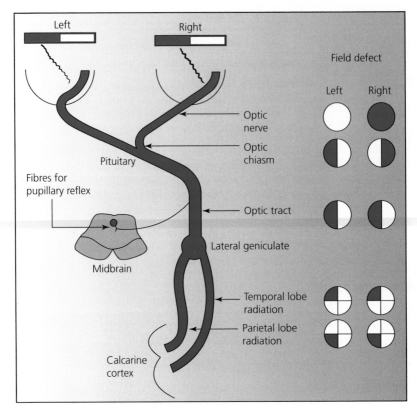

Figure 19.1 Visual pathway.
    The visual pathway. Characteristic field defects seen with lesions at various sites along the pathway are illustrated. The calcarine cortex in the occipital lobe is the location of the primary visual cortex. The occipital lobes are supplied by the posterior cerebral arteries, terminal branches of the basilar artery.
    The pupillary reflex is affected only if fibres proximal to the lateral geniculate body are damaged, or there is a lesion in the midbrain or of the III nerve.
    Source: Weiner HL, Levitt LP (1978). *Neurology for the house officer* 2e. William and Wilkins. Reproduced with permission of Wolters Kluwer Health.

    Monocular peripheral visual loss may be due to a retinal vascular event (e.g. branch retinal vein occlusion, branch retinal artery occlusion), other retinal disease (e.g. retinal detachment) or optic nerve disease (e.g. ischaemic optic neuropathy, optic neuritis, or asymmetric or monocular glaucoma).

Painful or painless?

Pain in the eye usually indicates anterior eye disease (e.g. keratitis, anterior uveitis, primary angle-closure glaucoma). Optic neuritis and giant cell arteritis can cause visual loss, which may or may not be associated with pain in the eye.
    Painless loss of vision is typical of cataract, retinal disorders and disorders of the visual pathway.

Drug history

A careful drug history is essential as many drugs can cause transient or persistent visual loss (Table 19.5).

Table 19.1 Focused assessment of the patient with visual loss.

History

See text: establish if the visual loss was:

- Sudden or gradual
- In one or both eyes
- Persistent or transient
- In the central or peripheral field
- Painful or painless; if painful, ache or gritty

Associated headache, nausea or vomiting?

Has the patient noticed 'floaters' or photopsia?

Other neuro-ophthalmic symptoms?

Symptoms suggestive of polymyalgia rheumatica/giant cell arteritis (malaise, lethargy, anorexia, weight loss, night sweats, headache, occipital pain, jaw claudication, scalp tenderness)?

Other systemic symptoms?

Cardiovascular risk factors?

Past eye history, for example cataract surgery or previous uveitis; refractive state, myopic or hypermetropic?

Past medical history: diabetes? Thyroid disease? Immunosuppression? Connective tissue disease?

Drug history

Family history

Social history, to include occupation and driving status

Examination

Perform a general examination, with particular attention to heart, blood pressure, carotid and temporal arteries.

Eyes

- Red eye, discharge, photophobia, watering?
- Pupillary abnormalities?
- Ptosis, eyelid swelling, eyelid erythema, proptosis = exophthalmos?
- Nystagmus?
- Eye movements and assessment for diplopia
- Fundoscopy

Visual acuity

Check the visual acuity using a Snellen chart, in each eye, with the patient wearing their glasses or contact lenses, or looking through a pinhole. If visual acuity is lower than can be measured by the Snellen chart, determine if the patient can count fingers (CF), detect hand movement (HM) or perceive light (PL).

Visual fields

Visual field respecting the horizontal midline (i.e. superior or inferior defects) are seen with retinal vascular or optic nerve disorders, or glaucoma. Defects respecting the vertical midline represent a neurological lesion such as a stroke or compressive lesions.

Central defects are caused primarily by age-related macular degeneration or other macular disease. In macular disease, the patient experiences a positive scotoma, that is, a 'spot' in the vision is seen and reported. Conversely, in optic nerve disease a negative scotoma is present, but not reported, that is, the defect is not 'seen' by the patient, but can be detected on examination.

Amsler grid

This is used to assess macular function. The Amsler grid is a $10\,cm^2$ grid, split into $5\,mm^2$ squares, with a central dot. The patient should wear their glasses or contact lenses with any reading correction, if worn. Hold the grid at eye level around 33 cm away in good lighting. Cover one eye and ask the patient to focus on the central dot with the uncovered eye, then repeat with the other eye. Distortion will be reported if there is macular pathology (age-related macular degeneration or macular oedema). A central scotoma may be detected in optic nerve disease.

Colour vision

Ask the patient to assess the colour quality of a bright red object (e.g. top of red pen). A relative difference between the eyes indicates pathology affecting the optic nerve (e.g. optic neuritis); the red is desaturated or 'washed out' in the affected eye.

Table 19.1 (*Continued*)

'Swinging flash light' test to detect a relative afferent pupillary defect (RAPD)
Normally, both pupils constrict symmetrically when a bright light is shone into one eye. When the torch is swung to the other eye, the pupils remain the same size. An RAPD is present if the pupil dilates, when the torch is swung to the affected eye. Both pupils constrict when the torch is swung back to the unaffected eye. A positive RAPD indicates severe retinal and/or optic nerve injury in the affected eye.

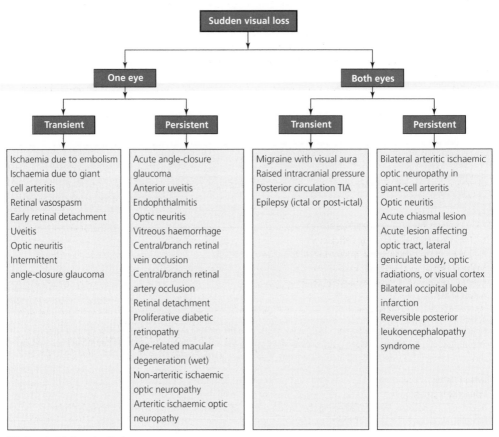

TIA, transient ischaemic attack

Figure 19.2 Analysis of sudden visual loss.

Further management

Visual loss due to suspected eye disease
Seek urgent advice from an ophthalmologist.

Suspected giant cell arteritis
If there is persistent visual loss, seek urgent advice from an ophthalmologist. Methylprednisolone IV can be given.

If there has been transient visual loss, give prednisolone 60 mg PO. The patient should be reviewed by an ophthalmologist the same day. In addition to prednisolone, start aspirin 75 mg daily, unless there are contraindications such as active peptic ulceration or a bleeding disorder. Start a proton pump inhibitor (e.g. omeprazole 20 mg daily) for gastrointestinal protection. Assess osteoporotic fracture risk, and prescribe bone protection therapy if indicated.

Table 19.2 Differential diagnosis of gradual visual loss.
(a) Painful

Cause	Features
Optic neuritis	Subacute but rapid profound visual loss, with gradual recovery over six weeks. May be pain on eye movements particularly convergence. RAPD, if unilateral, and reduced colour vision. Central or centrocecal visual field defect – central and including blindspot. May be history of multiple sclerosis.
Corneal epitheliopathy: herpes keratitis	Pain, watering, photophobia. Stains with fluorescein dye. Corneal sensation will be reduced.
Scleritis	Deep ache, beefy redness of the eye (best seen in daylight), which does not blanch with topical application of phenylephrine drops.
	May be a history of connective tissue disease, for example rheumatoid disease.

(b) Painless

Cause	Features
Keratoconus, corneal dystrophies	Blurring of vision and loss of acuity.
Cataract	Blurring of vision, foggy vision, glare and dazzle, gradual onset. No distortion.
Post-cataract surgery: cystoid macular oedema, posterior capsule opacification	Macula oedema: central smudge in vision that develops 4–6 weeks post-cataract surgery.
Age-related macular degeneration (dry)	Decreased vision with loss of clarity – may be some distortion.
Diabetic maculopathy (exudative, ischaemic)	Decreased visual acuity and blurry vision.
Macular problems: epiretinal membrane, macular hole	Decreased vision with loss of clarity – some distortion likely.
Compressive optic neuropathy	Tends to be unilateral. Insidious visual field loss that may become apparent when the good eye is covered.
	Can also be due to thyroid orbitopathy. As it is an optic neuropathy there will be an RAPD and variable loss of colour vision with associated field loss.
Drug-related: maculopathy, optic neuropathy	Decreased visual acuity and blurry vision.

AION, anterior ischaemic optic neuropathy; CF, counting fingers; CWS, cotton wool spot; HM, hand movements; NPL, no perception of light; PL, perception of light; RAPD, relative afferent pupillary defect.

Central and branch retinal artery occlusion

See urgent advice from an ophthalmologist.

Complete a full cardiovascular examination and record an ECG. Assess cardiovascular risk factors. Arrange an echocardiogram and carotid duplex scan to determine if there is an embolic source. Check full blood count, C-reactive protein ESR, blood glucose, biochemical profile and lipids.

Central and branch retinal vein occlusion

Complete a full cardiovascular examination and record an ECG.

Consider diabetes and hyperviscosity syndromes (check full blood count and serum protein electrophoresis). In younger patients consider thrombophilia (Table 56.1). Hypertension is the main risk factor but screen for other cardiovascular risk factors. Consider antiplatelet therapy if not contraindicated.

Arrange follow-up with an ophthalmologist.

Table 19.3 Differential diagnosis of sudden persistent visual loss.
(a) Painful

Cause	Features
Acute angle-closure glaucoma	Nausea and vomiting. Unwell, uncooperative. Congested eye with mid-dilated pupil. Iris details hazy due to corneal oedema. Periocular pain and headache. May be preceded by subacute attacks. High intraocular pressure, for example >35 mmHg. Clinical emergency.
Anterior uveitis	Brow ache, red eye, particularly perilimbal (around corneal limbus) injection. Pupil will likely be constricted. Hypopyon in severe cases.
Endophthalmitis	Post-operative endophthalmitis: within 2–14 days of surgery. Pain, lid swelling, loss of vision, hypopyon. Clinical emergency. Endogenous endophthalmitis: seek infective source, for example infected central venous cannula, septic focus. May be immunosuppressed. Less of a hot eye. Clinical emergency.
Optic neuritis	May affect one eye or both eyes. Pain is less of a feature than visual loss. Maybe pain on eye movements. RAPD, if unilateral. Subacute dramatic vision loss over 1–2 days. Swollen hyperaemic optic nerve when acute, optic disc pallor when established. Visual field loss. Uhthoff's sign – visual loss exacerbated by increased body temperature, for example hot bath. Frequently associated with multiple sclerosis (MS): 25–72% will develop MS at 15 years, depending on MRI findings.

(b) Painless
Affecting one eye

Cause	Features
Vitreous haemorrhage	Sudden onset of floaters and blurred vision. Red reflex may be absent if haemorrhage is significant. Will not cause RAPD. Caused by proliferative diabetic retinopathy, or retinal tear until proven otherwise in non-diabetics.
Central/branch retinal vein occlusion	Often presents in the morning with variable visual loss from mild to profound, depending on degree of ischaemia. RAPD if ischaemic. Dark blot haemorrhages in quadrants according to venous drainage involved, that is, supero-temporal if BRVO, whole fundus if CRVO; hemi-vein occlusion will cause haemorrhage in either superior or inferior retina. Respects horizontal meridian if not CRVO (in which case whole retinal involved).
Central/branch retinal artery occlusion	Retinal pallor and oedema with profound visual loss. May have cherry red spot if acute. Cattle trucking of blood cells in retinal arterioles (segmentation of blood column denoting impaired, sluggish circulation). RAPD. Must exclude giant cell arteritis.
Retinal detachment	May be preceded by flashes and floaters, symptomatic of posterior vitreous separation/detachment (PVD). PVD causes retinal tear(s) by traction on the retina, which may cause retinal detachment. Field loss commensurate with retinal elevation – supero-temporal detachment causing infero-nasal field loss. White billowing retina seen on ophthalmoscopy. Clinical emergency.
Proliferative diabetic retinopathy	May be asymptomatic until tractional retinal detachment or vitreous haemorrhage supervene. Venous new vessel proliferation at optic nerve or along arcades or in watershed (ischaemic) area nasal to the optic nerve. Other diabetic changes will be present. If markedly asymmetric, consider coexisting carotid disease.
Age-related macular degeneration (wet)	Central visual loss with haemorrhage +/- exudate in central macula. May be bilateral and may arise in dry macular degeneration. Variable visual loss from 6/6 to hand movement vision.
Non-arteritic ischaemic optic neuropathy (NAION)	Acute visual loss, typically in morning. Swollen disc with haemorrhagic component. RAPD and loss of colour vision and has associated field defect. Younger age group, 45–65.
Arteritic ischaemic optic neuropathy (AION)	As above but chalky white optic disc. Vision usually worse than NAION. Older age group >55, typically >75. May have associated symptoms and signs of giant-cell arteritis (but may be 'silent' GCA). If GCA suspected, treat with corticosteroid (see text).

Table 19.3 (*Continued*)

Cause	Features
Optic neuritis	May affect one eye or both eyes. Subacute visual loss with pain on ocular movement and RAPD with field loss. Colour vision profoundly affected. May have MS or develop MS. Neurology input required.

AION, anterior ischaemic optic neuropathy; CF, counting fingers; CWS, cotton wool spot; HM, hand movements; NPL, no perception of light; PL, perception of light; RAPD, relative afferent pupillary defect.

Affecting both eyes

Cause	Features
Bilateral arteritic ischaemic optic neuropathy (AION)	Chalky white optic discs. Vision usually worse than NAION. Older age group >55, typically >75. May have associated symptoms and signs of giant-cell arteritis (but may be 'silent' GCA). If GCA suspected, treat with corticosteroid (see text).
Optic neuritis	May affect both eyes. Subacute visual loss with pain on ocular movement and RAPD with field loss. Colour vision profoundly affected. May have MS or develop MS. Neurology input required.
Acute chiasmal lesion	May be infectious, inflammatory or vascular lesion. Pituitary apoplexy may complicate pituitary adenoma (Chapter 93). Typically results in bi-temporal hemianopia. III, IV or VI nerve palsies may be present if lesion extends into cavernous sinus.
Acute lesion affecting optic tract, the lateral geniculate body, the optic radiations, or the visual cortex	May be due to cerebral infarction or haemorrhage, or haemorrhage into brain tumour. Results in homonymous hemianopia.
Bilateral occipital lobe infarction	Due to posterior circulation stroke (see Chapter 65).
Reversible posterior leukoencephalopathy syndrome	Typically presents with seizures. Other features include headache, altered consciousness and visual abnormalities (e.g. blurred vision, homonymous hemianopia, cortical blindness).
Psychogenic	Diagnosis of exclusion.

Table 19.4 Differential diagnosis of transient visual loss.
Affecting one eye

Cause	Typical duration/characteristic features
Ischaemia due to atheroembolism from carotid artery disease or other source of embolism (amaurosis fugax)	1–10 min. Like a shutter coming down.
Ischaemia due to giant cell arteritis	Variable, may have preceding visual obscurations. May affect nerve (AION), retina (CRAO) or ocular circulation as a whole (ocular ischaemic syndrome). May also cause motility disturbance – cranial nerve palsies/extraocular muscles ischaemia.
Retinal vasospasm	Lasts 5–60 min, migrainous features such as aura and headache. Fortification spectra/scintillating scotoma are absent as they are cortical phenomena and relate to cephalic migraine.
Early retinal detachment	Variable – progressively worse, painless.
Uveitis	Variable – progressively worse and more painful.
Optic neuritis	Subacute visual loss with hyperaemic optic nerve and features of optic neuropathy: decreased colour vision, field loss and RAPD.

(*continued*)

Table 19.4 (*Continued*)

Cause	Typical duration/characteristic features
Intermittent angle-closure glaucoma Affecting both eyes	Brow ache and blurred vision – may get halos around lights and feel nauseous.

Cause	Typical duration/characteristic features
Migraine with visual aura	Lasts 10–30 min, migrainous features such as fortification spectra/scintillating scotoma and headache. Affects both eyes.
Raised intracranial pressure	Obscurations lasting seconds, which may be postural. Headache and other features of raised ICP. Bilateral disc swelling with preserved visual function (i.e. normal colour vision) in early stages. Enlarged blind spot in early stages.
Posterior circulation transient ischaemic attack affecting visual cortex	Lasts 1–10 min.
Epilepsy (ictal or post-ictal)	Ictal: 3–5 min. Post-ictal: 20 min.

Optic neuritis

Seek urgent advice from an ophthalmologist.

In most patients with optic neuritis complicating multiple sclerosis, symptoms resolve spontaneously, with recovery starting within ten days and usually complete by six weeks. Corticosteroid therapy (methylprednisolone IV) may accelerate recovery but does not alter long-term outcomes.

Amaurosis fugax

Complete a full cardiovascular examination and record an ECG. Assess cardiovascular risk factors. Arrange an echocardiogram and carotid duplex scan to determine if there is an embolic source. Check full blood count, C-reactive protein ESR, blood glucose, biochemical profile and lipids.

Consider/exclude giant cell arteritis (Chapter 99).

Give antiplatelet therapy if not contraindicated.

See Chapter 66 for further management of amaurosis fugax/transient ischaemic attack. Seek urgent advice from a stroke physician.

Table 19.5 Drugs causing visual symptoms.

Drug	Comment
Amiodarone	Corneal verticillata – asymptomatic, optic neuropathy rarely.
Corticosteroids	Raised intraocular pressure/glaucoma. Cataract.
Ethambutol	Toxic optic neuropathy.
Hydroxychloroquine	Maculopathy.
Isotretinoin	Dry eye, IIH.
Phenothiazines	Blurred vision from anticholinergic effect, pigment deposition in skin, cornea and lens. Pigmented retinopathy.
Sildenafil	Blue vision/NAION
Tamoxifen	Crystalline maculopathy.
Topiramate	Angle closure glaucoma, periorbital oedema, acute onset myopia.
Vigabatrin	Visual field defects.

Further reading

Biousse V, Newman NJ (2015) Ischemic optic neuropathies. *N Engl J Med* 372, 2428–2436. DOI: 10.1056/NEJMra1413352.

Lemos J, Eggenberger E (2015) Neuro-ophthalmological emergencies. *The Neurohospitalist* 5, 223–233.

Sawaya R, El Ayoubi N, Hamam R (2015) Acute neurological visual loss in young adults: causes, diagnosis and management. *Postgrad Med J* 91, 698–703. DOI: 10.1136/postgradmedj-2014-133071.

Abdominal

CHAPTER 20

Acute vomiting

Simon Anderson

Acute vomiting in an adult is usually due to gastrointestinal infection, or an adverse effect of medication or pregnancy, although it may be a feature of a broad range of disorders (Table 20.1). Management is summarized in Figure 20.1. The cause is usually apparent on clinical assessment (Table 20.2). Choice of tests should be guided by the duration and severity of vomiting, and associated symptoms. (Table 20.3).

Abdominal pain suggests a mechanical obstruction, particularly if the pain precedes vomiting. Other causes, such as acute pancreatitis or mesenteric ischaemia, also need to be considered in such circumstances (see Chapter 21). Vomiting with diarrhoea suggests a viral or bacterial gastroenteritis (see Chapter 22).

Pregnancy and diabetic ketoacidosis are important causes often overlooked. Always consider the latter in an unwell diabetic patient with vomiting.

Priorities

- Review the clinical observations and make a focused assessment (Table 20.2).
- In the patient with acute severe vomiting, put in an IV cannula, arrange urgent investigation (Table 20.3), give IV anti-emetic (Table 20.4), and start IV crystalloid.
- Further management is directed by the working diagnosis. If a 'surgical' cause is likely, insert a nasogastric tube, and seek urgent advice from the surgical team.

Acute Medicine: A Practical Guide to the Management of Medical Emergencies, Fifth Edition. Edited by David Sprigings and John B. Chambers.
© 2018 John Wiley & Sons Ltd. Published 2018 by John Wiley & Sons Ltd.

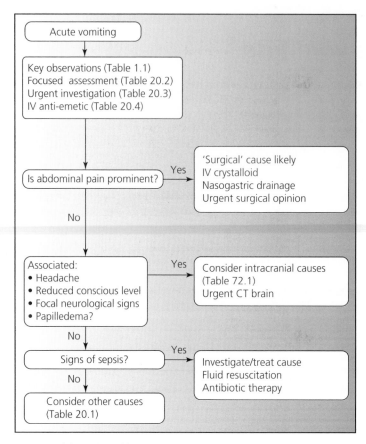

Figure 20.1 Management of the patient with acute vomiting.

Table 20.1 Causes of acute vomiting.

Infections

Gastroenteritis: viral (e.g. norovirus), bacterial (e.g. *Staphylococcus aureus, Bacillus cereus*)

Acute viral hepatitis

Systemic infections

Meningitis

Drugs and toxins

Chemotherapy: severe – cisplatinum, dacarbazine, nitrogen mustard nitrogen mustard compounds; moderate – etoposide, methotrexate, cytarabine; mild – fluorouracil, vinblastine, tamoxifen

NSAIDs, colchicine, antibiotics (erythromycin, tetracycline), azathioprine, theophylline, opioids

Alcohol, illicit drug use or drug overdose

Radiotherapy to upper abdomen or chest

Anaesthetic agents

Abdominal disorders

Mechanical obstruction: gastric outflow or small bowel

Functional disorders: idiopathic gastroparesis, chronic idiopathic pseudo-obstruction, non-ulcer dyspepsia, cyclical vomiting syndrome

Organic abdominal disorders: pancreatitis, peptic ulcer disease, cholelithiasis, mesenteric ischaemia, peritonitis

Neurological disorders
Migraine
Intracranial haemorrhage (subarachnoid haemorrhage, intracerebral haemorrhage, cerebellar haemorrhage)
Cerebellar infarction
Raised intracranial pressure (Chapter 72)
Labyrinthine disorders: vestibular neuritis, Ménière's disease

Psychiatric disorders
Psychogenic vomiting
Bulimia nervosa
Anxiety disorders

Metabolic and endocrine disorders
Pregnancy
Uraemia
Diabetic ketoacidosis (Chapter 83)
Hyper- or hypoparathyroidism
Adrenal insufficiency (Chapter 90)
Hyperthyroidism
Acute intermittent porphyria

Intrathoracic disorders
Inferior myocardial infarction

Table 20.2 Clinical assessment of the patient with vomiting.

History
Abdominal pain? Consider causes of an 'acute abdomen', specifically cholelithiasis, peptic ulcer disease, acute pancreatitis.
Early morning nausea and vomiting? Characteristic of pregnancy.
Abdominal pain with distension and tenderness? Suggests bowel obstruction, either mechanical (e.g. adhesions, strangulated hernia) or functional (pseudo-obstruction – Ogilvie's syndrome).
Headache? May indicate migraine. If worse with change in body position and associated with neurological signs (which may be subtle), suggests raised intracranial pressure due to, for example brain tumour or haemorrhage.
Nature of the vomitus? Vomiting food eaten several hours earlier indicates a gastric outflow obstruction or gastroparesis. Faeculent vomiting, usually with pain, suggests a complete small bowel obstruction or gastro-colic fistula.
Heartburn and nausea? May indicate gastro-oesophageal disease.
Vertigo, nystagmus, gait disturbance? Typical of vestibular neuritis, and if unilateral hearing deficit, labyrinthitis. Other cranial nerve deficits are typically absent in these conditions.
History of repeated episodes of stereotypical symptoms lasting 3–6 days, asymptomatic between events? Characteristic of cyclical vomiting syndrome. This usually occurs in school-age children but can occur in adults.

Examination
Are there signs of volume depletion or sepsis?
Are there signs pointing to a specific disorder (Table 20.1)? Check carefully for features of neurological disease. Consider bulimia if signs of dental enamel erosion, lanugo-like hair, parotid enlargement.

Table 20.3 Investigation of the patient with acute severe vomiting.

All patients
Blood glucose
Sodium, potassium, urea and creatinine
Liver function tests, albumin and calcium
Full blood count
Urinalysis

Depending on clinical setting
Arterial blood gases and pH; toxicology screen.
Chest X-ray
ECG
Abdominal X-ray if suspected intestinal obstruction/ileus (supine and erect or lateral decubitus)
Cranial CT
Blood culture

Table 20.4 Anti-emetic therapy.

Condition	Medication	Comments
Gastroenteritis	Metoclopramide 10 mg IV 8-hourly	Dopamine antagonist. May cause extrapyramidal side effects (ranging from mild restlessness, dystonia and rarely oculogyric crisis, particularly in children, women and elderly. Treat with procyclidine 5 mg IV.
	Domperidone 10 mg PO	Dopamine antagonist. Less likely to cause sedation and dystonic reaction. Small risk of cardiac adverse events (avoid in those >60 and/or on QT-prolonging medication)
	Ondansetron 4 mg IV 8-hourly as slow infusion over 15 min	5-HT3 antagonist. Second-line treatment, due to significant cost. Use with caution in those with prolonged QT-interval.
Pregnancy-induced vomiting	Metoclopramide 10 mg IV 8-hourly or Ondansetron 4 mg IV 8-hourly	Second-line treatment.
	Promethazine 25 mg IM or slow IV infusion	Antihistamine with anti-emetic and sedative properties.
	Vitamin B6 and ginger	For nausea.
Migraine with vomiting	Metoclopramide (see above) or Prochlorperazine 12.5 mg IM followed after 6 hours if needed with 10 mg PO	Phenothiazine.
Opioid-induced vomiting	Cyclizine 50 mg IV/IM or PO 8-hourly	Histamine H_1 – receptor antagonist.
	Prochlorperazine 12.5 mg IM	Both can also be used prophylactically.
Chemotherapy-induced vomiting	Ondansetron 8 mg IV (4 mg if >75 years old)	See above.
	Dexamethasone 8 mg IV OD.	Used as concomitant treatment with ondansetron.
	Prochloperazine or metoclopramide	Second-line agents.
Post-operative nausea and vomiting	Metoclopramide 10 mg IV 8-hourly	See above.
	Ondansetron 4–8mg IV 8-hourly	See above.
Vestibular neuritis	Prochlorperazine 12.5 mg IM followed after 6 hours with 10 mg PO if needed	
	Lorazepam 1 mg PO	Adjunctive treatment if needed.

Further reading

Furyk JS, Meek RA, Egerton-Warburton D. (2015) Drugs for the treatment of nausea and vomiting in adults in the emergency department setting. Cochrane Database of Systematic Reviews 2015, Issue 9. Art. No.: CD010106. DOI: 10.1002/14651858.CD010106.pub2.

Longstreth GF (2016) Approach to the adult with nausea and vomiting. UpToDate, last updated May 2016. https://www.uptodate.com/contents/approach-to-the-adult-with-nausea-and-vomiting.

CHAPTER 21

Acute abdominal pain

SIMON ANDERSON

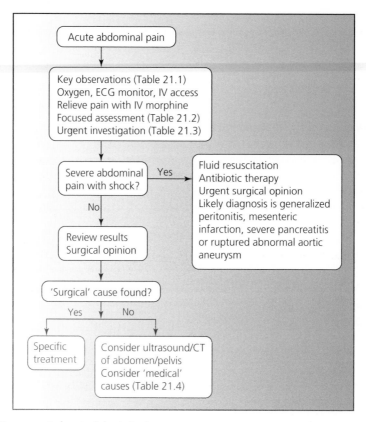

Figure 21.1 Management of acute abdominal pain.

Acute surgical causes of abdominal pain are typically due to gastro-intestinal obstruction, peritonitis or vascular emergencies.

- Visceral pain arising from the gut, biliary tract or pancreas is poorly localized to the body surface. In contrast, the pain of peritoneal irritation (due to inflammation or infection) is well localized (unless there is generalized peritonitis) and constant, and associated with abdominal tenderness.

Acute Medicine: A Practical Guide to the Management of Medical Emergencies, Fifth Edition. Edited by David Sprigings and John B. Chambers.
© 2018 John Wiley & Sons Ltd. Published 2018 by John Wiley & Sons Ltd.

Box 21.1 Acute abdominal pain – alerts.

> The most important initial decision is whether the cause is 'surgical' or 'medical'. Only after surgically-treatable causes have been excluded should other conditions be considered.
>
> A careful history is paramount as symptoms may evolve with time, for example evolution of peri-umbilical 'visceral' pain to right iliac fossa pain in acute appendicitis, or partial/intermittent intestinal obstruction progressing to complete bowel obstruction. In addition, patients on immunosuppressants (including corticosteroids) and with comorbidities (particularly renal disease, diabetes and atherosclerosis) and the elderly, may present with atypical signs.

- Gastro-intestinal obstruction usually manifests with pain, bloating, nausea and vomiting with absent or high-pitched bowel sounds.
- Peritonitis manifests as severe pain, often unresponsive to analgesia, with abdominal tenderness to light touch or movement and 'guarding'.

Priorities

1 If the patient has severe abdominal pain and is shocked (systolic BP <90 mmHg, tachycardia, cool peripheries), the likely diagnosis is generalized peritonitis, mesenteric infarction, acute severe pancreatitis or ruptured abdominal aortic aneurysm (Table 21.1). The patient will need:
- Vigorous fluid resuscitation, initially via a peripheral IV line and then guided by measurement of the central venous pressure (Chapter 116), with monitoring of the urine output by bladder catheter.
- Antibiotic therapy: start cefotaxime 1–2 g 6-hourly IV + metronidazole 500 mg 8-hourly IV.
- An urgent surgical opinion. If there are obvious signs of a ruptured abdominal aortic aneurysm (painful aortic pulsation and hypotension), emergency laparotomy is needed, before any radiological examination.

Table 21.1 Causes of acute severe abdominal pain with shock.

Cause	Pathologies	Comments
Generalized peritonitis	Perforation of viscus Mesenteric vascular occlusion leading to intestinal infarction and secondary peritonitis Inflammatory conditions with localized, followed by generalized peritonitis (e.g. appendicitis, cholecystitis, diverticulitis, Crohn's disease abscess, pancreatitis) Late intestinal obstruction (most commonly due to large bowel tumour, adhesions, hernia or volvulus)	Perforated duodenal ulcers are now relatively uncommon. Perforated colonic (or less commonly, small bowel) diverticula may be encountered. Most cases of perforation of the upper and lower GI tract are related to endoscopic procedures (e.g. polypectomy). Elderly patients and those on long-term corticosteroids may not manifest typical symptoms of peritonitis and signs may be misleadingly mild.
Mesenteric infarction	Thrombosis complicating atherosclerotic disease of the mesenteric arteries, polycythaemia, sickle cell disease, cryoglobulinaemia and amyloidosis Embolism from the heart (e.g. atrial fibrillation, endocarditis) Aortic dissection (Chapter 50)	Always consider a cardiac source of emboli in patients with atherosclerosis who present with features suggestive of acute mesenteric ischaemia.

(continued)

Table 21.1 (*Continued*)

Cause	Pathologies	Comments
	Vasculitis	Polyarteritis nodosa is often overlooked as a cause of vasculitic mesenteric infarction as the autoantibody screen is typically negative.
Acute severe pancreatitis	Common causes are gallstones (50% cases) and alcohol (20%) Less common causes include endoscopic retrograde cholangiopancreatography (ERCP) and severe hyperlipidaemias	See Chapter 79 for assessment and management of acute pancreatitis.
Ruptured abdominal aortic aneurysm	Atherosclerotic and inflammatory factors contribute to the pathogenesis of abdominal aortic aneurysm Risk of rupture greatly increased in male smokers >65 y and in aneurysms >5.5 cm in diameter	Typically causes acute severe abdominal, flank or back pain. Syncope without prominent pain can be a presentation. May also result in leg or spinal cord ischaemia.

2 History needs to establish the characteristics of the abdominal pain, and the patient's other medical problems (Table 21.2):
- When and how did the pain start – gradually or abruptly?
- Where is the pain felt, and has it moved since its onset?
- How severe is the pain?
- Has there been vomiting, and when did vomiting begin in relation to the onset of the pain?

Table 21.2 Focused assessment in acute abdominal pain.

History

When did the pain start and how did it start – gradually or abruptly?
Where is the pain, and has it moved since its onset? Visceral pain arising from the gut, biliary tract or pancreas is poorly localized. Peritoneal pain (due to inflammation or infection) is well localized (unless there is generalized peritonitis), constant and associated with abdominal tenderness.
How severe is the pain?
Has there been vomiting, and when did vomiting begin in relation to the onset of the pain?
Previous abdominal surgery, and if so what for?
Other medical problems?
Examination
Key observations
Abdominal distension?
Presence of abdominal scars? If present, check what operations have been done; adhesions from previous surgery may cause obstruction
Tenderness: localized or generalized?
Palpable organs, aorta or masses?
Hernial orifices (inguinal, femoral and umbilical) clear?
Femoral pulses present and symmetrical?
Bowel sounds
Rectal examination
Lungs: signs of basal pneumonia?

Table 21.3 Urgent investigation in acute abdominal pain.

All patients

Full blood count

Clotting screen if there is purpura or jaundice, prolonged oozing from puncture sites, or a low platelet count

C-reactive protein

Group and screen

Blood glucose

Sodium, potassium, urea and creatinine

Liver function tests, albumin and calcium

Serum amylase (raised in pancreatitis, perforated ulcer, mesenteric ischaemia and severe sepsis)

Other tests to confirm or exclude pancreatitis if indicated (serum lipase; urine dipstick test for trypsinogen-2 (which has a high negative predictive value))

Arterial gases and pH if hypotensive or oxygen saturation <94% breathing air (metabolic acidosis seen in generalized peritonitis, mesenteric infarction and severe pancreatitis)

Blood culture if febrile or suspected peritonitis

Urine: stick test, MC&S and pregnancy test

ECG if age >50 or known cardiac disease or unexplained upper abdominal pain

Chest X-ray – looking for free gas under the diaphragm, indicating perforation, and evidence of basal pneumonia

Abdominal X-ray (supine and erect or lateral decubitus) – looking for evidence of obstruction of large and/or small bowel; ischaemic bowel (dilated and thickened loops of small bowel); cholangitis (gas in biliary tree); radio-dense gallstones; radio-dense urinary tract stones

Selected patients

In suspected intestinal obstruction, CT scan of the abdomen is the most sensitive test.

Abdominal ultrasonography is the initial test of choice when there are signs of peritonitis, and can assess for appendicitis, abdominal abscess and pelvic abnormalities without radiation exposure. Ultrasonography is also the first-line investigation for right upper quadrant pain, to exclude gallstones and other biliary pathology.

- Has the patient had previous abdominal surgery and if so what for?
- Women of childbearing age should be asked about their pregnancy and menstrual history (last menstrual period, last normal menstrual period, previous menstrual period, cycle length) and use of contraception. A pregnancy test should be done. Establish if there has been vaginal discharge or bleeding, dyspareunia or dysmenorrhea.

3 As well as a careful examination of the abdomen (Table 21.2), you should:
- Check the temperature, pulse, JVP and blood pressure.
- Listen to the heart and over the lung bases.
- Give oxygen if the patient has severe pain, is breathless, or if oxygen saturation by pulse oximetry is <94%.
- Put in an IV cannula and take blood for urgent investigations (Table 21.3).
- Relieve severe pain with morphine 5–10 mg IV plus an antiemetic, for example prochlorperazine 12.5 mg IV.
- Start an infusion of crystalloid, at a rate determined by the volume status of the patient.
- Arrange appropriate imaging (Table 21.3).

Further management

Further management will be determined by the results of investigations and surgical assessment. 'Medical' causes of abdominal pain are summarized in Table 21.4.

Table 21.4 'Medical' causes of acute abdominal pain.

Site of pain	Pathologies to consider	Comment
Right upper quadrant	Right basal pneumonia (Chapters 62, 63) Pulmonary embolism Hepatic congestion due to congestive heart failure Alcoholic hepatitis (Chapter 78) Viral hepatitis Acute gonococcal perihepatitis (Fitz-Hugh-Curtis syndrome) Liver abscess Budd-Chiari syndrome Portal vein thrombosis	Always listen for basal lung signs (pleural rub, crackles) Fitz-Hugh-Curtis syndrome usually presents with right upper quadrant pain (which may radiate to the shoulder) and minimal pelvic signs. Think of Budd-Chiari syndrome in patients with acute or chronic upper abdominal pain, hepatomegaly and deranged liver enzymes.
Epigastric	Acute gastritis Gastroparesis Peptic ulcer disease Gastro-oesophageal reflux disease Acute inferior myocardial infarction (Chapter 45) Acute pericarditis (Chapter 53) Aortic dissection (Chapter 50) Acute pancreatitis (Chapter 79)	Pain in the distal oesophagus related to reflux oesophagitis can be difficult to distinguish from epigastric pain from gastric causes. An ECG should always be performed in patients with acute upper abdominal pain.
Left upper quadrant	Left basal pneumonia Pulmonary embolism Splenic infarction Splenic abscess	Splenic causes are relatively uncommon but should be considered in patients with haemoglobinopathies and in procoagulant states.
Lower abdomen	Ileitis: • Infections, for example Yersinia • Crohn's disease • NSAID-enteropathy Diverticulitis (usually causes left iliac fossa pain but may present with right iliac fossa pain) Ureteric obstruction or stones Cystitis In women: • Pelvic inflammatory disease • Adnexal disease (e.g. ectopic pregnancy, cysts, torsion) • Uterine disease (endometritis, complications of leiomyomas)	Ovarian cysts are commonly encountered on ultrasound and may not be the cause of pain. Always consider other causes such as appendicitis or ileitis.
Central or diffuse	Viral or bacterial gastroenteritis (Chapter 22) Acute inflammatory bowel disease (Chapter 76) Spontaneous bacterial peritonitis Diabetic ketoacidosis (Chapter 83) Acute adrenal insufficiency (Chapter 90) Aortic dissection (Chapter 50) Acute intermittent porphyria Vaso-occlusive crisis of sickle cell disease (Chapter 104) Henoch-Schonlein purpura (colicky pain with arthralgia, pupruric rash on buttocks and legs and sometimes bloody diarrhoea) Retroperitoneal haemorrhage (complicating anticoagulant therapy, bleeding disorder, leaking abdominal aortic aneurysm or vertebral fracture)	Crohn's disease can present with acute abdominal pain with minimal preceding symptoms. Spontaneous bacterial peritonitis can occur in patients with relatively mild ascites. Acute intermittent porphyria is rare but should be considered if recurrent unexplained generalized pain.

Further reading

Bhangu A, Søreide K, Di Saverio S, Hansson Assarsson J, Thurston Drake F. (2015) Acute appendicitis: modern understanding of pathogenesis, diagnosis, and management. *Lancet* 386, 1278–1287.

Clair DG, Beach JM. (2016) Mesenteric ischemia. *N Engl J Med* 374, 959–968.

Gans SL, Pols MA, Stoker J, Boermeester MA, on behalf of the expert steering group (2015) Guideline for the diagnostic pathway in patients with acute abdominal pain. *Dig Surg* 32, 23–31. http://www.karger.com/Article/FullText/371583.

Lankisch PG, Apte M, Banks P.A. (2015) Acute pancreatitis. *Lancet* 386, 85–96.

Badger SA, Harkin DW, Blair PH, Ellis PK, Kee F, Forster R. (2016) Endovascular repair or open repair for ruptured abdominal aortic aneurysm: a Cochrane systematic review. *BMJ Open* 6, e008391. DOI: 10.1136/bmjopen-2015-008391

CHAPTER 22

Acute diarrhoea

Simon Anderson

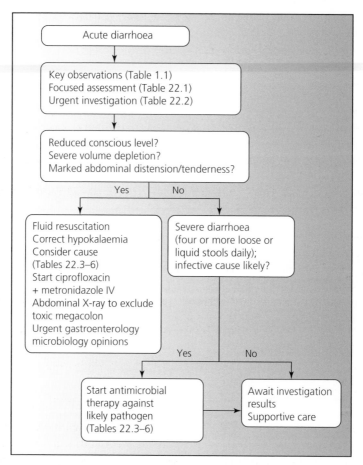

Figure 22.1 Management of acute diarrhoea.

Acute Medicine: A Practical Guide to the Management of Medical Emergencies, Fifth Edition. Edited by David Sprigings and John B. Chambers.
© 2018 John Wiley & Sons Ltd. Published 2018 by John Wiley & Sons Ltd.

Acute diarrhoea (Box 22.1) is usually due to intestinal infection or an adverse effect of medication. *Clostridium difficile* followed by norovirus infection are the main causes of fatal illness and should always be considered in hospitalized patients. Norovirus is the commonest cause overall (around 20% of all cases). The commonest bacterial causes are *Salmonella* and *Campylobacter*. Inflammatory bowel disease should be excluded if there is bloody diarrhoea (see Chapters 74 and 76).

Box 22.1 Acute diarrhoea – definitions.

Diarrhoea is the passage of loose or liquid stools (types 5, 6 or 7 (entirely liquid) on the Bristol Stool Chart). Severe diarrhoea is the passage of four or more loose or liquid stools daily.

Acute diarrhoea is ≤14 days, persistent diarrhoea 15–30 days, and chronic diarrhoea >30 days in duration.

Priorities

Establish the differential diagnosis from the history and examination (Table 22.1). Strict infection control protocols must be followed (including barrier nursing and hand-washing). Investigations needed urgently are given in Table 22.2.

- Features of community-acquired infective diarrhoea are given in Table 22.3 and hospital-acquired diarrhoea in Table 22.4.
- Particular causes to consider in the returning traveller are summarized in Table 22.5, and those in patients with HIV/ADS or immunosuppression in Table 22.6.

If the patient is severely ill (impaired consciousness level, severe volume depletion, marked abdominal distension or tenderness):

- Start vigorous fluid resuscitation with crystalloid, initially via a peripheral IV line, and correct electrolyte abnormalities.
- Start antibiotic therapy to cover the likely pathogens: ciprofloxacin 400 mg 12-hourly IV and metronidazole 500 mg 8-hourly IV (immunocompetent patients) or gentamicin 5 mg/kg IV (immunosuppressed patients).
- Obtain an abdominal X-ray to check for segmental or total colonic distension indicative of toxic megacolon.
- Seek urgent help from a microbiologist.
- Nurse the patient with standard isolation technique in a single room until the diagnosis is established.

All other patients:

- Further management will be determined by the results of microscopy and culture of the stool, and other investigations.
- If the patient has a fever, is dehydrated or is immunocompromised, start azithromycin 500 mg OD PO or ciprofloxacin PO or IV whilst awaiting the stool test results. The choice will depend upon your local antibiotic guidelines. (*Campylobacter* is currently the commonest bacterial cause and most strains are resistant to ciprofloxacin. Moreover azithromycin-resistent *Shigella* infections are common in certain high-risk patients.)
- Anti-motility drugs such as loperamide are best avoided but can be given for short-term symptomatic relief. They are absolutely contraindicated in patients with shigellosis or dysentery (bloody stools and fever) due to the risk of a toxic megacolon.

Further management

This is directed by the working diagnosis.

Table 22.1 Focused assessment of the patient with acute diarrhoea.

History

Mode of onset (abrupt, sub-acute or gradual) and duration.

Frequency and nature of the stools (watery or containing blood and mucus) (severe diarrhoea is defined as four or more stools daily; bloody stools are a common feature of shigellosis, salmonellosis, severe *Campylobacter* enteritis and ulcerative colitis, and are rare (5%) in *C.difficile* infection).

Have others in the same household or who have shared the same food also developed diarrhoea?

Other symptoms (malaise, fever, vomiting, abdominal pain)?

Current or recent hospital inpatient (at risk of *C. difficile* infection)?

Travel abroad in the past six months?

Previous significant gastro-intestinal symptoms or known GI diagnosis?

Medications (in particular antibiotics) taken in the six weeks before the onset of diarrhoea?

Any other medical problems?

HIV/AIDS or other immunosuppression? (Table 22.6)

Examination

Severity of illness and degree of volume depletion (mental state, temperature, heart rate, blood pressure lying and sitting).

Signs of toxic megacolon (marked abdominal distension and tenderness)? (May complicate many forms of infective colitis (including *C. difficile*) as well as colitis due to inflammatory bowel disease.)

Extra-abdominal features (e.g. rash, arthropathy, uveitis)?

Table 22.2 Urgent investigation in acute severe diarrhoea.

Stool microscopy and culture

Test for *Clostridium difficile* toxin in stool

Full blood count

C-reactive protein

Blood glucose

Sodium, potassium, urea and creatinine

Liver function tests, albumin

Blood culture if febrile

Sigmoidoscopy if bloody diarrhoea

Abdominal X-ray if marked distension or tenderness (toxic megacolon)

Always consider the possibility of *C. difficile* infection and norovirus – involve the Infectious Diseases team early.

A flexible sigmoidoscopy and biopsies are not routinely needed, but if a new presentation of IBD is a possibility, a gastroenterology opinion should be sought (see below).

Could this be inflammatory bowel disease?

- This should be considered if there is blood or if the diarrhoea is chronic or recurrent or if there are systemic signs (e.g. rash, arthropathy, uveitis).
- Ulcerative colitis may present with acute diarrhoea, usually bloody. Vomiting does not occur, and abdominal pain is not a prominent feature. Diagnosis is by exclusion of infective causes (particularily *C. dificile*) and typical histological appearances on rectal biopsy.

Table 22.3 Causes of community-acquired diarrhoea.

Cause	Clinical features	Diagnosis/treatment (if indicated)
Campylobacter enteritis (*C. jejuni*)	Incubation period 2–6 days. Associated fever and abdominal pain. Diarrhoea initially watery, later may contain blood and mucus. Usually self-limiting, lasting 2–5 days. May be followed after 1–3 weeks by Guillain-Barré syndrome (p. 434)	Culture of *C. jejuni* from stool. Azithromycin 500 mg od PO for 5 days or Erythromycin 500 mg 12-hourly PO for 5 days.
Non-typhoid salmonellosis (Salmonella species)	Incubation period 1–2 days. Associated fever, vomiting and abdominal pain. Diarrhoea may become bloody if colon involved. Usually self-limiting. More severe in immunosuppressed.	Culture of *Salmonella* species from stool. Ciprofloxacin 500 mg 12-hourly PO for 5 days or trimethoprim 200 mg 12-hourly PO for 5 days.
Escherichia coli O157:H7 (enterohaemorrhagic *E. coli*)	Incubation period 1–3 days. Associated vomiting and abdominal pain. May have low-grade fever. Watery diarrhoea which may become bloody. May be complicated by haemolytic uraemic syndrome from 2–14 (mean 7) days after onset of illness.	Culture of *E. coli* O157 from stool (using sorbitol MacConkey agar; missed by standard culture). Supportive treatment. Antibiotic therapy unhelpful.
Clostridium difficile colitis	Typically causes diarrhoea in hospital, but may occur in community. See Table 22.4.	
Norovirus	Usually short incubation time (1–2 days). Diarrhoea with vomiting is typical, with fever less common. Infections during outbreaks are more severe, with the elderly at particular risk of excess mortality.	The diagnosis is made by PCR analysis of stool and vomitus and the exclusion of other causes. Treatment is supportive.

Table 22.4 Causes of hospital-acquired diarrhoea.

Cause	Clinical features	Diagnosis/treatment
Clostridium difficile colitis	Diarrhoea usually begins within 4–10 days of antibiotic treatment, but may not appear for 4–6 weeks. Presentations range from mild self-limiting watery diarrhoea to (rarely) acute fulminating toxic megacolon. Low-grade fever and abdominal tenderness are common. Although the rectum and sigmoid colon are usually involved, in 10% of cases colitis is confined to the more proximal colon.	Diagnosis is based on detection of *C. difficile* toxins A and B in the stool. In severe colitis, sigmoidoscopy may show adherent yellow plaques (2–10 mm in diameter). Supportive treatment and isolation of the patient to reduce the risk of spread. Stop antibiotic therapy if possible. If diarrhoea mild (1–2 stools daily), symptoms may resolve within 1–2 weeks without further treatment. Refer to local treatment guidelines. In general, if moderate diarrhoea (three or more stools daily), give metronidazole 400 mg 8-hourly PO for 7–10 days. If severe infection (usually associated with hypoalbuminaemia), give vancomycin 125 mg 6-hourly PO.

(*continued*)

Table 22.4 (*Continued*)

Cause	Clinical features	Diagnosis/treatment
		Around 20% of patients will have a relapse after completing a course of metronidazole, due to germination of residual spores within the colon, re-infection with *C. difficile* or further antibiotic treatment: give either a further course of metronidazole or vancomycin 125 mg 6-hourly PO for 7–10 days.
		If the patient is severely ill and unable to take oral medication, give metronidazole 500 mg 8-hourly IV (IV vancomycin should not be used as significant excretion into the gut does not occur).
Drugs	Many drugs may cause diarrhoea, including chemotherapeutic agents, proton pump inhibitors and laxatives in excess.	Diarrhoea resolves after treatment completed or with withdrawal of the causative drug.
Norovirus	See Table 22.3.	See Table 22.3.

Table 22.5 Causes of acute diarrhoea following recent travel abroad.

Cause	Clinical features	Diagnosis/treatment
Giardiasis (*Giardia lamblia*)	Widespread distribution. Explosive onset of watery diarrhoea 1–3 weeks after exposure.	Identification of cysts or trophozoites in stool or jejunal biopsy. Metronidazole 400 mg 8-hourly PO for 5 days.
Amoebic dysentery (*Entamoeba histolytica*)	Mexico, South America, South Asia, West and South-East Africa. Diarrhoea may be severe with blood and mucus.	Identification of cysts in stools. Metronidazole 750 mg 8-hourly PO for 5 days.
Schistosomiasis (*S. mansoni* and *japonicum*)	*S. mansoni*: South America and Middle East; *S. japonicum*: China and the Philippines. Diarrhoea onset 2–6 weeks or longer after exposure.	Identification of ova in stool. Praziquantel (seek expert advice).
Shigellosis (*Shigella* species)	Incubation period 1–2 days. Associated fever and abdominal pain. Diarrhoea may be watery or bloody.	Culture of *Shigella* species from stool. Ciprofloxacin 500 mg 12-hourly PO for 5 days or Trimethoprim 200 mg 12-hourly PO for 5 days.
Non-typhoid salmonellosis	See Community-acquired diarrhoea, Table 22.3.	

Table 22.6 Acute diarrhoea in the immunosuppressed/HIV-positive patient: specific pathogens to consider.

Cause	Clinical features	Diagnosis/treatment
Cryptosporidiosis (***Cryptosporidium* species**)	Subacute onset Associated abdominal pain Severe diarrhoea	Identification of oocysts in stool Seek expert advice on treatment
Isosporiasis (***Isospora belli***)	Incubation period: one week Associated fever, abdominal pain, diarrhea with fatty stools	Identification of oocysts in stool, duodenal aspirate or jejunal biopsy Seek expert advice on treatment
Cytomegalovirus	Diarrhoea may be accompanied by systemic illness and hepatitis	Serological tests for cytomegalovirus Seek expert advice on treatment

- Crohn's disease is associated with less severe diarrhoea and blood is not prominent but there may be abdominal pain and tenderness particularly in the lower right quadrant.
- See Chapter 76 for further management of inflammatory bowel disease.

Could this be faecal impaction with overflow?

- This should be suspected in patients at risk of faecal impaction, for example the elderly, bed-bound, in those taking opioid analgesics.
- There is no vomiting or systemic illness. Rectal examination discloses hard impacted faeces.
- Treatment is with laxatives/enemas.

Further reading

DuPont HL (2014) Acute infectious diarrhea in immunocompetent adults. *N Engl J Med* 370, 1532–1540. DOI: 10.1056/NEJMra1301069

Leffler DA, Lamont JT (2015) *Clostridium difficile* infection. *N Engl J Med* 372: 1539–1548. DOI: 10.1056/ NEJMra1403772

Infectious Diseases Society of America. Practice guidelines for the management of infectious diarrhea. Update due late 2016.

CHAPTER 23

Acute jaundice

Ben Warner and Mark Wilkinson

Common causes for acute jaundice seen in the emergency department include decompensated chronic liver disease, alcoholic or viral hepatitis, and obstructive jaundice due to gallstones or malignancy. Vascular causes (e.g. acute Budd-Chiari syndrome) are rare but can be overlooked. Management is summarized in Figure 23.1.

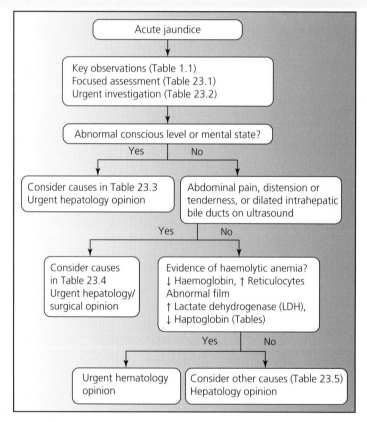

Figure 23.1 Assessment of the patient with acute jaundice.

Acute Medicine: A Practical Guide to the Management of Medical Emergencies, Fifth Edition. Edited by David Sprigings and John B. Chambers.
© 2018 John Wiley & Sons Ltd. Published 2018 by John Wiley & Sons Ltd.

Priorities

Make a focused clinical assessment (Table 23.1) and arrange urgent investigation (Table 23.2).

- If the jaundiced patient has signs of sepsis, give IV crystalloid, take blood (and ascitic fluid, if present) for culture, and start empirical IV antibiotic therapy to cover Gram-negative and anaerobic bacteria, in accordance with local guidelines (e.g. piperacillin-tazobactam or meropenem). Further management of sepsis is described in Chapter 35.
- The combination of jaundice and encephalopathy is characteristic of acute liver failure, but is also seen in other disorders (Table 23.3). If you suspect acute liver failure, seek urgent advice from a hepatologist. See Chapter 77 for further management of acute liver failure and decompensated chronic liver disease. Patients with suspected acute liver failure and grade 3 or 4 encephalopathy should be managed in an intensive care unit.
- Jaundice with abdominal pain, distension or tenderness may be seen in a range of medical and surgical disorders (Table 23.4). Obtain an urgent surgical opinion.

Table 23.1 Focused assessment of the jaundiced patient.

History

Duration and time course of jaundice and other symptoms (e.g. fever, abdominal pain)

Known liver or biliary tract disease?

Full drug history: including all non-prescription drugs, herbal remedies, dietary supplements, mushroom ingestion or khat, taken over the past year

Risk factors for viral hepatitis (foreign travel, IV drug use, men who have sex with men, multiple sexual partners, body piercing and tattoos, blood transfusion and blood products, needle-stick injury in health-care worker)?

Sexual history

Pregnancy?

Usual and recent alcohol intake?

Other medical problems (e.g. cardiovascular disease, transplant recipient, cancer, HIV/AIDS, haematological disease)?

Family history of jaundice/liver disease?

Examination

Physiological observations and systematic examination

Conscious level and mental state; grade of encephalopathy if present:

Grade of encephalopathy	Clinical features
Subclinical	Impaired work, personality change, sleep disturbance
	Abnormal findings on psychomotor testing
Grade 1	Mild confusion, agitation, apathy, oriented in time and place
	Fine tremor, asterixis
Grade 2	Drowsiness, lethargy, disoriented in time
	Asterixis, dysarthria
Grade 3	Sleepy but rousable, disoriented in time and place
	Hyperreflexia, hyperventilation
Grade 4	Responsive only to painful stimuli or unresponsive

Signs of chronic liver disease?

Right upper quadrant tenderness (Table 23.4)?

Liver enlargement (seen in early viral hepatitis, alcoholic hepatitis, malignant infiltration, congestive heart failure, acute Budd-Chiari syndrome)?

Splenomegaly?

Ascites (Chapter 24)?

Table 23.2 Urgent investigation in acute jaundice.

Full blood count and film (Chapter 100)
Coagulation screen (Chapter 102)
Blood glucose
Sodium, potassium, urea and creatinine
Liver function tests: bilirubin (total and unconjugated), aspartate aminotransferase, alanine aminotransferase, gamma-glutamyl transpeptidase, alkaline phosphatase, albumin
Paracetamol level (Appendix 36.1)
Serum lactate dehydrogenase (LDH) and haptoglobin if suspected haemolysis
Blood culture if febrile
Urine stick test, microscopy and culture
Markers of viral hepatitis (anti-HAV IgM, HBsAg, anti-HBc IgM, anti-HCV, anti-HEV, EBV)
Test for HIV
Autoimmune screen (ANA, AMA, SMA, ANCA and immunoglobulins)
Microscopy and culture of ascites if present (aspirate 10 mL for cell count (use EDTA tube) and culture (inoculate blood culture bottles) (see Chapter 24)
Ultrasound of liver, biliary tract and hepatic/portal veins
Pregnancy test in women of child-bearing age
Consider copper studies in young adults (Wilson disease, see Table 77.1)

EDTA, ethylene diaminetetra-acetic acid; HAV, hepatitis A virus; HBc, hepatitis B core; HBsAg, hepatitis B surface antigen; HCV, hepatitis C virus; HEV, hepatitis E virus; IgM, immunoglobulin M; HIV, human immunodeficiency virus; LDH, lactate dehydrogenase; EBV, Epstein-Barr Virus; ANA, anti-nuclear antibody; AMA, anti-mitochondrial antibody; SMA, smooth muscle antibody; ANCA, anti-neutrophil cytoplasmic antibody.

Table 23.3 Jaundice with abnormal conscious level/mental state.

Acute liver failure (Chapter 77)
Decompensated chronic liver disease (Chapter 77)
Alcoholic hepatitis (Chapter 78)
Sepsis with multiple organ failure
Severe acute cholangitis with septic encephalopathy
Severe heart failure with ischaemic hepatitis
Falciparum malaria (Chapter 33)

Table 23.4 Jaundice with abdominal pain, distension or tenderness.

Acute cholangitis (Charcot's triad of pain, fever and jaundice)
Intra-abdominal sepsis
Paracetamol poisoning (Appendix 36.1)
Severe heart failure
Liver abscess
Viral hepatitis
Alcoholic hepatitis (Chapter 78)
Acute pancreatitis (Chapter 79)
HELLP syndrome of pregnancy (haemolysis, elevated liver enzymes, low platelet count) (Chapter 32)
Budd-Chiari syndrome
Haemobilia (Sandblom's triad of gastrointestinal bleeding, biliary colic and jaundice)

- If there is evidence of haemolytic anaemia (anaemia with increased reticulocyte count, abnormal blood film (Chapter 100), elevated plasma lactate dehydrogenase (LDH) and low plasma haptoglobin), seek urgent advice from a haematologist.

Further management

Further management is directed by the working diagnosis.
- If ultrasonography demonstrates obstructive (post-hepatic) jaundice, early hepatobiliary intervention is needed: see Chapter 79. Causes of intrahepatic cholestasis are summarized in Table 23.5.
- Patients with presumed viral hepatitis can be discharged home with early clinic follow-up arranged, provided all the following criteria are met:
  - They are clinically stable and not encephalopathic.
  - Paracetamol poisoning, drug toxicity and other disorders which result in high AST/ALT levels have been considered and excluded (Table 23.6).
  - In women of child-bearing age, a pregnancy test is negative.

Table 23.5 Causes of intrahepatic cholestasis.

Viral hepatitis (some cases)
Alcoholic hepatitis
Drugs and toxins
Sepsis
Primary biliary cirrhosis
Primary sclerosing cholangitis
Liver infiltration (e.g. sarcoidosis, tuberculosis, lymphoma)
Intrahepatic cholestasis of pregnancy
Syphilitic hepatitis
End-stage liver disease

Table 23.6 Causes of plasma aspartate and alanine transaminase levels of more than 1000 units/L.

Common
Acute viral hepatitis
Ischaemic hepatitis
Acute drug or toxin-related liver injury (most commonly paracetamol)

Less common or rare
Acute exacerbation of autoimmune chronic active hepatitis
Reactivation of chronic hepatitis B
Acute Budd-Chiari syndrome
Veno-occlusive disease
HELLP syndrome of pregnancy (haemolysis, elevated liver enzymes, low platelet count)
Acute fatty liver of pregnancy
Hepatic infarction (may complicate HELLP syndrome)
Hepatitis delta in a chronic carrier of hepatitis B
Acute Wilson disease
Massive lymphomatous infiltration of the liver
Parasitic biliary obstruction

- Liver synthetic function is preserved (normal prothrombin time/international normalized ratio and serum albumin).
- Ultrasonography of the liver and biliary tract is normal.
- If the diagnosis is uncertain, contact your local gastroenterologist or hepatologist for advice.

Further reading

National Institute for Care and Health Excellence (2014) Gallstone disease: diagnosis and management Clinical guideline: https://www.nice.org.uk/guidance/cg188?unlid=10194680392016226172055.

Roy-Chowdhury N, Roy-Chowdhury J. (2016) Diagnostic approach to the adult with jaundice or asymptomatic hyperbilirubinemia. UpToDate https://www.uptodate.com/contents/diagnostic-approach-to-the-adult-with-jaundice-or-asymptomatic-hyperbilirubinemia?source=search_result&search=acute%20jaundice&selectedTitle=1~150.

Ryan DP, Hong TS, Bardeesy N. (2014) Pancreatic adenocarcinoma. *N Engl J Med* 371, 1039–1049. DOI: 10.1056/NEJMra1404198.

CHAPTER 24

Ascites

BEN WARNER AND MARK WILKINSON

Ascites is the accumulation of fluid within the peritoneal cavity. Assessment and management of the patient with ascites is summarized in Figure 24.1. The clinical features, together with findings on diagnostic paracentesis (of which the serum-to-ascites albumin gradient is of particular importance), will narrow the differential diagnosis and direct further investigation.

- The commonest causes for ascites seen in the emergency department are decompensated chronic liver disease, advanced heart failure and cancer.
- Patients who develop ascites as a complication of cirrhosis have a poor prognosis (two-year survival 50%), and should be referred to a hepatologist for consideration of liver transplantation.

Priorities

- Perform a diagnostic aspirate (30–50 mL) immediately on admission for new-onset ascites or if there is evidence of sepsis. The technique of diagnostic paracentesis is described in Box 24.1 Diagnostic tests on ascitic fluid are summarized in Table 24.1.
- If there is clinical or radiological evidence of cirrhosis, the cause of decompensation must be identified and treated: see Chapter 77.
- The management of spontaneous bacterial peritonitis is summarized in Appendix 24.1.
- Budd-Chiari syndrome is suspected in patients who present with sudden onset ascites in the absence of a known chronic liver disease. Presentation can range from asymptomatic to fulminant liver failure. Similarly, portal vein thrombosis can be asymptomatic, but typically presents with abdominal pain or features of portal hypertension such as varices or ascites. It is more common in patients with known chronic liver disease or who are in a hypercoagulable state. Duplex ultrasonography can be done if these are suspected, although CT and MRI are more diagnostic.
- Ascites may complicate cardiac disease (severe tricuspid regurgitation, other causes of right-sided heart failure, and constrictive pericarditis). If the jugular venous pressure is raised, or there are other features of heart disease, check plasma BNP/NT-proBNP and arrange echocardiography.
- Nephrotic syndrome as the cause of ascites can be confirmed or excluded by measurement of urinary protein excretion on a 24-hour urine collection (>3.5 g/day is nephrotic-range proteinuria) or by calculating the albumin-to-creatinine ratio (ACR) in a spot urine sample (ACR is usually >220 mg/mmol in nephrotic syndrome).

Further management of ascites due to cirrhosis

In all patients with ascites, avoid nephrotoxic drugs, including NSAIDs, ACE inhibitors and α-adrenergic blockers.

Acute Medicine: A Practical Guide to the Management of Medical Emergencies, Fifth Edition. Edited by David Sprigings and John B. Chambers.
© 2018 John Wiley & Sons Ltd. Published 2018 by John Wiley & Sons Ltd.

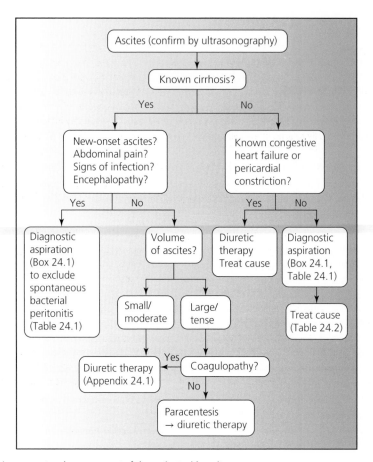

Figure 24.1 Assessment and management of the patient with ascites.

Grade 1 or 2 (mild or moderate) ascites

Unless the ascites is new or complicated, both of these grades of ascites can be managed as an outpatient.

Restrict dietary sodium intake to 80–120 mmol/day.

Start diuretic therapy with spironolactone 100 mg daily and increase by 100 mg weekly with monitoring of electrolytes and creatinine to a maximum of 400 mg daily. If spironolactone resistant, add in furosemide 40 mg daily and increase weekly by 40 mg to a maximum of 160 mg with biochemical monitoring.

Monitor daily weight. Target weight loss is 0.5 kg daily in patients without peripheral oedema and 1 kg daily in those with peripheral oedema.

Aim for the minimum dose of diuretics once ascites has resolved.

Complications from diuretics include gynaecomastia (amiloride 10–40 mg daily can be substituted for spironolactone), renal failure, hyperkalaemia (either reduce the spironolactone or add in furosemide), and encephalopathy. Stop diuretics if plasma sodium levels fall below 120 mmol/L as this may be consistent with diuretic-induced hypovolaemic hyponatraemia (Chapter 85).

Grade 3 (large volume) ascites, or diuretic-resistant ascites

Severe ascites can cause breathlessness and this can be alleviated by paracentesis. If there is tense ascites, consider a single paracentesis, followed by dietary sodium restriction and diuretic therapy. Human albumin

Box 24.1 Diagnostic aspiration of ascites.

1 Confirm the indications for aspiration of ascites. Explain the procedure to the patient and obtain consent. Deranged clotting (common in patients with cirrhosis and ascites) is not a contraindication, but ask advice from a haematologist if the patient has disseminated intravascular coagulation (p. 581). Complications of the procedure (haematoma, haemoperitoneum, infection) are rare. Inadvertent puncture of the intestine may occur but rarely leads to secondary infection.

2 The patient should lie relaxed in a supine position, having emptied the bladder. With guidance by ultrasonography, select a site for puncture in the right or left lower quadrant, away from scars and the inferior epigastric artery (whose surface marking is a line drawn from the femoral pulse to the umbilicus).

3 Put on gloves. Prepare the skin with chlorhexidine. Anaesthetize the skin with 2 mL of lidocaine 1% using a 25 G (orange) needle. Then infiltrate a further 5 mL of lidocaine along the planned needle path through the abdominal wall and down to the peritoneum.

4 Give the local anaesthetic time to work. Mount a 21 G (green) needle on a 50 mL syringe and then advance along the anaesthetized path. Aspirate as you advance. Having entered the peritoneal cavity, aspirate 30–50 mL of ascites. Remove the needle and place a small dressing over the puncture site.

5 Send samples for:
   • Albumin concentration (plain tube), if the aetiology is unknown
   • Total and differential white cell count (EDTA tube)
   • Bacterial culture (inoculate aerobic and anaerobic blood culture bottles with 10 mL each)
   • Other tests if indicated (Table 24.1)

6 Clear up and dispose of sharps safely. Write a note of the procedure in the patient's record: findings on ultrasonography/approach/appearance of ascites/volume aspirated/samples sent. Ensure the samples are sent promptly for analysis.

solution (100 mL of 20% HAS per 2 L of ascites removed) should be given IV during paracentesis. Seek advice from a hepatologist.

In the case of diuretic-resistant ascites and where the urinary sodium concentration remains below 30 mmol/L, the patient should be referred for a transjugular intrahepatic portosystemic shunt (TIPS) or consideration of liver transplantation.

Appendix 24.1 Spontaneous bacterial peritonitis (SBP)

Definition

Spontaneous bacterial peritonitis (SBP) is defined as infection of ascitic fluid without evidence of an intra-abdominal surgically treatable source; depending on the clinical context, imaging by CT may be needed to exclude such a source.

Background

SBP is a common complication of ascites due to cirrhosis; the lower the ascitic fluid albumin concentration (prior to infection), the higher the risk. Aerobic Gram-negative bacteria, especially *Escherichia coli*, are the commonest causative organisms. Features of SBP include fever (70%), abdominal pain (60%), abdominal tenderness (50%) and change in mental state (50%). It may be complicated by the hepatorenal syndrome (in up to 30%).

Table 24.1 Ascites: diagnostic tests.

Test	Comment
Visual inspection	Ascites due to cirrhosis is usually clear yellow, but may be cloudy when complicated by spontaneous bacterial peritonitis.
Albumin concentration	Measure the albumin concentration in ascites and serum and calculate the serum-to-ascites albumin gradient (SAAG) (serum minus ascitic albumin concentration).
	A SAAG of 11 g/L or greater indicates portal hypertension with 97% accuracy, while a SAAG of <11 g/L indicates the absence of portal hypertension.
	Causes of ascites according to the SAAG are given in Table 24.2.
Total and differential white cell count	Send a sample in an EDTA tube to the haematology laboratory for total and differential white cell count.
	In uncomplicated cirrhosis, the total white cell count is <500/mm^3 and neutrophil count <250/mm^3. Spontaneous bacterial peritonitis is associated with a neutrophil count of >250/mm^3.
	In peritoneal tuberculosis, the white cell count is usually 150–4000/mm^3, predominantly lymphocytes.
Bacterial culture	Send ascites for culture in patients with new-onset ascites or if you suspect infection (fever, abdominal pain, confusion, renal failure or acidosis)
	Inoculate aerobic and anaerobic blood culture bottles with 10 mL per bottle of ascites.
Cytology	Send a sample for cytology if you suspect malignancy or if the SAAG is <11 g/L.
	Cytology is usually positive in the presence of peritoneal metastases, but these are found in only about two-thirds of patients with ascites related to malignancy.
Other tests	Total protein
	Glucose
	LDH
	Gram stain
	Ziehl-Neelsen stain and testing for *Mycobacterium tuberculosis* DNA if suspected tuberculosis
	Amylase if suspected pancreatitis

EDTA, ethylene diaminetetra-acetic acid; LDH, lactate dehydrogenase.

Table 24.2 Causes of ascites according to the serum-to-ascites albumin gradient (SAAG).

High SAAG (≥ 11 g/L.) (associated with portal hypertension)

Cirrhosis
Alcoholic hepatitis
Hepatic outflow obstruction:
• Budd-Chiari syndrome (thrombosis of one or more of the large hepatic veins, the inferior vena cava, or both)
• Hepatic veno-occlusive disease
Cardiac ascites:
• Severe tricuspid regurgitation
• All causes of right-sided heart failure
• Constrictive pericarditis

Low SAAG (<11 g/L) (associated with peritoneal neoplasms, infection and inflammation)
Peritoneal carcinomatosis
Peritoneal tuberculosis
Pancreatitis
Serositis
Nephrotic syndrome
Chylous ascites (lymphatic vessel rupture)
Myxedema
Meig's syndrome

Diagnosis

The diagnosis of SBP is based on the finding of >250 neutrophils/mm^3 in ascitic fluid. If the neutrophil count is less than this, but there are features of sepsis, treatment should be given for SBP, pending the result of culture; if the patient is well, hold off antibiotic therapy and remeasure the cell count in 48 hours.

Management

- Treat with third-generation cephalosporin, for example cefotaxime 2 g 8-hourly IV for 5 days, followed by a quinolone PO for 5 days.
- If serum creatinine is >88 micromol/L, urea is >10.7 mmol/L, or bilirubin is >68 micromol/L, give human albumin solution 1.5 g/kg IV at diagnosis and 1 g/kg 48 h later to reduce the incidence of hepatorenal syndrome.
- Repeat diagnostic paracentesis at 48 hours: if the neutrophil count has not reduced by 25% or the patient has ongoing signs of sepsis, discuss changing the antibiotic regimen with your microbiologist.

Antibiotic prophylaxis

This is indicated for:

- Patients with cirrhosis who present with gastrointestinal bleeding (Chapters 73 and 74).
- Patients with cirrhosis and ascites, with ascitic fluid protein <10 g/L, who require hospital admission for another reason.
- Patients with cirrhosis and ascites, with ascitic fluid protein <15 g/L and:
  - Impaired renal function (serum creatinine >106 micromol/L or urea >8.9 mmol/L)
  - Low plasma sodium ≤130 mmol/L or
  - Liver failure (Child-Pugh score ≥9 and serum bilirubin ≥51 micromol/L
- Patients who have had one or more episodes of SBP, in whom the recurrence rate is up to 70% at one year. Discuss the choice of prophylaxis with a hepatologist or microbiologist.

Further reading

Hernaez R, Hamilton JP. (2016) Unexplained ascites. *Clinical Liver Disease* 7, 53–56. http://onlinelibrary.wiley .com/doi/10.1002/cld.537/full.

Pericleous M, Sarnowski A, Moore A, Fijten R, Zaman M. (2016). The clinical management of abdominal ascites, spontaneous bacterial peritonitis and hepatorenal syndrome: a review of current guidelines and recommendations. *Eur J Gastroenterol Hepatol*, 28, e10–18.

Solà E, Solé C, Ginès P. (2016) Management of uninfected and infected ascites in cirrhosis. *Liver Int* 36 (suppl 1), 109–115.

CHAPTER 25

Acute kidney injury

MARLIES OSTERMANN AND DAVID SPRIGINGS

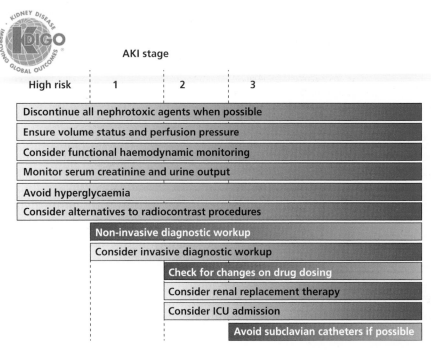

Figure 25.1 Stage-based management of acute kidney injury. Source: KDIGO Clinical Practice Guideline for Acute Kidney Injury. Kidney Int Suppl (2011). 2012 Mar; 2(1):6. Reproduced with permission of Elsevier.

Acute kidney injury (AKI), formerly known as acute renal failure, is a syndrome characterized by an abrupt (within hours to days) deterioration in renal function. It is defined by a rise in serum creatinine or reduction in urine output, or both (Box 25.1 and 25.2). AKI occurs in around 10–20% of patients admitted to hospital, and is most often due to hypovolaemia/hypotension, sepsis and nephrotoxins (Tables 25.1 and 25.2).

Acute Medicine: A Practical Guide to the Management of Medical Emergencies, Fifth Edition. Edited by David Sprigings and John B. Chambers.
© 2018 John Wiley & Sons Ltd. Published 2018 by John Wiley & Sons Ltd.

Box 25.1 Acute kidney injury (AKI).

AKI is defined by:
- A rise in serum creatinine by ≥27 µmol/L, in 48 h or less
- A >50% rise in serum creatinine from baseline, in 7 days, or
- A urine output of <0.5 mL/kg/h for >6 h.

AKI is staged by the magnitude of the rise in serum creatinine or decrease in urine output:

Stage of AKI	Serum creatinine	Urine output
1	Rise in serum creatinine ≥27 µmol/L in 48 h, or rise 1.5–1.9 times from baseline	<0.5 mL/kg/h for 6–12 h
2	Rise in serum creatinine 2.0–2.9 times from baseline	<0.5 mL/kg/h for ≥12 h
3	Rise in serum creatinine three times from baseline, or increase in serum creatinine to ≥354 µmol/L, or initiation of renal replacement therapy irrespective of serum creatinine	<0.3 mL/kg/h for ≥24 h or anuria for ≥12 h

Box 25.2 Acute kidney injury – alerts.

Contact your renal unit urgently about patients with acute kidney injury, if:
- The patient has a renal transplant or pre-existing chronic kidney disease stage 4 or 5; or
- Renal function continues to deteriorate despite correction of hypovolaemia/hypotension and removal of nephrotoxins

  or

- You suspect intrinsic renal disease (e.g. glomerulonephritis)

Priorities

Stage-based management of AKI is summarized in Figure 25.1. Consider and address potentially correctable causes or contributory factors (Tables 25.1 and 25.2):
- Obtain a full set of physiological observations.
- Review the medical record, and drug, observation and fluid balance charts.
- Make a focused clinical assessment (Table 25.3).
- Arrange urgent investigation (Table 25.4), which must include urinalysis and urine microscopy.

1 Correct hypovolaemia/hypotension
- Prompt and vigorous correction of hypovolaemia and hypotension will often reverse AKI. If there is clinically obvious hypovolaemia, give IV fluid (crystalloid or blood, as appropriate to the cause of hypovolaemia). A CVP line may be helpful (to avoid over-replacement of fluid), but the patient should be resuscitated first before this is placed.
- If the evidence for hypovolaemia is less certain, but there are no clinical signs of fluid overload, give a fluid challenge, ideally with monitoring of the CVP, especially if the JVP is difficult to assess. Target CVP is 5–10 cm water, measured from a mid-axillary line zero reference point (p. 662). Ultrasonography of the inferior vena cava is an alternative method of assessing the CVP.

Table 25.1 Causes of acute kidney injury: clinical features, typical findings on examination of the urine and confirmatory tests.

Cause of AKI	Clinical features suggesting diagnosis	Typical urinalysis/urine microscopy	Confirmatory tests
Hypovolaemia/ hypotension	Systolic BP <100 mmHg or a decrease in baseline BP of >40 mmHg or postural hypotension; low JVP	Normal urinalysis/hyaline casts	Resolution of AKI on correction of hypovolaemia/ hypotension
Sepsis	Fever or reduced body temperature (<36 °C) Clinical focus of infection	May be normal	Microbiological confirmation of infection
Nephrotoxic drugs and toxins	Exposure to known nephrotoxic drug or toxin (Table 25.2)	May be normal If there is acute tubular injury, epithelial cell casts and free renal tubular epithelial cells may be seen; eosinophiluria may be seen in drug-induced interstitial nephritis	Resolution of AKI on withdrawal of drug or toxin
Hepatorenal syndrome	Chronic or acute liver disease with liver failure and portal hypertension	Typically normal	Resolution of AKI with improvement in liver function
Diseases involving large renal vessels			
Renal artery thrombosis/ embolism/dissection	Flank pain	Mild proteinuria, haematuria	Renal artery duplex scan/ CT
Renal vein thrombosis	Background of nephrotic syndrome	Proteinuria, haematuria	Renal vein duplex scan/ CT
Diseases of small vessels and glomeruli			
Glomerulonephritis/ vasculitis	See Chapter 99 Evidence of multi-system disease	Proteinuria, haematuria	Renal biopsy
HUS/TTP	See Appendix 102.2 TTP may be associated with autoimmune disorders and with drugs	May be normal or mild proteinuria, haematuria	Renal biopsy
Severe hypertension with acute hypertensive nephrosclerosis	Severe hypertension, with retinal haemorrhages and exudates	Microscopic haematuria (75% of patients) or proteinuria	Renal biopsy
Scleroderma renal crisis (SRC)	Skin signs of scleroderma Moderate to severe hypertension, often with retinal haemorrhages and exudates	Proteinuria, if present, is usually mild The urine sediment is usually normal, with few cells or casts	Renal biopsy
Diseases of the tubulointerstitium			
Allergic interstitial nephritis	Recent drug exposure Fever, rash and arthralgia	Proteinuria White cell casts or eosinophiluria	Renal biopsy
Acute bilateral pyelonephritis	Fever, flank pain, renal tenderness	Proteinuria Pyuria Bacteriuria	Urine microscopy and culture
Urinary tract obstruction	Abdominal or flank pain	May be normal	Ultrasonography Non-contrast CT

AKI, acute kidney injury; CT, computed tomography; HUS/TTP, haemolytic uraemic syndrome/thrombocytopenic purpura; JVP, jugular venous pressure.

Table 25.2 Potentially correctable factors which may cause or contribute to acute kidney injury.

Hypovolaemia
Hypotension
Systemic sepsis
Urinary tract infection (especially of a single kidney)
Heart failure
Liver failure
Accelerated-phase hypertension
Hypercalcaemia
Urinary tract obstruction
Nephrotoxic drugs and toxins

Nephrotoxic drugs/exposures	Exogenous toxins	Endogenous toxins
Radiocontrast agents	*Amanita phalloides*	Free haemoglobin (intravascular haemolysis)
Aminoglycosides	Ethylene glycol	Free myoglobin (rhabdomyolysis (Appendix 25.1))
Amphotericin	Paracetamol poisoning	Free light chains (myeloma)
NSAIDs	Salicylate poisoning	
β-lactam antibiotics Sulphonamides		
Aciclovir		
Methotrexate		
Cisplatin		
Ciclosporin		
Tacrolimus		
ACE-inhibitors		
Angiotensin-receptor blockers		

ACE-inhibitor, angiotensin-converting-enzyme inhibitor.

- If the systolic BP remains <90 mmHg despite correction or exclusion of hypovolaemia, search for and treat other causes of hypotension, of which sepsis is the most likely (Chapter 35). If the BP remains low, inotropic-vasopressor therapy will be needed (p. 13 Table 2.7).

2 Search for and treat sepsis
- Suspect sepsis if AKI is associated with fever or reduced body temperature (<36°C), or there is an obvious focus of infection (e.g. signs of pneumonia or recent instrumentation of urinary or biliary tract). Bear in mind that many patients with neutropenic sepsis (Chapter 101) have no detectable clinical focus. Obtain a surgical opinion if you suspect an abdominal or pelvic source.
- The diagnosis and management of sepsis is described in Chapter 35. Start antibiotic therapy as soon as blood has been taken for culture and within one hour. Choice of antibiotic therapy should take account of the source of sepsis, if known, whether the infection is community or hospital acquired, results of previous isolates from the patient and the local pattern of antibiotic resistance.

3 Exclude urinary tract obstruction
- Ultrasonography should be performed within 24 h if obstruction is suspected or there is no identified cause of AKI. It should be performed as soon as possible in case of suspected pyonephrosis or obstruction of a solitary kidney. Non-contrast CT is an alternative to ultrasonography.
- AKI beginning in hospital is rarely due to urinary tract obstruction, once bladder outflow obstruction has been excluded by catheterization. The hallmark of obstruction is dilatation of the urinary tract above the obstruction, although this is not an invariable feature.

4 Treat immediate complications of AKI

Severe hyperkalaemia

- If there are ECG changes of hyperkalaemia, give 10 mL of 10% calcium gluconate 10% IV.
- If serum bicarbonate is <22 mmol/L and there is no fluid overload, give 500 mL of 1.26% sodium bicarbonate IV over 1–2 h.
- If plasma potassium is >6.5 mmol/L or there are ECG changes, give insulin 10 units in 50 mL of 50% glucose over 15 min; salbutamol 10 mg by nebulizer may also help (these measures will reduce plasma potassium for <4 h).
- Stop potassium supplements or any drugs (e.g. ACE-inhibitors, potassium-retaining diuretics) which may be contributing to hyperkalaemia.
- If renal function is not improving despite vigorous management of correctable factors, renal replacement therapy will be needed; discuss this with your renal unit or ICU early before any life-threatening complications of AKI occur.

Pulmonary oedema

- Sit the patient up and give oxygen 60–100%, aiming for an oxygen saturation >94%.
- Give furosemide 80 mg IV.
- If systolic BP is >110 mmHg, start a nitrate infusion.
- Look for underlying heart disease; investigation should include an ECG and echocardiogram.
- Further management of pulmonary oedema is described in Chapter 47.

Further management

Monitoring and supportive care in AKI is summarized in Table 25.5. Three common scenarios are encountered:

Corrected hypovolaemia/hypotension, with improving renal function

- Management is that of the underlying disorder, taking care to avoid hypovolaemia and nephrotoxic drugs (Table 25.2).
- Make sure all drug dosages are adjusted appropriately: consult the section on Prescribing in renal impairment in the *British National Formulary*.

Persisting/worsening AKI despite correction of hypovolaemia/hypotension and removal of nephrotoxins

- These patients should be discussed with your renal unit and/or intensive care unit. They need a definitive diagnosis, and may require renal replacement therapy. Indications for renal replacement therapy are summarized in Table 25.6.
- After haemodynamic resuscitation and removal of nephrotoxins, no specific therapy has been shown to be protective in AKI. Low-dose dopamine is not effective. Loop diuretics should only be used if there is fluid-overload.

Suspected urinary tract obstruction

- Ask advice from a urologist. A bladder catheter should be inserted if there is bladder outflow obstruction. Percutaneous nephrostomy drainage may be indicated if there is ureteric obstruction.

Table 25.3 Focused assessment in acute kidney injury.

Element	Comment
Has there been anuria, oliguria or polyuria?	Anuria is seen in severe hypotension or complete urinary tract obstruction. It is more rarely due to bilateral renal artery occlusion (e.g. with aortic dissection), renal cortical necrosis or necrotizing glomerular disease.
	Assume that anuria is due to bilateral urinary obstruction until proven otherwise.
Has the blood pressure been normal, high or low and, if low, for how long?	Hypertension and AKI: accelerated-phase hypertension, aortic dissection, pre-eclampsia, scleroderma renal crisis.
Is hypovolaemia likely?	Has there been haemorrhage, vomiting, diarrhoea, recent surgery or the use of diuretics? Are there signs of fluid depletion (tachycardia, low JVP with flat neck veins, hypotension or postural hypotension)?
Are there signs of fluid overload?	Signs include high JVP, triple cardiac rhythm, hypertension, lung crackles, pleural effusions, ascites and peripheral oedema.
Is systemic sepsis or urosepsis possible?	Are there predisposing factors? What are the results of recent blood, urine and other cultures?
Is there a past history of renal or urinary tract disease?	Are there previous biochemistry results to establish when renal function was last normal? Over how long has renal function been deteriorating? Patients with a renal transplant or pre-existing chronic kidney disease stage 4 or 5 should be discussed urgently with your renal unit.
Is there heart disease?	Acute heart failure (including decompensated chronic heart failure, Chapter 48) results in renal hypoperfusion or renal congestion, both of which may cause acute kidney injury. Patients with heart disease who have radiological procedures with administration of contrast are at risk of contrast nephropathy.
	Commonly used medications for heart disease (e.g. diuretics, ACE-inhibitors), may impair renal function, particularly in combination with other factors (e.g. concomitant administration of NSAIDs, sepsis).
	AKI may worsen heart function by mechanisms including hypertension, electrolyte derangements, acidosis, sodium and water retention, and the generation of cytokines.
Is there known arterial disease?	Peripheral arterial disease (commonly associated with atherosclerotic renal artery stenosis). Cardiac catheterization via femoral artery, with resulting cholesterolembolization.
Is there liver disease?	Hepatorenal syndrome, AKI from sepsis, paracentesis-induced hypovolaemia, diuretic-induced hypovolaemia, lactulose-induced hypovolaemia, cardiomyopathy, or any combination of these factors.
	Treatment of the trigger of deterioration and avoidance of hypovolaemia (preferably by albumin administration) can help to decrease the incidence of acute kidney injury. Terlipressin can improve glomerular filtration rate.
Is there diabetes or other multisystem disorder which can involve the kidneys?	Don't forget infective endocarditis and myeloma as causes of renal failure.
Has the patient been exposed to any nephrotoxic drugs or toxins?	Nephrotoxic drugs and toxins are summarized in Table 25.2. Consider occupational exposure to toxins.
Is there purpura?	AKI with purpura may be due to sepsis complicated by disseminated intravascular coagulation; meningococcal sepsis; thrombotic thrombocytopenic purpura; haemolytic-uraemic syndrome; Henoch-Schoenlein purpura and other vasculitides.
Is there jaundice?	AKI with jaundice may be due to hepatorenal syndrome; paracetamol poisoning; severe heart failure; severe sepsis; leptospirosis; incompatible blood transfusion; haemolytic–uraemic syndrome.

ACE-inhibitor, angiotensin-converting-enzyme inhibitor; AKI, acute kidney injury; NSAIDs, non-steroidal anti-inflammatory drugs.

Table 25.4 Investigation in acute kidney injury.

Needed urgently in all patients

Serum creatinine, urea, sodium, potassium, calcium and bicarbonate

Blood glucose

Arterial blood gases and lactate if venous bicarbonate low or there is evidence of severe hypoperfusion or sepsis

Full blood count

Coagulation screen, blood film, reticulocyte count and LDH if the patient has purpura or jaundice, or low platelet count

Blood culture if sepsis possible or cannot be excluded

Urine stick test for glucose, blood and protein

Urine protein to creatinine ratio if proteinuria detected by stick test

Urine microscopy and culture

ECG

Chest X-ray

Ultrasound of the kidneys and urinary tract if the cause of AKI is not known or obstruction of the urinary tract suspected

For later analysis

Full biochemical profile, including urate

Creatine kinase if suspected rhabdomyolysis (urine stick test positive for blood, but no red blood cells on microscopy; see Appendix 25.1)

Erythrocyte sedimentation rate and C-reactive protein

Serum and urine protein electrophoresis

Serum complement and other immunological tests (antinuclear antibodies, antineutrophil cytoplasmic antibodies, antiglomerular basement membrane antibodies) if suspected acute glomerulonephritis/vasculitis

Ultrasound of kidneys and urinary tract if not already done

Echocardiography if clinical cardiac abnormality, major ECG abnormality, or suspected endocarditis

Serology for HIV and hepatitis B and C if clinically indicated or dialysis is needed

Table 25.5 Criteria for initiation of renal replacement therapy in acute kidney injury.

Anuria (no or negligible urine output for >6 h)

Severe oliguria (urine output <200 mL over 12 h) and fluid overload

Hyperkalaemia (potassium concentration >6.5 mmol/L) and not responding to medical treatment

Severe metabolic acidosis (pH <7.2 despite normal or low partial pressure of carbon dioxide in arterial blood) not responding to supportive treatment

Volume-overload (especially pulmonary oedema unresponsive to diuretics)

Severe uraemia (serum urea concentration >30 mmol/L) or specific complications of uraemia (e.g. encephalopathy, pericarditis, neuropathy)

AKI due to dialyzable toxins/drugs

Table 25.6 Monitoring and supportive care in acute kidney injury.

Monitoring

Control hypertension/hypotension.

Correct electrolyte abnormalities.

Control acidemia.

Avoid fluid overload.

Monitor patients closely for cardiac complications.

Fluid balance

Keep the patient euvolaemic: avoid intravascular hypo- and hypervolaemia.

If euvolaemic: restrict the daily fluid intake to 500 mL plus the previous day's measured losses (urine, nasogastric drainage, etc.), allowing more if the patient is febrile (500 mL for each °C of fever).

The patient's fluid status should be assessed twice daily (by weighing and fluid balance chart) and the next 12 hours' fluids adjusted appropriately.

Diet

Aim for an energy intake 20–30 kcal/kg/d.

Restrict sodium and potassium content to <50 mmol/day.

Restrict dietary phosphate to <800 mg/day.

Protein intake should not be restricted.

Consider enteral or parenteral nutrition if renal failure is prolonged or the patient is hypercatabolic.

Potassium

Stop potassium supplements and potassium-retaining drugs.

Restrict dietary potassium intake to <50 mmol/day.

If plasma potassium rises above 6 mmol/L despite dietary restriction, start calcium resonium, which may be given orally (15 g 8-hourly PO) or by retention enema (30 g) (high risk of constipation, therefore add laxatives).

Infection

Patients with AKI are vulnerable to infection, especially pneumonia and urinary tract infection.

Urinary catheters and vascular lines should be removed wherever possible.

If the patient develops fever or unexplained hypotension, search for a focus of infection, send blood and urine for culture and start antibiotic therapy to cover both Gram-positive and negative organisms (e.g. third-generation cephalosporin).

Gastrointestinal bleeding

Gastrointestinal bleeding occurs in 10–30% of patients with AKI.

Start prophylactic therapy with a proton pump inhibitor or H2-receptor antagonist.

Drugs and contrast media

Make sure all drug dosages are adjusted appropriately: consult the section on Prescribing in renal impairment in the *British National Formulary*.

Appendix 25.1 Rhabdomyolysis

Element	Comment
Definition	Syndrome resulting from skeletal muscle injury with release of myocyte contents into plasma
Causes	
Traumatic causes	Trauma
	Crush injury
	Electrical injury (Chapter 109)
Non-traumatic causes	
Infection	Bacterial pyomyositis
	Legionella infection
	Viral infections
	Falciparum malaria
Electrolyte abnormalities	Hypokalaemia (Chapter 86)
	Hypocalcaemia (Chapter 87)
	Hypophosphataemia (Chapter 89)
	Hyponatraemia (Chapter 85)
Immune-mediated	Dermatomyositis
	Pyomyositis
Drugs	Medications: antipsychotics, statins, SSRI, lithium, colchicines, antihistamines
	Non-prescription drugs: heroin, cocaine, methadone
Metabolic disorders	Myophosphorylase deficiency
	Phosphofructase deficiency
	Carnitine palmitoyltransferase deficiency
Others	Status epilepticus (Chapter 16)
	Coma of any cause with muscle compression
	Hypothermia (Chapter 107)
	Diabetic ketoacidosis (Chapter 83)
	Hyperosmolar hyperglycaemic state (Chapter 84)
	Neuroleptic malignant syndrome (Appendix 69.2)
	Malignant hyperthermia
	Drowning (Chapter 108)
	Prolonged strenuous exercise
Investigation and management	
Biochemical markers	Raised plasma creatine kinase: levels >50,000 units/L are associated with an incidence of acute kidney injury of >50%
	Myoglobinuria: myoglobin gives positive result on stick test of urine for blood
Complications	Hypovolemia due to extravasation of fluid into muscle
	Acute kidney injury from hypovolemia and renal tubular obstruction, tubular damage and renal vasoconstriction
	Metabolic effects of muscle injury: hyperkalaemia, hypocalcaemia, hyperphosphataemia, hyperuricaemia
Management of severe rhabdomyolysis	Diagnose and treat underlying cause
	Vigorous fluid resuscitation with crystalloid
	Transfer the patient to high-dependency unit
	Put in a bladder catheter to monitor urine output and, in patients over 60 or with cardiac disease, a central venous catheter so that central venous pressure can be monitored to guide fluid replacement and avoid fluid overload
	Manage acute kidney injury along standard lines

Further reading

Floege J, Amann K (2016) Primary glomerulonephritides. *Lancet* 387, 2036–2048.

Kidney Disease: Improving Global Outcomes (KDIGO) Acute Kidney Injury Work Group. KDIGO (2012) Clinical Practice Guideline for Acute Kidney Injury. *Kidney Int* 2 (suppl 1), 1–138.

National Institute for Health and Care Excellence (2013) Acute kidney injury: prevention, detection and management. Clinical guideline (CG169). https://www.nice.org.uk/guidance/cg169?unlid=429931086201692925215.

Skin and Musculoskeletal

CHAPTER 26

Acute rash

Nemesha Desai and Ruth Lamb

'Rash' is a non-specific term for any abnormal skin finding:
- Acute rash develops over <4 weeks and is described by morphology and distribution (Box 26.1 and Figure 26.1). Acute rashes account for 3% of emergency department presentations. Causes are given in Table 26.1.
- Sub-acute rash develops over 4–6 weeks, Chronic rash is present for >6 weeks. Sometimes patients report itchiness. It is important to clarify if a rash preceded the itch or whether the eruption seen results from scratching a generalized itch with another cause.

Priorities

1 Assessment is summarised in Table 26.2 and urgent investigation in Table 26.3.
- Acute erythroderma, a dermatological emergency, is defined as >90% inflammation of the skin surface. Assess the cardiovascular system. See Chapter 96 for management.
- Examination of the skin includes mucosal membranes (oral/genital), the nails and scalp and must be performed in good lighting. Start with the hands; then the extensor surfaces of the elbows, moving on to the scalp, face, mucosal surfaces (eyes/mouth) followed by general and closer inspection of the trunk, limbs, other joints and genital skin if relevant. Assessment of morphology and distribution will inform the differential diagnosis (Figures 26.1 and 26.2).
- Additional examination depending on clinical suspicion includes examination for lymphadenopathy (seen in infection, inflammatory and malignant causes of rash), and other systems as appropriate, for example toxic erythema with pneumonia, splenomegaly with EBV infection.

2 **Address haemodynamic compromise**: fluid and electrolyte imbalance (see Chapters 1 and 2)
3 **Pain control:** erythematous, eroded skin is painful, and patients may require opioid analgesia.
4 **Assess for (bacterial and viral swabs) and treat suspected infection** (primary or superadded), according to local antibiotic policies.
5 **Stop any implicated drugs**.
6 **Seek dermatology advice** if the diagnosis or management are uncertain. Involvement of mucosal surfaces may require review by ENT/Ophthalmology to advise on supportive care (HSV/VZV/SJS).

Acute Medicine: A Practical Guide to the Management of Medical Emergencies, Fifth Edition. Edited by David Sprigings and John B. Chambers.
© 2018 John Wiley & Sons Ltd. Published 2018 by John Wiley & Sons Ltd.

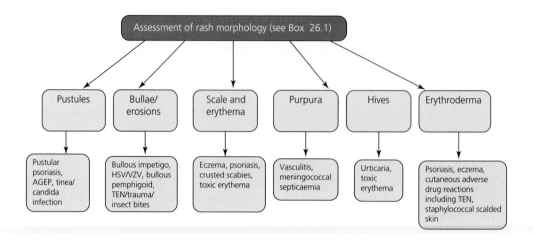

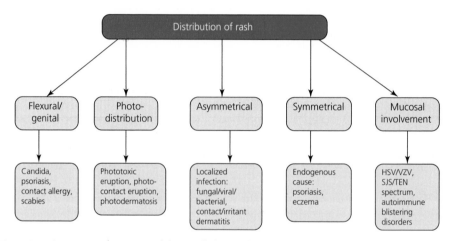

Figure 26.1 Assessment of an acute rash by morphology and distribution.

Box 26.1 Definition of skin abnormalities.

Skin abnormality	Definition
Macule	Flat skin lesion <10 mm diameter
Patch	Flat skin lesion >10 mm diameter
Papule	A raised/palpable lesion <10 mm diameter
Plaque	A raised/palpable lesion >20 mm diameter
Nodule	A larger, firm papule >10 mm diameter
Vesicle	A papule containing clear serous fluid <5 mm diameter
Bulla	A larger vesicle >5 mm diameter
Pustule	A papule containing purulent fluid
Wheal	An oedematous, erythematous elevation in the skin, often round in shape
Purpura	Non-blanching red-purple discolouration of the skin. May be palpable or non-palpable.

Table 26.1 Common eruptions seen acutely in the emergency department and in inpatients.

Aetiology	Localized	Widespread
Infectious:		
• **Any**	Cutaneous vasculitis	Toxic erythema
• **Viral**	Varicella zoster (VZV)	Eczema herpeticum (HSV)
	Eczema herpeticum	VZV
		Epstein Barr viral infection (+/- penicillin)
		Measles
		HIV seroconversion
		Erythema multiforme
• **Bacterial**	Impetigo	Meningococcemia
	Erysipelas	Staphylococcal scalded skin
	Cellulitis	Staphylococcal/Streptococcal toxic shock syndrome
	Necrotizing fasciitis	
• **Rickettsial**		Spotted fevers/typhus group
• **Treponemal**		Secondary syphilis
• **Other**	Tinea infection	Crusted scabies
Cutaneous adverse drug reactions	Cutaneous vasculitis	Stevens Johnson syndrome (SJS)
		Toxic epidermal necrolysis (TEN)
	Toxic erythema	Drug reaction with eosinophilia and systemic symptoms (DRESS)
		Acute generalized exanthematous pustulosis (AGEP)
		Phototoxic drug eruption
Inflammatory and autoimmune	Pompholyx	Infected exacerbation of atopic eczema
	Pyoderma gangrenosum	Psoriasis (including pustular variants)
		Pityriasis rubra pilaris
		Bullous pemphigoid
		Cutaneous lupus
Allergic		Contact dermatitis
		Urticaria +/− angioedema (see Chapter 27, Urticaria and angioedema)
Malignancy		Cutaneous T cell lymphoma and Sezary syndrome

Criteria for escalation of care

- Cutaneous adverse drug reactions lie on a spectrum and may progress over days from mild erythema to toxic epidermal necrolysis. Close monitoring is required. See Chapter 96 for further guidance.
- Patients with eczema herpeticum are at risk of aseptic/viral meningitis: assess frequently. If inflammation is widespread and/or infection affects periorbital skin then the patient is likely to require IV aciclovir and ophthalmology input.
- Any erythrodermic patient is at risk of haemodynamic decompensation and should be monitored in a high dependency unit.

Table 26.2 Focused assessment of the patient with acute rash.

	Key points to cover in history	Differential diagnosis
History of presenting complaint	Itch	Atopic eczema, scabies, contact dermatitis, urticaria
	Pain	Cutaneous adverse drug reaction, TEN, VZV, eczema herpeticum, unstable psoriasis
	Mucosal involvement? For example gritty eyes, mouth/genital ulceration?	SJS/TEN spectrum, HSV/VZV, Autoimmune bullous disorders
	Site of onset: Flexural, Extensor Dematomal	 Atopic eczema, flexural psoriasis Psoriasis VZV
	Associated systemic symptoms: Unwell in addition to rash? And/or pyrexia?	Infection/inflammatory/cutaneous Adverse drug reaction
	Joint symptoms	Inflammatory/autoimmune skin conditions, for example psoriasis, Behçet's disease, adult onset Still's disease.
	History of inflammatory skin condition	Inflammatory conditions: atopic eczema, psoriasis
Past medical history	Atopy (asthma/hayfever)	Atopic eczema
Family history	Inflammatory skin conditions	Atopic eczema, psoriasis
Medications	New medicines in the last 3–6 months: in particular antibiotics/ antiepileptics Dosage increase in existing drugs	Cutaneous adverse drug reactions
Social history	Foreign travel Occupational history Social circumstances	Tropical infections, phototoxic/sensitive eruptions Contact/irritant dermatitis Nursing home/institution: scabies At risk individuals: HIV seroconversion, secondary syphilis

Table 26.3 Urgent investigation in acute rash.

Swabs (bacterial and viral (VZV/HSV)) from eroded, crusted areas, blisters and pustules (use a sterile needle to burst vesicle/pustule)
Skin scrapings if fungal infection suspected
Blood culture if febrile
Full blood count (neutrophilia: infection/inflammation, eosinophilia: DRESS, allergic/atopic disease)
C-reactive protein
Blood glucose
Sodium, potassium, urea and creatinine
Liver function tests (deranged in cutaneous adverse drug reactions, erythroderma from any cause)
Urinalysis if vasculitic eruption suspected
Consider skin biopsy: consult Dermatology

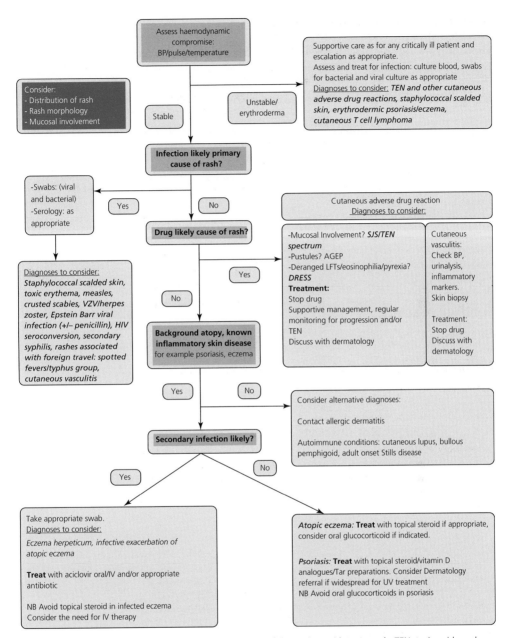

Figure 26.2 Approach to diagnosis and initial management of the patient with acute rash. TEN, toxic epidermal necrolysis; VZV, varicella-zoster virus; HIV, human immunodeficiency virus; SJS, Stevens-Johnson syndrome; AGEP, acute generalized exanthematous pustulosis; DRESS, drug reaction with eosinophilia and systemic symptoms; UV, ultraviolet.

Further management

Specific treatment is guided by the diagnosis. Often when a rash is seen in the early stages it can be difficult to diagnose with certainty. If the patient is systemically well, one approach is 'watch and wait'. In this situation, however, it is prudent to attempt to exclude exogenous causes (infection/drug) first and then treat symptomatically.

General principles of management include:
- Use of emollients to restore skin barrier function.
- Avoidance of soap/fragranced products that can further impair the skin barrier; use of soap substitutes.
- Avoid topical steroids and occlusion in patients with infected (bacterial/viral) skin.
- Consider early NG feeding to maintain protein losses, if patient has mucosal erosions preventing normal oral intake.
- Consider catheter insertion if patient compromised or has involvement of mucosal surfaces making passing urine painful.
- Photo-protection: for conditions exacerbated by ultraviolet light.
- Reassurance and psychological support.

Further reading

Baibergenova A, Shear NH. (2011) Skin conditions that bring patients to emergency departments. *Arch Dermatol* 147, 118–120.

CHAPTER 27

Urticaria and angioedema

Alexandra Croom

Urticaria (nettle rash, hives) arises from mast cell degranulation in the skin. Angioedema (tissue swelling) can accompany urticaria and is due to mast cell degranulation in deeper tissues. The clinical features of urticaria and angioedema are described in Box 27.1 and management in Box 27.2.

- Angioedema can cause life-threatening upper airway obstruction (Chapter 59) and airway management should be a priority (Chapter 112).
- Urticarial vasculitis may resemble urticaria in appearance but has distinct clinical features.
- Isolated angioedema can also occur without urticaria and independent of mast cell degranulation (refer to page 180).

Box 27.1 Clinical features of urticaria, angioedema and urticarial vasculitis.

Urticaria	**Weals**
	• Itchy, raised, central pallor with surrounding erythema
	• Variable size – pin prick to dinner plate
	• Single or multiple
	• Local or generalized
	• Individually may last few minutes to around 24 h
	• Rash may move around the body (flitting)
	• On resolution skin returns to normal (unless damaged by excoriation)
Angioedema	**Swelling**
	• Discrete swelling(s) – overlying skin may be normal in appearance or erythematous
	• May occur anywhere but favours distensible skin (eyelids, lips and genitalia); may involve mucosal surfaces (including oropharynx and gut)
	• Painful (due to tissue distension) rather than itchy
	• Resolution may take several days
Urticarial vasculitis	**Weals**
	• Tender rather than itchy
	• Individual weals may persist for days
	• Leaves bruising or discolouration on resolution
	• May be confined to skin or be part of a systemic process

Acute Medicine: A Practical Guide to the Management of Medical Emergencies, Fifth Edition. Edited by David Sprigings and John B. Chambers.
© 2018 John Wiley & Sons Ltd. Published 2018 by John Wiley & Sons Ltd.

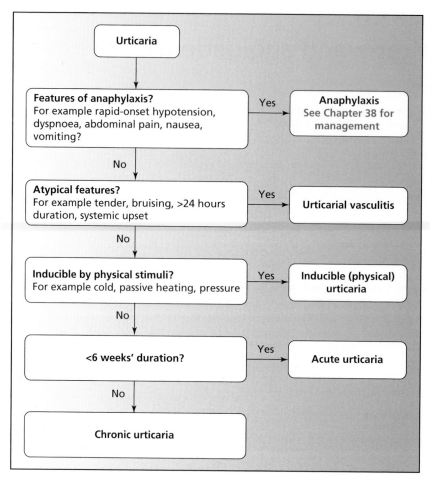

Figure 27.1 Assessment of urticaria.

Urticaria

For diagnostic purposes it is helpful to divide urticaria into two groups:
- Acute: symptoms of less than six weeks' duration
- Chronic: symptoms more or less daily for six weeks or more

The underlying causes of each group are different (Table 27.1). No cause is identified (idiopathic) in 50% of acute urticaria and 98% of chronic urticaria; chronic urticaria is rarely IgE mediated (but often perceived as being so).

Priorities

1 Search for the cause

Urticaria is a symptom rather than a diagnosis. Although most urticaria is idiopathic, an underlying cause may become apparent on clinical assessment (Table 27.2, Figure 27.1). Some patterns of symptoms are typical, for example the urticaria in an IgE mediated reaction is of rapid onset after

Box 27.2 Alert.

Angioedema can cause life-threatening upper airway obstruction (Chapter 59); early recognition and airway management should be a priority (Chapter 112).

If airway obstruction present or imminent alert anaesthetist; consider intervention early as advanced laryngeal oedema will distort anatomy and make intubation difficult.

If features of anaphylaxis are present (Chapter 38**)**

Give adrenaline 500 μgm IM into anterolateral thigh using a 23G needle (blue – length 25 mm); in morbidly obese use 21 G needle (green – length 38 mm) or administer to calf. Repeat every five minutes as needed.

Give hydrocortisone 200 mg IV and chlorphenamine 10 mg IV.

If features of anaphylaxis are absent
If mast cell mediated

Give hydrocortisone 200 mg IV and chlorphenamine 10 mg IV

Consider nebulized adrenaline (5 mL of 1:1000 solution)

Continue to observe for progression or biphasic reactions

If related to angiotensin-converting-enzyme inhibitor (ACEi)

Consider treatment with icatibant 30 mg SC

If hereditary angioedema (HAE) or acquired angioedema (AAE) known or likely

C1 inhibitor concentrate 20 units/kg (round up to nearest 500 units) IV slow infusion (1 mL/min)

Icatibant 30 mg SC (maximum 3 doses in 24 hours)

Discuss with on-call immunologist; consider repeat dose if no improvement within 30–60 min

exposure (within minutes) and peaks within two hours. Urticaria that evolves over hours or days is not allergic.

The investigations required for urticaria depend on its type and the suspected underlying cause.

In acute urticaria investigations are normally unnecessary other than for the identification of allergens in suspected IgE-mediated reactions (e.g. skin prick testing and/or spIgE assays (RASTs)).

Table 27.1 Causes of urticaria.

Acute urticaria	
IgE mediated	For example food allergy, drugs, latex
Drugs	For example betalactam antibiotics, NSAIDs
Infection	
Idiopathic	
Chronic urticaria	
Inducible (physical) urticaria	For example cold, exercise, solar, pressure, delayed vibration, aquagenic
Chronic infection	For example *H. pylori*, cholecystitis, parasitic infestation, hepatitis B and C, dental caries and gingivitis
Autoimmune	Antibody directed at FcεR1α or IgE on mast cells
	Thyroid autoimmunity (patient usually euthyroid)
Stress	
Miscellaneous	Urticaria pigmentosa
	CAPS (cryopyrin-associated autoinflammatory syndrome)
	Dietary pseudoallergens
Spontaneous (idiopathic)	

Table 27.2 Focused assessment in urticaria.

Duration and frequency of symptoms
Provoking factors
Relationship to food
Use of medications – prescribed, over the counter and naturopathic – regular and intermittent
Recent infective illness and/or vaccinations
Use of recreational drugs in particular cannabis
Comorbidities
Foreign travel
Occupation
Relationship to menses
Stress

These are usually deferred until after the acute event and done in specialist clinics. In chronic spontaneous urticaria, testing should be determined by the history and clinical findings, but as a minimum an FBC and ESR/CRP should be performed (as a screen for underlying inflammation as a driver for the urticaria).

Laboratory testing is not normally required for physical urticaria, with the exception of cold urticaria, which may be associated with the presence of cryoglobulins or cold agglutinins.

If a trigger is identified or suspected remove it and avoid it in the future. Where there is an underlying condition 'driving' the urticaria, treatment of that will be required before there is clinical improvement.

2 Give treatment

Antihistamines

These are the mainstay of treatment. Where rapid symptom control is required, for example anaphylaxis, use chlorphenamine 10 mg IV. Otherwise chlorphenamine (and other first-generation antihistamines) should, where possible, be avoided as it can cause sedation, and confusion and falls in the elderly. Second-generation antihistamines, for example cetirizine, loratidine and fexofenadine are mostly well tolerated. The onset of action of oral antihistamines is around 20–25 min.

Higher than licensed doses (e.g. cetirizine 10 mg 6–12-hourly) are recommended for chronic urticaria not responding to conventional doses.

Chlorphenamine is the antihistamine of first choice for pregnant women; loratidine is second choice and should be used if excessive sedation is a problem.

Corticosteroids

Corticosteroids may be used, particularly if angioedema dominates the clinical picture or urticaria does not immediately come under control with antihistamines. Short courses should be used (prednisolone 30–40 mg daily for 5–7 days). Avoid protracted courses (>2 weeks) as tachyphylaxis will result in diminishing efficacy and increasing adverse side effects. Specialist referral is required if steroid requirements persist.

There is no role for topical corticosteroids in urticaria.

Isolated angioedema

Angioedema that occurs without coexistent urticaria (either simultaneously or in the very recent past) is usually not due to mast cell degranulation and consequently responds poorly to antihistamines and corticosteroids. Causes are given in Table 27.3; most cases are idiopathic. Key features from the history are summarized in Table 27.4.

If urticaria is absent, the C1-inhibitor level and functional assay and complement levels should be checked.

Table 27.3 Causes of isolated angioedema.

Cause	Comment
Hereditary angioedema – type I, II and III	20% arise from spontaneous mutation
Acquired angioedema	Associated with lymphoproliferative and autoimmune conditions
Drugs	Angiotensin-converting-enzyme inhibitors
	Non-steroidal anti-inflammatory drugs
	Oral contraceptives
Idiopathic	

Table 27.4 Focused assessment in angioedema.

Presence/absence of urticaria (this episode or recently)
Speed of onset and duration
Sites affected by swelling
Symptoms (voice change, stridor with laryngeal swelling; vomiting and abdominal pain with gut involvement)
Precipating factors (drugs, trauma, menses, infection, stress)
Number of previous episodes
Age of onset
Family history
Response to treatment
General health and comorbidities

Hereditary angioedema (HAE)

This is due to low or dysfunctional C1-inhibitor. Clinical features suggestive of this group of conditions include:

• Repeated episodes of angioedema developing from childhood/adolescence
• Triggered by trauma, stress, OCP, menses and infection
• Non-painful, non-itchy swelling developing over a few hours and lasting 3–5 days
• Life-threatening laryngeal obstruction (30% mortality rate)
• Abdominal symptoms – vomiting, abdominal pain, hypotension, ascites; may be confused with acute abdomen

Acute episodes should be treated with plasma derived or recombinant human C1- inhibitor concentrate or icatibant (a bradykinin B2 receptor antagonist); supportive management of the airway may be necessary. FFP should only be used if none of these are available and patients should be counselled about risk of transmission of blood-borne disease. Androgens and antifibrinolytics are used long term for prophylaxis but have no role acutely.

Acquired angioedema (AAE)

This occurs in the context of autoimmune or lymphoproliferative disease. C1 inhibitor production is normal but functional activity is lost either due to increased catabolism of C1 inhibitor (type 1) or due to an autoantibody directed at C1 inhibitor (type 2). In contrast to HAE there is no family history and the onset is from middle age. AAE may improve as the underlying condition is treated. Acute episodes with life-threatening airway obstruction are rare but should be treated as per HAE.

Angiotensin-converting-enzyme inhibitor (ACEi) – associated angioedema

ACEi drugs may be a primary cause of angioedema or make coexisting angioedema worse. In the primary type, swelling is characteristically confined to the head; those of West African descent, women and smokers are at increased risk. The onset of swelling can be from months to years after initiation of treatment and can persist for several months after discontinuation of therapy. A switch to an angiotensin receptor blocking agent is normally well tolerated. Treatment is usually supportive but icatibant can be used if life-threatening airway obstruction occurs.

Further reading

Powell RJ, Leech SC, Till S, Huber PAJ, Nasser SM, Clark AT. (2015) BSACI guideline for the management of chronic urticaria and angioedema. *Clinical & Experimental Allergy* 45, 547–565. http://onlinelibrary.wiley.com/doi/10.1111/cea.12494/full.

CHAPTER 28

Acute arthritis

Kᴇʜɪɴᴅᴇ Sᴜɴᴍʙᴏʏᴇ

Arthralgia refers to joint pain without swelling, while arthritis signifies joint pain with swelling. In acute mono-arthritis, exclusion of septic arthritis is the immediate priority. Acute oligo- or polyarthritis has a broad differential diagnosis (Table 28.1), and if it has persisted >6 weeks, is unlikely to resolve spontaneously and needs urgent referral to a rheumatologist. Assessment of the patient with acute arthritis is summarized in Figure 28.1.

Table 28.1 Causes of acute arthritis.

Cause	Monoarthritis	Usually oligoarthritis (2–4 joints)	Usually polyarthritis (5 or more joints)
Common	Gout	Ankylosing spondylitis	Rheumatoid arthritis
	Pseudogout		Systemic lupus erythematosus
	Septic arthritis	Inflammatory bowel disease	
	Trauma*		Viral diseases (e.g. rubella, hepatitis B and C, infectious mononucleosis)
	Haemarthrosis secondary to warfarin anticoagulation	Reactive arthritis following gut or genitourinary infection	
	Flare of osteoarthritis (overuse or minor trauma)	Psoriatic arthritis	
		Endocarditis (acute synovitis or tenosynovitis)	
Uncommon or rare	Osteonecrosis	Sarcoidosis	Post-streptococcal infection
	Pigmented villonodular synovitis	Whipple disease	
			Leukaemia
			Vasculitis
	Tuberculosis		Syphilis
	Haemophilia		Adult Still's disease
	Palindromic rheumatism		Familial Mediterranean fever

* Causing internal derangement, haemarthrosis or fracture, or acute synovitis from penetrating injury.

Acute Medicine: A Practical Guide to the Management of Medical Emergencies, Fifth Edition. Edited by David Sprigings and John B. Chambers.
© 2018 John Wiley & Sons Ltd. Published 2018 by John Wiley & Sons Ltd.

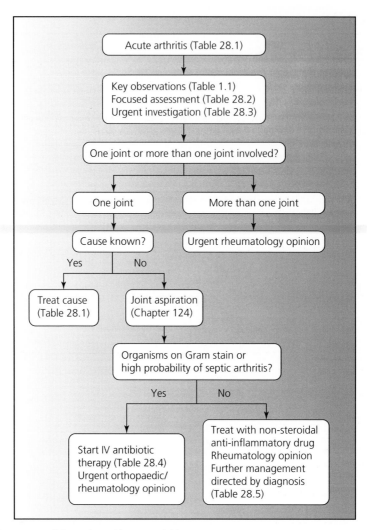

Figure 28.1 Assessment of the patient with acute arthritis.

Table 28.2 Focused assessment of acute arthritis.

History

- Duration and time course of arthritis and other symptoms (e.g. fever, rash, diarrhoea, urethritis, uveitis).
- Known arthritis or prosthetic joint?
- Previous similar attacks of arthritis?
- History of trauma?
- Possible septic arthritis? Septic arthritis usually follows a bacteraemia (e.g. from IV drug use) in a patient at risk because of rheumatoid arthritis, the presence of a prosthetic joint or immunocompromise.
- Risk of gonococcal arthritis?
- Other illness?
- Current medication

Examination

- Key observations plus systematic examination.
- Pattern of joint involvement: monoarthritis, oligoarthritis (two to four joints) or polyarthritis (five joints or more) (see Table 28.1).
- Arthritis or periarticular inflammation (bursitis, tendinitis or cellulitis)? Painful limitation of movement of the joint suggests arthritis.
- Extra-articular signs (e.g. fever, rash, mouth ulcers, anterior uveitis, urethritis).

Table 28.3 Urgent investigation in acute arthritis.

- Joint aspiration (Chapter 124)
- X-ray joint for baseline and to exclude osteomyelitis
- Blood glucose
- Creatinine and electrolytes
- Liver function tests
- Full blood count
- Erythrocyte sedimentation rate and C-reactive protein
- Viral serology if indicated
- Blood culture (×2)
- Urine stick test, microscopy and culture
- Swab of urethra, cervix and anorectum if gonococcal infection is possible

Table 28.4 Initial antibiotic therapy for suspected septic arthritis.

Organisms on Gram stain	Antibiotic therapy (IV, high dose)	
	Not allergic to penicillin	**Penicillin allergy**
Gram-positive cocci	Flucloxacillin	Clindamycin
Gram-negative cocci (gonococci)	Ceftriaxone	Minor allergy: ceftriaxone
		Major allergy: meropenem
Gram-negative rods	Ciprofloxacin + gentamicin	Ciprofloxacin and gentamicin
None seen: gonococcal infection unlikely	Flucloxacillin	Clindamycin
None seen: gonococcal infection likely	Ceftriaxone	Minor allergy: ceftriaxone
		Major allergy: meropenem

Table 28.5 Management of acute arthritis.

Cause of acute arthritis	Management
Septic arthritis See Chapter 98	Antibiotic therapy (Table 28.4) Joint drainage Seek advice from orthopedic surgeon/rheumatologist
Gout See Chapter 97	High-dose NSAID (consider PPI cover) Colchicine if NSAID contraindicated Oral corticosteroid (prednisolone 40 mg daily for 1–2 days, then tapered over 7–10 days) if NSAID/colchicine contraindicated or not tolerated Consider intra-articular corticosteroid in place or oral corticosteroid if only one joint affected
Pseudogout See Chapter 97	Joint drainage Intra-articular corticosteroid NSAID (consider PPI cover) Colchicine if NSAID contraindicated
Flare of rheumatoid arthritis	Seek advice from rheumatologist
Flare of osteoarthritis	NSAID (consider PPI cover) Intra-articular corticosteroid

NSAID, non-steroidal anti-inflammatory drug; PPI, proton pump inhibitor.

Further reading

Carlin E, Flew S. (2016) Sexually acquired reactive arthritis. *Clinical Medicine* 16, 193–196. http://www
.clinmed.rcpjournal.org/content/16/2/193.full.pdf+html.
Helfgott SM. (2015) Overview of monoarthritis in adults. UpToDate. https://www.uptodate.com/contents/
overview-of-monoarthritis-in-adults?source=search_result&search=acute%20arthritis&selectedTitle=2~150.
Smolen JS, Aletaha D, McInnes IB. (2016) Rheumatoid arthritis. *Lancet* 388, 2023–2038.

CHAPTER 29

Acute spinal pain

Michael Canty

Acute spinal pain represents a significant diagnostic challenge. Possible causes can range from benign musculoskeletal pain requiring little treatment, to a first presentation of malignant disease in a young person. While serious causes of spinal pain are uncommon, recognizing them early and intervening appropriately requires careful assessment of all such patients.

Lumbar spine, or low back pain, is the most common form of this presentation, and possibly the least likely to have a serious underlying cause. Low back pain will affect the majority of the population at some point during their lives, and is often short-lived. Cervical and thoracic spine pain are less common. They are more likely to have a sinister cause, although the majority of these patients again have a benign diagnosis.

Priorities

1 **Clinical assessment**

   Look for 'red flag' features indicative of serious pathology (Table 29.1). Examine the spine and perform a full neurological examination, including assessment of perineal and perianal sensation, and anal tone (Box 29.1).
   - Young patients rarely experience significant back pain and are unlikely to have established degenerative disease. Older patients will have conditions such as osteoporosis or primary cancers that predispose to serious spinal problems.
   - Spinal pain following trauma may represent an unstable fracture, or collapse in the presence of osteoporosis.
   - A primary cancer and nocturnal spinal pain are predictors of secondary spinal malignancy.
   - Thoracic spine pain is an unusual symptom and must always be taken seriously. In young patients it is particularly concerning and may be due to a sinister cause.
   - Systemic features such as fever, sepsis, or weight loss suggest a generalized illness such as cancer or infection, which may have begun to involve the spine.
   - Instability pain indicates a potential loss of spinal integrity, such as collapse, with resultant deformity secondary to malignancy, infection or benign fracture. It is characterized by pain present on mobilizing but usually absent at rest.
   - Perineal/perianal or 'saddle' numbness, is a hallmark of cauda equina syndrome and must never be ignored.
   - Bladder symptoms (especially inability to pass urine, or incontinence), and more rarely, bowel symptoms, may be due to cauda equina or spinal cord lesions.
   - Progressive limb neurology suggests significant nerve or cord compression and urgent investigation is required.
2 **If malignant spinal cord or cauda equina compression is suspected, arrange emergency MRI imaging of the entire spine.**

Acute Medicine: A Practical Guide to the Management of Medical Emergencies, Fifth Edition. Edited by David Sprigings and John B. Chambers.
© 2018 John Wiley & Sons Ltd. Published 2018 by John Wiley & Sons Ltd.

Box 29.1 Acute spinal pain – alerts.

Always consider potentially serious non-spinal causes of back or neck pain, including but not limited to ureteric colic, expanding abdominal aortic aneurysm, acute pancreatitis, aortic dissection and vertebral artery dissection.

A high index of suspicion and a low threshold for investigation should exist when considering spinal cord compression or cauda equina syndrome. The latter in particular is a clinical diagnosis. Emergency MRI imaging is needed and if delays are encountered, senior discussion should take place between the referring clinical specialty and Radiology immediately.

Always perform a perineal and perianal examination if you suspect spinal cord compression or cauda equina syndrome, for both clinical and medico-legal reasons. It is very useful and clinically prudent to document normal bladder motor function with a post-voiding bedside bladder scan.

In rectal examinations, references to 'reduced' anal tone are almost always extremely subjective and unhelpful; anal tone is better referred to as present or absent. It is also a very late sign of sacral nerve dysfunction. The absence of voluntary anal contraction is also unhelpful, as this occurs in many neurologically normal patients due to the unpleasant nature of the examination.

All patients requiring emergency MRI or CT scan may have a surgical diagnosis (e.g. cord compression, unstable spinal deformity) and should be kept nil by mouth pending their definitive imaging and discussion with a spinal surgeon. Keep the patient on bed rest; prescribe adequate analgesia; if there is significant sphincter involvement, particularly if in urinary retention, insert a bladder catheter.

Table 29.1 Focused assessment in acute spinal pain.

Red flags

While this term is overused and must be taken in context of the full assessment, the presence of one of these features may be the only indication of a significant underlying diagnosis.

History
Age younger than 20, or older than 55
Trauma
Known malignancy
Nocturnal pain
Thoracic pain
Systemic symptoms (fever, weight loss)
Significant pain on mobilizing that disappears at rest (may represent instability pain)
Perineal ('saddle') numbness
Bladder or bowel symptoms
Severe or progressive limb neurological deficit

Examination
Spinal deformity (e.g. kyphosis, 'step' in the posterior spine)
Bony spinal tenderness, particularly if thoracic
Significant weakness
Sensory level (i.e. a loss of sensation in all dermatomes below a certain level)
Upper motor neuron dysfunction (e.g. spasticity, brisk reflexes, extensor plantars)
Sacral dysfunction (e.g. absent anal tone, urinary retention, perineal/perianal numbness)

If MRI imaging is unavailable, discuss with Neurosurgery or Oncology whether referral for imaging elsewhere is indicated. Consider CT scanning of the spine.

3 **If cauda equina syndrome is present, even if not thought to be malignant, arrange emergency MRI imaging of the lumbosacral spine.**

   If MRI imaging is unavailable, discuss with the relevant spinal regional centre whether transfer for imaging is indicated.

4 **If a significant traumatic injury is suspected, or a spinal deformity due to any cause is present, imaging with either CT or MRI will be required.**
   - Discuss choice of imaging with Radiology.
   - Plain X-rays may confirm the diagnosis and expedite cross-sectional imaging, but they are not definitive.

5 **If spinal infection is suspected**, obtain urgent bloods for full blood count, C-reactive protein, creatinine and electrolytes and bone profile. Take blood cultures.
   - Look carefully for a primary source.
   - Arrange urgent MRI imaging of the relevant area of the spine. Consider imaging the entire spine.

6 **If nerve or cord compression is suspected**, but not thought to be acute or malignant (e.g. lumbar radiculopathy without features of cauda equina syndrome; degenerative cervical myelopathy), routine inpatient MRI is usually appropriate.

Further management

Patients with a confirmed diagnosis of **malignant spinal cord or cauda equina compression** should be referred immediately to Neurosurgery and/or Oncology.

Cauda equina compressions due to acute disc prolapse should also be referred immediately to Neurosurgery or the regional spinal service.

Traumatic spinal injuries and **spinal infections** should also be discussed with Neurosurgery or the regional spinal service, although many of these patients will be managed non-surgically and do not require transfer.

Patients with **lumbar radiculopathy** are usually managed on an outpatient basis by spinal surgeons. Discussion with the relevant specialty should take place if any uncertainty exists over the urgency of referral. **Cervical myelopathy** is also usually managed initially in outpatients, albeit on an expedited basis; it is prudent to discuss with the on-call specialty.

Osteoporotic collapse is managed by multiple modalities and specialties, but almost never by surgery. Vertebroplasty is advocated by some and may be appropriate in selected cases; it is usually provided by interventional radiologists.

Patients without a significant diagnosis following investigation usually have musculoskeletal pain and are managed by adequate analgesia, mobilization and physiotherapy. Some patients will have an underlying rheumatological cause such as an inflammatory arthropathy and should be discussed with Rheumatology for further advice and management.

Further reading

Berbari EF, Kanj SS, Kowalski TJ, *et al*. (2015) Infectious Diseases Society of America: clinical practice guidelines for the diagnosis and treatment of native vertebral osteomyelitis in adults. *Clinical Infectious Diseases* 61, e26–46. http://cid.oxfordjournals.org/content/early/2015/07/22/cid.civ482.full.

Della-Giustina D (2015) Evaluation and treatment of acute back pain in the emergency department. *Emerg Med Clin North Am* 33, 311–326.

CHAPTER 30

Acute limb pain

DAVID SPRIGINGS

Acute limb pain is a medical emergency: the cause may be a threat to life or the viability of the limb (Box 30.1).

Priorities

Make a focused assessment (Table 30.1). Investigation (Table 30.2) and further management are guided by the differential diagnosis.

Cellulitis
- Is characterized by painful swelling and erythema of the skin, with fever.
- If cellulitis is the likely diagnosis, having considered the differential diagnosis (Table 95.1), assess the severity of the illness on the basis of the clinical features and comorbidities, and manage the patient accordingly (Tables 95.3 and 95.4, Chapter 95).

Necrotizing fasciitis
- Should be suspected in an ill patient with severe pain and marked local tenderness of the skin. The skin may show blue-black discolouration and blistering.
- If necrotizing fasciitis is possible, give IV fluid, start antibiotic therapy (Table 95.4, Chapter 95) and seek urgent advice from an orthopaedic or plastic surgeon.

Deep vein thrombosis
- Should be considered in any patient with new-onset limb pain or swelling, especially if there are risk factors for venous thrombosis (Table 56.1). Upper-limb DVT is rare but may be seen in patients with axillary or subclavian venous catheters or cardiac-device leads, cancer or other thrombophilic states, anatomical abnormalities of the thoracic outlet, or may follow strenuous exercise involving the arm.
- See Chapter 56 for further management of DVT.

Acute limb ischaemia
- Is characterized by pain and paraesthesia, with absent arterial pulses. The skin distal to the occlusion is cool and may be pale or mottled.
- Causes of acute limb ischaemia include acute thrombosis of a limb artery or bypass graft, embolism from the heart or a proximal arterial aneurysm, aortic dissection with involvement of the limb artery and trauma (e.g. arterial puncture or cannulation).

Acute Medicine: A Practical Guide to the Management of Medical Emergencies, Fifth Edition. Edited by David Sprigings and John B. Chambers.
© 2018 John Wiley & Sons Ltd. Published 2018 by John Wiley & Sons Ltd.

Box 30.1 Differential diagnosis of acute limb pain.

Tissue/structure	Features indicating disease	Possible pathologies
Skin and subcutaneous tissues	Swelling; oedema; discolouration; rash; blister, ulcer or abscess formation; tenderness; induration; crepitus; temperature difference; lymphangitis	Erysipelas Cellulitis Necrotizing fasciitis Hypersensitivity reaction to insect sting or bite Contact dermatitis
Arteries	Arterial pulses reduced or absent; prolonged capillary refill; ischaemic lesions of the hands or feet	Acute ischaemia
Veins	Superficial thrombophlebitis; localized tenderness over the deep veins	Superficial thrombophlebitis Deep vein thrombosis
Nerves	Reduced muscle power and tendon reflexes; impaired light touch and pin-prick sensation	Acute neuropathies including Guillain-Barré syndrome Acute radiculopathies Herpes zoster
Muscles	Localized or diffuse swelling or tenderness; reduced muscle power	*Localized* Strain injury (partial tear) Contusion injury (direct impact) Intramuscular haematoma Intramuscular abscess Tendon rupture Compartment syndrome *Generalized* Systemic infection Acute myositis Acute vasculitis
Joints	Swelling around the joint; presence of effusion; increased temperature of the joint; reduced range of movement; instability; tenderness	Fracture Meniscal or ligamentous injury Acute arthritis Acute bursitis Ruptured Baker (popliteal) cyst (may complicate rheumatoid arthritis or osteoarthritis of the knee)
Bones	Abnormal alignment (angled or rotated); localized swelling; localized tenderness	Subperiosteal haematoma Fracture Primary or metastatic cancer Infection Stress fracture Medial tibial stress syndrome Loosened hip or knee replacement Osteomyelitis

Source: Oxford Clinical Diagnosis and Treatment eds Davey & Sprigings, OUP 2018. Reproduced with permission of Oxford University Press.

Table 30.1 Focused assessment in acute limb pain.

History

Is pain felt in one limb or both? What is the principal site of the pain? Is there associated weakness, sensory impairment, spinal pain or sphincter disturbance?

What is the time course of symptoms?

Has there been preceding trauma or fall?

Is there known arterial disease, diabetes or other systemic disease?

Are there risk factors for deep vein thrombosis (Table 56.1)?

Has the patient had previous joint, bone or other limb surgery?

Examination

Physiological observations and general examination

Systematic examination of the structures of the limb for signs of disease (Box 30.1)

- Findings on neurological examination (sensory loss/muscle weakness) and Doppler assessment of arterial and venous flow stratify the degree of ischaemia and guide further management.
- If acute limb ischaemia is suspected, give heparin 5000 units IV over 5 min IV, followed by an IV infusion (Chapter 103).
- Seek urgent advice from a vascular surgeon.

Table 30.2 Urgent investigation in acute limb pain.

Diagnostic tests are determined by the likely pathology (see below).
Additional tests needed may include:
Full blood count
C-reactive protein
Biochemical profile
Creatine kinase
Blood glucose
Blood culture if febrile

Suspected site of disease	Diagnostic tests to consider
Skin and subcutaneous tissues	Microscopy and culture of samples from areas of ulceration
	Plain radiography if suspected gas in tissue or underlying fracture, osteomyelitis or foreign body
	Ultrasonography, CT or MRI if suspected necrotizing fasciitis
Arteries	Duplex scan
	Angiography (CT or direct)
Veins	Duplex scan
	Plasma D-dimer
Nerves	Nerve conduction studies
	MRI of spine
Muscles	Ultrasonography
	MRI
	Plasma creatine kinase
Joints	Plain radiography (in anteroposterior and lateral views)
	Joint aspiration if effusion present
	CT or MRI if suspected fracture not revealed by plain radiographs
Bones	Plain radiography (in anteroposterior and lateral views)
	CT or MRI if suspected pathology not revealed by plain radiographs

CT, computed tomography; MRI, magnetic resonance imaging.

Compartment syndrome
- Is defined as increased pressure within a myofascial space (most often tibial), resulting in ischaemia.
- Typically follows trauma, particularly fractures, crush injuries and burns, but can also be caused by constricting casts or accidental pressurized intravenous or extravenous infusions.
- May complicate the nephrotic syndrome, rhabdomyolysis, bleeding disorders and limb infection.
- Suspect compartment syndrome if, in a patient at risk, there is pain which appears disproportionate to the injury, or is worse on stretching the muscles within the affected compartment.
- Seek urgent advice from an orthopaedic surgeon. The diagnosis can be confirmed by compartment pressure monitoring. If confirmed, treatment is decompression of the affected compartment by fasciotomy.

Bone and joint disease
- See Chapter 28 for the assessment of acute arthritis.
- If fracture is suspected or must be excluded, arrange plain radiography (in anteroposterior and lateral views). If fracture is still suspected despite non-diagnostic plain films (e.g. unable to weight-bear because of pain), arrange CT or MRI and seek an orthopaedic opinion.
- Pain arising from the long bones of the limbs is uncommon; it may be caused by primary or metastatic tumours, infection or stress fractures, and loosened hip or knee replacements. Arrange plain radiography (in anteroposterior and lateral views) and seek advice from an orthopaedic surgeon.

Neurological disorders
- Pain may be a feature of peripheral neuropathies due to diabetes and alcohol.
- Spinal disorders with referred pain should be considered if no pathology is evident in the leg.

Further reading

Falluji N, Mukherjee D (2014) Critical and acute limb ischaemia: an overview. *Angiology* 65, 137–146.
von Keudell AG, Weaver MJ, Appleton PT, *et al*. (2015) Diagnosis and treatment of acute extremity compartment syndrome. *Lancet* 386, 1299–1310.

Miscellaneous

CHAPTER 31

Comprehensive geriatric assessment

SIMON CONROY AND OJA PATHAK

Around 60–70% of inpatients are aged >65. The Comprehensive Geriatric Assessment (CGA) (Box 31.1 and Figure 31.1) assesses the whole patient, and can reduce length of stay and institutionalization, and improve quality of life. Geriatric syndromes such as falls, delirium or immobility can be used to stream patients towards CGA interventions.

Priorities

All the principles of early diagnosis and treatment apply as much to the frail older people as the young. However, assessment and management are harder because of:
- Non-specific presentations
- Communication barriers (requiring greater involvement of family, friends and carers)
- Multiple comorbidities
- More complex community care needs
    To resolve this, CGA produces a list of medical and non-medical problems, which can be constructed by any or all the members of the multidisciplinary care team. Common problems include:
- Cognition: differentiate delirium from dementia; see http://guidance.nice.org.uk/CG103. Is further investigation required? If so does it need to happen now or in a clinic?
- Continence:
    - Urinary incontinence is common and often misdiagnosed as urinary tract infection, which can precipitate acute incontinence but is rarely the explanation for long-standing incontinence. Consider detrusor

Box 31.1 Comprehensive Geriatric Assessment.

The Comprehensive Geriatric Assessment (CGA) is a multidimensional, interdisciplinary diagnostic process to determine the medical, psychological and functional capabilities of an older person in order to develop a coordinated and integrated plan for treatment and long-term follow-up.

Whilst integrating standard medical diagnostic evaluation, CGA emphasizes problem solving, functional status and prognosis, with the aim of restoring independence and alleviating distress.

Typically, CGA involves a team of people from various disciplines (geriatric medicine, physiotherapy, occupational therapy, nursing) or a combination of these, working towards a shared common goal using standardized assessment tools, pathways and documentation.

Acute Medicine: A Practical Guide to the Management of Medical Emergencies, Fifth Edition. Edited by David Sprigings and John B. Chambers.
© 2018 John Wiley & Sons Ltd. Published 2018 by John Wiley & Sons Ltd.

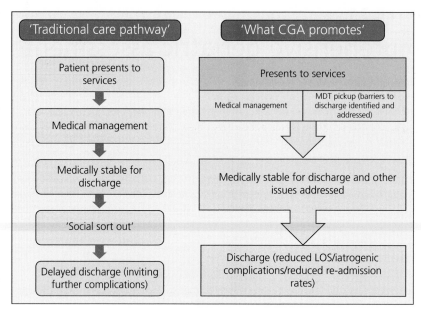

Figure 31.1 Comprehensive Geriatic Assessment (CGA).

instability, retention, stress and functional incontinence. Consider bladder scanning. If there is no immediately obvious cause on admission, ensure the community services are aware this issue needs addressing, as treating incontinence improves quality of life and can reduce admission to long-term care.
  • Are you sure you know how to diagnose urinary tract infection? See Chapter 80 and also NICE guidance (http://www.nice.org.uk/guidance/CG40). An abnormal urinalysis does not necessarily indicated infection. Malodorous urine may reflect dehydration rather than urosepsis.
  • Bowels: frequency/stool type/constipation – a common cause of 'coffee-ground vomitus'. A rectal examination is quicker, cheaper and usually more useful than an endoscopy or CT abdomen.
• Mobility: immobility, whether due to illness or institutionalization from hospital conservatism, can increase the risk of complications, such as chest infections and falls. All staff should seek opportunities to mobilize older people in hospital.

Assess mobility by the 'get up and go' test. Check the patient is able to stand (if they can straight leg raise in bed, they should be able to stand) and walk. Usual footwear should be worn, and usual walking aid used. Ask the patient to stand up from a standard chair, and walk a distance of at least 3 m, then turn and get back to the chair. There is no need to time the test (although >11 s indicates higher falls risk). People who cannot 'get up and go' unaided are at increased risk of future falls.
• Mood: depression is common in ill health and worsens outcomes. Ask simple questions like 'how is your mood?'. Note the patient's affect, and consider involving a mental health team if you are concerned about mood.
• Nutrition: ask about weight loss. What do they eat normally? Who shops/who cooks/who feeds? Are any modifications of food or drink required (e.g. pureed diet/thickened fluids)? Assess oral health: thrush/dentition/ulcers/dentures – do they fit?
• Activities of daily living. How do they transfer, for example in and out of bed? What aids to they need? Who washes/dresses? What about more advanced tasks: using a phone/driving? Minutes spent ascertaining this information up front and revising goals accordingly can save days later on in the patient journey.

- Medications: often medications are continued despite the original symptoms having subsided. Use a structured medication review process, for example STOPP/START criteria. Repeat offenders include the following which might be stopped/reduced:
  - NSAIDs (risk of GI bleeding/renal impairment)
  - Opioids (drowsiness/nausea/constipation)
  - Antihistamines (sedating)
  - Prochlorperazine (risk of extra-pyramidal side effects, ineffective for non-vestibular pathology)
  - Prophylactic antibiotics (there is little evidence that these prevent UTI; often increase resistance, making acute infection management more restrictive)
  - Anti-hypertensives (risk of postural hypotension)
  - Furosemide (risk of hypotension/fluid depletion/AKI: often erroneously started for dependent oedema)
- End-of-life care issues and ethics; is advance care planning indicated? Would you be surprised if this person was to die in the next 6–12 months? A third of frail older people discharged from AMU die within a year.

Further management

Once the initial assessment is complete, a problem list can be formulated (see Appendix 31.1 for an example). Anticipate future admissions. Often these are because of progressive disease, for example malignancy, severe heart failure, COPD or dementia. Other issues can be identified and addressed, such as:

- Incontinence, with referral to the relevant service.
- High falls risk. Management can include a falls care pathway for care homes/ambulance services to follow after a 'recurrent faller' has an event. This can guide what observations need to be done and which variance should prompt admission, as opposed to blanket admissions following all episodes.
- Risk of aspiration pneumonia in dementia. Discuss with family, community health professionals, care home staff that this is likely to recur. Address feeding issues (e.g. accepting spoon feeding with risk of aspiration) and avoid unnecessary speech and language therapy (SALT) assessments. Conveying the likely disease progression and prognosis can enable planning for end-of-life care.

Appendix 31.1 Formulation of a comprehensive problem list

The patient, an 86-year-old woman referred by Emergency Dept.

Presenting problem: found on floor: no meaningful history from patient as drowsy and not able to recall event.

From a residential care home, collateral: found on floor at 4 am. Last seen at 2 am in bed. Found right side and urinary incontinent at that time. Reduced appetite for last 24 hours and reports nausea. Bowels last opened two days ago.

Independently mobile. Requires supervision and prompting to feed self and wash and dress. Occasionally urinary incontinent and wears pads overnight. Continent with bowels. Usually disorientated but able to hold a conversation and answer aptly yes/no. But poor memory. Been at home for three years. No issues otherwise.

Past medical history: recurrent UTI/Alzheimer's dementia/hypertension/stroke

Medications: co-codamol 30/500 TT QDS (initiated two months ago following fall and right shoulder injury), bendroflumethiazide 2.5 mg, OD atenolol 50 mg, OD donepezil 10 mg OD, aspirin 75 mg OD, simvastatin 40 mg, OD trimethoprim 100 mg ON.

Examination: Clinically dehydrated (reduced skin turgor/dry mucous membranes) CVS: lying BP 105/64 mmHg. Too drowsy to stand. HR 54/min regular (confirmed on ECG). Neuro: alert and disorientated. Nil else focal. AMTS = 2/10. Resp: clear lung fields. GI: abdomen: soft, BS present: lower abdominal discomfort on palpation. PR: loaded rectum. Urinary: palpable bladder. Joint: bruised right shoulder, movement preserved in all four limbs. No bony/spinal tenderness. No sores seen.

Investigations: bladder scan: 710 mLs (post void residual) U&E: eGFR 24 (baseline 56). Urine dip +ve Previous MSU: resistant to trimethoprim. CK/Bone/LFT/FBC/TSH/Haematinics: normal ranges. CT head (fall and confusion): disproportionate hippocampal atrophy and moderate burden of small vessel disease. Mature infarct noted right temporoparietal lobe.

Problem list

1 **Multifactorial fall**
 • Poor cognition/dementia
 • Bradycardia (medications: atenolol/donepezil)
 • Neurological deficit (previous stroke)
 • Hypotension, medications and fluid depletion due to:
  • Reduced oral intake due to
  • Constipation due to
  • Opiates
2 **Urinary retention due to constipation/faecal impaction +/- donepezil causing:**
 • Recurrent UTI (multi drug resistance)
 • Acute (post-renal) kidney injury
3 **Polypharmacy (opioids/beta-blockade/thiazide)**
4 **Hypoactive delirium secondary to above issues**

Multiple issues have been identified as probable contributors to the fall. Now that these have been clearly identified they can be individually addressed: either immediately or over time.

Further reading

Clegg A, Young J, Iliffe S, Rikkert MO, Rockwood K (2013) Frailty in elderly people. *Lancet* 381, 752–762.
Ekdahl AW, Sjöstrand F, Ehrenberg A, *et al*. (2015) Frailty and comprehensive geriatric assessment organized as CGA-*ward* or CGA-*consult* for older adult patients in the acute care setting: A systematic review and meta-analysis. *European Geriatric Medicine* 6, 523–540.

CHAPTER 32

Acute medical problems in pregnancy

Lucy Mackillop and Charlotte Frise

Pregnant women may present with disorders specific to pregnancy; with problems related to chronic disorders exacerbated by pregnancy or with unrelated disorders. Achieving a good outcome for mother and fetus requires close collaboration between the medical and obstetric services.

Breathlessness (see Chapter 10)

Up to 70% of pregnant women will report breathlessness. The physiology of pregnancy predisposes to breathlessness. However, serious cardiorespiratory disorders may also occur (Table 32.1).

Priorities

- End of the bed assessment – if there is cyanosis, distress or a reduced conscious level, get help urgently.
  - Senior anaesthetist input at an early stage is required as intubation of a pregnant woman is particularly difficult.
  - An intensivist, obstetrician and neonatologist (if pregnancy >24 weeks or unsure of gestation) should be contacted.
  - Give high-flow oxygen.
  - Nurse the patient in the left lateral position to avoid vena caval compression by the gravid uterus.
- For women not in extremis, a detailed history should be taken including: the onset of symptoms and their relationship to the pregnancy; past medical and obstetric history.
- Use pregnancy-specific normal ranges for investigations so they are interpreted correctly (Table 32.2).
- Do not withhold critical investigations or treatment for fear of the effects on the fetus. A chest X-ray confers negligible radiation to the fetus at any gestation.

Chest pain/shock (see Chapters 2 and 7)

The pregnant patient with shock presents unique medical and management challenges. The differential diagnosis needs to include obstetric complications not often presenting to acute medical services, for example amniotic fluid embolus (Table 32.3). Furthermore, resuscitation of the pregnant woman carries particular challenges, including optimum position of the gravid uterus and potentially difficult airway management.

Acute Medicine: A Practical Guide to the Management of Medical Emergencies, Fifth Edition. Edited by David Sprigings and John B. Chambers.
© 2018 John Wiley & Sons Ltd. Published 2018 by John Wiley & Sons Ltd.

Table 32.1 Differential diagnosis of breathlessness in pregnancy.

Diagnosis	Key features	Management
Physiological breathlessness of pregnancy	Gradual onset in 2nd/3rd trimester. Worse on talking.	Exclude pathology and reassure.
Anaemia	Physiological haemodilution means anaemia is defined as Hb <105 g/L.	Exclude serious pathology. Check iron status. Iron supplements as required.
Cardiorespiratory causes		
Asthma	As in non-pregnant, but pregnancy may exacerbate the condition. Reflux can also exacerbate or mimic asthma symptoms.	Manage acute exacerbation as with non-pregnant patient (Chapter 60). Ensure compliance with prescribed medications.
Pneumonia	As in non-pregnant; however, some organisms are associated with particularly severe disease, for example H1N1, VZV.	As for non-pregnant. Lower threshold for admission. If VZV pneumonitis suspected – IV acyclovir. If delivery is within ten days – neonate needs ZIG.
Pneumothorax	Associated with the valsalva of second stage of labour.	Chest radiography.
Pulmonary embolus	~ 5-fold increase risk in pregnancy. ~ 25-fold increase risk immediately postnatal. Sudden onset CP and breathlessness. Signs of right heart strain. Classical clinical features of DVT are much less common in pregnancy therefore need high index of suspicion.	CXR, ECG, ABG. Make the diagnosis with available imaging. (Q scan or CTPA). Anticoagulate with LMWH. Consider IV heparin or thrombolysis if cardiovascular instability. Involve obstetricians with timing of delivery.
Pulmonary oedema	Rare but often missed. Associated with pre-eclampsia or peripartum cardiomyopathy.	If clinical suspicion, get urgent ECG, CXR and Echo. Off load with diuretics and liaise with obstetricians regarding timing and management around delivery.
Peripartum cardiomyopathy	Most common in 1st month after delivery in older, multiparous black women.	As per pulmonary oedema.
Pulmonary hypertension	Rare but is associated with 25% mortality in pregnancy; therefore needs to be excluded.	Refer to specialist pulmonary hypertension centre.
Heart valve disease	MS can present for the first time in pregnancy (usually in 2nd trimester) with breathlessness/palpitations, tachyarrhythmia, pulmonary oedema or stroke.	ECG, CXR, Echo. Treat failure, anticoagulate if in AF, β-blockers once failure treated. Liaise with obstetricians for management plan for delivery.
Other causes		
Amniotic fluid embolus	See chest pain/shock.	See chest pain/shock
Metabolic	Starvation ketoacidosis in 3rd trimester presents with breathlessness and often a short history of vomiting.	ABGs, ketones. Give glucose. Treat cause of vomiting. Re-establish oral intake.

MS, mitral stenosis.

Table 32.2 Interpreting investigations in pregnancy.

Investigations	Normal values	
	Pregnant	Non-pregnant
Haemoglobin g/dL	105–140	120–150
White cell count $\times 10^9/l$	6–16	4–11
Platelets $\times 10^9/l$	150–400*	150–400
Haematocrit	0.3–0.4	0.36–0.47
MCV fL	80–100	80–100
Sodium mmol/l	130–140	135–145
Potassium mmol/l	3.3–4.1	3.5–5.0
Urea mmol/l	2.4–4.1	2.5–7.5
Creatinine μmol/l	44–73	65–101
Bicarbonate mmol/l	18–22	22–28
C-reactive protein (CRP) g/l	0–7	0–7
ESR	Unreliable – high	0–10
D-dimer mg/L	Unreliable – high[†]	<0.5
pH	7.35–7.45	7.40–7.48
$PaCO_2$ kPa/mmHg	3.6–4.3/27–32	4.7–6.0/35–45
PaO_2 kPa/mmHg	12.6–14.0/94–105	10.6–14.0/80–105
Base excess	+2–2	+2–2
Peak expiratory flow (PEF)	No change	
Forced expiratory volume in 1 second (FEV1)	No change	

* A 10% fall in platelet count maybe expected during pregnancy.
† Difference especially marked in late pregnancy.

Priorities

- Institute advanced life support (Chapter 6).
- Call a senior anaesthetist, intensivist, obstetrician and neonatologist.
- Nurse in left lateral position to avoid vena caval compression by the gravid uterus.
- Give high-flow oxygen and gain intravenous access with large-bore cannulae.
- If output is lost, return patient to the supine position to initiate chest compressions.
- Peri-mortem caesarean section should be considered to aid maternal resuscitation.

Headache/seizures (see Chapters 15 and 16)

Headache is a common symptom reported by pregnant women and although benign in most cases, awareness of warning symptoms is required so that important pathology is not missed (Table 32.4).

Seizures are uncommon in pregnancy, but when they occur, are potentially life threatening to both mother and fetus (Table 32.5).

Priorities

- In addition to a thorough medical history, an obstetric history should be obtained: establish the details of present and previous pregnancies, and whether any complications arose.
- Examination should include blood pressure, urinalysis and neurological examination, including fundoscopy.
- Pregnancy is not a contra-indication to CT, MRI or lumbar puncture.

Table 32.3 Differential diagnosis of chest pain/shock in pregnancy.

Diagnosis	Key features	Management
Pulmonary embolism	See breathlessness.	
Myocardial infarction • **ACS from atherosclerosis** • **Coronary artery dissection**	As in non-pregnant (atypical presentations more common in women).	ECG, troponin (not altered by pregnancy). Medical management as in non-pregnant, that is, primary PCI, except avoid IIb/IIIa inhibitors and statins.
Stroke CVT/SAH/ICH/infarction	As in non-pregnant.	Appropriate imaging depends on availability and most likely cause of symptoms, but MRI is usually preferred after the 1st trimester Aspirin and other antiplatelet agents can be given in pregnancy as can UFH and LMWH.
Aortic dissection	Associated with pregnancy particularly in women with Marfan syndrome, Ehlers-Danlos type IV or coarctation of the aorta.	CXR, CT Combined caesarean section and surgical repair if type A and viable fetus.
Amniotic fluid embolism	Shock. Respiratory distress and cyanosis. Early and severe bleeding (DIC).	CXR. FBC, PT, APTT. High flow oxygen and respiratory and circulatory support.
Septic shock	Often rapid onset. Temp >38 or <36°C. HR >100/min. RR >20 resps/min. WBC <4 or >17 × 10^9/L. Clinical signs – fever, rigors, abdominal pain, vomiting, headache, confusion, offensive vaginal discharge.	Blood cultures, plasma lactate, FBC, U&Es. IV fluids. Antibiotics. HVS/LVS and MSU. Early transfer to level two critical care. Of note – group A strep is increasing in prevalence.
Anaphylactic shock	As in non-pregnant.	Need senior anaesthetist early, as intubation in pregnancy is difficult.

Pre-eclampsia and acute fatty liver of pregnancy

Each year on average 2 women in the UK die from eclampsia or pre-eclampsia and one from acute fatty liver of pregnancy (MBRRACE-UK report 2016).

Pre-eclampsia is defined as new hypertension and proteinuria after 20 weeks of gestation, and can lead to complications including seizures (eclampsia) and HELLP syndrome (Haemolysis, Elevated Liver enzymes, Low Platelets) (Table 32.6). Pre-eclampsia complicates 3–5% of all pregnancies and its course is unpredictable.

Women with pre-eclampsia often present to maternity services. However, pre-eclampsia should be considered in any woman presenting to acute care services with signs and symptoms suggestive, as undiagnosed or concealed pregnancy is not uncommon.

Acute fatty liver of pregnancy (AFLP) is a distinct condition but it is likely to be related (Table 32.7). AFLP is rare but can cause fulminant liver failure (Chapter 77).

Table 32.4 Differential diagnosis of headache in pregnancy.

Diagnosis	Key features	Management
Meningitis	As in non-pregnant population	Bloods: FBC, CRP, blood cultures Urgent antibiotics Antivirals, that is acyclovir if suspicion of viral encephalitis
Subarachnoid haemorrhage	As in non-pregnant population	CT head Lumbar puncture to look for xanthochromia if CT head negative
Space occupying lesion Benign intracranial hypertension	As in non-pregnant population Papilloedema and raised intracranial pressure (ICP) in the absence of another explanation This can present for the first time in pregnancy	Depends on lesion and the presentation Imaging to exclude another cause for raised intracranial pressure Lumbar puncture to measure pressure and can be repeated for symptom relief Regular assessment of visual acuity and fields To reduce ICP, thiazides and acetazolamide (avoid 1st trimester)
Migraine	Features as in non-pregnant population (see Chapter 15) Classical migraine may improve in pregnancy Can be different in nature to the migraines experienced when not pregnant, that is, aura without headache, or new aura	Analgesia (not NSAIDs) Antiemetics Triptans can be used sporadically if they are the only successful treatment for an acute event Prophylaxis: low dose aspirin or propranolol Avoid ergotamine, pizotifen, valproate, gabapentin and topiramate
Pre-eclampsia or hypertension	Hypertension and proteinuria Other symptoms: visual disturbance, epigastric/right upper quadrant pain MRI may show posterior reversible encephalopathy syndrome (PRES)	Bloods: platelet count, renal and liver function Antihypertensives IV magnesium sulphate if severe disease present (Table 32.8) Delivery depends on gestation and severity
Intracranial haemorrhage	Sudden onset headache Risk factors include pre-eclampsia or hypertension, trauma, vascular or coagulation abnormalities	Bloods: FBC and coagulation Imaging – CT or MRI Management is neurosurgical and depends on nature of the haemorrhage and underlying aetiology
Cerebral venous thrombosis	Is associated with pregnancy and can occur in any trimester or post-partum May be associated with vomiting, photophobia, reduced conscious level, seizures or signs of raised intracranial pressure On examination focal signs may be present; a low grade fever is also common	Bloods may show a raised white cell count Imaging – CT or MRI, and venography Thrombophilia screen LMWH or UFH can be used safely in pregnancy and during breastfeeding
Drug-related headache	May be caused by regular analgesic use, vasodilators such as calcium antagonists (e.g. nifedipine used in treatment of hypertension in pregnancy)	Review use of the likely causative drug
Post-dural puncture headache	Headache occurs within 1–7 days of dural puncture Usually postural and is relieved on lying flat Other symptoms: neck stiffness, visual symptoms or seizures (rare)	Conservative management – analgesia, bed rest, maintain good hydration or a blood patch

Table 32.5 Differential diagnosis of seizures in pregnancy.

Diagnosis	Key features	Management
Epilepsy	Seizures may occur at increased frequency even if epilepsy previously well controlled, as a result of: Dose reduction because of concern about teratogenicity Increased metabolism of AEDs Precipitants such as sleep deprivation	Consider drug level to help guide dose adjustment Management of status epilepticus as in non-pregnant patient
Eclampsia	May not have been preceded by hypertension, proteinuria or symptoms of pre-eclampsia	
Cerebral venous thrombosis	See headache section	
Intracranial haemorrhage	See headache section	
Thrombotic thrombocytopenic purpura	Features: microangiopathic haemolytic anaemia (MAHA), fever, renal impairment, neurological symptoms and low platelets, but often not all features are present	Initiation of plasma exchange should be considered in all patients with MAHA and low platelets without another obvious cause
Hypoglycaemia	Usually in women taking exogenous insulin Less commonly: acute fatty liver of pregnancy, adrenal or pituitary disease, insulinomas	Parenteral glucose
Hypocalcaemia	Can be associated with magnesium sulphate therapy or hypoparathyroidism	Intravenous calcium
Drug or alcohol withdrawal	As in non-pregnant population	

Table 32.6 Pre-eclampsia and HELLP syndrome (Haemolysis, Elevated Liver enzymes, Low Platelets).

Element	Comment
Risk factors	First pregnancy, multiple pregnancy, family history, medical conditions such as renal disease
Symptoms	Headache, epigastric or right upper quadrant pain, oedema of face or limbs
Examination findings	Blood pressure >140/90 mmHg, proteinuria either dipstick ≥1+, urinary protein:creatinine ratio >30 mg/mmol, or 24-h urinary protein >300 mg, oedema, RUQ/epigastric discomfort, hyperreflexia (NB: hypertension and proteinuria may be absent in HELLP syndrome)
Blood tests	Pre-eclampsia: raised uric acid, mild elevation in transaminases, mild elevation in creatinine HELLP (all or some): haemolysis (reduced Hb, increased reticulocytes, reduced haptoglobins, fragments on blood film), low platelets, raised transaminases +/- bilirubin, renal impairment, elevated LDH
Markers of severity	BP: SBP >160 mmHg or DBP >110 mmHg CNS: Seizures, visual disturbance, severe headache or >3 beats clonus Hepatic: RUQ/epigastric pain, nausea/vomiting, transaminases > twice ULN CVS: pulmonary oedema Renal: creatinine >100 umol/L; urine output <10 mL/h

Table 32.7 Acute fatty liver of pregnancy.

Element	Comment
Symptoms	Gradual onset of nausea, anorexia and malaise, severe vomiting and/or abdominal pain, polyuria, polydipsia
Examination findings	Hypertension and proteinuria usually mild, RUQ/epigastric discomfort, jaundice or ascites
Blood tests	Leukocytosis, coagulopathy, acute kidney injury, elevated transaminases, hypoglycaemia, elevated urate, elevated ammonia
Swansea criteria for diagnosis	The presence of six or more features (in the absence of an alternative diagnosis):

Vomiting	Leucocytosis
Abdominal pain	Elevated transaminases
Polydipsia/polyuria	Acute kidney injury
Encephalopathy	Elevated ammonia
Elevated bilirubin	Hypoglycaemia
Elevated urate	Coagulopathy
Ascites or bright liver on ultrasound	Microvesicular steatosis on liver biopsy

Priorities

Patients with pre-eclampsia or acute fatty liver of pregnancy should be admitted to hospital. If they show features of severe disease (Table 32.6), they should be managed on a high-dependency unit.

Fluid balance – women with pre-eclampsia are often transiently oliguric but are at increased risk of pulmonary oedema, therefore use caution with fluid resuscitation.

Antihypertensive treatment – hypertension tends to peak 3–5 days post-partum. Calcium channel blockers, beta blockers and the ACE inhibitor enalapril can all be used while breastfeeding.

Organ dysfunction – in severe disease, organ support such as haemofiltration may be required, but renal function usually recovers. In acute liver impairment (i.e. AFLP) N-acetyl cysteine can be used.

Blood products – may be required depending on the severity of the anaemia, thrombocytopenia or coagulopathy.

Seizure prophylaxis – IV magnesium sulphate as treatment and prophylaxis for eclampsia (see Table 32.8).

Table 32.8 Use of intravenous magnesium sulphate.

Element	Comment
Loading dose	Magnesium sulphate 4 g by slow IV bolus over 5–10 min
Maintenance infusion	1 g/h magnesium sulphate for 24 h, or 24 h after last seizure Omit maintenance infusion if oligo-anuric
Therapeutic level	Aim for Mg level of 2–4 mmol/L
Caution	Caution with concurrent use of calcium antagonists as the use of both can lead to profound hypotension
Observation during infusion	Check reflexes (upper and lower limb) – before treatment, every 30 min for first two hours and then every hour
Management of suspected overdose	Overdose causes muscle weakness, and so if reflexes are absent the infusion should be stopped and a Mg level checked
Antidote	Calcium gluconate 1 g IV

Delivery – this is the only curative intervention for these conditions and should be expedited but only once the mother has been medically stablized with coagulopathy corrected and blood pressure controlled.

Long-term issues – lifetime risk of cardiovascular disease is increased in women who develop pre-eclampsia.

Further reading

Edlow JA, Caplan LR, O'Brien K, Tibbles CD (2013) Diagnosis of acute neurological emergencies in pregnant and post-partum women. *Lancet Neurol* 12, 175–185.

McNamara DM, Elkayam U, Alharethi R, *et al.* (2015) Clinical outcomes for peripartum cardiomyopathy in North America: Results of the IPAC study (Investigations of Pregnancy-Associated Cardiomyopathy). *J Am Coll Cardiol* 66, 905–914.

Mol BWJ, Roberts CT, Thangaratinam S, Magee LA, de Groot CJM, Hofmeyr GJ (2016) Pre-eclampsia. *Lancet* 387, 999–1011.

Moussa HN, Arian SE, Sibai BM (2014) Management of hypertensive disorders in pregnancy. *Women's Health (Lond Engl)* 10, 385–404.

Westbrook RH, Dusheiko G, Williamson C (2016) Pregnancy and liver disease. *Journal of Hepatology* 64, 933–945.

CHAPTER 33

Fever on return from abroad

NICK BEECHING AND MIKE BEADSWORTH

The management of the patient with a febrile illness within two months of travel abroad is summarized in Figure 33.1. See Box 33.1 for sources of advice on the diagnosis and management of infectious diseases acquired abroad.

- Malaria must be excluded if there has been travel through an endemic area (most of Africa, Asia, Central and South America). Malaria is the most common single cause of fever requiring admission to hospital after travel to the tropics, accounting for 40–60% of cases from sub-Saharan and West Africa and about 10% from Southeast Asia. Its clinical features are non-specific, and diagnosis requires examination of blood films for parasites, supplemented by rapid diagnostic tests. Chemoprophylaxis against malaria does not ensure full protection and may prolong the incubation period.
- Other common causes of fever in travellers include respiratory and gastrointestinal infections. Arboviruses such as dengue, chikungunya and Zika virus infections are widespread, and enteric fevers (typhoid and paratyphoid) are common, particularly in Asia and the Indian subcontinent. Tick typhus is common in visitors to Africa.
- For travellers who have returned within 21 days from rural west Africa and central Eurasia (especially Afghanistan and rural Pakistan), a viral haemorrhagic fever must be considered. Isolate the patient and follow local and national protocols for investigation. Seek advice from local infection and public health specialists and consult the national Imported Fever Service in the UK.
- Consider other causes of febrile illness unrelated to travel, such as influenza, community-acquired pneumonia (Chapter 62) and urinary tract infection (Chapter 80)

Priorities

- Admit to a single room and nurse with standard isolation technique until the diagnosis is established.
- The focused assessment of the patient with fever on return from abroad is given in Table 33.1, and typical incubation periods for selected tropical infections in Table 33.2. Clinical features of malaria and enteric fever are summarized in Appendices 33.1 and 33.2.
- Investigations needed urgently are given in Table 33.3.

Further management

This will depend on the clinical syndrome and likely pathogens.

Acute Medicine: A Practical Guide to the Management of Medical Emergencies, Fifth Edition. Edited by David Sprigings and John B. Chambers.
© 2018 John Wiley & Sons Ltd. Published 2018 by John Wiley & Sons Ltd.

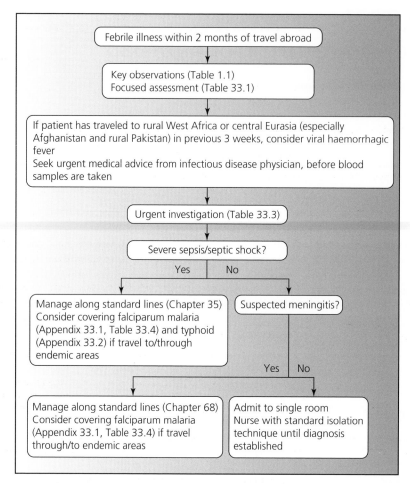

Figure 33.1 Management of the patient with a febrile illness within two months of travel abroad.

Box 33.1 Advice on management of infectious diseases acquired abroad.

Imported Fever Service: 24-h advice on clinical management, diagnostic tests and public health aspects of imported infection. Call the service on 0844 778 8990 after first obtaining advice from local infection specialists (infectious diseases or microbiology). Provides all VHF screening for England and Wales

    https://www.gov.uk/guidance/imported-fever-service-ifs

National Travel Health Network and Centre (NaTHNaC): detailed pre-travel advice and frequent intelligence reports on outbreaks overseas that may be imported to the UK

    http://travelhealthpro.org.uk/

Malaria Guidelines: UK Government website providing access to current UK standards of diagnosis, treatment and prevention of malaria

    https://www.gov.uk/government/collections/malaria-guidance-data-and-analysis

British Infection Association: publishes numerous guidelines on infection, including imported diseases, with free access to these from

    http://www.britishinfection.org/guidelines-resources/

Table 33.1 Focused assessment of the patient with a febrile illness after travel abroad.

History

Which countries traveled to and through? Travel in urban or rural areas or both? Precise localities and dates essential

Immunizations before travel

Malaria prophylaxis taken as prescribed? Insect bite avoidance measures taken?

When did symptoms first appear (Table 33.2)?

Treatments taken?

Known or possible occupational or recreational exposure to infection (including sexually transmitted diseases)?

Exposure	Potential infection or disease
Raw or undercooked foods	Enteric infections, hepatitis A and E, trichinosis
Drinking untreated water; milk, cheese	Gastroenteritis, enteric fever, hepatitis A and E, brucellosis, tularaemia
Fresh water swimming	Schistosomiasis, leptospirosis
Sexual contact	HIV, syphilis, hepatitis B, gonococcaemia
Insect bites	Malaria, chikungunya, dengue and Zika (mosquitoes); tick typhus, Crimean-Congo haemorrhagic fever, borreliosis, tularaemia (ticks); scrub typhus (mites); Chagas' disease (triatomine bugs); African trypanosomiasis (tse tse flies)
Animal exposure or bites	Rabies, Q fever, tularaemia, borreliosis, viral haemorrhagic fevers, plague, MERS CoV
Exposure to infected persons	Influenza, measles, viral hepatitis, viral haemorrhagic fevers, meningococcemia

Examination Sign	Potential infection or disease
Rash	Chikungunya, dengue and Zika virus, typhoid, tick-borne, endemic or scrub typhus, syphilis, gonorrhoea, measles, viral haemorrhagic fever
Jaundice	Hepatitis A, B and E (patients usually afebrile when jaundice appears), malaria, yellow fever, leptospirosis, relapsing fever, cytomegalovirus and Epstein-Barr virus infection
Lymphadenopathy	Rickettsial infections, brucellosis, dengue fever, HIV, tuberculosis, visceral leishmaniasis, toxoplasmosis, EBV infection
Hepatomegaly	Amoebiasis, malaria, typhoid, hepatitis, leptospirosis, most arboviruses
Splenomegaly	Malaria, relapsing fever, trypanosomiasis, typhoid, brucellosis, kala-azar, typhus, chikungunya, dengue and Zika
Eschar (crusted ulcer with black centre and erythematous margin)	Typhus (tick-borne or scrub), borreliosis, Crimean-Congo haemorrhagic fever, cutaneous anthrax (relatively painless oedema as well)
Haemorrhage	Severe dengue; meninococcaemia; epidemic louse borne typhus; Rocky Mountain spotted fever, viral haemorrhagic fevers

Septic shock

- Initial antimicrobial therapy for patients who have travelled in endemic regions may need to cover falciparum malaria (Appendix 33.1) and enteric fever (Appendix 33.2). Typhoid, paratyphoid and many other bacterial infections acquired in the tropics are increasingly resistant to many antimicrobials, particularly if the traveller has been in the Middle East or Asia and/or in contact with healthcare settings while travelling. Quinolone resistance is common in Gram-negative organisms and resistance to cefalosporins and carbapenems is rapidly increasing, so local sepsis treatment policies may not be appropriate and infection specialists should be consulted to advise on empirical treatment until results of cultures and sensitivity patterns become available.
- Empirical treatment for suspected enteric fever or gastroenteritis severe enough to merit antimicrobials is currently with azithromycin, or ceftriaxone for severe enteric fever.
- Patients with severe falciparum malaria and hypotension should also receive antibiotics to cover Gram-negative infection, as mixed infections may occur. See Chapter 35 for the management of sepsis and septic shock.

Table 33.2 Indicative incubation periods for selected tropical infections.

Short (<10 days)
Arboviral infections (including chikungunya, dengue and Zika virus)
Enteric bacterial infections
Malaria (minimum six days)
Plague
Scrub typhus, Q fever, spotted fever group, for example tick typhus (louse-borne, flea-borne)
Typhoid and paratyphoid
Viral haemorrhagic fever (VHF) (Lassa, Marburg, Crimean-Congo haemorrhagic fever, Ebola, Rift Valley)

Medium (10–21 days)
African trypanosomiasis
Brucellosis
Leptospirosis
Malaria
Scrub typhus, Q fever, spotted fever group, for example tick typhus
Typhoid and paratyphoid

Long (>21 days)
Amoebic liver abscess
Filariasis
HIV
Malaria
Schistosomiasis (Katayama fever)
Tuberculosis
Viral hepatitis
Visceral leishmaniasis

Table 33.3 Urgent investigation of the patient with a febrile illness after travel abroad.

Full blood count and differential white count
Blood films and rapid diagnostic tests for malarial parasites if travel to or through an endemic area; the intensity of the parasitaemia is variable in malaria. If the diagnosis is suspected but the film and RDT are negative, repeat blood films three times over 24–48 hours.
Blood culture × 2
C-reactive protein
Blood glucose
Sodium, potassium, urea and creatinine
Liver function tests
Throat swab
Urine stick test, microscopy and culture
Stool microscopy and culture
Serology as appropriate, for example for suspected viral hepatitis, Legionella pneumonia, typhoid, amoebic liver abscess, leptospirosis (save serum initially if diagnosis uncertain)
Chest X-ray and ultrasound liver if clinical suspicion
Lumbar puncture if neck stiffness present (preceded by CT only if indicated) (Chapter 68)

Appendix 33.1 Falciparum malaria.

Element	Comment
Clinical features	Prodromal symptoms of malaise, headache, myalgia, anorexia and mild fever.
	Paroxysms of fever lasting 8–12 h but classical cyclical fever patterns rarely present in early infection.
	Dry cough, abdominal discomfort, diarrhoea and vomiting common.
	Moderate tender hepatosplenomegaly (without lymphadenopathy).
	Jaundice may occur.
Cerebral malaria	Reduced conscious level.
	Focal or generalized fits.
	Abnormal neurological signs may be present (including opisthotonos, extensor posturing of decorticate or decerebrate pattern, sustained posturing of limbs, conjugate deviation of the eyes, nystagmus, dysconjugate eye movements, bruxism, extensor plantar responses, generalized flaccidity).
	Retinal haemorrhages common (papilloedema may be present but is unusual).
	Abnormal patterns of breathing common (including irregular periods of apnoea and hyperventilation). Tachypnoea may be due to acidosis or adult respiratory distress syndrome.
Blood results	Neutropenia
	Thrombocytopenia
	Low pH, raised lactate
	Haemolysis and anaemia
	Hypoxaemia
	Hypoglycaemia
	Renal failure
	Disseminated intravascular coagulation
	Abnormal transaminases
	Hyperbilirubinaemia and sometimes hyperbilirubinuria
Diagnosis	Microscopy of Giemsa-stained thick and thin blood films and rapid diagnostic tests (RDT) for malaria. RDT and thick films are more sensitive for detection of malaria and the thin film allows species identification and quantification of the percentage of parasitized red cells.
Treatment	Supportive management as for severe sepsis; early admission to high dependency or intensive care facility.
	Chemotherapy: see Table 33.4.
	Seek advice from an infectious disease or tropical physician.
Management of complications	See Table 33.5.

Appendix 33.2 Enteric fever (typhoid and paratyphoid).

Element	Comment
Clinical features	Insidious onset with malaise, headache, myalgia,
	dry cough, anorexia and fever
	Abdominal pain, distension and tenderness
	Sustained high fever
	Diarrhoea early and late, constipation in mid course of illness
	Ileal perforation (due to necrosis of Peyer patch in bowel wall) resulting in peritonitis in ~2%
	Gastrointestinal bleeding (due to erosion of Peyer patch into vessel) in ~15%
	Encephalopathy in ~10%
	Liver and spleen often palpable after first week

(*Continued*)

Element	Comment
	Erythematous macular rash (rose spots) on upper
	abdomen and anterior chest (may occur during second week) in ~25%
Blood results	Raised white cell count
	Mild thrombocytopenia
	Abnormal liver function tests
Diagnosis	Blood culture positive in 40–80%
	Stool and urine culture positive after first week
	Laboratory should test isolates for fluoroquinolone resistance (common)
Treatment	Supportive management as for severe sepsis
	Antibiotic therapy with azithromycin or ceftriaxone

Table 33.4 Chemotherapy of falciparum malaria (see guidelines and *British National Formulary*).

Patient seriously ill or unable to take tablets

IV artesunate is treatment of choice, but if not immediately available start with IV quinine. There is no added benefit from giving both agents.

Artesunate regimen: 2.4 mg/kg given as an intravenous injection at 0, 12 and 24 h, then daily thereafter. After completion of a minimum of 24 h therapy (maximum five days), a full course of an oral ACT should be taken when the patient can tolerate oral medication.

All patients receiving artesunate or ACT in hospital should have follow up full blood count 2 weeks later for possible anaemia.

OR

IV quinine: loading dose of 20 mg/kg quinine dihydrochloride in 5% dextrose or dextrose saline over 4 h (usual maximum dose 1.4 g), followed by 10 mg/kg (usual maximum 700 mg) every 8 h for first 48 h (or until patient can swallow). Frequency of dosing should be reduced to 12 hourly if intravenous quinine continues for more than 48 hours. Omit high loading dose if quinine, quinidine or mefloquine given within the previous 12 h.

Parenteral quinine therapy should be continued until the patient can take oral therapy, when quinine sulphate 600 mg should be given three times a day to complete five to seven days of quinine in total.

Quinine treatment should always be accompanied by a second drug: doxycycline 200 mg (or clindamycin 450 mg three times a day for children or pregnant women), given orally for total of seven days from when the patient can swallow.

Patient not seriously ill and able to swallow tablets

Artemether with lumefantrine (Riamet): if weight is over 35 kg, give four tablets initially, followed by five further doses of four tablets at 8, 24, 36, 48 and 60 h (total 24 tablets over 60 h).

or

Dihydroartemisinin-piperaquine (DHA-PPQ) is another co-artem combination that may be used: if 36–60 kg, 3 tablets daily for 3 days; if >60 kg 4 tablets daily for 3 days. See product literature cautions, especially in patients with cardiac conditions and/or taking agents that prolong QT interval.

or

Atovaquone with proguanil (Malarone) four tablets once daily for three days.

or

Quinine 600 mg of quinine salt 8-hourly PO for 5–7 days, PLUS doxycycline 200 mg daily PO (or clindamycin 450 mg 8-hourly) for 7 days (start these as soon as possible with the quinine).

It is not necessary to give doxycycline or clindamycin with or after treatment with agents other than quinine.

Table 33.5 Management of complications of falciparum malaria.

Complication	Management
Hypotension	Transfer to high dependency unit.
	Give IV fluids to maintain blood pressure but caution against fluid overload.
	Maintain adequate oxygenation.
	Start inotropic vasopressor therapy if systolic BP remains <90 mmHg despite fluids (Chapter 2).
	Start antibiotic therapy for possible coexistent Gram-negative sepsis after taking blood cultures (Chapter 35).
Hypoglycaemia	This is a common complication.
	Blood glucose should be checked 4-hourly, or 2-hourly while on IV quinine, or whenever conscious level deteriorates or if seizures occur.
	If blood glucose is <4 mmol/L, give 100 mL of glucose 20% IV and start an IV infusion of glucose 10% (initially 1 L 12-hourly) via a large peripheral or central vein.
Seizures	Recheck blood glucose.
	Manage along standard lines (Chapter 16).
	Exclude coexistent bacterial meningitis by CSF examination (NB lumbar puncture should not be done within 1 h of a major seizure).
Pulmonary oedema	May occur from excessive IV fluid or ARDS (Chapter 47).
	Manage along standard lines (Chapter 47).
Renal failure and acidosis	Haemofiltration may be needed for renal failure or control of acidosis or fluid/electrolyte imbalance.
Anaemia and thrombocytopenia	Both improve after several days of malaria chemotherapy. Anaemia is haemolytic and transfusion is only required for severe symptomatic anaemia. Thrombocytopenia is common and may be profound but platelet transfusions are not usually indicated.

ARDS, acute respiratory distress syndrome; CSF, cerebrospinal fluid.

Chest X-ray shadowing

Consider pulmonary tuberculosis, SARS and MERS CoV, and Legionnaires' disease, in addition to the common causes of community-acquired pneumonia (Chapter 62).

Meningism

- See Chapter 68 for the management of suspected bacterial meningitis, and Chapter 69 for suspected encephalitis.
- Perform a lumbar puncture, preceded by CT only if indicated.
- If the CSF shows no organisms but a high lymphocyte count, consider tuberculous meningitis (Appendix 68.1), leptospirosis or brucellosis.
- If there are other features suggesting leptospirosis (haemorrhagic rash, conjunctivitis, renal failure, jaundice), give ceftriaxone or benzyl penicillin or doxycycline.

Jaundice

- See Chapter 23 for the assessment of the patient with acute jaundice.
- Always consider falciparum malaria. Others causes are viral hepatitis A, B and E (but with these infections patients are usually afebrile when jaundice appears), leptospirosis, cytomegalovirus and Epstein-Barr virus infection, in addition to non-infectious causes, including drug and alcohol toxicity.

Diarrhoea

- See Chapter 22 for the management of the patient with acute diarrhoea.
- Causes to consider following recent travel abroad are given in Table 22.5.

Eosinophilia

The presence of eosinophilia in association with fever in returned travellers usually indicates an invasive helminth infection, but exclude other causes, especially atopy and drug reactions. Causes include filariasis (clues nocturnal or diurnal fever pattern); early phase of strongyloides and hookworm infections (abdominal pain, diarrhoea); hookworm and roundworm pneumonitis (cough, wheeze); early schistosomiasis (freshwater exposure especially in Africa/Middle East, urticarial rash, wheeze, altered semen); and loiasis (travel to Africa, transient peripheral skin swellings). Seek expert advice on special investigations needed.

Further reading

Beeching NJ, Fletcher TE, Wijaya L (2013). Health problems in returned travellers. *In Principles and Practice of Travel Medicine*, 2nd edn. Ed. Jane N. Zuckerman. Blackwell Publishing Ltd. pp 260–286.

Centers for Disease Control and Prevention: *Traveler's Health*. https://www.cdc.gov/

Checkley AM, Chiodini PL, Dockrell DH, et al, for British Infection Society and Hospital for Tropical Diseases. Eosinophilia in returning travellers and migrants from the tropics: UK recommendations for investigation and initial management (2010). *Journal of Infection*, 60, 1–20.

Johnston V, Stockley JM, Dockrell D, et al, for British Infection Society and the Hospital for Tropical Diseases Fever in returned travellers presenting in the United Kingdom: recommendations for investigation and initial management (2009). *Journal of Infection*, 59, 1–18.

Kularatne SAM (2015). Dengue fever. *BMJ* 351, h4661. DOI: 10.1136/bmj.h4661.

Lalloo DG, Shingadia D, Bell DJ, Beeching NJ, Whitty CJM, Chiodini PL, for the PHE Advisory Committee on Malaria Prevention in UK Travellers (2016). *UK malaria treatment guidelines. Journal of Infection* 72, 635–649.

Thwaites GE, Day NP (2017). Approach to fever in the returning traveler. *New England Journal of Medicine*, 376, 548–560.

CHAPTER 34

Acute medical problems in the HIV-positive patient

Mas Chaponda and Nick Beeching

Human immunodeficiency virus (HIV) positive patients get common diseases as well as those that reflect their immune deficiency. The spectrum of HIV infection is summarized in Box 34.1.

* Establish from the patient who knows about the HIV diagnosis among the patient's relatives and friends: be sensitive to their needs and respect the patient's right to confidentiality.

Box 34.1 Spectrum of HIV infection.

Group 1	Acute infection or primary HIV infection (a mononucleosis-like syndrome associated with sero-conversion)
Group 2	Asymptomatic infection
Group 3	Symptomatic disease
Group 4	Advanced disease: CD4 count $<200 \times 10^6$/L)

Constitutional disease (e.g. fever, weight loss, diarrhoea)*
Neurological disease (HIV encephalopathy, opportunistic infection, central nervous system lymphoma)
Secondary infectious diseases:
* Pneumocystis pneumonia
* Cytomegalovirus chorioretinitis, colitis, pneumonitis or adrenalitis
* *Candida albicans*: oral thrush*, oesophagitis
* *Mycobacterium avium-intracellulare*: localized or disseminated infection
* *Mycobacterium tuberculosis* infection*
* *Cryptococcus neoformans*: meningitis or disseminated infection
* *Toxoplasma gondii*: encephalitis or intracerebral mass lesions
* Herpes simplex virus: severe mucocutaneous lesions, oesophagitis
* *Cryptosporidium* spp. diarrhoea
* *Cystoisospora belli* diarrhoea
Secondary neoplasms:
* Kaposi's sarcoma (cutaneous and visceral)
* Lymphoma (brain, bone marrow, gut)
Other conditions (thrombocytopenia, non-specific interstitial pneumonitis)*
AIDS is diagnosed in an HIV-positive patient with group 4 disease, except those marked*

Acute Medicine: A Practical Guide to the Management of Medical Emergencies, Fifth Edition. Edited by David Sprigings and John B. Chambers.
© 2018 John Wiley & Sons Ltd. Published 2018 by John Wiley & Sons Ltd.

- Take appropriate safety precautions when handling any body fluid and label specimens according to local policies.
- The management of acute medical problems in the patient with HIV/AIDS is often complex, and you should seek advice from an infectious disease (ID) physician early on.

Breathlessness (see also Chapter 10)

Pulmonary infection (especially with *Pneumocystis jirovecii* pneumonia) remains the most common acute presentation of HIV-positive patients. Causes to consider are given in Table 34.1. Management is summarized in Figure 34.1.

1 Attach a pulse oximeter and check arterial blood gases: the patient may be severely hypoxaemic with minimal lung signs. Give oxygen to maintain arterial oxygen saturation >90%. Investigations needed urgently are given in Table 34.2.

2 Your clinical assessment and the chest X-ray appearance may provide clues to the likely diagnosis (Table 34.3).
- Dual pathology is relatively frequent, and definitive diagnosis depends on microbiological findings.
- Initial treatment for suspected *Pneumocystis jirovecii* pneumonia (PCP) is given in Table 34.4.
- Seek advice from a chest physician and ID physician on further management. Examination of induced sputum and/or bronchoscopic alveolar lavage fluid are often helpful in making a diagnosis.

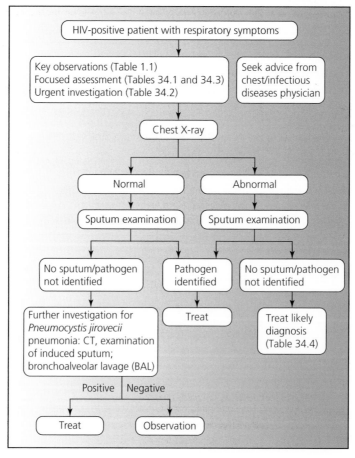

Figure 34.1 Assessment and management of the HIV-positive patient with respiratory symptoms.

Table 34.1 Respiratory symptoms in the HIV-positive patient.

CD4 T cell count (×10⁶/L)		
>500	**200–500**	**<200**
Usual causes	Usual causes	Usual causes
Mycobacterium tuberculosis infection	*M. tuberculosis* infection	*Pneumocystis jirovecii* pneumonia
		M. tuberculosis infection
		M. avium-intracellulare infection
		Cytomegalovirus pneumonitis
		Fungal pneumonia
		Kaposi's sarcoma

Table 34.2 Urgent investigation of the HIV-positive patient with respiratory symptoms.

Chest X-ray
Arterial blood gases and pH
Full blood count and differential white count
CD4 T cell count and HIV viral load
Blood culture (positive in most patients with *Mycobacterium avium-intracellulare* infection: use specific myobacterial culture bottles)
Blood glucose
Sodium and potassium, urea and creatinine
Liver function tests
Lactate dehydrogenase (raised in *Pneumocystis jirovecii* pneumonia)
Expectorated sputum if available for Gram and Ziehl-Neelsen stains and culture
Induced sputum (using hypertonic saline via nebulizer) for staining or PCR for *Pneumocystis jirovecii* and mycobacterial stains and culture
Consider fibre-optic bronchoscopy (for bronchoalveolar lavage or transbronchial biopsy)

Table 34.3 Diagnostic clues in the HIV-positive patient with respiratory symptoms.

Diagnosis	Clinical features	Chest X-ray features
***Pneumocystis* (*jirovecii*) pneumonia (PCP)**	Dyspnoea, often of slow onset Dry cough Lungs clear, or sparse basal crackles Fever See Table 34.4	Perihilar haze: diffuse bilateral interstitial or alveolar shadowing Lobar consolidation rare Pleural effusion rare Pneumothorax may occur See Table 34.4
***Mycobacterium tuberculosis* infection**	Cough Haemoptysis Fever	More often typical of tuberculosis if CD4 count is >200: multiple areas of consolidation, often with cavitation, in one or both upper lobes
***Mycobacterium avium-intracellulare* infection**	Cough Dyspnoea Fever	Often normal
Bacterial pneumonia (Chapter 62)	Commoner in smokers Productive cough Focal signs Fever	Focal consolidation
Cytomegalovirus pneumonitis	Clinically indistinguishable from PCP (dual infection may occur)	Diffuse bilateral interstitial shadowing
Fungal pneumonia	Fever Cough Weight loss Systemic features of fungal infection may be present (skin lesions, lymphadenopathy, hepatosplenomegaly)	Diffuse bilateral interstitial shadowing in ~50% Focal shadowing, nodules, cavities, pleural effusion and hilar adenopathy may be seen
Kaposi's sarcoma	No fever Dyspnoea May be associated with cutaneous Kaposi's sarcoma	Diffuse bilateral interstitial shadowing, more nodular than PCP May be unilateral and associated with hilar adenopathy Pleural effusion strongly suggestive

Table 34.4 *Pneumocystis jirovecii* pneumonia (PCP): diagnosis and management.

Element	Comment
Patients at risk	Newly diagnosed HIV infection with advanced disease (CD4 count <200)
	Patients with previous PCP or CD4 count <200 who are not taking prophylaxis
Clinical features	Subacute onset
	Fever (~90%)
	Cough (~95%), usually non-productive Progressive breathlessness (~95%)
	Tachypnoea (~60%)
	Chest examination normal in ~50%
Chest X-ray features	Initially normal in up to 25%
	Commonest abnormalities are diffuse bilateral interstitial or alveolar shadowing
	Lobar consolidation rare. Pleural effusion rare. Pneumothorax may occur
Induced sputum	Staining of induced sputum for *P. jirovecii* trophic forms and cysts
	Specificity ~100%, sensitivity 50–90%
	PCR Sensitivity 98%, specificity 80–98%
Bronchoscopy with bronchoalveolar lavage	Indicated if PCP is suspected but induced sputum is non-diagnostic or cannot be done
	Specificity ~100%, sensitivity ~80–90%
Antimicrobial therapy	First choice: co-trimoxazole PO or IV for 21 days. Causes haemolysis in glucose-6-phosphate dehydrogenase-deficient patients (African/Mediterranean). Other side effects include nausea, vomiting, fever, rash, marrow suppression and raised transaminases.
	Alternative regimens: primaquine + clindamycin; atovaquone; pentamidine
Adjuvant steroid therapy	Start immediately if severe PCP (breathless at rest; PaO2 breathing air <8 kPa; extensive interstitial shadowing on chest X-ray)
	Give prednisolone 40 mg twice daily PO for 5 days, followed by prednisolone 40 mg daily PO for 5 days, then prednisolone 20 mg daily PO for 11 days

Neuro-ophthalmic problems (see also Chapter 14)

With improved PCP prophylaxis, HIV-positive patients are presenting more frequently with neuro-ophthalmic problems (Table 34.5).

Table 34.5 Headache/delirium/focal neurological signs in the HIV-positive patient.

CD4 T cell count (×10⁶/L)		
>500	**200–500**	**<200**
Usual causes	Usual causes	Usual causes
(see also Chapters 4, 14 and 15)	HIV encephalopathy	Primary CNS lymphoma
	Tuberculous meningitis (Appendix 68.1)	Tuberculous meningitis (Appendix 68.1)
		Toxoplasmosis
		Cryptococcal meningitis (Appendix 68.2)
		Progressive multifocal leucoencephalopathy

Delirium with or without headache (see also Chapters 4 and 15)

Consider toxoplasmosis, cryptococcal meningitis (Appendix 68.2), cerebral lymphoma and progressive multifocal leucoencephalopathy. HIV encephalopathy is diagnosed by exclusion of other causes.

- Arrange urgent cranial CT or MR scan.
- Perform a lumbar puncture (LP) if the scan is normal. Send CSF for cell count; protein concentration; glucose (fluoride tube, together with blood glucose at same time); Gram, Ziehl–Neelsen and India ink stains; and culture and specific tests for *Cryptococcus* spp., *Toxoplasma gondii* and mycobacteria.
- If no specific diagnosis can be made, consider giving empirical treatment for toxoplasmosis with pyrimethamine and sulphadiazine, and repeat the scan after 2–3 weeks.
- Seek advice from an ID physician and neurologist.

Focal upper motor neuron signs

- Consider toxoplasmosis or lymphoma.
- Arrange urgent cranial CT or MRI.
- Perform a LP if the scan is normal, and send CSF for investigation as above.
- If focal lesions (ring-enhancing, with surrounding oedema on CT), treat as toxoplasmosis.
- Seek advice from an ID physician and neurologist.
- Consider sterotactic biopsy.

Impaired vision (see also Chapter 19)

Ophthalmic complications are more likely in advanced HIV and CD4 T cell count <50, particularly cytomegalovirus (CMV) retinitis and toxoplasmosis. Syphilis and tuberculosis may also affect the eye and may occur at any CD4 count.

- Suspect CMV retinitis: fundoscopy shows characteristic infiltrates, similar in appearance to soft exudates.
- Seek advice from an opthalmologist.
- Treatment is with ganciclovir (or cidofovir or foscarnet if ganciclovir is contraindicated; both are nephrotoxic). Gancicovir and its oral form valganciclovir can cause severe marrow depression which must be monitored.

Acute diarrhoea (see also Chapter 22)

See Chapter 22 for the assessment and management of the patient with acute diarrhoea.

Establish the differential diagnosis from the history and examination (Table 22.1). Strict infection control protocols must be followed (including barrier nursing and hand-washing). Investigations needed urgently are given in Table 22.2.

- Features of community-acquired infective diarrhoea are given in Table 22.3 and hospital-acquired diarrhoea in Table 22.4.
- Particular pathogens to consider in the patient with HIV/AIDS are given in Table 34.6.
- Seek advice from an ID physician and gastroenterologist.

Table 34.6 Chronic diarrhoea in the HIV-positive patient: specific pathogens to consider (in addition to other causes: see Chapter 22).

Cause	Clinical features	Diagnosis/treatment
Cryptosporidiosis (*Cryptosporidium* species)	Subacute onset Associated abdominal pain Severe diarrhoea	Identification of oocysts in stool Seek expert advice on treatment
Cystoisosporiasis (*Cystoisospora belli*)	Incubation period One week Associated fever, abdominal pain, diarrhoea with fatty stools	Identification of oocysts in stool, duodenal aspirate or jejunal biopsy Seek expert advice on treatment
Cytomegalovirus (CMV)	Diarrhoea may be accompanied by systemic illness and hepatitis	Serology and/or blood PCR for CMV; consider large bowel endoscopy and biopsy Seek expert advice on management

Further reading

British Association for Sexual Health and HIV Guidelines https://www.bashh.org/guidelines

British HIV Association (BHIVA) Guidelines http://www.bhiva.org/guidelines.aspx

European AIDS Clinical Society Guidelines. Version 8.1 October 2016. http://www.eacsociety.org/files/guidelines_8.1-english.pdf.

Maartens G, Celum C, Lewin SR (2014). HIV infection: epidemiology, pathogenesis, treatment, and prevention. *Lancet* 384, 258–271.

World Health Organization. Consolidated guidelines on HIV prevention, diagnosis, treatment and care for key populations; 2016 update. http://apps.who.int/iris/bitstream/10665/246200/1/9789241511124-eng.pdf?ua=1.

Syndromes and Disorders

General

CHAPTER 35

Sepsis

GUY GLOVER AND MANU SHANKAR-HARI

- Make a working diagnosis of sepsis (Box 35.1) if a patient has organ dysfunction in the context of suspected or proven infection. Because infection may be occult consider the diagnosis whenever organ dysfunction is unexplained.

Box 35.1 Definitions and criteria.

Term	Definition	Clinical criteria
Sepsis	Life-threatening organ dysfunction caused by a dysregulated host response to infection	Suspected or proven infection with total SOFA score ≥2
Septic shock	Subset of sepsis in which underlying circulatory, cellular and metabolic abnormalities are associated with a greater risk of mortality than sepsis alone	Sepsis with persisting hypotension requiring vasopressor therapy to maintain mean arterial pressure ≥65 mmHg and having a serum lactate level >2 mmol/L, despite adequate volume resuscitation.
Organ dysfunction	Organ dysfunction is identified using SOFA score. If previous baseline organ dysfunction is not known, for the purposes of the initial diagnosis baseline SOFA could be assumed as 0.	Please refer to Table 35.6
qSOFA	Consists of three variables Presence of two or more of these abnormalities in patients with suspected infection identifies higher risk of developing adverse outcomes often associated with sepsis.	Systolic blood pressure <100 mmHg Acute change in mentation (GCS ≥13) Respiratory rate >22/min

Definition refers to the illness concept and Criteria refers to the clinical variables used to identify a case of sepsis or septic shock.

Acute Medicine: A Practical Guide to the Management of Medical Emergencies, Fifth Edition. Edited by David Sprigings and John B. Chambers.
© 2018 John Wiley & Sons Ltd. Published 2018 by John Wiley & Sons Ltd.

Box 35.2 Sepsis Care Bundle: quality standards.

To be completed within three hours
- Measure lactate level
- Obtain 2 or more blood cultures prior to administration of antibiotics
- Administer broad spectrum antibiotics
- Administer 30 mL/kg crystalloid for hypotension or lactate ≥ 4 mmol/L

To be completed within six hours
- Start vasopressor therapy for hypotension that does not respond to initial fluid resuscitation, to maintain a mean arterial pressure (MAP) >65 mmHg.
- In the event of persistent hypotension after initial fluid administration (MAP < 65 mmHg) or if initial lactate was ≥ 4 mmol/L, re-assess volume status and tissue perfusion and document findings with:
  - EITHER:
    Repeat focused exam (after initial fluid resuscitation) including vital signs, capillary refill, pulse, and skin findings.
  - OR TWO OF THE FOLLOWING
    - Measure CVP
    - Measure ScvO$_2$
    - Bedside cardiovascular ultrasound
    - Dynamic assessment of fluid responsiveness with passive leg raise or fluid challenge
- Re-measure lactate if initial lactate was elevated

- Septic shock (Box 35.1) is a subset of sepsis in which underlying circulatory, cellular and metabolic abnormalities are associated with a greater risk of mortality than sepsis alone.
- *Escherichia coli*, *Staphylococcus aureus* and *Streptococcus pneumoniae* (pneumococcus) are the commonest pathogens.

  A good outcome depends on prompt diagnosis, adequate fluid resuscitation, timely administration of appropriate initial antibiotic therapy, and drainage of any infected collection. An overview of the principles of clinical management is shown in Box 35.2.

Priorities

Manage patients with sepsis according to a sepsis bundle, for example Surviving Sepsis Campaign Bundle (Box 35.2**) or the United Kingdom 'Sepsis 6'.**

1 If systolic BP is <100 mmHg and/or the serum lactate is elevated, give crystalloid IV 500 mL over 15 min using one, if necessary two, large bore (16 G or larger) cannulae. Give further IV fluid up to at least 30 mL/kg if hypotension or hyperlactataemia persists. Give high flow oxygen by mask initially, adjusted as needed to maintain arterial oxygen saturation >94% once adequate monitoring is in place.

2 Examine for a focus of infection (Table 35.1).
- The clinical setting may make it obvious, for example signs of pneumonia (Chapters 62, 63) or meningitis (Chapter 68) or recent instrumentation of the urinary or biliary tract.
- Check for neck stiffness, focal lung crackles or bronchial breathing, heart murmur, abdominal tenderness or guarding, acute arthritis, cellulitis, soft tissue abscess and signs of infection at the site of IV lines.
- Obtain a surgical opinion if you suspect an abdominal or pelvic source of sepsis.
- Many patients with neutropenic sepsis (Chapter 101) have no detectable clinical focus.

3 Investigations required urgently are given in Tables 35.2 and 35.3.

Table 35.1 Clinical assessment of the patient with suspected sepsis.

History

Context: age, sex, comorbidities, medications, hospital or community acquired

Current major symptoms and their time course

Risk factors for sepsis? Consider immunosuppressive therapy, HIV-AIDS, cancer, renal failure, liver failure, diabetes, malnutrition, splenectomy, IV drug use, prosthetic heart valve, other prosthetic material, peripheral IV cannula, central venous cannula, bladder catheter

Recent culture results?

Recent surgery or invasive procedures?

Recent foreign travel?

Contact with infectious disease?

Examination

Physiological observations

Head and neck: Neck stiffness? Jaundice? Mouth, teeth and sinuses: focus of infection? Lymphadenopathy?

Chest: Focal lung crackles/bronchial breathing? Pleural/pericardial rub? Heart murmur? Prosthetic heart valve? Pacemaker/ICD?

Abdomen and pelvis: Distension? Ascites? Tenderness/guarding? Bladder catheter? Perineal/perianal abscess?

Limbs: Acute arthritis? Prosthetic joint? Abscess?

Skin and soft tissues: Rash/purpura? Pressure ulceration? Cellulitis? Soft-tissue infection? IV cannula/tunnelled line?

- Early confirmation of infection is from microscopy or Gram staining or PCR panels or antigen detection tests. Take blood cultures and cultures from other relevant sites urgently in sepsis.
- A raised lactate is an important marker of septic shock and is associated with increased mortality (other causes include liver dysfunction, seizures, metformin and salbutamol).

4 Start antibiotic therapy as soon as blood has been taken for culture and well within one hour. Mortality rises with any delay.

Table 35.2 Urgent investigation of the patient with sepsis.

Blood tests

Full blood count (the white cell count may be low in overwhelming bacterial sepsis; a low platelet count may reflect disseminated intravascular coagulation)

Clotting screen if purpura or jaundice, prolonged oozing from puncture sites, bleeding from surgical wounds or low platelet count

C-reactive protein

Sodium, potassium, urea and creatinine

Blood glucose (hypoglycaemia can complicate sepsis, especially in patients with liver disease)

Liver function tests

Amylase

Arterial gases, pH and lactate

Microbiological tests (Table 35.3)

Imaging

Chest X-ray

Other imaging as directed by the clinical picture

Other tests

ECG if aged >50, history of cardiac disease or suspicion of arrythmia

Table 35.3 Microbiological tests in suspected sepsis.

Blood cultures – two sets drawn before administration of antimicrobials provided it will not lead to significant delays in therapy (positive in 30–50% and then associated with a worse outcome)

If a vascular catheter is suspected as the source then either:

1. Take paired cultures from peripheral stab and from each lumen of the catheter (this technique may be associated with a high rate of contamination) or

2. Remove the catheter and request MC&S on the tip – this latter is recommended if the patient is in septic shock and deteriorating.

Sputum culture – once intubated a deep, non-directed, or bronchoscopic directed washing has greater sensitivity and specificity

Mid-stream urine for urinalysis and MC&S

Invasive sampling/drainage of fluid collections in otherwise sterile spaces, for example joint aspiration if suspected septic arthritis (P. 701), pleural or ascitic fluid aspiration for microscopy and culture (P. 679 and 688), lumbar picture for CSF examination if suspected meningitis (P. 696)

Stool MC&S, CDT (if diarrhoea or recent foreign travel)

Bacterial swabs of any inflamed or discharging soft tissue areas or wounds

Molecular or antigen based tests, for example urinary antigens for legionella, pneumococcus, nasopharyngeal swabs for respiratory viral panel

Malarial film if appropriate travel history (P. 211)

HIV test

- Principles of good antibody practice are given in Table 35.4. The antibiotic used should be guided by a hospital protocol or an infection specialist based on the likely organism, taking account of the source of sepsis if known (Table 35.5), whether the infection is community or hospital-acquired, results of previous isolates from the patient and the local pattern of antibiotic resistance in patients.
- Gentamicin levels need to be monitored and doses should be reduced in renal impairment (consult the *British National Formulary*).
- Substitute amikacin for gentamicin if gentamicin resistance is prevalent.
- Substitute vancomycin for flucloxacillin if methicillin-resistant *Staphylococcus aureus* (MRSA) infection is possible. Serum levels of vancomycin should be measured.

5 'Red flag' signs:
- Systolic blood pressure <90 mmHg (or >40 mmHg fall from baseline)
- Heart rate >130/min
- Oxygen saturations <91%
- Respiratory rate >25/min
- Responds only to voice or pain/unresponsive
- Lactate >2.0 mmol/L

  Presence of one or more of red flag signs is an emergency. Refer to the Critical Care Outreach Team for further management of these patients in an intensive care or high-dependency unit.

6 Patients with sepsis are at risk of rapid deterioration and should be monitored closely every 30–60 min:
- Heart rate
- Blood pressure
- Respiratory rate
- Arterial oxygen saturation
- Temperature
- Conscious level
- Fluid balance including hourly urine output

Table 35.4 Good practice in antimicrobial prescribing for sepsis.

Antibiotics should be administered within one hour of diagnosis

Antibiotics should be 'broad spectrum', covering all of the likely pathogens (Table 35.5)

Consider whether the infection is community acquired or healthcare associated, any previously known culture results and the patient's allergy status when selecting antimicrobials

The first dose should prescribed as a timed 'stat' and the need for urgent administration should be communicated to nursing staff

The indication for the antibiotics should be documented as well as a review and stop date

Antibiotics should be de-escalated as soon as it is safe to do so by narrowing the spectrum and converting to oral therapy

Table 35.5 An example of initial antibiotic therapy regime for adult sepsis (excludes penicillin allergic patients). Always seek local guidance and check doses in the *British National Formulary*.

Suspected source of sepsis	Initial antibiotic therapy (IV, high dose if septic shock)
Bacterial meningitis	Ceftriaxone 4 g IV as a single dose on day 1, then 2 g IV OD thereafter. If immunocompromised or age >60 y consider amoxicillin 2 g IV q 4-hourly to cover listeria
Community-acquired pneumonia	Severe (CURB 65 ≥2): co-amoxiclav 1.2 g IV tds, plus doxycycline 200 mg PO OD
Hospital-acquired pneumonia	Co-amoxiclav 1.2 g IV tds, plus gentamicin 5 mg/kg IV (if late >3 days after admission)
Infective endocarditis	Take 3 sets of cultures, ideally 2–4 hours apart. Discuss with Infection prior to starting antibiotics see Table 52.7 P. 336
Urinary tract infection	Complicated/healthcare associated/pyelonephritis: co-amoxiclav 1 g IV tds
Intra-abdominal sepsis, for example appendicitis, peritonitis. Seek advice for other conditons, for example spontaneous bacterial peritonitis.	Cefuroxime 1.5 g IV tds plus metronidazole 500 mg IV tds
Suspected vascular catheter related bloodstream infection	Vancomycin IV plus gentamicin 5 mg/kg IV
Septic arthritis (native joint) Seek advice for prosthetic joint or metalwork infection	Flucloxacillin 2 g IV qds
Cellulitis	Flucloxacillin 2 g IV qds
Necrotizing fasciitis Discuss urgently with Infection/plastic surgeon	Cefuroxime 1.5 g IV tds plus gentamicin 5 mg/kg IV plus metronidazole 500 mg IV tds
No localizing signs: neutropenic	Meropenem 1 g IV tds
No localizing signs: not neutropenic	Community associated: cefuroxime 1.5g IV tds plus gentamicin 5 mg/kg IV plus metronidazole 500 mg IV tds Healthcare associated: co-amoxiclav 1.2 g IV tds plus gentamicin 5 mg/kg IV

Further management

Hypotension and organ dysfunction

Management requires invasive monitoring and critical care expertise.

Arterial and central venous monitoring will be required if the patient is in septic shock or once in the ICU but placement should not delay initial priorities.

The first priority is adequate fluid resuscitation, using a balanced crystalloid (e.g. Hartmann's solution). This should be guided by a clinical assessment of the circulation and tissue perfusion. A CVP of +8–12 (12–15 mmHg in mechanically ventilated patients) has been proposed as a target to guide fluid resuscitation, although more sophisticated measures may also be used which include response to passive leg raising, echocardiography or cardiac output monitoring.

If the patient remains hypotensive despite adequate fluid correction, start norepinephrine (dose range 0.05–1.0 µgm/kg/min). This must be administered via a central line. Aim for mean arterial pressure >65 mmHg. The goal is to restore tissue perfusion. Monitor with:

- Vital signs, capillary refill time, pulse and skin findings
- Urine output (aim for >0.5 mL/kg/hr)
- Arterial lactate (aim for normalization)
- Central venous O_2 saturation ($ScvO_2$) (aim for $\geq 70\%$)

If evidence of end organ hypoperfusion persists, perform a bedside echocardiogram and / or measure the cardiac output. Consider measures to improve oxygen delivery, such as transfusion of packed red cells or adding inotropic therapy, for example dobutamine.

Respiratory support

Mechanical ventilation in sepsis is indicated for:

- Severe acidosis
- Multi-organ failure
- Reduced consciousness
- Respiratory failure, for example due to pneumonia or the acute respiratory distress syndrome (ARDS). ARDS is characterized by acute-onset hypoxia and bilateral pulmonary infiltrates in the absence of a cardiac cause (excluded by pulmonary artery occlusion pressure measurement or echocardiography).
  The principles of ARDS management include:
- Mechanical ventilation with positive end expiratory pressure (PEEP) and low tidal volumes (6 mL/kg predicted body weight)
- A conservative fluid regimen
- Ventilation in the prone position for moderate or severe ARDS
- Neuromuscular blocking drugs for severe ARDS

Acute kidney injury (see Chapter 25)

Acute kidney injury (AKI) is common in sepsis and is associated with a worse outcome. The principles of treatment of AKI in sepsis are:

- Rule out additional obstruction
- Optimize fluid replacement and correction of tissue perfusion
- Consider renal replacement (usually with continuous veno-venous haemofiltration or haemodialysis) for refractory oliguria, fluid overload, acidosis, hyperkalaemia or azotaemia

Source control

When a persisting source of sepsis exists it is unlikely that antibiotics alone will be effective. Consider empyema, appendicitis, pyelonephrosis, necrotizing fasciitis. Indwelling cannulae, especially central venous lines, should be removed (and the tip sent for culture)

Antibiotic de-escalation and stewardship

Once the pathogenic organism is known the spectrum should be narrowed. Change to oral therapy once the patient is improved and apyrexial for >24 h. Most guidelines recommend a 7–10 day course but a shorter course (e.g. 5 days) may be safe if clinical resolution has occurred. In some situations, prolonged courses are necessary, for example infective endocarditis, lung abscess or bone infection: seek advice from a microbiologist. To avoid the development of resistance and the development of health-care associated infection (e.g. *Clostridium difficile* diarrhoea) antibiotics should not be overused:

- Document the indication for the drug
- Review the need for continuing antibiotics early and repeatedly
- If the diagnosis of sepsis is refuted the antibiotic should be stopped

Problems

Sepsis in the neutropenic patient (see Chapter 101)

Patients with neutrophil counts $<0.5 \times 10^9$/L are at high risk of bacterial infection, particularly from Gram-negative rods and *Staphylococcus aureus* and *epidermidis*. If the neutropenic patient has a single temperature $>38°C$, or two spikes of fever of $>37.5°C$ during a 24-h period, the likely cause is bacterial infection and empiric broad spectrum antibiotic therapy should be started. Search for a focus of infection. Examination should include the entire skin including the perineum and perianal region, indwelling IV line and other IV sites, and the mouth, teeth and sinuses. Investigations required urgently are given in Tables 35.2 and 35.3. Several antibiotic regimens have been shown to be effective in neutropenic patients without localizing signs:

- Antipseudomonal penicillin plus an aminoglycoside (e.g. azlocillin and gentamicin) or
- Monotherapy with a third-generation cephalosporin (e.g. ceftazidime) or aztreonam.
  Ask for advice from a haematologist.

Sepsis associated with IV drug use

Several causes of fever must be considered (Table 35.7). Right-sided endocarditis may not give rise to abnormal cardiac signs. Antibiotic therapy must cover staphylococci.

Table 35.6 Sequential (sepsis-related) organ failure assessment score.

Organ system	Variable (units)	Dysfunction		Failure	
		1	**2**	**3**	**4**
Respiratory system	PaO$_2$/FiO$_2$ ratio (kPa)	<53.3	<40	<26.7 and ventilation	<13.3 and ventilation
Cardiovascular system	MAP (mmHg) or vasoactive drugs μgm/Kg/min	MAP <70	Dopamine <5 or Dobutamine	Epinephrine or norepinephrine <0.1	Epinephrine or norepinephrine >0.1
Central nervous system	Glasgow coma score	13–14	10–12	6–9	<6
Coagulation	Platelets	<150	<100	<50	<20
Renal	Creatinine (μmol/L) OR Urine output (mL/24 hr)	110–170	171–299	300–440 <500 mLs/24 hours	>400 <200 hours
Liver	Bilirubin μmol/L	30–32	33–101	102–204	>204

Table 35.7 Possible causes of fever associated with IV drug use.

Infection at injection sites
Thrombophlebitis
Endocarditis (especially right-sided) (which may be complicated by septic pulmonary embolism)
Pulmonary tuberculosis
Hepatitis B or C
Septic arthritis
Pyrogen reaction
AIDS-related infection, for example cryptococcal meningitis, *Pneumocystis carinii* pneumonia

Disseminated intravascular coagulation

Disseminated intravascular coagulation (DIC) is a complication of sepsis (as well as a number of non-infective disorders). This should be suspected in patients with sepsis and also in patients with septic shock who develop purpura, prolonged oozing from puncture sites, bleeding from surgical wounds or bleeding from the gastro-intestinal and respiratory tracts. Confirm by a low platelet count ($<100 \times 10^{12}$/L), prolonged prothrombin and activated partial thromboplastin times, and a high plasma concentration of fibrin degradation products. Ask advice on management from a haematologist.

If there is active bleeding or a significant invasive procedure (i.e. surgery or radiological drainage) is needed, give fresh frozen plasma and platelet concentrates, although this is not usually necessary for invasive lines in the ICU (seek senior advice). There is no conclusive evidence for the use of heparin in the treatment of DIC, but this should be considered if there is thromboembolism. Give vitamin K 10 mg IV to reverse possible vitamin K deficiency which may contribute to the coagulopathy, although there is no evidence base addressing this specific question in sepsis.

Further reading

Long B, Koyfman A (2016) Clinical mimics: An Emergency Medicine–focused review of sepsis mimics. *Journal of Emergency Medicine*. 52, 34–42.

Seymour CW, Liu VX, Iwashyna TJ, *et al*. (2016) Assessment of clinical criteria for sepsis: For the Third International Consensus definitions for sepsis and septic shock (Sepsis-3). *JAMA* 315, 762–774.

Shankar-Hari M, Phillips GS, Levy ML, *et al*. (2016) Developing a new definition and assessing new clinical criteria for septic shock: For the Third International Consensus definitions for sepsis and septic shock (Sepsis-3). *JAMA* 315, 775–787.

Singer M, Deutschman CS, Seymour CW, *et al*. (2016) The Third International Consensus definitions for sepsis and septic shock (Sepsis-3). *JAMA* 315, 801–810.

Surviving Sepsis Campaign Guidelines. http://www.survivingsepsis.org/Guidelines/Pages/default.aspx.

Vincent J-L, Mira J-P, Antonelli M. (2016) Sepsis: older and newer concepts. *Lancet Respir Med* 4, 237–240.

CHAPTER 36

Poisoning

NIGEL LANGFORD AND DAVID SPRIGINGS

- In the UK, if you need advice about the management of a patient with severe or complex poisoning (e.g. multiple medications taken, pregnancy or major comorbidities), contact the National Poisons Information Service (NPIS) for advice (24-hour phone line, 0344 892 0111).
- Information on poisons and the management of poisoning is also available at the TOXBASE website (www.toxbase.org) (the primary clinical toxicology database of the NPIS; user name and password needed).
- Management of the patient with suspected poisoning is summarized in Figure 36.1.

Priorities

The unconscious patient with suspected poisoning

1 Stabilize the airway, breathing and circulation
- For detailed guidance, see Chapters 1, 59, 112 (airway management), 11 and 113 (management of respiratory failure) and 2 (management of hypotension and shock).
- If carbon monoxide poisoning is suspected (Appendix 36.2), give oxygen 10 L/min by a tightly fitting facemask with a circuit which minimizes rebreathing.

2 Exclude and correct hypoglycaemia
- If blood glucose is <4.0 mmol/L, give 100 mL of 20% glucose or 200 mL of 10% glucose over 15–30 min IV, or glucagon 1 mg IV/IM/SC.
- Recheck blood glucose after 10 min: if still <4.0 mmol/L, repeat the above IV glucose treatment.
- In patients with malnourishment or alcohol-use disorder, there is a remote risk of precipitating Wernicke encephalopathy by a glucose load: prevent this by giving thiamine 100 mg IV before or shortly after glucose administration.
- See Chapter 81 for further management of hypoglycaemia.

3 Treat prolonged or recurrent major seizures
- Take into account pre-hospital treatment. Give **lorazepam** (which is less likely to cause respiratory suppression) 0.1 mg/kg (typically 4–8 mg) IV over 5–10 min (Table 16.2), **midazolam** 10 mg buccally (NICE-recommended, but only licensed in patients <18 years), or **diazepam** 10–20 mg IV at a rate of <2.5 mg/min (faster injection rates carry the risk of sudden apnoea).
- If the seizure does not terminate, give a second dose, to a maximum total dose of lorazepam 8 mg or diazepam 40 mg.
- See Chapter 16 for further management of seizures/status epilepticus.

4 Give naloxone, if opioid poisoning is possible or must be excluded
- If the respiratory rate is <12/min, or the pupils are pinpoint, or there is other reason to suspect opioid poisoning, give naloxone 800 µgm IV every 2–3 min up to a total dose of 4000 µgm or until the respiratory rate is >15/min. Large doses may be required in a severely poisoned patient or if synthetic opioids have been taken. Aim for reversal of respiratory depression, not full reversal of consciousness.

Acute Medicine: A Practical Guide to the Management of Medical Emergencies, Fifth Edition. Edited by David Sprigings and John B. Chambers.
© 2018 John Wiley & Sons Ltd. Published 2018 by John Wiley & Sons Ltd.

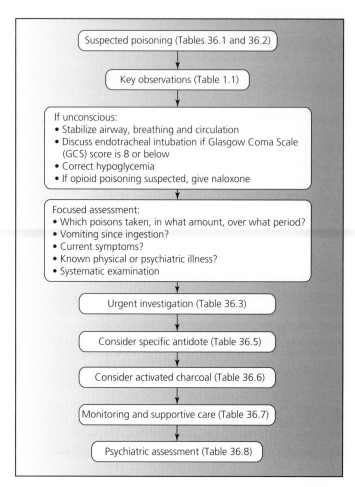

Figure 36.1 Management of the patient with suspected poisoning.

- If there is a response to bolus naloxone, start an IV infusion: make up a naloxone solution with 10 mg naloxone (25 vials) made up to a final volume of 50 mL with glucose 5% (200 μgm/mL) and infuse using an IV pump. Start the infusion at 60% of the initial dose required for resuscitation per hour, and titrate against the respiratory rate and conscious level.
- In patients who have taken partial opioid agonists such as buprenorphine, methadone and tramadol, repeated large (1200 μgm) doses of naloxone may be required to achieve a satisfactory response.
- If there is no response to naloxone, this suggests that another CNS depressant has been taken or brain injury has occurred.

5 **Obtain the history**

The history should be obtained from all available sources: ambulance personnel, friends and family, primary care and hospital records.

6 **Make a systematic examination**
- The clinical features may provide clues to the poison (Tables 36.1 and 36.2). Mixed poisoning is common.
- Bear in mind the possibility of multiple pathology (e.g. poisoning followed by head injury; poisoning on a background of chronic liver disease). Points to cover in the neurological examination of the unconscious patient are given on p. 18.

Table 36.1 Clues to the poison (1): clinical and biochemical features.

Feature	Poisons to consider
Coma	Barbiturates, benzodiazepines, ethanol, opioids, trichloroethanol, tricyclics
Fits	Amphetamines, cocaine, dextropropoxyphene, insulin, oral hypoglycaemics, phenothiazines, theophylline, tricyclics, lead
Constricted pupils	Opioids, organophosphates, trichloroethanol
Dilated pupils	Amphetamines, cocaine, phenothiazines, quinine, sympathomimetics, tricyclics
Arrhythmias	Anti-arrhythmics, anticholinergics, phenothiazines, quinine, sympathomimetics, tricyclics
Hypertension	Amphetamines, cocaine
Pulmonary oedema	Carbon monoxide, ethylene glycol, irritant gases, opioids, organophosphates, paraquat, salicylates, tricyclics
Ketones on breath	Ethanol, isopropyl alcohol, alcoholic or starvation ketoacidosis
Hypothermia	Barbiturates, ethanol, opioids, tricyclics
Hyperthermia	Amphetamines and MDMA, anticholinergics, cocaine, monoamine oxidase inhibitors
Hypoglycaemia	Insulin, oral hypoglycaemics, ethanol, salicylates
Hyperglycaemia	Theophylline, organophosphates, salbutamol
Acute kidney injury	Amanita phalloides, ethylene glycol, paracetamol, salicylates, prolonged hypotension, rhabdomyolysis (Appendix 25.1)
Hypokalaemia	Salbutamol, salicylates, theophylline
Metabolic acidosis	Carbon monoxide, ethanol, ethylene glycol, methanol, paracetamol, salicylates, tricyclics
Raised plasma osmolality	Ethanol, ethylene glycol, isopropyl alcohol, methanol
Rhabdomyolysis	Carbon monoxide, ethanol, opioids, solvents

MDMA, 3,4-methylenedioxy-methamphetamine ('ecstasy').

- Is there evidence of IV substance use? Check for needle marks in the antecubital fossae, neck, supra-clavicular areas, groins, dorsum of feet and under the tongue. IV substance use may be complicated by venous thrombosis, cellulitis and, rarely, botulism.
- Check for possible complications of coma (hypothermia, pressure necrosis of skin or muscle, corneal abrasions, inhalation pneumonia).

7 Investigations

These are needed urgently and are given in Table 36.3. The results may provide further clues to the poison. Urine is preferable to blood for qualitative analysis as toxins are concentrated in the urine.

8 Discuss management with an intensivist and arrange admission to ICU if:

- The Glasgow Coma Scale score is 8 or below, or there are recurrent seizures.
- There is respiratory failure despite administration of antidotes, or an endotracheal tube has been placed.
- There are major arrhythmias or the patient is at high risk of arrhythmias (e.g. tricyclic poisoning with broad QRS complex).
- There is hypotension or severe acidosis (pH <7.2) not responding to fluid resuscitation.

The conscious patient with poisoning

1 Check baseline observations

Document conscious level (fully orientated or confused – use AVPU score), pulse, blood pressure, respiratory rate, arterial oxygen saturation, temperature and blood glucose.

2 Establish:

- Which poisons were taken, in what amount and over what period.
- If the patient has vomited since ingestion, and when (unlikely to have eliminated significant amounts of poison if over an hour from ingestion).

Table 36.2 Clues to the poison (2): toxidromes.

Toxidrome	Example	Heart rate	Blood pressure	Respiratory rate	Conscious level	Pupil size	Sweating	Temperature	Comments
Sympathomimetic	Cocaine, cathinones, amphetamines, some novel psychoactive substances (legal highs)	↑	↑	↑	↑	↑	↑	↑	Electrolyte disturbances and muscle breakdown
Anticholinergic	Hyoscine, antidepressants, diphenhydramine, antipsychotics	↑	(↑)	↓	↑	↑	↓	↑	Urinary retention
Cholinergic	Organophosphorous sarin, VX	↓	No change	No change	(No change)	↓	↑	(No change)	Emesis, diarrhoea, urinary incontinence, hypersalivation
Opioid	Morphine, fentanyl, oxycodone, codeine, methadone, buprenorphine	↓	↓	↓	↓	↓	↓	↓	Classical triad not always present Monitor GCS/AVPU as naloxone only short acting
Sedative hypnotic	Benzodiazepines, "Z" hypnotics	↓	↓	↓	↓	(↑)	↓	↓	Monitor GCS/AVPU
Serotonin syndrome	SSRI, SNRI lithium	↑	↑	↑	↑	↑	↑	↑	Check for myoclonus
Neuroleptic malignant syndrome	Antipsychotics	↑	(↑)	No change	↓	(↑)	↑	↑	Short onset and duration of events ↑ muscle tone and CK Takes five or more days to resolve
Alcohol withdrawal	Alcohol	↑	No change	(No change)	(↑)	↑	↑	(↑)	Consider using **CIWA-Ar/ GMAWS** to objectively monitor and respond to withdrawal
Opioid withdrawal	Opioids	↑	(No change)	(↑)	(↑)	↑	↑	(↑)	Consider using **COWS** to objectively monitor and respond to withdrawal

↓ reduction in effect

() qualified change in effect

↑ increase in effect

Sources: Sullivan JT, Sykora K, Schneiderman J, Naranjo CA, Sellers EM (1989) Assessment of alcohol withdrawal: The revised Clinical Institute Withdrawal Assessment for Alcohol scale (**CIWA-Ar**). *British Journal of Addiction* 84, 1353–1357.

Wesson DR, Ling W (2003) The Clinical Opiate Withdrawal Scale (**COWS**). *J Psychoactive Drugs* 35, 253–259.

Table 36.3 Urgent investigation of the patient with poisoning.

Tests requested should take into account poison(s) taken, physiological status and comorbidities
Blood glucose, sodium, potassium, urea and creatinine
Plasma osmolality*
Paracetamol level if paracetamol poisoning is known or possible
Full blood count
Urinalysis (myoglobinuria due to rhabdomyolysis gives a positive stick test for blood)
Arterial blood gases and pH
Chest X-ray
ECG if there is hypotension, coexistent heart disease or suspected ingestion of cardiotoxic drugs (e.g. anti-arrhythmics, tricyclics)
If the substance ingested is not known, save serum (10 mL) and urine (50 mL) at 4°C in case later analysis is needed

*The normal range of plasma osmolality is 280–300 mOsmol/kg. If the measured plasma osmolality (by freezing-point depression method) exceeds calculated osmolality (from the formula [2(Na + K) + urea + glucose]) by 10 mOsmol/kg or more, consider poisoning with ethanol, ethylene glycol, isopropyl alcohol or methanol.

- Current symptoms.
- Associated physical or psychiatric illness.

3 **Investigations** needed will depend on the poisons and the presence of other physical illness. After poisoning with some drugs (Table 36.4), plasma levels should be checked.

4 **If the patient is at risk of harm but refuses treatment**
  Ask the help of a senior colleague and a psychiatrist. Issues of mental capacity and consent to treatment are discussed in Chapter 111.

Table 36.4 Poisoning in which plasma levels should be measured.
NB: Always check the units of measurement used by your laboratory.

Poison	Plasma level at which specific treatment is indicated	Treatment
Aspirin and other salicylates	250–500 mg/L (mild poisoning)	Fluids
	500–750 mg/L (moderate poisoning)	Urinary alkalinization
	750–1000 mg/L (severe poisoning)	HD
	>1000 mg/L (massive poisoning)	HD
Digoxin	>4 ng/mL	Digoxin-specific antibody fragments
Ethylene glycol	>500 mg/L	Ethanol or 4-methyl pyrazole, HD
Iron*	>3.5 mg/L	Desferrioxamine
Lithium (send sample in plain tube)	>5 mmol/L	HD
Methanol	>500 mg/L	Ethanol or 4-methyl pyrazole, HD
Paracetamol	See Appendix 36.1	Acetylcysteine
Theophylline	>50 mg/L	RAC, HD
Carbamazepine	>40 mg/L (170 micromol/L)	MDAC, consider lipid emulsion for cardiac toxicity

HD, haemodialysis; RAC, repeated oral activated charcoal.
*Also measure plasma iron level if clinical evidence of severe iron toxicity (hypotension, nausea, vomiting, diarrhoea) or after massive ingestion (>20 mg elemental iron/kg body weight; one 20 mg tablet of ferrous sulphate contains 6 mg elemental iron).

Table 36.5 Specific antidotes.
NB: Discuss the case with a Poisons Centre first, unless you are familiar with the poison and its antidote, as some antidotes may be harmful if given inappropriately.

Poison	Antidote
Anticholinergic agents	Physostigmine
Arsenic	Dimercaprol
Benzodiazepines	Flumazenil
Beta-blockers	Glucagon
Calcium antagonists	Calcium gluconate
Cyanide	Dicobalt edetate alone or sodium nitrite + sodium thiosulphate
Dabigatrin	Idarucizumab
Digoxin	Digoxin-specific antibody fragments
Ethylene glycol	Ethanol or 4-methylpyrazole
Fluoride	Calcium gluconate
Buproprion, local anaesthetics	Lipid emulsion (Intralipid®)
Iron	Desferrioxamine
Lead	Dimercaprol or penicillamine
Mercury	Dimercaprol or penicillamine
Methanol	Ethanol or 4-methylpyrazole
Opioids	Naloxone
Organophosphates	Atropine
Paracetamol	Acetylcysteine (Appendix 36.1)
Thallium	Berlin blue
Warfarin	Vitamin K or fresh frozen plasma or prothrombin complex concentrate (see p. 591)

Further management

Is a specific antidote or treatment indicated?
- See Table 36.5. Discuss the case with a Poisons Centre first, unless you are familiar with the poison and its antidote, as some antidotes may be harmful if given inappropriately.
- The management of paracetamol and carbon monoxide poisoning is given in Appendices 36.1 and 36.2.

Reducing absorption
Activated charcoal (50 g mixed with 200 mL of water) should be given if a significant amount of any poison has been ingested within 1 h (or longer if modified-release preparations or drugs with anticholinergic effects have been taken), and oral antidotes are not indicated (Table 36.6). Exceptions to this are poisoning with substances which are poorly absorbed by charcoal. Because of the risk of inhalation, activated charcoal should not be given to a patient with a reduced conscious level unless the airway is protected by a cuffed endotracheal tube.

  Gastric lavage should **not** be employed in the management of poisoned patients, as the risks of complications outweigh any benefits.

Increasing elimination
- Drugs whose elimination can be increased by repeated dosing with activated charcoal are given in Table 36.6. Give 50 g initially then 25 g 4-hourly by mouth or nasogastric tube until recovery or until plasma drug levels have fallen to within the safe range. Laxatives may also be required.
- Other methods (e.g. haemodialysis) may be indicated in selected cases, after discussion with a Poisons Centre.

Table 36.6 Charcoal administration after poisoning.

Repeated dosing indicated	Single dose indicated (only within the first hour after presentation)	Charcoal not indicated
Barbiturates	Antihistamines	Acids
Carbamazepine	Paracetamol	Alkalis
Dapsone	Salicylates	Carbamate
Digoxin	Tricyclics	Cyanide
Phenytoin	Other poisons unless charcoal contraindicated	Ethanol
Quinine		Ethylene glycol
Sustained-release preparations		Hydrocarbons
Theophylline		Iron
		Lithium
		Methanol
		Organophosphates

Monitoring

In all patients with severe poisoning, monitor:

- Conscious level (initially hourly).
- Respiratory rate (initially every 15 min).
- Oxygen saturation by pulse oximeter (continuous display).
- ECG monitor (continuous display).
- Blood pressure (initially every 15 min).
- Temperature (initially hourly).
- Urine output (put in a bladder catheter if the poison is potentially nephrotoxic, the patient is unconscious or there is significant haemodynamic collapse).
- Arterial blood gases and pH (initially 2-hourly) if the poison can cause metabolic acidosis (Table 36.1) or there is suspected acute respiratory distress syndrome or after inhalation injury.
- Blood glucose if the poison may cause hypo- or hyperglycaemia (initially hourly) or in paracetamol poisoning presenting after 16 h (initially 4-hourly).

   Monitoring should be continued until the time symptoms are likely to develop has passed or until the patient has recovered. Specific times for individual drugs can be found in TOXBASE. Prolonged observation may be required for patients who have taken sustained release medication.

Supportive care

- Unconscious patients not requiring endotracheal intubation or transfer to ICU (see above) should be nursed in the recovery position in a high-dependency area (level 2).
- Management of problems commonly seen after poisoning is summarized in Table 36.7.

Psychiatric assessment

All patients with deliberate self-poisoning should have a psychiatric assessment, performed when recovered from the physical effects of the poisoning. Points to be covered include:

- The circumstances of the overdose: carefully planned, indecisive or impulsive; taken alone or in the presence of another person; action taken to avoid intervention or discovery; suicidal intent admitted?
- Past history of self-poisoning or self-injury; psychiatric history or contact with psychiatric services; alcohol or substance use disorder.
- Family history of depression or suicide.

Table 36.7 Problems encountered in the patient with poisoning.

Problem	Comment and management
Coma	If associated with focal neurological signs or evidence of head injury, CT must be done to exclude intracranial haematoma.
Cerebral oedema	May occur after cardiac arrest, in severe carbon monoxide poisoning, in acute liver failure from paracetamol (Chapter 77), and in MDMA poisoning, due to hyponatraemia. Results in hypertension and dilated pupils. Give mannitol 20% 100–200 mL (0.5 g/kg) IV over 10 min, provided urine output is >30 mL/h. Check plasma osmolality: further mannitol may be given until plasma osmolality is 320 mOsmol/kg Hyperventilate to a $PaCO_2$ of 4 kPa (30 mmHg)
Seizures	Due to toxin or metabolic complications. Check blood glucose, arterial gases and pH, plasma sodium, potassium, calcium and magnesium. Treat prolonged or recurrent major fits with diazepam IV up to 20 mg. See Chapter 16 for further management.
Respiratory depression	Half-life of most opioids is longer than that of naloxone and repeated doses or an infusion may be required. Elective ventilation may be preferable.
Inhalation pneumonia	Treatment includes tracheobronchial suction, consideration of bronchoscopy to remove particulate matter from the airways, physiotherapy and antibiotic therapy (Chapter 63).
Hypotension	Usually reflects vasodilatation, but always consider other causes (e.g. gastrointestinal bleeding). Obtain an ECG if the patient has taken a cardiotoxic poison, has known cardiac disease, if hypotension does not respond to IV fluids.
Arrhythmias	Due to toxin or metabolic complications. Check arterial gases and pH, and plasma potassium, calcium and magnesium. See Chapter 39 for further management.
Acute kidney injury	May be due to prolonged hypotension, nephrotoxic poison, haemolysis or rhabdomyolysis. See p. 160 for further management.
Gastric stasis	Place a nasogastric tube in comatose patients to reduce the risk of regurgitation and inhalation.
Hypothermia	Usually managed by passive rewarming. See Chapter 107.

MDMA, 3,4-methylenedioxy-methamphetamine ('ecstasy').

Table 36.8 Patients with self-poisoning at high risk of suicide.

Middle-aged or elderly male
Widowed/divorced/separated
Unemployed
Living alone
Chronic physical illness
Psychiatric illness, especially depression
Alcohol or substance abuse
Circumstances of poisoning: massive; planned; taken alone; timed so that intervention or discovery unlikely
Suicide note written or suicidal intent admitted

- Social circumstances.
- Mental state: evidence of depression or psychosis?

Patients at increased risk of suicide (Table 36.8) and those with overt psychiatric illness should be discussed with a psychiatrist. Follow-up by the primary care physician or psychiatric services should be arranged before discharge.

Appendix 36.1 Paracetamol poisoning

Hepatotoxicity may occur after a single ingestion of more than 150 mg/kg paracetamol taken in less than 1 h, though rarely ingestions as low as 75 mg/kg have produced hepatotoxicity. Hepatotoxicity is more likely if there is hepatic enzyme induction due to chronic alcohol use or drug therapy (carbamazepine, phenobarbitone, phenytoin, rifampicin), or if there is depletion of hepatic glutathione as in anorexia or AIDS. Acetylcysteine (AC) replenishes hepatic glutathione and is the preferred antidote.

- For patients weighing more than 110 kg who are obese (body mass index >30), use a body weight of 110 kg rather than actual body weight when calculating dose of paracetamol ingested (in mg/kg).
- The plasma paracetamol level is a poor guide to the risk of hepatotoxicity in patients with staggered poisoning (overdose taken over a period of longer than 1 h or multiple ingestions within a 24-h period). If the total amount taken is >150 mg/kg in a 24-h period, or the patient is at increased risk of liver damage, acetylcysteine should be given.

Management (Figure 36.2)

Patient seen within 8 h after poisoning

- Give activated charcoal 50 g if <1 h since ingestion and >75 mg/kg paracetamol has been ingested.
- Take blood for plasma paracetamol level at or after 4 h since ingestion.
- If the plasma paracetamol concentration at four or more hours post ingestion is less than the paracetamol treatment line, the patient is asymptomatic and the investigations are normal, there is no risk of serious complications, the patient may be discharged following psychiatric assessment.
- Start acetylcysteine (AC) (Table 36.9) if the plasma paracetamol level is above the treatment line (Figure 36.2).
- If the plasma paracetamol level is not available by 8 h, begin AC if >75 mg/kg of paracetamol has been taken.
- Discontinue AC if the plasma paracetamol level is below the treatment line.
- On completion of AC treatment, check the prothrombin time, alanine transaminase/aspartate transaminase activities and plasma creatinine.
- If the patient is asymptomatic post AC treatment and the investigation results are normal (INR <1.3, ALT <2 × upper limit normal, creatinine normal), there is no risk of serious complications and the patient may be discharged (with appropriate written advice), after psychiatric assessment.

Patient seen 8–24 h after poisoning

- Take blood for plasma paracetamol level, prothrombin time, alanine transaminase/aspartate transaminase activities, plasma creatinine and bilirubin, acid-base status (venous sample) and full blood count.
- Start AC immediately (Table 36.9) if >75 mg/kg paracetamol has been taken.
- Discontinue AC if the plasma paracetamol level is below the treatment line (Figure 36.3).
- On completion of AC treatment repeat above investigations (except paracetamol level).
- If the investigations are abnormal or if the patient is symptomatic, consider continuing AC treatment (100 mg/kg in 1 L 5% glucose over 16 h, repeated until recovery (INR less than or equal to 1.3 or falling on two consecutive blood tests and is less than 3.0)). Repeat investigations as appropriate.
- If the patient is asymptomatic following treatment and the investigation results are normal (INR <1.3, ALT <2 × upper limit normal, creatinine normal), there is little risk of serious complications. The patient may be discharged (with appropriate written advice), after psychiatric assessment.

Patient seen >24 h after overdose

- Take blood on admission for plasma paracetamol level, prothrombin time, alanine transaminase/aspartate transaminase activities, plasma creatinine, bilirubin and phosphate, acid-base status (venous sample), glucose and full blood count.
- If the patient has taken >150 mg/kg paracetamol, is symptomatic, or has abnormal investigation results, give a standard course of AC (Table 36.9).
- Repeat the above investigations at the end of the AC course.
- Normal blood tests at 24 hours indicate that serious liver toxicity has not occurred and treatment can be discontinued. Patient may be discharged (with appropriate written advice), after psychiatric assessment.

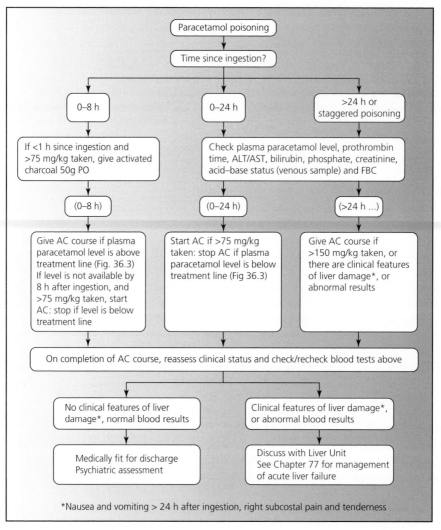

Figure 36.2 Management of paracetamol poisoning.

Severe hepatotoxicity

Make early contact with a Liver Unit if the patient has evidence of severe hepatotoxicity (Table 36.10). In such patients (before transfer):

- Start a course of acetylcysteine if not previously administered.
- Give glucose 10% 1 L 12-hourly IV to prevent hypoglycaemia, and monitor blood glucose 4-hourly.
- Monitor conscious level 4-hourly.
- Monitor CVP and urine output: correct hypovolaemia with crystalloid.
- Check prothrombin time 12-hourly and plasma creatinine daily.
- Start prophylaxis against gastric stress ulceration with omeprazole 40 mg daily IV by mouth or by nasogastric tube.
- See Chapter 77 for other aspects of the management of acute liver failure.

Table 36.9 Acetylcysteine (AC) regimen in paracetamol poisoning.

150 mg/kg in 200 mL glucose 5% IV over 1 h, then
50 mg/kg in 500 mL glucose 5% IV over 4 h, then
100 mg/kg in 1 L glucose 5% IV over 16 h

Minor reactions to acetylcysteine (nausea, flushing, urticaria and pruritus) are relatively common, and usually settle when the peak rate of infusion is passed. If there is a severe reaction (angioedema, wheezing, respiratory distress, hypotension or hypertension), stop the infusion and give an antihistamine (chlorphenamine 10 mg IV over 10 min). Then re-start the acetylcysteine infusion at the lowest rate (100 mg/kg in 1 L glucose 5% IV over 16 h).

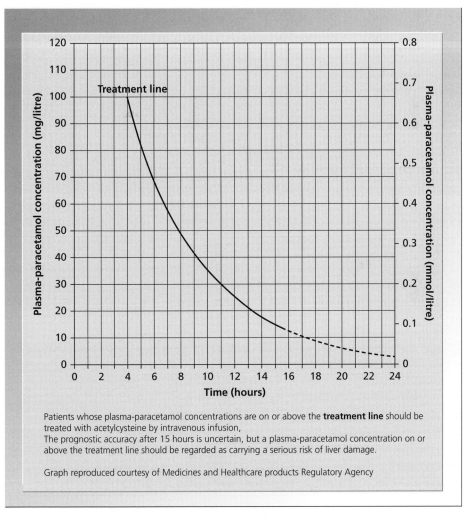

Patients whose plasma-paracetamol concentrations are on or above the **treatment line** should be treated with acetylcysteine by intravenous infusion,
The prognostic accuracy after 15 hours is uncertain, but a plasma-paracetamol concentration on or above the treatment line should be regarded as carrying a serious risk of liver damage.

Graph reproduced courtesy of Medicines and Healthcare products Regulatory Agency

Figure 36.3 Treatment threshold after paracetamol poisoning. Source: http://webarchive.nationalarchives.gov.uk/ 20141205150130/ http://www.mhra.gov.uk/Safetyinformation/Safetywarningsalertsandrecalls/ Safetywarningsandmessagesformedicines/CON178225. Accessed November 2016. This Crown copyright material is reproduced by permission of the Medicines and Healthcare products Regulatory Agency (MHRA) under delegated authority from the Controller of HMSO.

Table 36.10 Paracetamol poisoning: indications of severe hepatotoxicity.

Rapid development of grade 2 encephalopathy (confused but able to answer questions)
Prothrombin time >20 s at 24 h, >45 s at 48 h or >50 s at 72 h
Increasing plasma bilirubin
Increasing plasma creatinine
Falling plasma phosphate
Arterial pH <7.3 more than 24 h after ingestion

Appendix 36.2 Carbon monoxide poisoning

- May occur from inhalation of car exhaust fumes, fumes from inadequately maintained or ventilated heating systems (including those using natural gas), smoke from all types of fires and methylene chloride in paint strippers (by hepatic metabolism).
- The severity of poisoning depends on the concentration of carbon monoxide in the inspired air, the length of exposure and the presence of anaemia or cardiorespiratory disease. Clinical features of acute poisoning are given in Table 36.11.

Management (Figure 36.4)

1 If carbon monoxide poisoning is suspected, give 100% oxygen (10 L/min) using a tightly fitting facemask with a circuit which minimizes rebreathing. Unconscious patients should be intubated and ventilated mechanically with 100% oxygen. Cerebral oedema may occur and is treated with mannitol and mild hyperventilation (Table 36.7).

2 Attach an ECG monitor and record a 12-lead ECG. Severe poisoning may result in myocardial ischaemia, with anginal chest pain, ST segment depression and arrhythmias. Check arterial blood gases and pH (metabolic acidosis is usually present) and arrange a chest X-ray.

3 Check the carboxyhaemoglobin (COHb) level in blood (heparinized sample) (most arterial blood gas analysers will do this). If acute carbon monoxide poisoning is confirmed (COHb >10%), recheck 2-hourly and continue 100% oxygen until two consecutive samples contain <5%.

4 Although its effectiveness is disputed, generally accepted indications for hyperbaric oxygen therapy are:
- Carboxyhaemoglobin level >40% at any time
- Coma
- Neurological symptoms or signs other than mild headache
- Evidence of myocardial ischaemia or arrhythmias
- Pregnancy

Table 36.11 Acute carbon monoxide poisoning: clinical features.

Blood carboxyhaemoglobin (%)	Clinical features which may be seen
<10	No symptoms – acute poisoning excluded if exposure was within 4 h
10–50	Headache, nausea, vomiting, tachycardia, tachypnoea
>50	Coma, fits, cardiorespiratory arrest

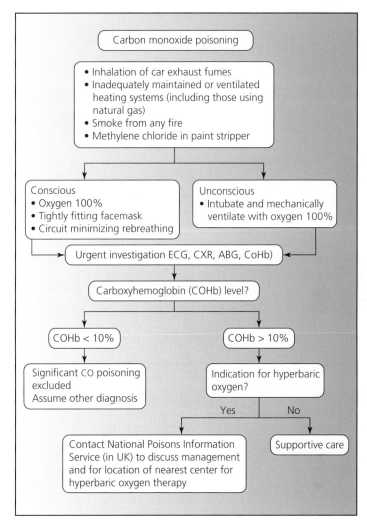

Figure 36.4 Management of carbon monoxide poisoning.

Contact a Poisons Centre to discuss the management of severe poisoning and for the location of the nearest centre which can provide hyperbaric oxygen therapy.

Further reading

Chen H-Y, Albertson TE, Olson KR (2015) Treatment of drug-induced seizures. *Br J Clin Pharmacol* 81, 412–419. http://onlinelibrary.wiley.com/doi/10.1111/bcp.12720/pdf.

National Institute for Health and Care Excellence (2016) Self-harm: long-term management. Clinical guideline (CG133). https://www.nice.org.uk/guidance/cg133.

CHAPTER 37

Acid-base disorders

NICK TALBOT

Arterial pH is tightly regulated (Box 37.1). Disorders of arterial pH are commonly encountered in acute medicine; arterial blood gases and pH should be measured in any patient with critical illness. Abnormalities of acid-base balance can be identified as acidosis or alkalosis, noting the severity and potential adverse features (Tables 37.1–37.3; Figure 37.1). The physiological and pathological consequences of acid-base disorders are summarized in Table 37.4.

- An effective approach to understanding an acid-base disorder is to look at the relationship between arterial pH (or hydrogen ion concentration) and $PaCO_2$ (Figure 37.1). When the primary disturbance is metabolic, the $PaCO_2$ will generally be either normal or out of keeping with the pH, that is, low in metabolic acidosis and high in metabolic alkalosis. When the primary disturbance is respiratory, the $PaCO_2$ will be in keeping with the pH, that is, high in respiratory acidosis, and low in respiratory alkalosis.

Box 37.1 Compensation for acid-base disturbances.

Several homeostatic mechanisms defend against extracellular pH disturbance:
- Excess plasma hydrogen ions are buffered rapidly by other blood constituents. In particular, negatively charged proteins such as albumin and haemoglobin have a large capacity for binding hydrogen ions. The concentration of these proteins therefore influences the buffering capacity of the blood.
- Hydrogen ions may be taken up across cell membranes, often in exchange for potassium ions.
- Through sensing of the hydrogen ion concentration by arterial and central chemoreceptors, metabolic acid-base disturbances often result in respiratory compensation. This typically starts within minutes and can lead to profound changes in alveolar ventilation, particularly in the setting of acidosis.
- Metabolic compensation for acid-base disturbance can be mediated through changes in bicarbonate handling within the kidney. Changes in the plasma bicarbonate concentration may begin within hours, but typically progress over several days, so the presence of significant metabolic compensation is a marker of chronicity in acid-base disturbances.

In some cases, compensation for acid-base disturbance will be partial, such that the pH remains abnormal. Alternatively, a disturbance may be fully compensated. The latter is common, for example, in patients with longstanding type 2 respiratory failure due to chronic obstructive pulmonary disease (COPD), in whom the arterial partial pressure of CO_2 ($PaCO_2$) is likely to be chronically elevated, but the pH normal, due to a compensatory rise in plasma bicarbonate. Beware of attributing any pH disturbance to overcompensation, which is much less likely than a mixed disturbance.

Acute Medicine: A Practical Guide to the Management of Medical Emergencies, Fifth Edition. Edited by David Sprigings and John B. Chambers.
© 2018 John Wiley & Sons Ltd. Published 2018 by John Wiley & Sons Ltd.

Table 37.1 Acidity of arterial blood: conversion of pH units to hydrogen ion concentration (nmol/L).

	0	1	2	3	4	5	6	7	8	9
7.0	100	98	95	93	91	89	87	85	83	81
7.1	79	78	76	74	72	71	69	68	66	65
7.2	63	62	60	59	58	56	55	54	52	51
7.3	50	49	48	47	46	45	44	43	42	41
7.4	40	39	38	37	36	35	35	34	33	32
7.5	31	31	30	30	29	28	28	27	26	26
7.6	25	25	24	23	23	22	22	21	21	20

Source: Fiorica V (1968) A table for converting pH to hydrogen ion concentration over the range 5–9. Available online at: http://www.faa.gov/data_research/research/med_humanfacs/oamtechreports/1960s/media/am68-23.pdf.

Table 37.2 Classification and examples of acid-base disorders according to arterial hydrogen ion concentration/pH and PCO_2 (Figure 37.1).

Arterial PCO_2 (kPa)	Arterial hydrogen ion concentration (nmol/L) or pH		
	[H+] >45 pH < 7.35	35–45 7.35–7.45	<35 >7.45
<4.7	Metabolic acidosis with partial respiratory compensation *or* Metabolic acidosis plus respiratory alkalosis, for example: • Pulmonary oedema • Salicylate poisoning • Hepatorenal syndrome	Respiratory alkalosis with metabolic compensation	Respiratory alkalosis *or* Respiratory alkalosis plus metabolic alkalosis, for example: • Acute liver failure with vomiting, nasogastric drainage or severe hypokalaemia • Peritoneal dialysis for chronic renal failure
4.7–6.0	Metabolic acidosis	Normal acid-base status	Metabolic alkalosis
>6.0	Respiratory acidosis *or* Respiratory acidosis plus metabolic acidosis, for example: • Cardiopulmonary arrest • COPD complicated by circulatory failure or sepsis • Severe pulmonary oedema • Combined respiratory and renal failure • Severe tricyclic poisoning	Respiratory acidosis with metabolic compensation, for example: • COPD with chronic CO_2 retention	Metabolic alkalosis plus respiratory acidosis, for example: • Diuretic therapy plus COPD with chronic CO_2 retention

COPD, chronic obstructive pulmonary disease.

Table 37.3 Grading of severity of acid-base disorders.

Arterial pH	Acid-base status	Arterial hydrogen ion concentration (nmol/L)
<7.2	Severe acidosis	>60
7.2–7.3	Moderate acidosis	50–60
7.3–7.35	Mild acidosis	45–50
7.35–7.45	Normal range	35–45
7.45–7.5	Mild alkalosis	30–35
7.5–7.6	Moderate alkalosis	20–30
>7.6	Severe alkalosis	<20

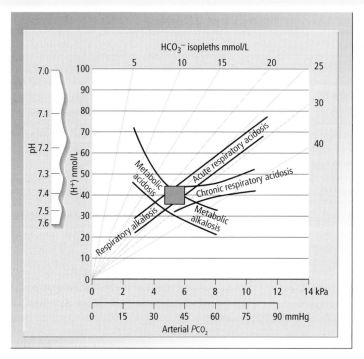

Figure 37.1 Acid-base diagram relating arterial pH or hydrogen ion concentration to PaCO$_2$.
The shaded rectangle is the normal range. The 95% confidence limits of hydrogen ion concentration/PaCO$_2$ relationships in single disturbances of acid-base balance are shown. Source: Flenley DC (1971) *Lancet* 1, 961. Reproduced with permission of Elsevier.

- Note that hyperkalaemia commonly accompanies both acute and chronic extracellular acidosis, so the plasma potassium concentration should be measured early in acidotic patients. Hyperkalaemia often results from impaired potassium excretion in renal failure, but extracellular acidosis of any cause may also lead to hyperkalaemia through the uptake of hydrogen ions into cells, in exchange for potassium. In extracellular alkalosis, the direction of exchange is reversed, so hypokalaemia may result.
- Common causes of the four primary acid-base disturbances are given in Tables 37.5–37.8.

Table 37.4 Consequences of acid-base disorders.

Acidosis	Alkalosis
Physiological	**Physiological**
Systemic vasodilatation	Peripheral vasoconstriction
Pulmonary vasoconstriction	Pulmonary vasodilatation
Hyperventilation	Hypoventilation
Renal ammoniagenesis	Renal bicarbonate secretion
Pathological	**Pathological**
Hyperkalaemia	Hypokalaemia
Impaired cardiac contractility	Reduced coronary blood flow
Bone demineralization	Reduced cerebral blood flow
Cardiac arrhythmia	Decreased ionized plasma calcium
Drowsiness and coma	Paraesthesia and muscle cramps

Table 37.5 Causes of metabolic acidosis.

With increased anion gap

Ketoacidosis

- Diabetic ketoacidosis
- Alcoholic ketoacidosis*
- Starvation ketoacidosis

Lactic acidosis

- Inadequate tissue perfusion due to hypotension, low cardiac output or sepsis
- Prolonged hypoxemia
- Muscle contraction: status epilepticus
- Metformin

Renal failure

- Chronic uraemic acidosis
- Acute renal failure

Toxins

- Ethylene glycol
- Methanol
- Salicylates
- Toluene

With normal anion gap (hyperchloraemic acidosis)

Renal

- Renal tubular acidosis
- Carbonic anhydrase inhibitors

Gastrointestinal

- Severe diarrhoea
- Obstructed ileal conduit
- Small bowel fistula
- Uretero-enterostomy
- Drainage of pancreatic or biliary secretions
- Small bowel fistula

Others

- Recovery from ketoacidosis
- Infusion of normal saline

* Alcoholic ketoacidosis is due to alcohol binge plus starvation, and is often associated with pancreatitis; hyperglycaemia may occur but is mild (<15 mmol/L).

Table 37.6 Causes of respiratory acidosis (inadequate alveolar ventilation resulting in a raised arterial PCO_2).*

Brain
Stroke
Mass lesion with brainstem compression
Encephalitis
Sedative drugs
Status epilepticus
Spinal cord
Cord compression
Transverse myelitis
Poliomyelitis
Motor neuron disease
Rabies
Peripheral nerve
Guillain-Barré syndrome
Critical illness polyneuropathy
Toxins
Acute intermittent porphyria
Vasculitis
Diphtheria
Neuromuscular junction
Myasthenia gravis
Eaton-Lambert syndrome
Botulism
Toxins
Muscle
Myotonic dystrophy
Muscular dystrophy
Hypokalaemia
Hypophosphatemia
Rhabdomyolysis
Thoracic cage and pleura
Crushed chest
Morbid obesity
Kyphoscoliosis
Ankylosing spondylitis
Large pleural effusion
Lungs and airways
Upper airway obstruction
Severe acute asthma
Chronic obstructive pulmonary disease
Severe pneumonia
Severe pulmonary oedema

*Ventilatory failure commonly results from a combination of factors, for example pneumonia in an obese patient with chronic obstructive pulmonary disease; see Chapter 11.

- Causes of metabolic acidosis can be subdivided according to the size of the so-called 'anion gap'. This value represents the difference between the sum of the concentration of major plasma cations (sodium and potassium), and the sum of the concentration of major plasma anions (chloride and bicarbonate):

$$\text{Anion gap} = ([Na^+] + [K^+]) - ([Cl^-] + [HCO_3^-])$$

Table 37.7 Causes of metabolic alkalosis.

Loss of gastric acid:
• Prolonged vomiting
• Gastric aspiration
Diuretic therapy
Severe and prolonged potassium deficiency
Mineralocorticoid and glucocorticoid excess
Post-hypercapnic alkalosis*

* Typically in patients with subacute-on-chronic respiratory acidosis, in whom $PaCO_2$ is rapidly reduced through ventilatory support. The plasma bicarbonate falls back to baseline more slowly, leading to a transient metabolic alkalosis.

Table 37.8 Causes of respiratory alkalosis.

Pulmonary disorders with hyperventilation:
• Acute asthma
• Pneumonia
• Pulmonary embolism
• Pulmonary oedema
Hyperventilation syndrome
Anxiety and pain
Central nervous system disorders, for example stroke, bacterial meningitis
Liver failure
Sepsis
Salicylate poisoning

A normal anion gap is around 10–18 mmol/L, but the reference range can vary considerably according to laboratory. It is an estimate of the unmeasured anions in the plasma. A high anion gap implies excess unmeasured plasma anions, which may be the cause of metabolic acidosis.

• When the primary pathology is not clear, consider a mixed disturbance, with two or more contributing factors (Table 37.2). This is distinct from a single disturbance with compensation (Box 37.1). Common examples include respiratory and metabolic acidosis in the setting of severe pneumonia and sepsis, or combined metabolic alkalosis and metabolic acidosis in a patient with vomiting and chronic renal failure.

Further reading

Berend K, de Vries APJ, Gans ROB (2014) Physiological approach to assessment of acid-base disturbances. *N Engl J Med* 371, 1434–1445.
Seifter JL (2014) Integration of acid-base and electrolyte disorders. *N Engl J Med* 371, 1821–1831.

CHAPTER 38

Anaphylaxis

ALEXANDRA CROOM

Suspect anaphylaxis if, after an IV or IM injection, insect sting or exposure to a potential allergen, the patient develops breathlessness and wheeze, or hypotension/shock. The potential manifestations of anaphylaxis are shown in Table 38.1; not all features will occur in every patient. Wheeze is more common in food-induced anaphylaxis, as coexistent asthma is more frequent.

Causes of anaphylactic reaction are given in Table 38.2. Symptoms usually start within minutes of exposure to a trigger, and most reactions will occur within 60 min. The route of allergen exposure influences the rapidity of symptom onset; allergens encountered parenterally and insect stings produce a more rapid clinical deterioration than ingested allergens. Delayed onset reactions (beyond 60 min) are recognized with food-dependent exercise-induced anaphylaxis (FDEIA) and meat allergy.

The management of anaphylaxis is summarized in Figure 38.1. Prompt administration of adrenaline IM is the key element of treatment.

Priorities

Is this anaphylaxis?

The rapid onset of breathlessness and wheeze (due to upper airway obstruction or bronchospasm) or hypotension/shock, associated with itch, flushing or urticaria, suggest anaphylaxis and you should consider immediate treatment with adrenaline IM.

- There should be a high index of suspicion if there has been exposure to a possible allergen, for example administration of IV medication, or after eating by a person known to have food allergy.
- Skin changes are not essential to the diagnosis of anaphylaxis, and adrenaline should not be withheld in their absence if the diagnosis is suspected.
- The differential diagnosis of anaphylaxis includes any condition that can cause the rapid onset of dyspnoea or hypotension, as well as those which cause urticaria and angioedema (Chapter 27). See Table 38.3 for a list of the most common differential diagnoses.

Suspected severe anaphylactic reaction (anaphylactic shock)

1 Call for assistance. If there is cardiorespiratory arrest, start resuscitation.
2 Remove the trigger allergen if possible (e.g. stop IV infusion of antibiotic; remove the stinger after a bee sting). Do not induce vomiting.
3 Unless contraindicated because of breathlessness, lay the patient flat and raise the foot of the bed. This position should be maintained; resuming an upright position before the volume shifts in shock have improved can lead to cardiac arrest.

Acute Medicine: A Practical Guide to the Management of Medical Emergencies, Fifth Edition. Edited by David Sprigings and John B. Chambers.
© 2018 John Wiley & Sons Ltd. Published 2018 by John Wiley & Sons Ltd.

Suspect anaphylaxis if there is:
Rapid development of stridor and/or wheeze and/or hypotension
associated with itch, skin and mucosal angioedema and urticaria
following exposure to potential trigger (see Table 38.2 for causes)

Remove allergen if possible[1]
Lay patient flat with legs elevated[2]
Call for additional help

Administer IM adrenaline – anterolateral aspect of thigh
using 25 mm needle: 500 μgm (0.5 mL 1:1000 solution).
Further doses at 5–10 min intervals if no improvement

Insert large bore cannula
High flow O_2

Airway/breathing
For wheeze nebulized
salbutamol 2.5–5 mg;
treat asthma as per
BTS guidelines.
(Figure 60.1 p. 378)
Upper airways
obstruction may
require endotracheal
intubation or
tracheostomy

Circulation
Give IV fluid
challenge over 10 min[3]
Repeat challenge if
BP remains <100 mmHg;
if no improvement seek
specialist supervision
of IV adrenaline and
other vasopressors

Monitor:
BP
ECG[4]
Pulse oximetry

Give second line drugs:
Chlorphenamine 10 mg slow
IV push
Hydrocortisone 200 mg IV

Check serum tryptase (see
Table 38.4)

Post reaction care
Observe for biphasic reaction
If drug implicated mark notes, drug charts and issue patient with 'alert' wrist band
Continue oral steroids prednisolone 30–40 mg daily for 3 days (longer course if asthma)
and antihistamines – cetirizine 10 mg daily or chlorphenamine 4 mg tds

Pre-discharge care
Assess risk of further anaphylaxis and requirement of adrenaline autoinjector
Advise on future allergen avoidance
Refer for specialist investigation

1. Stop any infusions including colloids. Vomiting should NOT be induced when allergens
   have been ingested.
2. Lying flat increases respiratory effort and should not be forced in patients in whom
   airway problems predominate.
3. If there is hypotension, give 1 L normal saline or Hartmann's solution IV over
   10 mins. If normotensive, give 500 mL; if heart failure, give 250 mL and monitor for signs
   of fluid overload. Consider CVP monitoring.
4. Myocardial ischaemia may occur even with unobstructed coronary arteries.

Figure 38.1 Management of anaphylaxis.

Table 38.1 Manifestations of anaphylaxis and anaphylactoid reactions.

Flushing
Itch
Urticaria
Angioedema
Nausea and vomiting
Diarrhoea
Abdominal pain (may be due to gut or uterine cramping)
Stridor
Wheeze
Dyspnoea
Dizziness
Syncope
Chest pain due to myocardial ischaemia (may occur with normal coronary arteries)
Sense of impending doom or panic
Confusion
Cardiac or respiratory arrest

Table 38.2 Causes of anaphylactic and anaphylactoid reactions.

Drugs*
Antibiotics – most commonly of beta-lactam group
Non-steroidal anti-inflammatory drugs (NSAIDs)
Neuromuscular blocking agents
Cytotoxic agents
Radiocontrast media
Therapeutic monoclonal antibodies

Foods[†]

Insect venom[‡]

Other causes
Exercise (with or without food allergy)
Latex
Plasma expanders
Blood products
Seminal fluid

Idiopathic (20%)

*50% fatal anaphylaxis in UK is iatrogenic. Beta-lactam antibiotics are the commonest cause of medication-induced anaphylaxis. Drugs may cause mast cell degranulation through both IgE-mediated (allergic) mechanisms or direct mast cell activation. The latter reactions, sometimes termed anaphylactoid, are clinically indistinguishable from IgE-mediated reactions but may occur without previous exposure, that is, first dose reactions.

[†] Peanuts and tree nuts (e.g. Brazil nuts, cashew nuts and walnuts) are the commonest causes of food anaphylaxis, and along with wheat, egg, fish, seafood, soya and milk are responsible for over 90% of reactions. Cofactors are increasingly recognized as being important in food anaphylaxis: in their absence a foodstuff will be tolerated but in their presence a reaction will occur. Recognized cofactors include exercise, NSAIDs and alcohol. Food-dependent exercise-induced anaphylaxis (FDEIA) requires the presence of the trigger food and exercise and may occur even if exercise is taken up to 4 h after the foodstuff is ingested.

[‡] Responsible insect varies worldwide – bee and wasp in UK.

Table 38.3 Differential diagnosis of anaphylaxis.

Diagnosis	Comment
Chronic spontaneous urticaria and angioedema	Background of symptoms daily for >6 weeks
	Rapid development of symptoms rare
	Stridor may develop due to laryngeal oedema
	Hypotension and wheeze not typical
ACE-inhibitor-induced angioedema	Swelling affects head and neck only
	Stridor may develop due to laryngeal oedema; if life-threatening airways obstruction treat with icatibant
	No urticaria or hypotension
	May develop days to years after starting ACE-inhibitor; may persist for some weeks after ACEI discontinuation
Hereditary angioedema	Urticaria and hypotension absent
	Stridor (due to laryngeal oedema) rather than wheeze
	Usually personal or family history
	Treat with C1-esterase inhibitor (either plasma-derived or recombinant human C1 inhibitor or icatibant; fresh frozen plasma may be used if neither of these available)
Acute asthma	No itch, urticaria or angioedema
	Hypotension late feature
Acute heart failure	No itch, urticaria or angioedema
Scombrotoxin poisoning	Caused by bacterial overgrowth in improperly stored dark-meat fish (e.g. tuna, mackerel)
	Symptoms appear within 30 min of eating spoiled fish: urticarial, nausea, vomiting, diarrhoea, headache, metallic taste
	Treat with antihistamine
Vasovagal reaction	No itch, urticaria or angioedema
Acute panic disorder	No itch, urticaria, angioedema, hypoxia or hypotension
	Functional stridor may develop as a result of forced adduction of vocal cords

ACE, angiotensin-converting enzyme.

4 **Adrenaline** is the first-line drug in anaphylaxis; absent or delayed use is associated with fatal outcome.
  - In the first instance administration should be IM in the anterolateral aspect of the thigh (where skin to muscle depth is least). A 23 G needle (blue – length 25 mm) should be used to ensure that muscle is reached; in the morbidly obese consider a 21 G (green – needle length 38 mm) or administration into the calf. Subcutaneous or deltoid muscle administration is NOT recommended. A dose of 500 µgm adrenaline should be given IM. If a second dose of IM adrenaline is required it should be given at a separate site (usually the contralateral thigh).
  - Nebulized adrenaline (5 mL of 1:1000 solution) may be of some use where there is significant laryngeal obstruction due to angioedema.
5 If there is respiratory distress, call an anaesthetist. This may be due to upper airway obstruction from oedema of the larynx or epiglottis, and may require endotracheal intubation or emergency tracheotomy.

  If there is bronchospasm, give nebulized salbutamol. IV aminophylline (Chapter 116) can be added if needed.
6 Start an IV infusion of crystalloid, 500 mL to 1 L over 15 min (the higher rate if systolic BP is <90 mmHg). If there is heart failure, give 250 mL over 15 min. Monitor for signs of fluid overload.
7 Give chlorphenamine 10–20 mg IV over 1 min and hydrocortisone 200 mg IV.
8 Take timed blood samples for mast cell tryptase testing as follows: a sample as soon as possible after emergency treatment has started, a second sample ideally within 1–2 h (but no later than 4 h) from the onset of

Table 38.4 Serum mast cell tryptase.

May be of use when diagnostic uncertainty
Peaks at 60–120 min after onset of symptoms
Take samples at onset of symptoms then 2–4 h and >24 h (baseline) thereafter; label sample time clearly on request form
Two-fold increase (even within the reference range) indicative of anaphylaxis
Poor negative predictive value – rise often absent in food anaphylaxis
Baseline elevated >20 µgm/L may be due to mast cell disorders including mastocytosis

symptoms. A raised serum mast cell tryptase (see Table 38.4) may be used to confirm that anaphylaxis has taken place but has a poor negative predictive value.

9 If systolic BP remains <100 mmHg:
- Arrange transfer to the ICU.
- Give adrenaline 0.5–1 mg (0.5–1 mL of 1 in 1000 solution) IM every 10 min.
- Continue IV crystalloid infusion, giving a further 500 mL over 30 min. When the patient's condition is stable, put in a CVP line to guide fluid management (p. 13, Table 2.7).
- If multiple doses of adrenaline are needed, consider starting an infusion (which must be given via a central line) (p. 657).
- If the patient has been taking a non-cardioselective beta blocker and is resistant to adrenaline, give glucagon (50 µgm/kg by IV bolus followed by an infusion of 1–5 mg/h) or salbutamol by IV infusion (p. 379).

Further management

1 Admit to hospital. In up to 20% of cases, biphasic reactions occur between 1 and 8 h after the onset of symptoms; rarely the second phase of the reaction may be more severe than the first. There are no features of anaphylaxis predictive of a biphasic reaction occurring, other than the individual having had one during a previous episode.
2 Give hydrocortisone 200 mg 6-hourly IV for 2–4 doses and chlorphenamine 8 mg 8-hourly PO for 24–48 h. Warn patients about potential sedative side effects of chlorphenamine.
3 Inform the patient of the allergen responsible for the reaction. The advice given by non-specialists on allergen avoidance should be over-inclusive (e.g. avoid all nuts when only one type appears implicated): this can be revised in specialist care. Recommend a medical ID bracelet engraved with trigger allergens (this may be deferred until after specialist review). Put patients in contact with patient support groups (e.g. Anaphylaxis Campaign).
   - Patients at high risk of anaphylaxis should carry adrenaline for self-injection in the event of further exposure to allergen. Consult the *British National Formulary* for a suitable device. Adrenaline should be prescribed where an allergen is not predictably avoidable or is unknown. Prescription should not be deferred until specialist review. Prescribing and training for adrenaline autoinjectors is device specific.
   - If anaphylaxis was due to a drug, report the reaction to the Committee on Safety of Medicines (see the Adverse Reactions to Drugs section of the *British National Formulary*). Mark clinical notes clearly with the drug implicated; inform the patient's GP and other involved health professionals.
   - Specific allergen immunotherapy (desensitization) is indicated in the case of severe anaphylactic reaction to bee or wasp stings: seek advice from a clinical immunologist or allergist.
   - Poorly controlled asthma increases the risk of life-threatening and fatal anaphylaxis. Assess ongoing asthma control (nocturnal disturbance, frequency of use of rescue medication, oral corticosteroid use) and intensify treatment as appropriate.

- Beta blockers will antagonize the effects of adrenaline (a beta agonist) and may make anaphylaxis difficult to treat. Risk assess their continued use and discontinue if the benefit does not outweigh that risk.
- Refer to an allergy clinic for specialist assessment if new presentation; consider referral if previously diagnosed and taking high-risk behaviour or if a new allergen is implicated.

4 Where there have been recurrent episodes of apparently idiopathic anaphylaxis (or reactions thought to be anaphylaxis) consider mastocytosis and carcinoid syndrome (in which asthma is associated with flushing rather than itch).

Allergic reaction without anaphylaxis

Not all allergic reactions progress to anaphylaxis. Patients in whom symptoms are confined to the skin or at the point of allergen contact (e.g. oral itch with a food) should receive chlorphenamine and hydrocortisone and remain under close monitoring until their symptoms have abated.

Further reading

Lieberman PL (2014) Recognition and first-line treatment of anaphylaxis. *Am J Medicine* 127, S6–S11.

National Institute for Health and Care Excellence (2016) Anaphylaxis: assessment and referral after emergency treatment. Clinical guideline (CG134). https://www.nice.org.uk/guidance/cg134?unlid=639094620201610 645435.

Simons FER, Ebisawa M, Sanchez-Borges M, *et al.* (2015) Update of the evidence base: World Allergy Organization anaphylaxis guidelines. *World Allergy Organization Journal* 8, 32 (Open access) 10.1186/ s40413-015-0080-1.

Cardiovascular

CHAPTER 39

Acute arrhythmias: general principles of management

DAVID SPRIGINGS AND JOHN B. CHAMBERS

Priorities

If there is imminent cardiac arrest, call the arrest team and manage along standard lines (see Chapter 6).

If there is a reduced level of consciousness, severe pulmonary oedema, or the systolic BP is <90 mmHg:

- Record a 12-lead ECG (if possible) for later analysis.
- If the heart rate is >150/min, call an anaesthetist in preparation for DC cardioversion starting at 200 J (Chapter 121).
- If the heart rate is <40/min, give atropine 0.6–1.2 mg IV, with further doses at 5-min intervals up to a total dose of 3 mg if the heart rate remains below 60/min. If the bradycardia is unresponsive or recurs, use an external cardiac pacing system or put in a temporary transvenous pacemaker (Chapter 119).

If the patient is haemodynamically stable, there is time to make a working diagnosis and plan management. Clinical assessment in summarized in Table 39.1 and urgent investigation in Table 39.2. Record a 12-lead electrocardiogram and a long rhythm strip. Further management is determined by the type of arrhythmia.

Regular broad complex tachycardia (see Chapter 40):

- The diagnosis is usually ventricular tachycardia (VT). Haemodynamic stability does not exclude VT.
- If there is ischaemic heart disease or cardiomyopathy, the diagnosis is virtually always VT.
- Suspect diagnoses other than VT in young patients (age <40 years), or with known Wolff-Parkinson-White or bundle branch block. If there is doubt, assess the effect of adenosine (Table 42.3).

Irregular broad complex tachycardia (see Chapter 41):

- This is likely to be atrial fibrillation with bundle branch block or, less commonly, pre-excited atrial fibrillation (Figure 41.1). The difference between the maximum and minimum instantaneous heart rates calculated from the shortest and longest RR intervals is usually >30/min.
- The differential diagnosis is polymorphic ventricular tachycardia. This is usually due to therapy with anti-arrhythmic and other drugs which prolong the QT interval (e.g. amiodarone, sotalol), especially in patients with hypokalaemia or hypomagnesaemia.

Regular narrow complex tachycardia (see Chapter 42):

- The differential diagnosis is given in Table 39.4.
- Vagotonic manoeuvres increase AV block and may terminate the arrhythmia if it involves the AV node, or reveal atrial activity. Ask the patient to perform a Valsalva manoeuvre (attempting to blow the plunger from a 10 mL syringe, while semi-recumbent, is an effective method of generating the necessary intrathoracic pressure) or try carotid sinus massage. If vagotonic manoeuvres do not restore sinus rhythm, give adenosine (Table 42.3).

Acute Medicine: A Practical Guide to the Management of Medical Emergencies, Fifth Edition. Edited by David Sprigings and John B. Chambers.
© 2018 John Wiley & Sons Ltd. Published 2018 by John Wiley & Sons Ltd.

Table 39.1 Focused assessment of the patient with an acute arrhythmia.

Symptoms?
- Of arrhythmia (palpitations, presyncope, syncope)
- Of underlying cardiac disease (chest pain, breathlessness)

Haemodynamically stable? Signs of instability are:
- Heart rate <40/min or >150/min
- Bradycardia with pauses >3 s
- Systolic BP <90 mmHg
- Reduced conscious level
- Chest pain
- Pulmonary oedema

Known arrhythmia?
- How diagnosed?
- Previous management?
- Current therapy?

Evidence of ischaemic or other structural heart disease (e.g. history of ACS, Q waves on ECG)?
- This makes ventricular tachycardia almost certainly the diagnosis if there is a regular broad complex tachycardia
- Flecainide should be avoided for cardioversion or preventing atrial fibrillation because of the risk of precipitating ventricular arrhythmias

Could LV systolic function be significantly impaired (e.g. exertional breathlessness, large cardiac silhouette on chest X-ray, LV ejection fraction <40% on previous echocardiography)?
- If so, avoid high-dose beta-blocker and flecainide

Is there Wolff-Parkinson-White syndrome? This may cause:
- AV re-entrant tachycardia (narrow complex, regular) (conduction forward through the AV node and back via the accessory pathway)
- Fast conduction of atrial fibrillation down the accessory pathway (broad complex, irregular)
- Antidromic tachycardia (broad complex, regular) (conduction forward down the accessory pathway and back via the AV node)

Associated acute or chronic illness?
- Acute atrial fibrillation commonly complicates pneumonia and other infection
- Electrolyte disorders (especially of potassium, calcium and magnesium) should be excluded/corrected

ACS, acute coronary syndrome; AV, atrioventricular; LV, left ventricular.

Table 39.2 Urgent investigation of the patient with an acute arrhythmia.

12-lead ECG and long rhythm strip during the arrhythmia and after resolution (heart rate, delta wave, AV conduction abnormality, bundle branch block, Q waves, evidence of LV hypertrophy, QT interval, ST/T abnormalities)

Electrolytes (if on diuretic, include magnesium) and creatinine

Blood glucose

Thyroid function (for later analysis)

Plasma digoxin level if taking digoxin (at least 8 h after digoxin last taken)

Plasma troponin

Chest X-ray (heart size, evidence of raised left atrial pressure, coexistent pathology, for example pneumonia?)

Echocardiogram (for LV function, RV function, valve disease, pericardial effusion) if there is VT. Can be done the next day for other primary arrhythmias. May not be indicated if AF or flutter complicates pneumonia and the patient has no historical symptoms or signs of cardiac disease.

LV, left ventricular; RV, right ventricular.

Table 39.3 Differential diagnosis of bradycardia and AV block.

Diagnosis	ECG features
Sinus bradycardia	Constant PR interval <200 ms
	QRS regular
Junctional bradycardia	P wave absent or position constant either after, immediately before or hidden in the QRS complex
First-degree AV block	Constant PR interval >200 ms
Second-degree AV block, Mobitz type 1	Progressively lengthening PR interval followed by dropped beat
Second-degree AV block, Mobitz type 2	Constant PR interval with dropped beats
Third-degree (complete) AV block	Relationship of P wave to QRS varies randomly

AV, atrioventricular.

- Suspect atrial flutter with 2:1 AV conduction rather than sinus tachycardia if the rate is around 150/min.
- Suspect atrial tachycardia or junctional tachycardia if digoxin toxicity is possible. Digoxin toxicity is likely if plasma digoxin level is >3.0 ng/mL (>3.8 nmol/L), especially if there is hypokalaemia (<3.5 mmol/L), hypomagnesaemia or hypercalcaemia. Systemic features include nausea, vomiting, diarrhoea and delirium.

Irregular narrow complex tachycardia (see Chapters 42 and 43)
- The diagnosis is usually atrial fibrillation (AF).
- Other possibilities are sinus rhythm with frequent supraventricular extrasystoles or multifocal atrial tachycardia (the rhythm looks half-way between sinus and AF).

Bradycardia (rate <60/min) (see Chapter 44)
- The differential diagnosis is given in Table 39.3. Look carefully at the PR interval and the relationship between the P wave and QRS complex
- A regular ventricular rate <50/min in a patient with atrial fibrillation indicates complete heart block (not 'slow AF'); always consider digoxin toxicity.

Table 39.4 Differential diagnosis of narrow complex tachycardia.

Arrhythmia	QRS rate (per min)	Atrial rate (per min)	Regular QRS?	Atrial activity	Effect of vagotonic manoeuvres or adenosine
Sinus tachycardia	100–200	100–200	Y	P wave precedes QRS	*
SVT	150–250	150–250	Y	Usually not seen or inverted P after QRS	†
Atrial tachycardia	100–200	120–250	Y	Abnormal shaped P wave, may outnumber QRS	‡
Atrial flutter	75–175	250–350	Y	'Saw-tooth' in the inferior leads/V1	‡
Atrial fibrillation	<200	350–600	N	Chaotic (f waves)	‡
MAT	100–130	100–130	N	P waves of three or more morphologies	*

SVT, supraventricular tachycardia (re-entrant tachycardia involving the AV node or an accessory pathway); MAT, multifocal atrial tachycardia.
* No effect or slight slowing.
† May terminate tachycardia.
‡ Slowing of ventricular rate.

Further reading

European Resuscitation Council Guidelines (2015). https://cprguidelines.eu/.

Gale CP, Camm AJ (2016) Assessment of palpitations. *BMJ* 352, h5649. http://dx.doi.org/10.1136/bmj.h5649.

Priori SG, Wilde AA, Horie M, *et al.* (2013) HRS/EHRA/APHRS Expert consensus statement on the diagnosis and management of patients with inherited primary arrhythmia syndromes. *Heart Rhythm* 10, 1933–1958.

Raviele A, Giarda F, Bergfeldt L, *et al.* (2011) Management of patients with palpitations: a position paper from the European Heart Rhythm Association. *Europace* 13, 920–934. http://dx.doi.org/10.1093/europace/eur130.

Resuscitation Guidelines. Resuscitation Council (UK): https://www.resus.org.uk/resuscitation-guidelines/.

CHAPTER 40

Regular broad complex tachycardia

Michael Cooklin and David Sprigings

The approach to the patient with regular broad complex tachycardia (Table 40.1) is summarized in Figure 40.1.

Table 40.1 Regular broad complex tachycardia: differential diagnosis and management.

Arrhythmia	Comment	Management
Monomorphic ventricular tachycardia (Figure 40.2)	Commonest cause and should be the default diagnosis (especially if there is a history of previous myocardial infarction or other structural heart disease) Restore sinus rhythm as soon as possible, even in haemodynamically stable patients, as sudden deterioration may occur	DC cardioversion (Chapter 121) if there is haemodynamic instability or other measures are ineffective In stable patient, DC cardioversion, IV antiarrhythmic therapy (Table 40.2), or antitachycardia pacing Refer to a cardiologist
Supraventricular tachycardia (SVT) with bundle branch block	Confirm with adenosine test (Table 42.3)	DC cardioversion (Chapter 121) if there is haemodynamic instability or other measures are ineffective In stable patient, IV adenosine, verapamil or beta blocker (Table 42.3) Record 12-lead ECG after sinus rhythm restored to check for pre-excitation (WPW syndrome) Refer to a cardiologist if episodes are frequent or severe or if pre-excitation is found
Antidromic tachycardia or pre-excited atrial flutter in WPW syndrome	These are rarely seen but should be considered in a young patient with known WPW syndrome who does not have structural heart disease	DC cardioversion Refer to a cardiologist
Pseudoventricular tachycardia (Figure 40.3)	Caused by body movement and intermittent skin-electrode contact ('toothbrush tachycardia') No haemodynamic change during apparent ventricular arrhythmia	No action needed It is important to avoid misdiagnosis as ventricular tachycardia

WPW, Wolff-Parkinson-White.

Acute Medicine: A Practical Guide to the Management of Medical Emergencies, Fifth Edition. Edited by David Sprigings and John B. Chambers.
© 2018 John Wiley & Sons Ltd. Published 2018 by John Wiley & Sons Ltd.

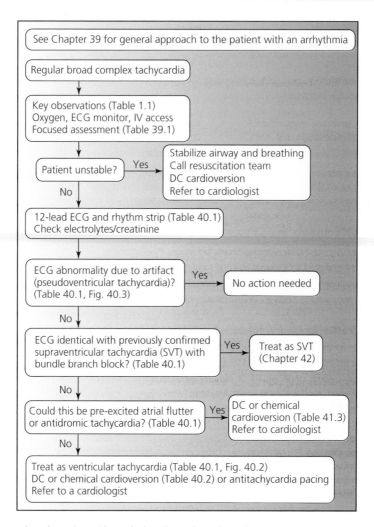

Figure 40.1 Approach to the patient with regular broad complex tachycardia.

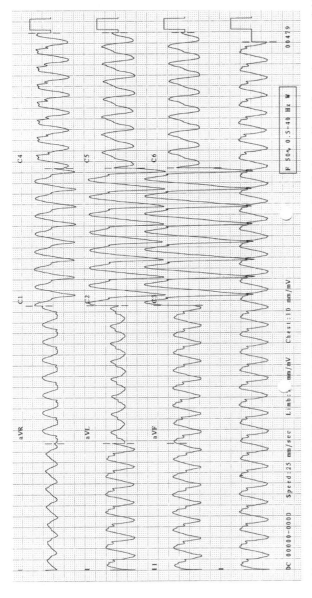

Figure 40.2 Monomorphic ventricular tachycardia (VT). VT is almost certain if there is a broad complex tachycardia with structural heart disease (e.g. myocardial infarction). Specific ECG features strongly suggestive of VT are the QRS width (approx 200 ms) and the 'North-West axis' (positive QRS in lead aVR). Evidence of ventriculo-atrial dissociation, capture or fusion beats are specific findings strongly suggestive of VT, but often not seen, including in this trace.

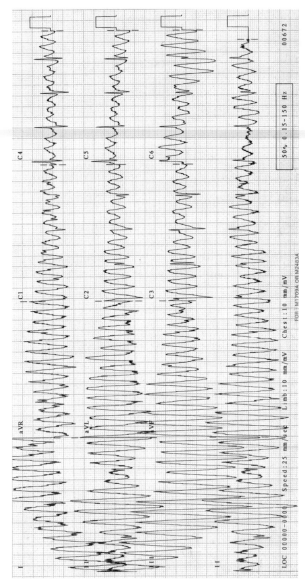

Figure 40.3 Pseudoventricular tachycardia. There are native QRS complexes at the cycle length of the baseline rhythm within the artifact, best seen in C4 and C5.

Table 40.2 Drug therapy of haemodynamically stable monomorphic ventricular tachycardia.

Drug	Comment	Dose (IV)
Amiodarone	Efficacy in converting VT uncertain Major role is in suppression of recurrent episodes Needs to be given via central vein to avoid thrombophlebitis	Loading: 300 mg, diluted in 5% glucose to a volume of 20–50 mL, infused over 20 min via a central vein Maintenance: 900–1200 mg over 24 h Supplementary doses of 150 mg can be given as necessary every 10 min for recurrent or resistant VT to a maximum total daily dose of 2.2 g
Lidocaine	Converts ~30% Appropriate when VT is due to myocardial ischaemia or infarction May cause hypotension and neurological side effects	Loading: 1.5 mg/kg over 2 min Maintenance: 1–4 mg/min

VT, ventricular tachycardia.

Further reading

National Institute for Health and Care Excellence (2014) Implantable cardioverter defibrillators and cardiac resynchronization therapy for arrhythmias and heart failure. Technology appraisal guidance (TA314). https://www.nice.org.uk/guidance/ta314.

The Task Force for the management of patients with ventricular arrhythmias and the prevention of sudden cardiac death of the European Society of Cardiology (ESC). (2015) 2015 ESC Guidelines for the management of patients with ventricular arrhythmias and the prevention of sudden cardiac death. *Eur Heart J* 36, 2793–2867. DOI: 10.1093/eurheartj/ehv316.

CHAPTER 41

Irregular broad complex tachycardia

MICHAEL COOKLIN AND DAVID SPRIGINGS

The approach to the patient with irregular broad complex tachycardia (Table 41.1) is summarized in Figure 41.1.

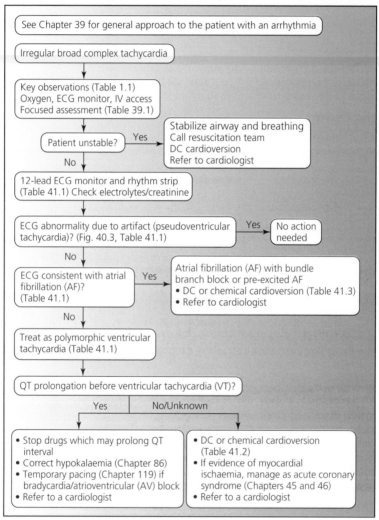

Figure 41.1 Approach to the patient with irregular broad complex tachycardia.

Acute Medicine: A Practical Guide to the Management of Medical Emergencies, Fifth Edition. Edited by David Sprigings and John B. Chambers.
© 2018 John Wiley & Sons Ltd. Published 2018 by John Wiley & Sons Ltd.

Table **41.1** Irregular broad complex tachycardia: differential diagnosis and management.

Arrhythmia	Comment	Management
Atrial fibrillation with bundle branch block	Difference between maximum and minimum instantaneous heart rates, calculated from the shortest and longest RR intervals is usually >30/min, with QRS showing typical LBBB or RBBB morphology	DC cardioversion (Chapter 121) if there is haemodynamic instability or other measures are ineffective In stable patient, DC cardioversion or antiarrhythmic therapy (see Chapter 43)
Polymorphic ventricular tachycardia		
With preceding QT prolongation (torsade de pointes)	Usually due to therapy with antiarrhythmic and other drugs which prolong the QT interval (e.g. amiodarone, sotalol, erythromycin, psychotropic drugs), especially in patients with hypokalaemia and/or bradycardia Rarely congenital long QT syndrome (possible family history)	DC cardioversion if there is haemodynamic instability or other measures are ineffective Stop drugs which may prolong QT interval Correct hypokalaemia (target potassium 4.5–5 mmol/l) If there is bradycardia/AV block, use temporary pacing at 90/min (Chapter 119 p. 673)
	Also advanced conduction system disease with block	If due to long QT syndrome, give magnesium sulfate 2 g IV bolus over 2–3 min, repeated if necessary, and followed by an infusion of 2–8 mg/min Refer to a cardiologist
Without preceding QT prolongation	Usually due to myocardial ischaemia in the setting of acute coronary syndrome Other causes include acute myocarditis, cardiomyopathies (e.g. arrhythmogenic right ventricular cardiomyopathy) and Brugada syndrome (VT/VF with RBBB and precordial ST elevation)	DC cardioversion if there is haemodynamic instability or other measures are ineffective In stable patient, DC cardioversion or antiarrhythmic therapy with IV amiodarone or beta-blocker (Table 41.2) Manage as acute coronary syndrome (Chapters 45 and 46) with urgent coronary angiography and revascularization if ischaemia is suspected or cannot be excluded Refer to a cardiologist
Pre-excited atrial fibrillation (AF) in WPW syndrome (Figure 41.2)	AF conducted variably over accessory pathway Ventricular rate typically 200–300/min QRS morphology shows beat to beat variation in degree of pre-excitation	DC cardioversion if there is haemodynamic instability or other measures are ineffective In stable patient, DC in cardioversion or antiarrhythmic therapy with flecainide or amiodarone (Tables 41.2 and 41.3) Refer to a cardiologist
Pseudoventricular tachycardia (Figure 40.3)	Caused by skin-electrode contact ('toothbrush tachycardia') No haemodynamic change during apparent ventricular arrhythmia	No action needed The importance of recognition is to prevent misdiagnosis as VT

AV, atrioventricular; LBBB, left bundle branch block; RBBB, right bundle branch block; VF, ventricular fibrillation; VT, ventricular tachycardia; WPW, Wolff-Parkinson-White.

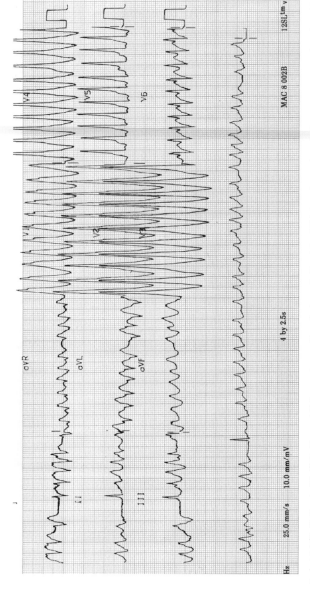

Figure 41.2 Pre-excited atrial fibrillation in Wolff-Parkinson-White syndrome. Despite irregularity of the RR interval over the whole trace, some sections (e.g. V_{1-6}) look regular. By contrast, in atrial flutter the tachycardia is usually regular and in antidromic tachycardia, it is reproducibly regular.

Table 41.2 Drug therapy of haemodynamically stable polymorphic ventricular tachycardia (VT) without preceding QT prolongation.

Drug	Comment	Dose (IV)
Amiodarone	Needs to be given via central vein to avoid thrombophlebitis	Loading: 300 mg, diluted in 5% glucose to a volume of 20–50 mL, infused over 20 min via a central vein Maintenance: 900–1200 mg over 24 h Supplementary doses of 150 mg can be given as necessary every 10 min for recurrent or resistant VT to a maximum total daily dose of 2.2 g

Table 41.3 Drug therapy of haemodynamically stable pre-excited atrial fibrillation.

Drug	Comment	Dose (IV)
Flecainide	May cause hypotension Avoid if known structural heart disease	2 mg/kg (to a maximum of 150 mg) over 20 min
Amiodarone	Needs to be given via central vein to avoid thrombophlebitis	300 mg, diluted in 5% glucose to a volume of 50 mL, infused over 20 min via a central vein

Further reading

National Institute for Health and Care Excellence (2014) Implantable cardioverter defibrillators and cardiac resynchronisation therapy for arrhythmias and heart failure. Technology appraisal guidance (TA314). https://www.nice.org.uk/guidance/ta314.

The Task Force for the management of patients with ventricular arrhythmias and the prevention of sudden cardiac death of the European Society of Cardiology (ESC) (2015) 2015 ESC Guidelines for the management of patients with ventricular arrhythmias and the prevention of sudden cardiac death. *Eur Heart J* 36, 2793–2867. DOI: 10.1093/eurheartj/ehv316.

CHAPTER 42

Narrow complex tachycardia

Michael Cooklin and David Sprigings

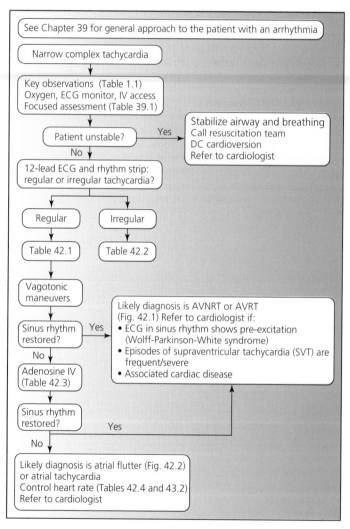

Approach to the patient with narrow complex tachycardia.

Acute Medicine: A Practical Guide to the Management of Medical Emergencies, Fifth Edition. Edited by
David Sprigings and John B. Chambers.
© 2018 John Wiley & Sons Ltd. Published 2018 by John Wiley & Sons Ltd.

Table **42.1** Differential diagnosis and management of narrow complex regular tachycardia.

Arrhythmia	Comment	Management
Sinus tachycardia	May sometimes be difficult to distinguish from other causes of tachycardia Adenosine causes gradual deceleration of sinus rate followed by acceleration, with or without AV block	Identify and treat the underlying cause IV adenosine (Table 42.3) may be appropriate to exclude other causes of narrow- complex regular tachycardia if in doubt
AV nodal re-entrant tachycardia (AVNRT)	The commonest cause of paroxysmal SVT Typically presents in teenagers or young adults with no underlying cardiac disease, though may present at any age Retrograde P wave usually hidden within or inscribed at the end of the QRS complex (simulating S wave in inferior leads, partial RBBB in V1) Heart rate usually 140–200/min	DC cardioversion if there is haemodynamic instability (uncommon) or other measures are ineffective In stable patient try vagotonic manoeuvres. If these fail, use IV adenosine, or verapamil* if adenosine is not tolerated or is contraindicated (Table 42.3) Record 12-lead ECG after sinus rhythm restored to check for pre-excitation (WPW syndrome) Refer to a cardiologist if episodes are frequent or severe or if pre-excitation is found
AV re-entrant tachycardia involving accessory pathway (AVRT) (Fig. 42.1)	Typically presents in children, teenagers or young adults with no underlying cardiac present Retrograde P wave may be seen inscribed in the ST segment or the ascending limb of the T wave Heart rate usually 140–230/min	DC cardioversion if there is haemodynamic instability or other measures are ineffective In stable patient try vagotonic manoeuvres. If these fail, use IV adenosine, or verapamil* if adenosine is not tolerated or is contraindicated (Table 42.3) Record 12-lead ECG after sinus rhythm restored to check for pre-excitation (WPW syndrome) Refer to a cardiologist if episodes are frequent or severe or if pre-excitation is found
Atrial flutter (Figure 42.2)	Suspect atrial flutter with 2:1 block when the rate is 150/min Often associated with structural heart disease Vagotonic manoeuvres and adenosine slow the ventricular rate to reveal flutter waves	See Chapter 43 DC cardioversion if there is haemodynamic instability or other measures are ineffective In stable patient, aim for rate control with AV node-blocking drugs (Table 42.4) Discuss further management with a cardiologist
Atrial tachycardia	Caused by discrete focus of electrical activity P wave usually of abnormal morphology, at a rate 130–300/min, conducted with varying degree of AV block May be associated with structural heart disease in older patients	DC cardioversion if there is haemodynamic instability or other measures are ineffective In stable patient, aim for rate control with AV node-blocking drugs (Table 42.4) Discuss further management with a cardiologist

AV, atrioventricular; RBBB, right bundle branch block; SVT, supraventricular tachycardia; WPW, Wolff-Parkinson-White.
ALERT Atrial flutter and atrial tachycardia may be irregular if there is variable AV conduction.
NOTE: 1. In up to 50% of patients with AVRT the accessory pathway is concealed and a delta wave is never present in sinus rhythm. These patients do not have Wolff-Parkinson-White syndrome.
2. It may be impossible to distinguish AVRT from AVNRT on the surface ECG. Initial treatment is identical.
* Avoid if patient already taking an oral beta blocker.

Table 42.2 Differential diagnosis and management of narrow complex irregular tachycardia.

Arrhythmia	Comment	Management
Atrial fibrillation	Difference between maximum and minimum instantaneous heart rates, calculated from the shortest and longest RR intervals is usually >30/min No organized atrial activity evident: fibrillation waves of varying amplitude may be seen	See Chapter 43
Atrial flutter with variable AV conduction	Often associated with structural heart disease Vagotonic manoeuvres and adenosine slow the ventricular rate to reveal flutter waves ('saw-tooth' flutter waves in inferior limb leads)	See Chapter 43 DC cardioversion if there is haemodynamic instability. In stable patient, aim for rate control with AV node-blocking drugs (Table 42.4) Discuss further management with a cardiologist
Multifocal atrial tachycardia	Irregular tachycardia, typically 100–130/min, with P waves of three or more morphologies and irregular PP interval Most commonly seen in COPD	Treatment is directed at the underlying disorder and correction of hypoxia/hypercapnia Consider verapamil if the heart rate is consistently over 110/min DC cardioversion is ineffective

AV, atrioioventricular; COPD, chronic obstructive pulmonary disease.

Table 42.3 Intravenous therapy to terminate supraventricular tachycardia (AV nodal re-entrant tachycardia and AV re-entrant tachycardia).

Drug	Comment	Dose
Adenosine	May cause facial flushing, chest pain, hypotension, bronchospasm May cause brief asystole, atrial fibrillation and non-sustained ventricular tachycardia Use with caution in patients with severe airways disease Contraindicated in patients with heart transplant	6 mg IV bolus through large bore cannula, followed by rapid saline flush. Repeat as necessary, if no response within 2 min, with 12, 18 and 24 mg boluses
Verapamil	May cause hypotension Contraindicated in patients taking beta blockers or in heart failure	5 mg IV over 5 min, to maximum dose of 15 mg
Esmolol	Short-acting (half-life 8 min) beta-1 selective beta blocker	500 µgm/kg over 1 min, followed by 200 µgm/kg over 4 min
Metoprolol	May cause hypotension	5 mg IV over 5 min, to maximum dose of 15 mg

Table 42.4 Intravenous therapy for rate control in atrial fibrillation, atrial flutter and atrial tachycardia.

Drug	Comment	Dose (IV)
Esmolol	Short-acting (half-life 8 min) beta-1 selective beta blocker	500 µgm/kg over 1 min, followed by 200 µgm/kg over 4 min
Metoprolol	May cause hypotension	5 mg over 5 min, to maximum dose of 15 mg
Verapamil	May cause hypotension Contraindicated in patients taking beta blockers or in heart failure	5 mg over 5 min, to maximum dose of 15 mg
Digoxin	Use if there is heart failure	500–1000 µgm in 50 mL saline over 1 h
Amiodarone	May be combined with digoxin for rate control in haemodynamically unstable patients	Loading: 300 mg, diluted in 5% glucose to a volume of 20–50 mL, infused over 20 min via a central vein Maintenance: 900–1200 mg over 24 h

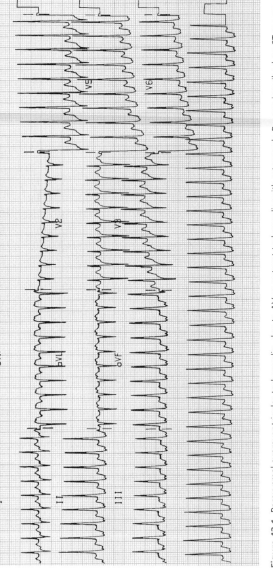

Figure 42.1 Paroxysmal supraventricular tachycardia, due to AV re-entrant tachycardia with retrograde P wave inscribed on ST segment.

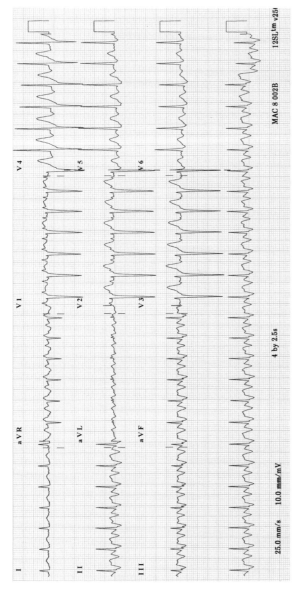

Figure 42.2 Atrial flutter with 2:1 conduction.

Further reading

Appelboam A, Reuben A, Mann C, *et al.*, on behalf of the REVERT trial collaborators (2015) Postural modification to the standard Valsalva manoeuvre for emergency treatment of supraventricular tachycardias (REVERT): a randomised controlled trial. *Lancet* 386, 1747–1753.

Page RL, Joglar JA, Caldwell MA, *et al.* (2016) 2015 ACC/AHA/HRS guideline for the management of adult patients with supraventricular tachycardia: a report of the American College of Cardiology/American Heart Association Task Force on Clinical Practice Guidelines and the Heart Rhythm Society. *J Am Coll Cardiol* 67, e27–115.

CHAPTER 43

Atrial fibrillation and flutter

MICHAEL COOKLIN AND DAVID SPRIGINGS

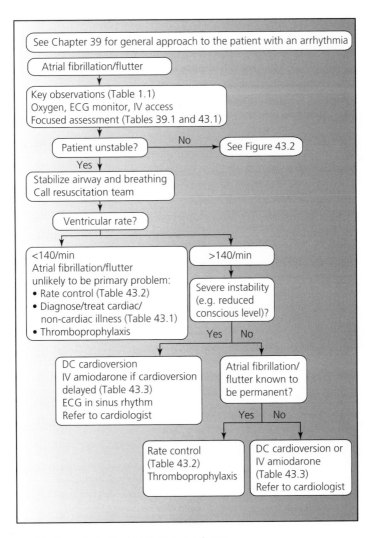

Figure 43.1 Approach to the patient with atrial fibrillation or flutter.

Acute Medicine: A Practical Guide to the Management of Medical Emergencies, Fifth Edition. Edited by David Sprigings and John B. Chambers.
© 2018 John Wiley & Sons Ltd. Published 2018 by John Wiley & Sons Ltd.

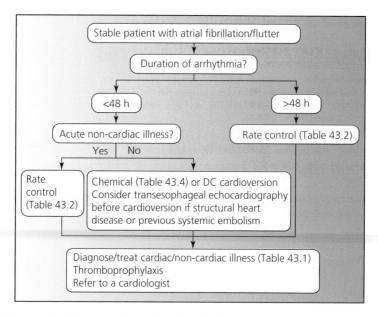

Figure 43.2 Management of the stable patient with atrial fibrillation or flutter.

Table 43.1 Disorders associated with atrial fibrillation.

Cardiovascular disorders
- Hypertension
- Coronary artery disease: previous myocardial infarction or acute coronary syndrome
- Cardiomyopathy
- Valve disease
- Any cause of heart failure (with resultant atrial hypertension/dilatation)
- Wolff-Parkinson-White syndrome
- Pulmonary embolism
- Acute pericarditis
- Cardiac surgery

Systemic disorders
- Sepsis, especially pneumonia
- Acute exacerbation of chronic obstructive pulmonary disease
- Alcohol binge
- Thyrotoxicosis
- Severe hypokalaemia
- Non-cardiac surgery

Table 43.2 Rate control in atrial fibrillation and flutter.

Drug	Comment	Dose (IV)	Dose (oral)
Esmolol	Short-acting (half-life 2–9 min) beta-1 selective beta blocker	500 µgm/kg over 1 min, followed by 200 µgm/kg over 4 min	Not available
Metoprolol	May cause hypotension	5 mg over 5 min, to maximum dose of 15 mg	25–100 mg 12-hourly
Verapamil	May cause hypotension Contraindicated in patients taking beta blockers or in heart failure	5 mg over 5 min, to maximum dose of 15 mg	40–80 mg 8-hourly
Digoxin	Use if there is heart failure Verapamil and amiodarone increase plasma digoxin level	500–1000 µgm in 50 mL saline over 1 h	Maintenance dose 62.5–250 µg daily, according to renal function/age
Amiodarone	May be combined with digoxin for rate control in haemodynamically unstable patients	Loading: 300 mg, diluted in 5% glucose to a volume of 20–50 mL, infused over 20 min via a central vein Maintenance: 900–1200 mg over 24 h	200 mg 8-hourly for one week, then 200 mg 12-hourly for one week, then 200 mg daily

Table 43.3 Drug therapy of atrial fibrillation or flutter: medication to restore sinus rhythm (chemical cardioversion).

Drug	Comment	Dose
Flecainide	May cause hypotension Avoid if known/possible structural or coronary heart disease	IV 2 mg/kg (to a maximum of 150 mg) over 10–30 min or PO 200–300 mg stat
Amiodarone	Needs to be given via central vein to avoid thrombophlebitis	IV 300 mg, diluted in 5% glucose to a volume of 20–50 mL, infused over 20 min via a central vein

Further reading

Atrial fibrillation: management. (2014) NICE (National Institutue for Health and Care Excellence). *Clinical guideline* [CG180]. Available at www.nice.org.uk

Bun S-S, Latcu DG, Marchlinski F, Nadir Saoudi N. (2015) Atrial flutter: more than just one of a kind. *European Heart Journal* 36, 2356–2363.

Freedman B, Potpara TS, Lip GYH. (2016) Stroke prevention in atrial fibrillation. *Lancet* 388, 806–817.

Piccini JP, Laurent Fauchie L. (2016) Rhythm control in atrial fibrillation. *Lancet* 388, 829–840.

The Task Force for the management of atrial fibrillation of the European Society of Cardiology (ESC) (2016) 2016 ESC Guidelines for the management of atrial fibrillation developed in collaboration with EACTS. *European Heart Journal*. Update citation at proof stage.

Van Gelder IC, Rienstra M, Crijns HJGM, Olshansky O. (2016) Rate control in atrial fibrillation. *Lancet* 388, 818–828.

CHAPTER 44

Bradycardia and atrioventricular block

MICHAEL COOKLIN AND DAVID SPRIGINGS

The approach to the patient with bradycardia or atrioventricular block (Table 44.1) is summarized in Figure 44.1.

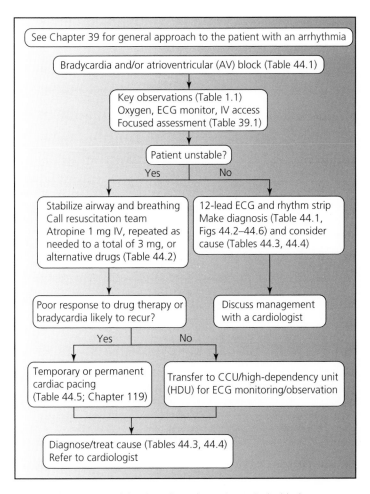

Figure 44.1 Approach to the patient with bradycardia and/or atrioventricular block.

Acute Medicine: A Practical Guide to the Management of Medical Emergencies, Fifth Edition. Edited by David Sprigings and John B. Chambers.
© 2018 John Wiley & Sons Ltd. Published 2018 by John Wiley & Sons Ltd.

Table 44.1 Classification of bradycardia and atrioventricular (AV) block.

Bradycardia (sinus node disease and atrioventricular block)
- Sinus bradycardia (see Table 44.3 for causes)
- Second-degree sino-atrial exit block
- Junctional escape secondary to profound sinus bradycardia or complete sino-atrial exit block or sinus arrest (Figure 44.2)
- Atrial fibrillation with slow ventricular rate (distinguished from atrial fibrillation with complete AV block by irregular RR interval)
- Atrial flutter/atrial tachycardia with high grade AV block
- Complete AV block with junctional or ventricular escape rhythm (Figure 44.6)

Atrioventricular block (see Table 44.4 for causes)
- First degree AV block (constant PR interval >200 ms)
- Second degree AV block, Mobitz type 1 (Wenckebach) (Figure 44.3)
- 2:1 second degree AV block (Figure 44.4)
- Second degree AV block, Mobitz type 2 (Figure 44.5)
- High grade AV block (e.g. 4;1 or 5:1 AV block)
- Third degree/complete AV block with junctional or ventricular escape rhythm (Figure 44.6)

Table 44.2 Drug therapy of bradycardia.

Drug	Comment	Dose (IV)
Atropine	Inhibition of vagal tone	Bolus of 500–1000 µgm, with further doses at 5 min intervals up to a total dose of 3 mg to achieve target heart rate
Dobutamine	Cardiac beta-1 receptor stimulation	Start infusion at 10 µgm/kg/min
	High doses may provoke ventricular arrhythmias	Adjust rate of infusion to achieve target heart rate
Glucagon	To reverse beta blockade	Bolus of 2–10 mg followed by infusion of 50 µgm/kg/h

Table 44.3 Causes of sinus bradycardia.

Cardiovascular
- Chronic sinus node dysfunction (due to idiopathic degenerative/fibrotic change in sinus node)
- Acute sinus node dysfunction due to ischaemia (typically in inferior myocardial infarction; sinus node artery arises from right coronary artery in ~90%)
- Manoeuvres triggering high vagal tone, for example suctioning of airway
- Vasovagal syncope
- Carotid sinus hypersensitivity

Systemic
- Drugs (beta blockers, digoxin, diltiazem, verapamil, other antiarrhythmic drugs)
- Hypothermia
- Hypothyroidism
- Hypokalaemia, hyperkalaemia
- Raised intracranial pressure

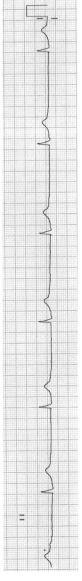

Figure 44.2 Junctional bradycardia secondary to sinus node disease. Heart rate 30–60/min with P wave absent or position constant either after, immediately before or hidden in QRS complex. Occurs when junctional pacemaker overtakes slow sinus node pacemaker or with complete sino-atrial exit block or sinus arrest.

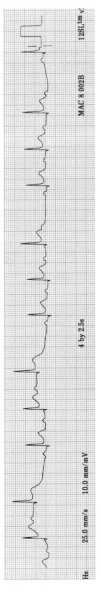

Figure 44.3 Second-degree atrioventricular block, Mobitz type 1 (Wenckebach). Progressively lengthening PR interval followed by dropped beat.

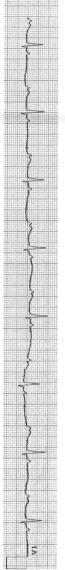

Figure 44.4 2:1 Second-degree atrioventricular (AV) block: alternate P waves non-conducted. May be due to disease in the AV node or below. If due to His-Purkinje disease often progresses to complete AV block.

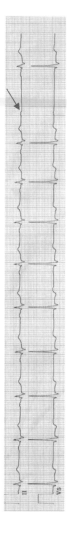

Figure 44.5 Second-degree atrioventricular (AV) block, Mobitz type 2. Constant PP interval and PR interval, with sudden dropped beat (non-conducted P wave, arrow). Usually due to disorder of His-Purkinje system and often progresses to complete AV block, frequently with an unreliable escape rhythm.

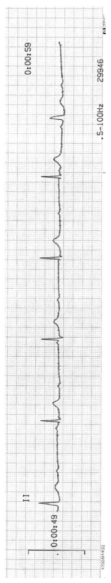

Figure 44.6 Complete atrioventricular block. Relationship of P wave to QRS varies randomly. P waves are absent if there is atrial fibrillation. Escape rhythm may be junctional (narrow complex) or ventricular (broad complex). Even in asymptomatic patients, this carries a risk of sudden death due to ventricular standstill or polymorphic ventricular tachycardia/ventricular fibrillation. The escape rhythm is usually slower and less reliable when it is ventricular.

Table 44.4 Causes of atrioventricular (AV) block.

Acute
- High vagal tone (may cause Mobitz type 1 second-degree AV block, but not Mobitz type 2 or complete AV block)
- Myocardial ischaemia/infarction
- Drugs (beta blockers, digoxin, diltiazem, verapamil, other antiarrhythmic drugs)
- Hyperkalaemia
- Infections: Lyme disease
- Myocarditis
- Infective endocarditis with aortic root abscess

Chronic
- Idiopathic conducting system fibrosis
- Congenital complete AV block
- Cardiomyopathy

Table 44.5 Temporary cardiac pacing: indications, contraindications and potential complications (for technique, see Chapter 119).*

Indications
- Bradycardia/asystole (sinus or junctional bradycardia or second/third-degree AV block) associated with haemodynamic compromise and unresponsive to atropine
- After cardiac arrest due to bradycardia/asystole
- To prevent perioperative bradycardia. Temporary pacing is indicated in:
  - Second degree Mobitz type 2 AV block or complete heart block *or*
  - Sinus/junctional bradycardia or second degree Mobitz type I (Wenckebach) AV block or bundle branch block (including bifascicular and trifascicular block) only if history of syncope or presyncope
- Atrial or ventricular overdrive pacing to prevent recurrent monomorphic ventricular tachycardia or polymorphic ventricular tachycardia with preceding QT prolongation (torsade de pointes)

Contraindications
- Risks of temporary pacing outweigh benefits, for example rare symptomatic sinus pauses, or complete heart block with a stable escape rhythm and no haemodynamic compromise. Discuss management with a cardiologist. Consider using standby external pacing system instead of transvenous pacing.
- Prosthetic tricuspid valve.

Complications
- Complications of central vein cannulation, especially bleeding in patients with acute coronary syndromes treated with thrombolytic therapy (reduced with ultrasound-guided approach)
- Cardiac perforation by pacing lead (may rarely result in cardiac tamponade)
- Arrhythmias (including ventricular fibrillation) during placement of pacing lead
- Infection of pacing lead

*Always discuss first with a cardiologist. Where possible, temporary pacing should be avoided, because of the high risk of complications. When bradycardia is likely to be reversible or contraindications to early permanent pacing are present (e.g. sepsis), temporary cardiac pacing may be indicated.
AV, atrioventricular.

Further reading

The Task Force on cardiac pacing and resynchronization therapy of the European Society of Cardiology (ESC) (2013) 2013 ESC Guidelines on cardiac pacing and cardiac resynchronization therapy. *European Heart Journal* 34, 2281–2329.

CHAPTER 45

Acute coronary syndromes (1): ST-segment elevation

Jim Newton and John B. Chambers

Acute coronary syndrome should be considered in any patient with central chest pain. Other presentations include epigastric pain, hypotension, pulmonary oedema and arrhythmia. If the presentation is consistent with acute myocardial ischaemia and the ECG shows persisting ST-segment elevation in two or more adjacent leads, or complete left bundle branch block not known to be old, immediate treatment to open the occluded epicardial coronary artery is needed.

Management of suspected ST-segment-elevation acute coronary syndrome (STE-ACS) is summarized in Figure 45.1.

Priorities

Many emergency departments will have a specific protocol for the management of STE-ACS, consisting of:
- Focused clinical assessment (Figure 45.1) and observations, using an ABCDE protocol:
  - Time, onset and character of pain
  - Past history and risk factors for coronary disease
  - Bleeding risk
  - Consider alternative diagnoses – could pulmonary embolism or aortic dissection be possible?
- 12-lead ECG (repeated every 15 min if not initially diagnostic and chest pain persists) and other urgent investigation (Table 45.1). Evaluate carefully for:
  - ST-segment elevation >1 mm in 2 or more adjacent leads or
  - Complete left bundle branch block not known to be old
- Oxygen therapy if indicated:
  - Monitor arterial oxygen saturation, aiming for >92%
  - Give high-flow oxygen if oxygen saturation is <92% or there is evident respiratory distress or pulmonary oedema
- Put in an IV cannula and give opioid analgesia:
  - 5 mg morphine IV (2.5 mg if elderly or frail) over 3–5 min, with further doses at 15-min intervals as needed to relieve pain
  - Co-administer an antiemetic, for example metoclopramide 10 mg IV

Acute Medicine: A Practical Guide to the Management of Medical Emergencies, Fifth Edition. Edited by David Sprigings and John B. Chambers.
© 2018 John Wiley & Sons Ltd. Published 2018 by John Wiley & Sons Ltd.

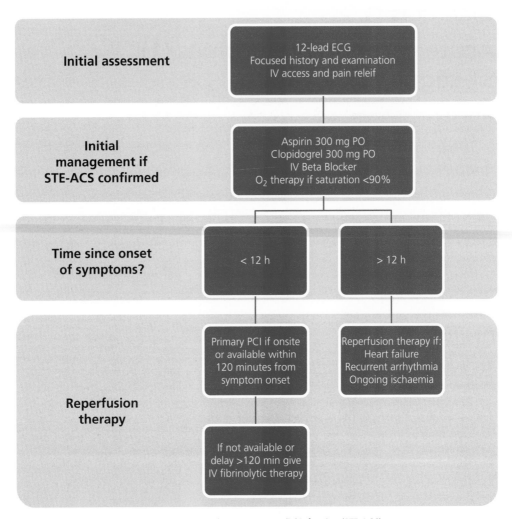

Figure 45.1 Management of acute ST-segment elevation myocardial infarction (STE-ACS).

Table 45.1 Investigation in suspected ST-segment elevation ACS.

Needed urgently

ECG (repeated every 15 min if not initially diagnostic and chest pain persists)

Chest X-ray

Creatinine and electrolytes (recheck potassium if significant arrhythmia occurs or after large diuresis)

Blood glucose (blood glucose >10 mmol/L should be managed by insulin infusion (Chapter 82)

Troponin level (repeat after 3 h if high-sensitivity assay, after 12 h if standard assay)

Echocardiography if diagnosis is uncertain, murmur, hypotension or pulmonary oedema

For later analysis

Full blood count

Lipid profile (cholesterol value is representative if checked within 24 h of infarction and enables patients with hypercholesterolaemia to be identified before discharge)

Table 45.2 Thrombolytic therapy: contraindications.

Absolute

Active internal bleeding
Suspected aortic dissection
Prolonged or traumatic cardiopulmonary resuscitation
Recent head trauma or known intracranial neoplasm
Trauma or surgery within the previous two weeks, which could be a source of rebleeding
Diabetic haemorrhagic retinopathy or other haemorrhagic ophthalmic condition
Pregnancy
Recorded blood pressure >200/120 mmHg
History of cerebrovascular accident known to be haemorrhagic

Relative

Recent trauma or surgery (>2 weeks)
History of chronic severe hypertension with or without drug therapy
Active peptic ulcer
History of cerebrovascular accident
Known bleeding diathesis or current use of anticoagulants
Significant liver dysfunction

If there are one or more relative contraindications to thrombolytic therapy, you must weigh the risks and benefits of therapy for the individual before deciding whether or not it should be given

If the clinical presentation and ECG are consistent with STE-ACS:
- Give aspirin 300 mg PO unless already administered.
- Give a beta blocker (e.g. atenolol 5–10 mg or metoprolol 5–10 mg) IV unless there is pulmonary oedema, or systolic BP is <100 mmHg, or the heart rate is <60/min.
- Is primary percutaneous coronary intervention (pPCI) available within 90 min? If so:
  - Give an additional antiplatelet agent – clopidogrel, ticagrelor or prasugrel, depending on local protocol
  - Transfer the patient to the cardiac catheterization laboratory for immediate angiography and follow-on pPCI
- If pPCI not available, assess eligibility for reperfusion therapy:
  - Less than 12 h since the onset of symptoms?
  - Other causes for ST-segment elevation (pericarditis, early repolarization, acute aortic dissection; see Chapter 7) considered and excluded?
  - Contraindications to reperfusion therapy absent? (Table 45.2)
- Give thrombolysis if appropriate (Table 45.3):
  - Problems encountered with thrombolysis are as shown in Table 45.4.
  - Repeat a 12-lead ECG 60 min after start of lytic therapy. If there is persisting ST-segment elevation, transfer for immediate coronary angiography. If ST segment has resolved, and the patient is clinically stable, discuss with a cardiologist inpatient coronary angiography during the same hospital admission.

Problems in the acute phase

Delayed presentation of STE-ACS

The benefits of reperfusion therapy fall if the diagnosis of STE-ACS is made more than 12 h after the onset of symptoms, but should still be considered if there is:
- Severe heart failure
- Haemodynamic disturbance
- Recurrent ventricular arrhythmia
- Persistent ischaemic pain

Table 45.3 Thrombolytic therapy.

Streptokinase
Suitable for the majority of patients
Adjunctive heparin not needed
Give streptokinase 1.5 MU as an IV infusion over 1 h

Alteplase (tissue plasminogen activator (tPA)): standard regimen
Use if the patient has received streptokinase within the previous 4 days to 12 months
Adjunctive heparin and antiplatelet therapy should be given
Give alteplase 1.5 mg/kg as an IV infusion over 3 h
Give heparin 5000 U IV bolus, followed by a continuous IV infusion to maintain APTT 1.5–2.5 times control (Chapter 103) for at least 2 days

Alteplase: accelerated regimen
May be of additional benefit in patients aged <50 with large anterior infarcts presenting within 4 h who are normotensive (systolic BP <140 mmHg), that is, low risk of haemorrhagic stroke
Adjunctive heparin and antiplatelet therapy should be given
Give alteplase 15 mg IV bolus, followed by 0.75 mg/kg (maximum 50 mg) over 30 min, and followed by 0.5 mg/kg (maximum 35 mg) over the next 60 min
Give heparin 5000 U IV bolus, followed by a continuous IV infusion to maintain APTT 1.5–2.5 times control (Chapter 103) for at least 2 days

If on-site primary PCI is not available, then the decision over reperfusion therapy depends on the time required for transfer and initiation of PCI. Ideally, this should be less than 90 min from diagnosis of STEMI to restoration of flow in the occluded vessel. If it is likely to be longer than 120 min, then fibrinolytic therapy and follow-on angiography maybe more appropriate.

Table 45.4 Thrombolytic therapy: problems.

Hypotension during streptokinase infusion
Usually reversed by elevating the foot of the bed or slowing the infusion

Allergic reaction to streptokinase
Give chlorpheniramine 10 mg IV and hydrocortisone 100 mg IV (prophylactic treatment not needed)

Oozing from puncture sites
If venepuncture is necessary, use a 22 G (blue) needle and compress the puncture site for 10 min
Central venous lines should be inserted via an antecubital fossa vein
For arterial puncture, use a 23 G (orange) needle in the radial or brachial artery and compress the puncture site for at least 10 min

Uncontrollable bleeding
Stop the infusion of thrombolytic
Transfuse whole fresh blood if available or fresh frozen plasma: seek advice from a haematologist
As a last resort, give tranexamic acid 1 g (10 mg/kg) IV over 10 min

Symptomatic bradycardia unresponsive to atropine
If temporary pacing is required within 24 h of thrombolytic therapy, the lead should ideally be placed via an antecubital fossa vein
If there is no suitable superficial vein, place via the femoral or internal jugular vein with ultrasound guidance (Chapter 116)

Diagnosis of ST-segment-elevation ACS but normal coronary anatomy

Consider stress cardiomyopathy (Takotsubo syndrome) (Table 45.5). This typically occurs in a female aged >65 following an emotional shock. The diagnosis is suggested by echocardiography showing the wall motion abnormality extending from the apex to the midcavity and crossing more than one arterial territory. Coronary angiography is required to exclude coronary disease, although it is recognized that bystander coronary disease may occur. Other possibilities are myocarditis, resolution of plaque rupture, coronary embolism and coronary spasm (e.g. caused by cocaine).

Hypotension without pulmonary oedema

Hypotension is not always due to cardiac dysfunction. Carefully evaluate for evidence of hypovolaemia which may be due to vomiting or bleeding following percutaneous coronary intervention. If there is no evidence of pulmonary oedema, consider a fluid challenge.

- Check the JVP, which will be low in hypovolaemia and high in right ventricular (RV) infarction.
- An echocardiogram (Chapter 114) will show:
  - RV size and function
  - An inferior vena cava, flat in hypovolaemia and engorged in right ventricular infarction
- For both hypovolaemia and right ventricular infarction initial treatment is with IV fluid. Give crystalloid 500 mL IV over 15–30 min followed by a further 500 mL over 30–60 min if systolic BP remains <100 mmHg and there is no pulmonary oedema.
- If BP remains low start an infusion of dobutamine (Table 2.7 page 13).
- If hypotension persists, consider placement of a pulmonary artery catheter to guide further therapy. In right ventricular infarction, the right atrial pressure will be high (12–20 mmHg) and equal or greater than the wedge pressure.
- Give more fluid to raise the wedge/pulmonary artery diastolic pressure to 15 mmHg. You can risk pulmonary oedema giving IV fluids without monitoring if there is an associated large inferior infarct.

Hypotension with pulmonary oedema

Review for signs of cardiogenic shock (Chapter 49):
- Systolic pressure <90 mmHg
- Heart rate either >100 or <40/min
- Hypoxaemia (arterial oxygen saturation <90%) or tachypnoea (respiratory rate >30/min)
- Poor peripheral perfusion
- Sweating and agitation
- Oliguria
  Cardiogenic shock carries a poor prognosis and is an indication for PCI. Discuss with a cardiologist.
- Increase the inspired oxygen concentration, aiming for oxygen saturation >92% (PaO_2 >8 kPa).
- Consider a continuous positive airway pressure (CPAP) system if this target is not achieved (Chapter 113).
- Start inotrope/vasopressor therapy (Table 45.6) if hypotension persists.

Table 45.5 Features of stress (Takotsubo) cardiomyopathy.

- Transient hypokinesis, akinesis or dyskinesis of the left ventricular mid-segments with or without apical involvement
- The regional wall motion abnormalities extend beyond a single epicardial vascular distribution
- Absence of obstructive coronary disease* or angiographic evidence of acute plaque rupture
- New electrocardiographic abnormalities (either ST-segment elevation and/or T-wave inversion) and/or modest elevation in cardiac troponin
- Absence of phaeochromocytoma (Chapter 94) or myocarditis

*May rarely coexist with obstructive coronary disease.

Table 45.6 Choice of inotropic/vasopressor therapy in cardiogenic shock due to myocardial infarction.

Systolic BP (mmHg)	Choice of therapy
>90	Dobutamine
80–90	Dopamine
<80	Noradrenaline

- Use intravenous nitrates if systolic BP >100 mmHg.
- Place a bladder catheter and aim for a urine output >30 mL/h.
- Arrange urgent echocardiography to assess ventricular function and assess for structural complications.
- For pulmonary oedema without significant hypotension:
  - Give furosemide 40–80 mg IV
  - Start a nitrate infusion

Arrhythmias
Bradycardia (Chapter 44)
- Give IV atropine 0.6–1.2 mg IV if symptomatic bradycardia <40/min.
- Temporary pacing is occasionally indicated (Table 45.7): discuss with a cardiologist. The procedure risks perforation of infarcted myocardium and triggering of ventricular arrhythmia.

Tachyarrhythmia (Chapters 39–43)
- Broad complex tachycardia should be treated as ventricular tachycardia. If there is haemodynamic compromise, DC cardioversion should be done promptly (Chapter 121).
- Ensure serum potassium is maintained between 4 and 5 mmol/L.

Further management

General supportive care
- Bed/chair rest for 24 h, then mobilization.
- Oxygen is not required if normal oxygen saturation and clear chest X-ray.

Table 45.7 Indications for temporary pacing in acute myocardial infarction.

Asystole (after restoration of spontaneous rhythm)
Complete heart block
Right bundle branch block with new left anterior hemiblock or left posterior hemiblock*
New left bundle branch block
Mobitz type II second-degree AV block
Mobitz type I (Wenckebach) second-degree AV block with hypotension not responsive to atropine
Sinus bradycardia with hypotension or recurrent sinus pauses not responsive to atropine
Atrial or ventricular overdrive pacing for recurrent ventricular tachycardia (seek advice from a cardiologist)

* Left anterior hemiblock gives left axis deviation (S wave > R in lead II); left posterior hemiblock gives right axis deviation (S wave > R in lead I).

Table 45.8 Fever after myocardial infarction.

Due to the infarct itself
Pericarditis
Thrombophlebitis at cannula site
Infection related to central line or temporary pacing lead
Deep vein thrombosis
Urinary tract infection
Pneumonia (consider inhalation pneumonia after resuscitation)

- Fever and leucocytosis are common in response to infarction, but ensure no evidence of thrombophlebitis, pericarditis or lower respiratory tract infection complicating resolving pulmonary oedema (Table 45.8).
- Continuous ECG monitoring (by bedside monitor or telemetry) for 48 h.
- Thromboprophylaxis with low-molecular-weight heparin.
- Cardiopulmonary examination at least daily. Causes of a murmur are given in Table 45.9.
- Review all usual medication and stop any drugs that are contraindicated post-infarction:
  - Non-steroidal anti-inflammatory drugs should be avoided as increased bleeding risk
  - Pro-arrhythmic agents including some antidepressant and anti-epileptic drugs
  - Drugs that may depress myocardial function, for example calcium channel blockers

Drug therapy
- Aspirin 75 mg daily for life.
- Second antiplatelet agent (P2Y$_{12}$ inhibitor, e.g. clopidogrel) in addition to aspirin for one year.
- Oral beta blocker the next day:
  - Delay if heart failure
  - Caution if low cardiac output
  - Delay or avoid if high risk for heart block
  - Contraindicated in true reactive asthma (but not COPD)
- An ACE inhibitor should be started on the morning of the day after admission unless there is a contraindication:
  - Highest value in patients with anterior infarction
  - Prognostic value if LV ejection fraction <40%
  - Can be replaced by angiotensin receptor blocker if required, but not in addition
- High-dose statin therapy should be commenced in all patients irrespective of initial lipid profiles – dose and agent can be modified in the recovery phase if required.

Table 45.9 Complications of myocardial infarction and their management.

Complication	Management
Tachyarryhthmia	See Chapters 39–43
Bradyarrhythmia	See Chapter 44
Myocardial rupture of:	
Papillary muscle, causing severe mitral regurgitation	Cardiac surgery
Ventricular septum, causing ventricular septal rupture	Cardiac surgery
Free wall, causing tamponade or a pseudoaneurysm	Surgery for pseudoaneurysm
True aneurysm	Heart failure therapy, occasionally LV reduction surgery or percutaneous devices
Pericarditis	NSAID; see Chapter 53
LV thrombus	Anticoagulation with warfarin

Glycaemic control

- In patients with known diabetes or an elevated blood glucose on arrival (>10 umol/L) start a variable rate insulin infusion (Chapter 82).
- Post-infarction treatment with subcutaneous insulin is preferred unless prior glycaemic control (and an HbA1c measurement) was excellent on oral hypoglycaemia agents. Input and education from a specialist diabetes team should be requested.

Managing recurrent pain

- Chest soreness is common after infarction and can be severe following cardiopulmonary resuscitation, which may result in rib fracture.
- Pericarditis occurs in 20% of patients and can cause pain similar to infarction but less severe, and usually postural and affected by respiration. Treat with higher dose aspirin or non-steroidal anti-inflammatory agents with gastro-protection.
- Re-infarction presenting with recurrence of infarct symptoms and new ST elevation should be managed as acute STE-ACS with urgent revascularization unless contraindicated.

New murmur

- A pericardial friction rub may be mistaken for a murmur.
- Request an echocardiogram for all murmurs, either electively or as an emergency, if there is hypotension or pulmonary oedema:
  - Soft systolic murmurs are usually benign, but may occasionally result from an early ventricular septal rupture, while still limited or from significant mitral regurgitation with an eccentric jet.
  - A loud systolic murmur suggests aortic stenosis and the murmur may become obvious as LV function improves.
  - Pan systolic murmurs may be due to ventricular septal rupture or mitral regurgitation, which may be chronic, but can be acute following papillary muscle disruption or rupture.

Rehabilitation and secondary prevention

- Give advice on diet, exercise and driving/work implications.
- Smoking cessation advice and nicotine replacement therapy if needed.
- Seek advice on management of diabetes from the specialist diabetes team.
- Treat hypertension aiming for BP <140/85 or <130/80 mmHg if diabetic.
- Continue high-dose statin; if the initial lipid profile showed severe hypercholesterolaemia or hypertriglyceridaemia, refer to a lipid specialist.
- Involve hospital rehabilitation team and enrol in post-discharge support programme.
- Psychological support may be needed.

Assessment of LV systolic function

Echocardiography to assess LV systolic function should be done before discharge. If LV ejection fraction is <40%, seek advice on management from a cardiologist prior to discharge.

Testing for inducible myocardial ischaemia

- As the majority of patients will undergo reperfusion with primary PCI and the culprit lesion treated with a stent there is no requirement for pre-discharge stress testing unless multivessel disease was identified with significant bystander disease.
- Exercise electrocardiography is safe if there are no recurrent symptoms and no arrhythmia for 72 h prior to the test. Pharmacological stress testing with assessment of ischaemia by non-invasive imaging (e.g. stress echocardiography or myocardial perfusion scintigraphy) is also safe and can be performed pre-discharge or in the recovery period to help guide the need for further revascularization.

Table 45.10 Discharge checklist after myocardial infarction.

Aspirin 75 mg daily lifelong
Clopidogrel 75 mg daily for 12 months (or prasugrel/ticagrelor)
Beta blocker unless contraindicated
ACE-inhibitor if there has been clinical heart failure or LVEF is <40%
High-dose statin (e.g. atorvastatin 80 mg daily)
Advice on smoking cessation, diet, lifestyle and work
Exercise rehabilitation arranged
Echocardiography done
Testing for inducible myocardial ischaemia done, or arranged if not fully revascularized

Discharge checklist

See Table 45.10.

Further reading

Eisen E, Giugliano RP, Braunwald E. (2016) Updates on acute coronary syndrome: a review. *JAMA Cardiol.*
    DOI: 10.1001/jamacardio.2016.2049. Update citation at proof stage.
Reed GW, Rossi J, Cannon CP. (2016) Acute myocardial infarction. *Lancet.* Update citation at proof stage.
The Task Force on the management of ST-segment elevation acute myocardial infarction of the European
    Society of Cardiology (ESC) (2012) ESC Guidelines for the management of acute myocardial infarction in
    patients presenting with ST-segment elevation. *European Heart Journal* 33, 2569–2619.

CHAPTER 46

Acute coronary syndromes (2): Non-ST-segment elevation

JIM NEWTON AND JOHN B. CHAMBERS

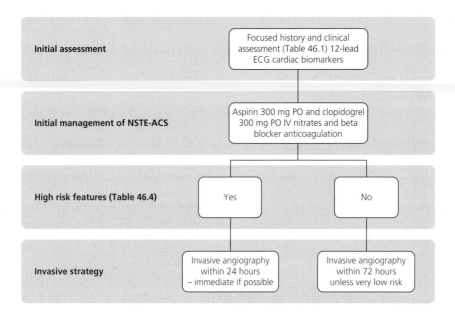

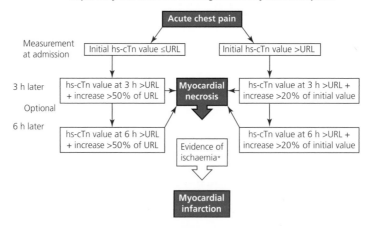

Figure 46.1 Management of suspected non-ST-segment elevation acute coronary syndrome (NSTE-ACS).

Acute Medicine: A Practical Guide to the Management of Medical Emergencies, Fifth Edition. Edited by David Sprigings and John B. Chambers.
© 2018 John Wiley & Sons Ltd. Published 2018 by John Wiley & Sons Ltd.

Non-ST-segment-elevation acute coronary syndrome (NSTE-ACS) occurs as a result of transient or partial occlusion of an epicardial coronary artery. A variety of ECG changes may occur, and importantly the ECG may be entirely normal: a high index of suspicion and serial assessment is key to ensuring correct diagnosis and management. Patients presenting with NSTE-ACS have a poor prognosis if not identified and treated appropriately. Management of suspected NSTE-ACS is summarized in Figure 45.1.

Priorities

The initial assessment of acute chest pain is dominated by the ECG. If this does not show ST-segment elevation or new left bundle branch block, pain characteristics, coronary risk scoring and troponin concentration are used to make the diagnosis of non-ST-segment elevation ACS and to guide further management. Investigations required urgently are given in Table 46.1.

Chest pain characteristics

Typical cardiac chest pain is retrosternal pressure or heaviness/tightness radiating to the left arm (occasionally right or both arms) or to the neck or jaw and sometimes associated with sweating and nausea.

Atypical symptoms occur more commonly in the elderly, female patients, those with diabetes and renal failure and can include:

- Epigastric pain
- Dyspeptic symptoms
- Breathlessness
- Delirium

The likelihood of cardiac ischaemia causing the pain is increased if there has been previous similar exertional pain or there is known coronary artery disease. Response to nitrate administration is not specific to cardiac ischaemia. The differential diagnosis of acute chest pain is discussed in Chapter 7.

The 12-lead ECG

This may be entirely normal, particularly if pain has resolved. If there is a high clinical suspicion or chest pain persists, repeat every 15 minutes and include modified leads (lateral and right-sided leads) as left circumflex coronary territory or right ventricular ischaemia may not appear with standard lead positions.

Table 46.1 Investigation in suspected non-ST-segment-elevation ACS.

Needed urgently

ECG (repeated every 15 min if not initially diagnostic and chest pain persists)
Chest X-ray
Creatinine and electrolytes (recheck potassium if significant arrhythmia occurs or after large diuresis)
Blood glucose (blood glucose >10 mmol/L should be managed by insulin infusion (Chapter 82)
Troponin level (repeat after 3 hours if high-sensitivity assay, after 12 hours if standard assay)
Echocardiography if diagnosis is uncertain, murmur, hypotension or pulmonary oedema

For later analysis
Full blood count
Lipid profile (cholesterol value is representative if checked within 24 h of infarction and enables patients with hypercholesterolaemia to be identified before discharge)

Typical ECG findings are:
- ST depression >0.05 mV in two or more contiguous leads
- T wave changes:
  - Inversion
  - Flattened T waves
  - Pseudo-normalization of inverted T waves

Plasma troponin

- The measurement of plasma troponin (released during myocardial ischaemia) complements but does not supplant the history, examination and ECG findings.
- Measurement of plasma troponin using a high-sensitivity assay is recommended, as increases in plasma troponin can be detected within 1–2 hours of symptom onset. Point-of-care assays are less sensitive and may take several more hours to become abnormal.
- The universal definition of myocardial infarction is given in Table 46.2. For spontaneous non-ST-segment-elevation myocardial infarction, or infarction as a result of low coronary perfusion (e.g. prolonged syncope or hypotension), one troponin level above the 99th centile for a normal person is abnormal. If the baseline level is raised, a >20% rise in 3 hours is required.
- A similar definition applies to Types 4b and 4c. Type 4a requires one level >5 times the 99th centile or a new rise by >20%. Type 5 requires a level >10 times the 99th centile
- Many conditions are associated with a raised plasma troponin, and should be considered in the differential diagnosis (Table 46.3).
  - Avoid unnecessary measurement of troponin or other biomarkers to 'rule-out' ACS without consideration of the history and serial ECGs.
  - The recognition of a NSTE-ACS requires the additional presence of chest pain or other significant symptom or an acute change in the 12-lead ECG.

Risk assessment in NSTE-ACS

If the diagnosis of NSTE-ACS is confirmed by the history, ECG findings and plasma troponin results, the risk of mortality in hospital and at six months can be calculated and used to guide further management. A number of risk models are available; the GRACE 2.0 risk calculator is widely preferred and is based on the following clinical factors:
- Age
- Systolic blood pressure
- Heart rate
- Serum creatinine
- Killip class:
  - I – no evidence of pulmonary oedema
  - II – audible crepitation, raised venous pressure, third heart sound

Table 46.2 Universal classification of myocardial infarction and injury.

Type 1	Spontaneous infarction due to plaque rupture
Type 2	Myocardial injury secondary to either increased oxygen demand or reduced supply, for example coronary spasm or embolism, arrhythmia, hypotension, anaemia, hypertension, respiratory failure
Type 3	Sudden unexpected cardiac death associated with ECG changes or fresh thrombus in the coronary artery but occurring before an elevation in cardiac biomarkers
Type 4	Associated with intervention either percutaneous (4a) or stent thrombosis (4b) or restenosis (4c)
Type 5	Associated with coronary artery by-pass grafting (CABG)

Table 46.3 Causes of raised troponin concentration not due to acute coronary syndrome.

Cardiac

Stress (Takotsubo) cardiomyopathy
Myocarditis
Arrhythmia
Severe aortic stenosis
Contusion or other trauma (e.g. radiofrequency ablation, pacing)
Infiltration (e.g. amyloid)
Hypertrophic cardiomyopathy
Cardiogenic shock of any cause

Non-cardiac
Pulmonary embolism or severe pulmonary hypertension
Subarachnoid haemorrhage
Sepsis
Strenuous exercise
Respiratory failure
Acute kidney injury or advanced chronic kidney disease
Other causes of shock (hypovolaemic, septic, anaphylactic)

- III – acute pulmonary oedema
- IV – cardiogenic shock
- Cardiac arrest at admission to hospital
- Elevated cardiac biomarkers
- ST segment deviation
  The GRACE calculator is available online at: http://gracescore.org/WebSite/WebVersion.aspx.

Treatment of confirmed or suspected NSTE-ACS
- Insert an IV cannula and relief pain with IV morphine
- Give oxygen therapy if saturations <92% or obvious respiratory distress
- Intravenous nitrates therapy with close blood pressure monitoring:
  - More effective than sublingual nitrates
  - Contraindicated if recent intake of phosphodiesterase type-5 inhibitors (e.g. sildenafil)
- Start a beta blocker, oral or IV unless:
  - Risk of cardiogenic shock – heart rate >110/min and systolic <120 mmHg
  - Bronchospasm
  - Ischaemia due to vasospasm or cocaine intake (unopposed alpha-mediated vasoconstriction)
- Give antiplatelet agents and continue for one year, unless there is excessive risk of bleeding:
  - Aspirin 300 mg orally unless already administered (lifelong at a dose of 75 mg daily)
  - Clopidogrel 300 mg or alternative $P2Y_{12}$ inhibitor, for example prasugrel 60 mg or ticagrelor 180 mg

Assessment of bleeding risk
Clinical factors that may influence bleeding risk include:
- Increasing age
- Female gender
- Low body weight, for example <65 kg
- Diabetes

- Peripheral vascular disease
- Renal function
- Prior bleeding

Anticoagulation

Combining dual anti-platelet therapy with anticoagulation to reduce thrombin generation or activation is more effective than antiplatelet or anticoagulant therapy alone. Protocols vary by institution but typically recommend the addition of **one** of the following:

- Intravenous unfractionated heparin, for example 60 IU/kg bolus and 12–15 IU/kg infusion
- Subcutaneous low molecular weight heparin, for example enoxaparin 1 mg/kg twice daily
- Subcutaneous factor Xa inhibitor, for example fondaparinux 2.5 mg/day
- Intravenous thrombin inhibitor, for example bivalirudin 0.75 mg/kg bolus and 1.75 mg/kg/h infusion

Anticoagulation should not be continued indefinitely alongside dual antiplatelet therapy as there is a marked increase in bleeding risk. Triple therapy should be avoided in all but highly selected cases with a clear indication for both anticoagulation and dual antiplatelet therapy at high risk of thrombotic complications if discontinued. This should be discussed with cardiology and a management plan agreed before coronary intervention.

Invasive coronary angiography

Risk factors mandating invasive management are summarized in Table 46.4.

Non-invasive assessment

Patients with no high risk features, and without diabetes, renal impairment, LV systolic dysfunction or prior revascularization who settle on medical therapy with no on-going symptoms can be managed with non-invasive assessment of ischaemia. If this shows a significant volume of ischaemia (>10% of viable myocardium) then invasive angiography is indicated. If ischaemia is absent or confined to a small volume then medical therapy is appropriate.

NSTE-ACS with normal coronary arteries

Up to 10% of patients presenting with NSTE-ACS will not have a culprit lesion identified at angiography. Cardiac causes are given in Chapter 45. Always revisit the initial diagnosis and ensure an alternative major pathology has not been missed and consider computed tomography to exclude aortic dissection or pulmonary embolism.

Further management

General supportive care

As for ST-elevation ACS: see p. 294–7

Drug therapy

- Aspirin 75 mg daily for life
- Second antiplatelet agent (P2Y$_{12}$ inhibitor, e.g. clopidogrel) in addition to aspirin for one year
- Oral beta blocker the next day:
  - Delay if heart failure
  - Caution if low cardiac output
  - Delay or avoid if high risk for heart block
  - Contraindicated in true reactive asthma (but not COPD)

Table 46.4 Risk criteria mandating an invasive strategy in non-ST-elevation acute coronary syndrome.

Very-high-risk criteria
• Haemodynamic instability or cardiogenic shock
• Recurrent or ongoing chest pain refractory to medical treatment
• Life-threatening arrhythmias or cardiac arrest
• Mechanical complications of MI
• Acute heart failure
• Recurrent dynamic ST-T wave changes, particularly with intermittent ST-elevation
High-risk criteria
• Rise or fall in cardiac troponin compatible with MI
• Dynamic ST- or T-wave changes (symptomatic or silent)
• GRACE score > 140
Intermediate-risk criteria
• Diabetes mellitus
• Renal insufficiency (eGFR <60 mL/min/1.73 m^2)
• LVEF <40% or congestive heart failure
• Early post-infarction angina
• Prior PCI
• Prior CABG
• GRACE risk score >109 and <140
Low-risk criteria
• Any characteristics not mentioned above

CABG = coronary artery bypass graft eGFR = estimated glomerular filtration rate: GRACE = Glotxal Registry of Acute Coronary Events: LVEF = left ventricular election fraction, PCI = percutaneous coronary intervention, MI = myocardial infarction.

CABG, coronary artery bypass grafting; eGFR, estimated glomerular filtration rate; GRACE, Global Registry of Acute Coronary Events (see text); LVEF, left ventricular ejection fraction; PCI, percutaneous coronary intervention; MI, myocardial infarction.

Reproduced with permission from: 2015 ESC Guidelines for the management of acute coronary syndromes in patients presenting without persistent ST-segment elevation (2016) *European Heart Journal* 37, 267–315.

- An ACE inhibitor should be started on the morning of the day after admission unless there is a contraindication:
  - Highest value in patients with anterior infarction
  - Prognostic value if LV ejection fraction <40%
  - Can be replaced by angiotensin receptor blocker if required, but not in addition
- High-dose statin therapy should be commenced in all patients irrespective of initial lipid profiles – dose and agent can be modified in the recovery phase if required

Rehabilitation and secondary prevention
- Give advice on diet, exercise and driving/work implications
- Smoking cessation advice and nicotine replacement therapy if needed

- Seek advice on management of diabetes from the specialist diabetes team
- Treat hypertension, aiming for BP <140/85 or <130/80 mmHg if diabetic
- Continue high-dose statin; if the initial lipid profile showed severe hypercholesterolaemia or hypertriglyceridaemia, refer to a lipid specialist
- Involve hospital rehabilitation team and enrol in post-discharge support programme
- Psychological support may be needed – particularly for younger men

Assessment of LV systolic function

Echocardiography to assess LV systolic function should be done before discharge. If LV ejection fraction is <40%, seek advice on management from a cardiologist prior to discharge.

Testing for inducible myocardial ischaemia

- As the majority of patients will undergo reperfusion with primary PCI and the culprit lesion will be treated with a stent there is no requirement for pre-discharge stress testing unless multivessel disease was identified with significant bystander disease.
- Exercise electrocardiography is safe if there are no recurrent symptoms and no arrhythmia for 72 hours prior to the test. Pharmacological stress testing with assessment of ischaemia by non-invasive imaging (e.g. stress echocardiography or myocardial perfusion scintigraphy) is also safe and can be performed pre-discharge or in the recovery period to help guide the need for further revascularization.

Discharge checklist

As for ST-elevation ACS: see Table 45.10.

Further reading

Eisen E, Giugliano RP, Braunwald E. (2016) Updates on acute coronary syndrome: a review. *JAMA Cardiol.* 1(6):718–730. doi:10.1001/jamacardio.2016.2049

Reed GW, Rossi J, Cannon C.P. (2017) Acute myocardial infarction. *Lancet*; 389(10065):197–210. PMID: 27502078.

The Task Force for the management of acute coronary syndromes in patients presenting without persistent ST-segment elevation of the European Society of Cardiology (ESC) 2015. ESC guidelines for the management of acute coronary syndromes in patients presenting without persistent ST-segment elevation. http://eurheartj.oxfordjournals.org/content/early/2015/08/28/eurheartj.ehv320.

CHAPTER 47

Acute pulmonary oedema

Davⁱᴅ Sᴘʀɪɢɪɴɢꜱ ᴀɴᴅ Jᴏʜɴ B. Cʜᴀᴍʙᴇʀꜱ

DAVID SPRIGINGS AND JOHN B. CHAMBERS

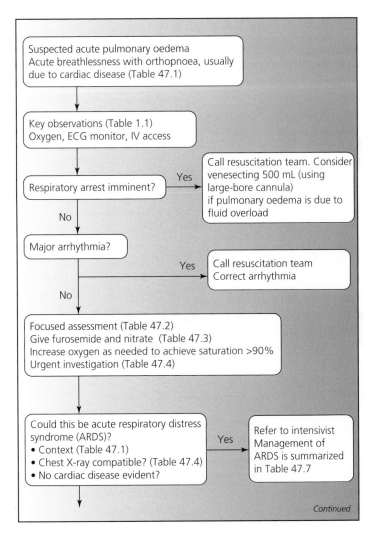

Figure 47.1 Approach to the patient with suspected pulmonary oedema.

Acute Medicine: A Practical Guide to the Management of Medical Emergencies, Fifth Edition. Edited by David Sprigings and John B. Chambers.
© 2018 John Wiley & Sons Ltd. Published 2018 by John Wiley & Sons Ltd.

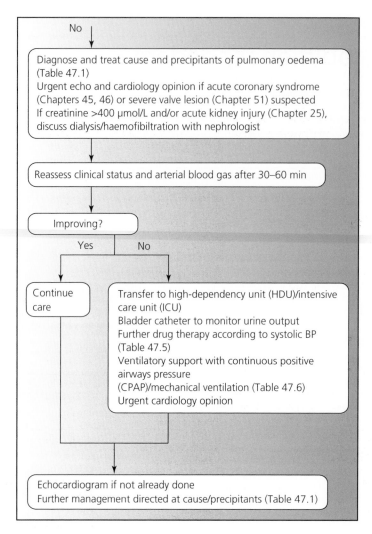

Figure 47.1 (*Continued*)

Table 47.1 Causes of acute pulmonary oedema.

Causes due to elevated pressure in the pulmonary capillaries

Cardiac disease, new presentation:

- Acute myocardial infarction or severe myocardial ischaemia
- Acute myocarditis
- Severe aortic or mitral stenosis
- Acute aortic regurgitation (aortic dissection, infective endocarditis, chest trauma)
- Acute mitral regurgitation (infective endocarditis, ruptured chordae or papillary muscle, chest trauma)
- Ventricular septal rupture after myocardial infarction
- Left atrial myxoma

Precipitants of pulmonary oedema in patients with previously stable valve or left ventricular disease:

- Acute myocardial infarction or myocardial ischaemia
- Arrhythmia
- Poor compliance with diuretic therapy
- Drugs causing fluid retention (e.g. NSAIDs, steroids)
- Iatrogenic fluid overload
- Infective endocarditis
- Progression of disease
- Intercurrent illness (e.g. pneumonia, anaemia)

Renal disease:

- Acute kidney injury or advanced chronic kidney disease
- Renal artery stenosis

Iatrogenic fluid overload

Subarachnoid haemorrhage

Negative-pressure pulmonary oedema (Table 47.8)

Causes due to increased pulmonary capillary permeability

(acute lung injury/ARDS); for management see Table 47.7

Direct lung injury	**Indirect lung injury**
Common causes	
Pneumonia (viral or bacterial)	Sepsis
Aspiration of gastric contents	Severe trauma with shock and multiple transfusions
Less common causes	
Pulmonary contusion	Cardiopulmonary by-pass
Fat emboli	Drug overdose
Drowning	Acute pancreatitis
Inhalational injury	Transfusions of blood
Reperfusion pulmonary oedema after lung transplantation or pulmonary embolectomy	products

ARDS, acute respiratory distress syndrome; NSAIDs, non-steroidal anti- inflammatory drugs.

Table 47.2 Focused assessment in acute pulmonary oedema.

What is the cause of the pulmonary oedema?

- Usually cardiac disease (Table 47.1), less often acute kidney injury
- Pulmonary oedema developing in hospital is often due to fluid overload in patients with pre-existing cardiac or renal disease
- Consider acute respiratory distress syndrome in patients without evidence of cardiac disease (Table 47.1)
- In post-operative patients, negative-pressure pulmonary oedema is occasionally seen (Table 47.8)
- Neurogenic pulmonary oedema may complicate subarachnoid haemorrhage (Chapter 67)

Table 47.3 Initial drug therapy in acute pulmonary oedema.

Drug	Comment
Oxygen	Give oxygen 60–100%.
	Pulse oximetry may be unreliable due to peripheral vasoconstriction.
	Check arterial blood gases if the patient is hypotensive or there is no improvement within 30 min.
	Target oxygen saturation >92%, PaO_2 >8 kPa.
Furosemide	Give furosemide 40 mg IV if plasma creatinine is <150 μmol/L and 80 mg if 150–200 μmol/L.
	In patients with plasma creatinine >200 μmol/L, standard doses of furosemide are often ineffective. Try a furosemide infusion (100 mg IV over 60 min by syringe pump).
Nitrate	Give nitrate (sublingual, buccal or IV infusion).

Table 47.4 Urgent investigation in acute pulmonary oedema.

- ECG Arrhythmia? Evidence of acute myocardial infarction or ischaemia? Evidence of other cardiac disease, e.g. left ventricular hypertrophy, left bundle branch block?
- Chest X-ray (to confirm the clinical diagnosis and exclude other causes of breathlessness). With non-cardiogenic pulmonary oedema, the heart size is usually normal; septal lines and pleural effusions are usually absent; and air bronchograms are usually present.
- Arterial blood gases and pH.
- Blood glucose.
- Creatinine, sodium and potassium.
- Full blood count.
- Erythrocyte sedimentation rate (ESR) or C-reactive protein.
- Transthoracic echocardiography, in all newly diagnosed cases especially if acute valve lesion or ventricular septal rupture is suspected, or distinction between cardiogenic/non-cardiogenic pulmonary oedema is uncertain (in other patients, echocardiography should be done within 24 h).
- Cardiac biomarkers: plasma troponin and brain natriuretic peptide.

Table 47.5 Further drug therapy of acute cardiogenic pulmonary oedema.

Systolic blood pressure	Action
>110 mmHg	Give another dose of furosemide 40–80 mg IV
	Start a nitrate infusion
90–110 mmHg	Start a dobutamine infusion at 5 μgm/kg/min; this can be given via a peripheral line
	Increase the dose by 2.5 μgm/kg/min every 10 min until systolic BP is >110 mmHg or a maximum dose of 20 μgm/kg/min has been reached
	A nitrate infusion can be added if systolic BP is maintained at >110 mmHg
80–90 mmHg	Start a dopamine infusion at 10 μgm/kg/min; this must be given via a central line
	Increase the dose by 5 μgm/kg/min every 10 min until systolic BP is >110 mmHg
	If systolic BP remains <90 mmHg despite dopamine 20 μgm/kg/min, use norepinephrine instead
	A nitrate infusion can be added if systolic BP is maintained at >110 mmHg
<80 mmHg	Start a norepinephrine infusion at 2.5 μgm/kg/min; this must be given via a central line
	Increase the dose by 2.5 μgm/kg/min every 10 min until systolic BP is >110 mmHg
	A nitrate infusion can be added if systolic BP is maintained at >110 mmHg

Table 47.6 Ventilatory support for respiratory failure due to cardiogenic pulmonary oedema.

Mode of ventilation	Indications	Contraindications	Disadvantages and complications
Non-invasive ventilatory support with continuous positive airways pressure (CPAP)	Oxygenation failure: oxygen saturation <92% despite FiO_2 >40% Ventilatory failure: mild to moderate respiratory acidosis, arterial pH 7.25–7.35	Recent facial, upper airway or upper gastrointestinal tract surgery Vomiting or bowel obstruction Copious secretions Haemodynamic instability Impaired consciousness, confusion or agitation	Discomfort from tightly fitting facemask Discourages coughing and clearing of secretions
Endotracheal intubation and mechanical ventilation	Upper airway obstruction Impending respiratory arrest Airway at risk because of neurological disease or coma (GCS 8 or lower) Oxygenation failure: PaO_2 <7.5–8 kPa despite supplemental oxygen/NIV Ventilatory failure: moderate to severe respiratory acidosis, arterial pH <7.25	Severely impaired functional capacity and/or severe comorbidity Cardiac disorder not remediable Patient has expressed wish not to be ventilated	Adverse haemodynamic effects Pharyngeal, laryngeal and tracheal injury Pneumonia Ventilator-induced lung injury (e.g. pneumothorax) Complications of sedation and neuromuscular blockade

GCS, Glasgow Coma Scale score.

Table 47.7 Management of acute respiratory distress syndrome (ARDS).

Element	Comment
Transfer to ICU	ARDS is usually part of multiorgan failure
Oxygenation	Increase inspired oxygen, target PaO_2 >8 kPa
	Ventilation will be needed if PaO_2 is <8 kPa despite FiO_2 60%
	Ventilation in the prone position improves oxygenation
	Haemoglobin should be kept around 10 g/dl (to give the optimum balance between oxygen-carrying capacity and blood viscosity)
Fluid balance	Acute kidney injury is commonly associated with ARDS
	Consider early haemofiltration
Prevention and treatment of sepsis	Sepsis is a common cause and complication of ARDS
	Culture blood, tracheobronchial aspirate and urine daily
	Treat presumed infection with broad-spectrum antibiotic therapy
Nutrition	Enteral feeding if possible, via nasogastric tube if ventilation needed
DVT prophylaxis	Give DVT prophylaxis with stockings and LMW heparin
Prophylaxis against gastric stress ulceration	Give proton pump inhibitor

DVT, deep vein thrombosis; ICU, intensive care unit; LMW, low molecular weight.

Table 47.8 Negative-pressure pulmonary oedema.

- Seen in the early postoperative period
- Due to forced inspiration in the presence of upper airway obstruction (e.g. from laryngospasm after extubation)
- After relief of laryngospasm, patients develop clinical and radiological features of pulmonary oedema
- Typically resolves over the course of a few hours with supportive care
- Cardiogenic pulmonary oedema should be excluded by clinical assessment, ECG and echocardiography

Further reading

Busl KM, Bleck TP. (2015) Concise definitive review: Neurogenic pulmonary edema. *Critical Care Medicine* 43, 1710–1715. DOI: 10.1097/CCM.0000000000001101.

Mac Sweeney R, McAuley DF. (2016) Acute respiratory distress syndrome. *Lancet* 388, 2416–2430.

The Task Force for the diagnosis and treatment of acute and chronic heart failure of the European Society of Cardiology (ESC) (2016) 2016 ESC Guidelines for the diagnosis and treatment of acute and chronic heart failure. *European Heart Journal* 37, 2129–2200. http://eurheartj.oxfordjournals.org/content/ehj/early/2016/05/19/eurheartj.ehw128.full.pdf.

CHAPTER 48

Acute heart failure and decompensated chronic heart failure

JOHN B. CHAMBERS AND DAVID SPRIGINGS

This may present with acute pulmonary oedema or cardiogenic shock, but more often presents sub-acutely, with sodium and water retention causing progressive breathlessness and oedema.

- About 20% of patients with a presumed exacerbation of chronic obstructive pulmonary disease (Chapter 61) have left ventricular failure as the correct or coexistent diagnosis.
- Patients with suspected acute heart failure should have measurement of plasma B-type natriuretic peptide (BNP) or N-terminal pro-BNP (NT-pro-BNP) at presentation. The finding of a normal level of plasma BNP or NT-pro-BNP effectively excludes heart failure.
- If the clinical/ECG features or natriuretic peptide level indicate acute heart failure or decompensated chronic heart failure, transthoracic echocardiography should be done within 48 hours of admission.

Priorities

If there is acute pulmonary oedema, see Chapter 47, or if cardiogenic shock, see Chapter 49. If the patient is clinically stable, complete your assessment (Table 48.1). Investigations needed urgently are given in Table 48.2.

Make a formulation, addressing the following points:

- Is this new heart failure or decompensated chronic heart failure?
- What is the underlying cause of the heart failure (e.g. recent myocardial infarction, hypertensive heart disease, severe aortic stenosis)? Other causes to consider are given in Table 48.3.
- Are there precipitating or aggravating events? These include:
  - Poor compliance with medication
  - New onset of atrial fibrillation
  - Intercurrent illness (e.g. pneumonia or urinary tract infection)
  - Pulmonary embolism
  - Medication causing fluid retention (e.g. NSAID, steroid)
  - Acute coronary syndrome
  - Worsening functional mitral regurgitation
- Are there points of concern for treatment? These include heart rate and rhythm, blood pressure, plasma potassium and renal function (Table 48.4).

Acute Medicine: A Practical Guide to the Management of Medical Emergencies, Fifth Edition. Edited by David Sprigings and John B. Chambers.
© 2018 John Wiley & Sons Ltd. Published 2018 by John Wiley & Sons Ltd.

Table 48.1 Focused assessment of the patient with acute heart failure or decompensated chronic heart failure.

History

Total duration of symptoms and of acute deterioration

Degree of exertional breathlessness (after how many steps or stairs, on the flat or slopes or hills; see Box for NYHA functional classification)

New York Heart Association (NYHA) functional classification

Class 1 Can manage ordinary physical activity without undue fatigue or breathlessness

Class 2 Slight limitation of ordinary activity by fatigue or breathlessness

Class 3 Marked limitation of ordinary activity by fatigue or breathlessness

Class 4 Cannot manage any activity without fatigue or breathlessness, and may have symptoms at rest

---

Orthopnoea or paroxysmal nocturnal dyspnoea?

Is heart failure or a cardiomyopathy known? What investigations have been done? Who normally manages care?

Is there a history of hypertension or coronary artery disease?

Drug history including any recent change and evidence for compliance?

Any change in diet, for example increase in salt intake?

Examination

General appearance

Body mass index (cachexia?)

Heart rate and blood pressure

Jugular venous pressure, peripheral oedema, ascites

Respiratory rate, arterial oxygen saturation, inspiratory crackles, signs of pleural effusion

Murmurs, third heart sound, apex displacement

Further management

Establish and treat the cause and precipitants of heart failure

- Heart failure may be caused by myocardial, valvular or pericardial disease, or metabolic disorders (e.g. thyrotoxicosis). Clinical assessment, ECG and echocardiography will usually identify the likely diagnosis. Further investigation (e.g. coronary angiography or cardiac magnetic resonance imaging) may be needed for definitive diagnosis.
- Heart failure (HF) due to left ventricular (LV) dysfunction is categorized by the LV ejection fraction (EF) as HF with preserved EF ($\geq$50%) (HFpEF), HF with reduced EF (<40%) (HFrEF), and HF with mid-range EF (40-49%) (HFmrEF).
- In patients with decompensated chronic heart failure, consider and exclude the precipitating or aggravating factors listed above.

Seek advice from the specialist heart failure team. Input from a cardiologist is particularly important if:

- This is a new presentation of heart failure.
- Echocardiography shows more than mild heart valve disease or a heavily thickened and immobile aortic valve, even with a low transvalvular gradient: the gradient in severe aortic stenosis may be low in the presence of heart failure.
- There is an LV ejection fraction <35%, as cardiac resynchronization therapy (CRT) or an implantable cardioverter-defibrillator (ICD) may be indicated.

Table 48.2 Urgent investigation of the patient with acute heart failure or decompensated chronic heart failure.

ECG

Look for:

- Abnormal rhythm
- QRS duration (relevant to consideration of cardiac resynchronization therapy (biventricular pacing))
- Evidence of LV hypertrophy (aortic valve disease? hypertrophic cardiomyopathy?)
- Pathological Q waves indicative of previous myocardial infarction
- Low QRS voltage (pericardial effusion? cardiac amyloidosis?)

Chest X-ray

Look for:

- Evidence of raised LA pressure
- Pleural effusion (may contribute to breathlessness)
- Pulmonary consolidation

Arterial blood gases, pH and lactate

Echocardiogram

Assess:

- LV size, geometry, regional and global systolic function, ejection fraction and diastolic function
- RV size and systolic function
- Estimated right atrial pressure (from inferior vena caval size and respiratory variation)
- Estimated pulmonary artery pressures
- Valve disease (present in 29% in EuroHeart Failure survey)
- Pericardial effusion

Plasma brain natriuretic peptide (BNP) or N-terminal pro-BNP (NT-pro-BNP)

- For patients with suspected acute heart failure the optimal cut-points for excluding the diagnosis are:
  - BNP <100 pg/mL (29 pmol/L)
  - NT-pro-BNP <300 pg/mL (35 pmol/L)
- BNP/NT-pro-BNP may be lowered by obesity (body mass index >30) and by heart failure treatment.
- BNP/NT-pro-BNP may be raised in LV hypertrophy, COPD without RV dilatation, diabetes, age, liver cirrhosis, hypoxia of any cause, tachycardia.
- Raised plasma BNP/NT-pro-BNP with clinical features of heart failure in the presence of an apparently normal LV on echocardiography raises the possibility of diastolic heart failure, which is suggested by:
  - LV hypertrophy or left atrial dilatation
  - Diastolic dysfunction using echocardiographic indices (e.g. E' <9 cm/s, E/E' ratio >15)

Other blood tests

Sodium, potassium, urea and creatinine (including eGFR)

Albumin and liver function including INR (liver congestion)

Thyroid function

Full blood count

C-reactive protein if coexistent infection suspected

Glucose (undiagnosed diabetes common)

Plasma troponin if acute coronary syndrome possible

Correct sodium and water retention

- If new-onset heart failure or no previous diuretic therapy, give furosemide 40 mg IV bolus (or equivalent dose of another loop diuretic).
- If decompensated chronic heart failure, give furosemide IV bolus at least equivalent to the usual oral dose.
- If there is no significant diuresis in response to this initial IV bolus, consider an infusion (e.g. furosemide 250 mg over 24 h).

Table **48.3** Causes of acute heart failure.

Myocardial ischaemia infarction
- Acute coronary syndrome (due to atherosclerotic or non-atherosclerotic coronary disease (e.g. coronary artery dissection or embolism)
- Mechanical complication of myocardial infarction

Stress cardiomyopathy (Takotsubo syndrome)

Acute myocarditis

Global left ventricular hypokinesis from other causes
- Related to persistent tachyarrhythmia
- Severe hypertension
- Dilated cardiomyopathy/end-stage hypertrophic cardiomyopathy
- Septic cardiomyopathy
- Post-cardiac arrest
- Complicating multi-organ failure

Severe valve disease (see Chapter 51)
- Severe aortic/mitral stenosis
- Acute severe aortic/mitral regurgitation

- Monitor with a weight chart and check electrolyte and creatinine levels daily.
- For selected patients with diuretic-resistant fluid retention, haemofiltration may be an option: discuss with a cardiologist and nephrologist.

Vasodilator therapy
- Start or up-titrate ACE-inhibitor/angiotensin-receptor blocker (ARB) therapy if there is HF with reduced LV ejection fraction (EF <40%) and systolic BP is >90 mmHg, plasma potassium <5 mmol/L and eGFR >30 mL/min.
- If ACE-inhibitor/ARB contraindicated (e.g. bilateral renal artery stenosis, eGFR <30 mL/min), use hydralazine (initially 25 mg 12-hourly PO) and isosorbide mononitrate (initially 10 mg 12-hourly PO).

Mineralocorticoid receptor antagonist (MRA) therapy
- Start spironolactone or eplerenone if there is reduced LV ejection fraction (EF <40%) and plasma potassium is <5 mmol/L.
- Stop MRA if plasma potassium is >5.5 mmol/L or eGFR <30 mL/min.

Heart rate and rhythm control
- If in atrial fibrillation, control the ventricular rate with a beta blocker initially, adding digoxin if heart rate remains >100/min. See Chapter 43.
- If in sinus rhythm, start or up-titrate beta-blocker therapy (bisoprolol or carvedilol) unless there is bradycardia or AV block, or systolic BP is <90 mmHg.
- Consider ivabradine for patients in sinus rhythm with contraindications to beta blockade.

Thromboprophylaxis against systemic and venous thromboembolism
- Treatment-dose, low-molecular-weight heparin or oral anticoagulation if paroxysmal, persistent or permanent atrial fibrillation/flutter, or LV thrombus on echocardiography. See Chapter 103.
- Prophylactic-dose low-molecular-weight heparin for other patients.

Table 48.4 Management of oral therapy for acute heart failure in the first 48 h.

	Hypotension			Low heart rate		Potassium		Renal impairment	
	Normotension/ Hypertension	85–100 mmHg	<85 mmHg	<60 ≥50/min	<50/min	≤3.5 mg/dl	>5.5 mg/dl	Cr <2.5, eGFR >30	Cr >2.5, eGFR <30
ACE-I/ARB	Review/Increase	Reduce/Stop	Stop	No change	No change	Review/Increase	Stop	Review	Stop
Beta blocker	No change	Reduce/Stop	Stop	Reduce	Stop	No change	No change	No change	No change
MRA	No change	No change	Stop	No change	No change	Review/Increase	Stop	Reduce	Stop
Diuretics	Increase	Reduce	Stop	No change	No change	Review/ No change	Review/Increase	No change	Review
Other vasodilarors (nitrates)	Increase	Reduce/Stop	Stop	No change	No change	No change	No change	No change	No change
Other heart rate slowing drugs (amiodarone, CCB, Ivabradine)	Review	Reduce/Stop	Stop	Reduce/Stop	Stop	Review/Stop (*)	No change	No change	No change

Legends: CCB, calcium channel blockers; Cr, creatinine blood level (mg/dl); eGFR, estimated glomerular filtration rate mL/min/1.73 m², MRA, mineralocorticoid receptor antagonist; (*) amiodarone.

Source: Mebazaa A, Yilmaz MB, Levy P, et al. (2015) Recommendations on pre-hospital and early hospital management of acute heart failure: a consensus paper from the Heart Failure Association of the European Society of Cardiology, the European Society of Emergency Medicine and the Society of Academic Emergency Medicine. European Journal of Heart Failure 17, 544–558. Reproduced with permission of John Wiley & Sons.

Drugs to avoid

Avoid the following drugs which may cause harm:

- Glitazones which can exacerbate existing HF and increase the risk of new-onset HF
- Calcium channel blockers (except amlodipine and felodipine), which have a negative inotropic effect
- NSAIDs and COX-2 inhibitors, which cause sodium and water retention
- Angiotensin-receptor blocker, if already taking an ACE-inhibitor and a mineralocorticoid antagonist, because of the risk of hyperkalaemia

Problems

Heart failure with mid-range and preserved LV ejection fraction (EF ≥40%)

- Treat congestion with a diuretic.
- Maintain sinus rhythm. If persistent/permanent atrial fibrillation, aim for a resting heart rate <100/min.
- Treat systolic hypertension, aiming for systolic BP <130–140 mmHg.
- Seek advice from a cardiologist regarding further investigation for coronary artery disease.
- Avoid medications which can exacerbate heart failure (see above Drugs to avoid)

Palliative care

Judging when palliative care (Chapter 110) is appropriate may be difficult. It should be considered for patients in whom transplantation, circulatory support or other definitive treatment including heart valve surgery has been ruled out and:

- In whom palliation has already been discussed and agreed as part of a chronic care plan
- With severe recurrent and progressive heart failure despite maximally tolerated therapy
- With multi-organ failure not responding to therapy
- With a chronically poor quality of life and NYHA class 4 symptoms

Further reading

Harjola V-P, Mebazaa A, Celutkiene J, *et al*. (2016) Contemporary management of acute right ventricular failure: a statement from the Heart Failure Association and the Working Group on pulmonary circulation and right ventricular function of the European Society of Cardiology. *European Journal of Heart Failure* 18, 226–241.

Page RL, O'Bryant CL, Cheng D, *et al*. (2016) Drugs that may cause or exacerbate heart failure. A scientific statement from the American Heart Association. *Circulation* 134, e32–e69. http://dx.doi.org/10.1161/CIR.0000000000000426.

The Task Force for the diagnosis and treatment of acute and chronic heart failure of the European Society of Cardiology (ESC) (2016) 2016 ESC Guidelines for the diagnosis and treatment of acute and chronic heart failure. *European Heart Journal* 37, 2129–2200.

CHAPTER 49

Cardiogenic shock

JOHN B. CHAMBERS AND DAVID SPRIGINGS

Cardiogenic shock is defined by persistent hypotension (systolic BP <90 mmHg) with severely reduced cardiac output, reflected in cool extremities, low urine output and changes in the mental state. Often there is pulmonary oedema.

- Cardiogenic shock may be due to a range of cardiac disorders (Table 49.1). In 75% of cases, the cause is acute myocardial infarction with left ventricular failure, or, less commonly, ventricular septal rupture, papillary muscle rupture, free wall rupture or right ventricular infarction.
- The mortality of cardiogenic shock is high. In patients at particularly high risk of death because of advanced age (>80 years) or severe comorbidities, aggressive management may not be appropriate.

Priorities

See Chapter 2 for the initial assessment and management of the patient with hypotension and shock. Focused clinical assessment and investigation in suspected cardiogenic shock are summarized in Tables 49.2 and 49.3. Seek urgent advice from a cardiologist.

- Correct major arrhythmias (Chapters 39–44).
- If there is ECG evidence of ST-segment-elevation acute coronary syndrome, consider primary angioplasty if feasible (Chapter 45).
- If there is no clinical evidence of pulmonary oedema, give a fluid challenge (500 mL crystalloid over 15 min), repeated once if systolic BP remains <90 mmHg without evidence of pulmonary oedema.
- Arrange urgent echocardiography to assess left and right ventricular function and to exclude ventricular septal rupture, cardiac tamponade (Chapter 54) and acute aortic or mitral regurgitation (Chapters 51 and 52) (Table 49.4).
- Increase the inspired oxygen, aiming for an oxygen saturation of >90%/arterial PO_2 >8 kPa. If these targets are not met despite an inspired oxygen concentration of 60%, use a continuous positive airway pressure system (Chapter 113). Intubation and mechanical ventilation may be appropriate in some patients: discuss this with an intensivist and cardiologist.
- Start inotropic/vasopressor therapy (Tables 2.6 and 2.7) if systolic BP remains <90 mmHg despite correction of major arrhythmias, and fluid challenge if indicated.

    Diuretics are relatively ineffective in patients with cardiogenic shock, but can be used in case of fluid overload once the cardiac output has increased (as shown by improvement in the patient's mental state and skin perfusion): if renal function is normal, give furosemide 40 mg IV.
- Providing the systolic BP has increased to at least 100 mmHg, start a nitrate infusion, initially at low dose (e.g. isosorbide dinitrate 2 mg/h).

Acute Medicine: A Practical Guide to the Management of Medical Emergencies, Fifth Edition. Edited by David Sprigings and John B. Chambers.
© 2018 John Wiley & Sons Ltd. Published 2018 by John Wiley & Sons Ltd.

Table 49.1 Causes of cardiogenic shock and their management.

Cause	Pulmonary oedema	Management
Acute myocardial infarction (MI) (typically STE-ACS, but may occur in NSTE-ACS)	Usually present, except when due to right ventricular infarction	Reperfusion with percutaneous coronary intervention (PCI) Coronary artery bypass grafting may be considered for chronic total occlusions untreatable by PCI
Ventricular septal rupture complicating myocardial infarction	Often present	Surgical repair, sometimes with a period of stabilization using intra-aortic balloon counterpulsation and/or left ventricular assist device
Papillary muscle rupture complicating myocardial infarction	Always present	Surgical repair
Right ventricular infarction (typically occurs in association with inferior myocardial infarction)	Usually absent	Reperfusion with PCI if appropriate Optimization of heart rate and AV conduction Optimization of right atrial (central venous) pressure Inotropic-vasopressor therapy if needed
Stress (Takotsubo) cardiomyopathy	Often present	Inotropic-vasopressor therapy if needed
Acute myocarditis	Often present	Mechanical circulatory support may indicated for some patients
Other causes of left ventricular disease Related to persistent tachyarrhythmia Severe hypertension Dilated cardiomyopathy/end-stage hypertrophic cardiomyopathy Septic cardiomyopathy Post-cardiac arrest Complicating multi-organ failure	Often present	Treat underlying disease
Acute tachyarrhythmia (Chapters 40–43)	Typically present when associated with valve disorder, for example severe aortic stenosis, or severely impaired left ventricular function	Cardioversion to restore sinus rhythm or control of ventricular rate (if atrial fibrillation/flutter with rapid ventricular response)
Critical aortic or mitral stenosis (Chapter 51)	Usually present	Surgery or a transcatheter procedure including balloon valvotomy (for mitral stenosis or aortic stenosis) or a transcatheter valve implant (aortic stenosis)
Acute aortic or mitral regurgitation (Chapter 51)	Always present	Surgical valve replacement (for aortic or mitral regurgitation) or percutaneous procedure (some patients with mitral regurgitation)
Acute major pulmonary embolism (Chapter 57)	Not present	Thrombolysis
Cardiac tamponade (Chapter 54)	Not present	Pericardiocentesis

Table 49.2 Focused assessment in suspected cardiogenic shock.

History
Context: is there known cardiac disease (Table 49.1)?
Associated chest pain? (If so, consider acute coronary syndrome, pulmonary embolism or acute aortic syndrome)
Associated breathlessness?
Comorbidities?

Examination
Mental status
Skin perfusion, sweating
Heart rate and blood pressure
Jugular venous pressure (elevated in pulmonary embolism with shock, cardiac tamponade and right ventricular infarction)
Arterial pulses
Murmurs (often absent even with critical valve disease, if there is low cardiac output)
Respiratory rate
Arterial oxygen saturation
Signs of pulmonary oedema

- If the patient is not improving, consider haemodynamic monitoring using pulse contour or thermodilution techniques to allow more accurate titration of therapy. Adjust the doses of inotropic/vasopressor and nitrate therapy, aiming for normalization of tissue perfusion parameters (serum lactate, urine output, skin perfusion).

Further management

- Transfer the patient to HDU/ICU, place arterial and central venous lines and a bladder catheter.
- See Chapter 2 for general aspects of the management of the patient with shock.
- Specific management is directed at the underlying cause (Table 49.1).
- Pending definitive treatment, systemic blood pressure and organ perfusion must be maintained by inotropic/vasopressor therapy. For some patients with refractory cardiogenic shock complicating left ventricular disease, mechanical circulatory support (with intra-aortic balloon counterpulsation or left ventricular assist device) may be indicated.

Table 49.3 Urgent investigation in suspected cardiogenic shock.

ECG
Chest X-ray
Arterial blood gases, pH and lactate
Transthoracic echocardiography
Plasma troponin
Blood glucose
Electrolytes and creatinine
Liver function tests
Full blood count
C-reactive protein
Blood culture, if infective endocarditis possible (Chapter 52)

Table 49.4 Echocardiographic findings in cardiogenic shock.

Cause	IVC	LV size	LV contraction	RV size	RV contraction
LV dysfunction due to ischaemia	Normal or dilated	Large	Reduced regionally or globally	Normal	Normal (unless associated RV infarction)
Acute major pulmonary embolism	Dilated	Normal or small	Normal or increased	Large	Reduced
Cardiac tamponade	Dilated	Normal	Normal or increased	Normal	Diastolic free wall collapse
RV infarction	Dilated	Normal or large if associated LV inferior infarction	Normal or reduced if associated inferior infarction	Large	Reduced

IVC, inferior vena cava; LV, left ventricular; RV, right ventricular.

Further reading

Harjola V-P, Mebazaa A, Celutkiene J. (2016) Contemporary management of acute right ventricular failure: a statement from the Heart Failure Association and the Working Group on pulmonary circulation and right ventricular function of the European Society of Cardiology. *European Journal of Heart Failure* 18, 226–241.

Levy B, Bastien O, Bendjelid K (2015) Experts' recommendations for the management of adult patients with cardiogenic shock. *Annals of Intensive Care* 5, 17. (Open access). DOI: 10.1186/s13613-015-0052-1.

Van Herck JL, Claeys MJ, De Paep R, Van Herck PL, Vrints CJ, Jorens PG (2015) Management of cardiogenic shock complicating acute myocardial infarction. *European Heart Journal: Acute Cardiovascular Care* 4, 278–297.

CHAPTER 50

Aortic dissection and other acute aortic syndromes

JOHN B. CHAMBERS

Consider acute aortic syndrome in any patient with chest, back or upper abdominal pain of abrupt onset. Aortic dissection is the most common acute aortic syndrome and is classified as proximal (Type A; involving the ascending thoracic aorta) or distal (Type B; only involving the descending thoracic aorta) (Figure 50.1). The risk of death is very high in the first few hours, so immediate discussion with an aortic surgical centre is vital. Management of suspected aortic dissection is summarized in Figure 50.2.

Priorities

- Put in an IV cannula and relieve pain with morphine 5–10 mg IV (2.5–5 mg in the small or elderly) with further doses every 15 min as required. Obtain an ECG to exclude acute myocardial infarction as an alternative cause for the pain. Very rarely, aortic dissection can involve the right coronary artery, causing inferior infarction (p. 326).
- Complete your clinical assessment (Table 50.1). Urgent investigations are given in Table 50.2.
    Review the chest X-ray. Abnormalities which may be seen are shown in Table 50.3.
    - A PA film alone is normal in around 50% of cases.
    - AP (anteroposterior) films commonly show apparent widening of the mediastinum in normal subjects and this feature in isolation should not be given undue weight.

If immediately available, transthoracic echocardiography (Table 50.3) should be done, looking for: a diagnostic intimal flap (seen in 80% of proximal and 50% of distal dissections); suggestive signs (dilatation of the ascending aorta, aortic regurgitation not associated with thickening of the aortic valve, pericardial fluid (which is an ominous sign signifying retrograde extension into the pericardial space); evidence of high-risk (impaired LV or RV function).

The working diagnosis is aortic dissection if (Table 50.4):
- The pain was severe and of instantaneous onset and
- There is a high-risk condition or high-risk abnormality on examination (Table 50.2) or
- There is an abnormal echocardiogram or characteristic abnormality on chest X-ray (Table 50.3)

Acute Medicine: A Practical Guide to the Management of Medical Emergencies, Fifth Edition. Edited by David Springings and John B. Chambers.
© 2018 John Wiley & Sons Ltd. Published 2018 by John Wiley & Sons Ltd.

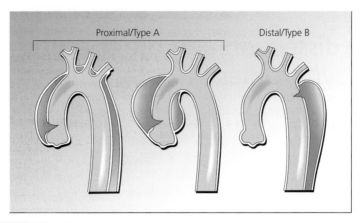

Figure 50.1 Classification of aortic dissection.

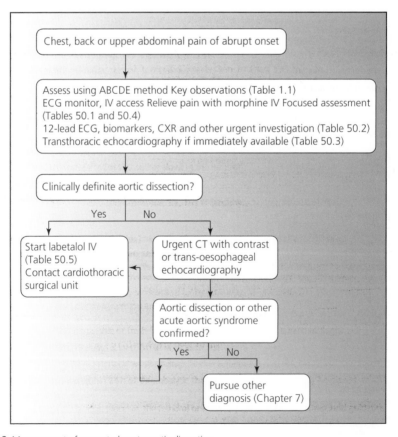

Figure 50.2 Management of suspected acute aortic dissection.

Table 50.1 Clinical assessment in suspected dissection.

History

Was the pain instantaneous in onset (like a hammer-blow or a light turning on)?

Did the pain radiate along the course of the aorta or its major branches?

Were there associated neurological symptoms (e.g. transient blurring of vision) (in 15–40% cases)?

Was there syncope (in 15% dissections)?

Is the patient at increased risk of dissection because of:

- A congenital predisposition (Marfan, Ehlers-Danlos, Turner or Loeys-Dietz syndromes or to a lesser degree a bicuspid aortic valve)
- Pregnancy
- Dilated aorta
- Family history of dissection or sudden premature death?
- Recent cardiac surgery or cardiac catheterization?

Has there been cocaine use?

Examination

Blood pressure in both arms (the normal difference in systolic pressure is <20 mmHg).

Elevation of the JVP and arterial paradox as signs of tamponade.

Presence and symmetry of the peripheral pulses.

Early diastolic murmur of aortic regurgitation (due to distortion or dilatation of the aortic root).

Limb power and tendon reflexes.

Evidence of Marfan syndrome or other collagen abnormality.

Further management

1 Working diagnosis of aortic dissection

- Make sure adequate analgesia has been given.
- Start hypotensive treatment (Table 50.5).
  - Put in a bladder catheter to monitor urine output.
  - Aim to reduce systolic blood pressure to 100–120 mmHg, providing the urine output remains >30 mL/h.
- Discuss further management with a cardiothoracic surgeon at your regional aortic centre.
- Patients with clinically definite or a high suspicion of dissection should be transferred immediately for further investigation, unless they would not be candidates for surgery, for example because of advanced age or severe comorbidity.
  - Proximal dissections require urgent repair.
  - The early death rate is very high and time should not be lost arranging investigation locally.
  - Distal dissections will usually be managed medically unless there are complications.

Table 50.2 Urgent investigation in suspected aortic dissection.

ECG

Chest X-ray

Transthoracic echocardiography

Full blood count

Plasma D-dimer level

Plasma troponin

Blood glucose

Sodium, potassium and creatinine

Table 50.3 Chest X-ray and echocardiographic findings in aortic dissection.

Chest X-ray

Widened mediastinum (caused by mediastinal haematoma)

Widened or double lumen to aortic knuckle

Irregular aortic contour

Discrepancy in diameter of ascending and descending thoracic aorta (lateral film)

Displacement of calcified intima

Small left pleural effusion (15–20% Type A or B dissections) resulting from inflammation

Large left pleural effusion as a sign of rupture

Transthoracic echocardiography

Dissection flap

Dilated aorta

Aortic regurgitation

Pericardial effusion

Transoesophageal echocardiography

As for transthoracic echocardiography but better definition of dissection flap with imaging of true and false lumen and entry tears

Intramural haematoma:

- Aortic wall >5 mm thick.
- Echolucencies caused by blood in the aortic wall.
- Fascial planes in the aortic wall which 'shear' during systole.

Penetrating ulcer:

- Usually descending thoracic aorta
- Crater-like outpouching through intima
- Extensive atheroma

2 Aortic dissection is likely clinically but there is no dissection flap on transthoracic echocardiography

- Other causes of an acute aortic syndrome are:
  - Intramural haematoma (15–25% acute aortic syndromes)
  - Penetrating ulcer (occur in 2–7% acute aortic syndromes)
  - Aortic pseudoaneurysm
  - Free or contained rupture
- Pseudoaneurysms and free or contained rupture should be suspected after deceleration injuries or cardiac catheterization or cardiac surgery

Table 50.4 Clinical scoring in suspected acute aortic syndrome.

Aortic dissection is likely if there are ≥2 of:

- Instantanous onset chest or back pain
- One high-risk condition from:
  - A congenital predisposition (Marfan, Ehlers-Danlos, Turner's or Loeys-Dietz syndromes)
  - Pregnancy
  - Aortic valve disease or
  - Dilated aorta or
  - Recent cardiac surgery or cardiac catheterization
  - Family history of dissection or sudden premature death
- One high-risk sign from:
  - Asymmetric major pulses or blood pressure
  - Focal neurological deficit
  - Hypotension

Table 50.5 Hypotensive therapy for acute aortic dissection.

The patient should be managed in a high dependency or intensive care unit.
- Make sure adequate analgesia has been given, as pain will contribute to hypertension.
- Consider placement of an arterial cannula to allow continuous BP monitoring. Put in a bladder catheter to monitor urine output.
- Start labetalol IV. Give a bolus of 20 mg over 2 min, followed by an infusion of 1–6 mg/min, increasing the infusion rate every 10 min as needed to achieve target systolic BP.
- Target systolic BP is 100–120 mmHg within 20–30 min, providing urine output remains >30 mL/h, and there is no other clinical evidence of organ ischaemia.
- If target BP is not achieved with labetalol 6 mg/min, add a nitrate infusion, for example isosorbide dinitrate 2–12 mg/h.
- Start or increase oral anti-hypertensive therapy.

- The differential diagnosis is made with a CT scan or TOE. A scan without contrast shows an intramural haematoma and with contrast shows a dissection flap or leakage into a pseudoaneurysm or rupture. The CT must be ECG gated and must have sufficiently frequent cuts. A CT pulmonary angiogram may not detect an abnormal aorta.
- The treatment for all acute aortic syndromes is surgery, except for intramural haematoma of the descending thoracic aorta which is initially treated medically.

3 The diagnosis is clinically uncertain
- If the clinical suspicion is low, a normal plasma D-dimer level (within 24 h of onset of symptoms) is a good rule-out for aortic dissection as well as pulmonary embolism. It may rarely be normal with intramural haematoma or localized dissections.
- Very high D-dimer level favours dissection over pulmonary embolism.
- If the chest X-ray is normal and expert emergency transthoracic echocardiography is not available, and if an acute aortic syndrome remains a clinical possibility with no alternative cause for pain (e.g. pleurisy, vertebral crush fracture), further investigation is needed: either CT or transoesophageal echocardiography as available.
- Pitfalls of CT to be aware of are:
  - An intimal flap can be missed if the contrast is too dense.
  - Failure to gate to the ECG may cause artefacts resembling a dissection flap.
  - CT scans with a small number of cuts (as performed for detecting pulmonary emboli) may miss a localized dissection.
  - Views without contrast may be needed to show an intramural haematoma.
- Transoesophageal echocardiography in trained hands detects aortic dissection and intramural haematoma (Table 50.3).
- If dissection remains highly likely clinically but the initial CT or TOE is normal, consider the alternative test or magnetic resonance imaging.

4 Confirmed distal aortic dissection
- If, after discussion, the decision is to manage locally, this means that the patient has a dissection unequivocally involving only the descending thoracic aorta. Emergency endovascular stent implantation for a stable Type B dissection is not routine and not definitely better than medical therapy.
- Transfer the patient to an ICU or CCU, and continue IV hypotensive therapy. Start oral therapy, which should include a beta blocker (with ACE-inhibitor/angiotensin receptor blocker added later) unless there are major contraindications.
- Maintain adequate pain relief (initially with a combination of opiate and non-steroidal anti-inflammatory drug).
- Monitor for evidence of complications (Table 50.6)

Table 50.6 Monitoring in distal (Type B) dissection.

Pain score

Blood pressure

Heart rate and rhythm (continuous ECG monitoring)

Clinical assessment for evidence of:

- Brain or spinal cord ischaemia
- Myocardial ischaemia
- Renal ischaemia (creatinine, eGFR, urine output)
- Mesenteric ischaemia (abdominal pain which is frequently non-specific, with bloody diarrhoea, rising lactate)
- Limb ischaemia (distal pulses)

- Discuss with a cardiothoracic surgeon if the dissection becomes complicated as defined by one or more of:
  - Severe pain continues or recurs.
  - Signs of rupture (large pleural effusion, increasing para-aortic or mediastinal haematoma).
  - The urine output falls. If not due to excessive hypotensive therapy or hypovolaemia, this suggests involvement of the renal arteries and is an ominous sign.
  - There is evidence of other branch artery involvement (e.g. abdominal pain with bloody diarrhoea due to ischaemic colitis).
  - Refractory hypertension.
  - Early aortic expansion.
- The preferred treatment of a complicated Type B dissection is with an endovascular stent, which has better outcomes than surgery (30-day mortality 8%, stroke 8% and spinal cord ischaemia 2%).

Problems

The patient is hypotensive

- Check for clinical evidence of a large left pleural effusion (as a sign of constrained rupture).
- Review the CT scan for evidence of a contained rupture or extensive mediastinal or abdominal haematoma.
- On the transthoracic echo cardiogram look for:
  - Pericardial tamponade
  - Impaired LV function either pre-existing or secondary to acute myocardial ischaemia
  - Severe aortic regurgitation
  - Evidence of hypovolaemia (flat IVC, small RV and LV cavities)
- If hypovolaemic, give a fluid challenge.
- If evidence of contained rupture, pericardial tamponade or severe aortic regurgitation discuss immediately with a cardiac surgeon.

Clinically dissection is possible but there is inferior ST elevation on ECG

- Coronary disease is the overwhelming cause of inferior infarction. Only about 3% of dissections involve the right coronary artery and acute dissection occurs at a frequency about 1% of an ACS.
- However, if the pain was of instantaneous onset and there are other reasons for concern (e.g. Marfan syndrome, widened mediastinum), investigate further for dissection before starting reperfusion therapy.
- The troponin level is raised in 25% acute dissections and therefore will not be helpful in distinguishing between dissection and ACS.
- If a dissection flap is not definitely visible on transthoracic echocardiography arrange an urgent CT scan with contrast.
- If the diagnosis is confirmed the management is as for dissection. The coronary artery should not be treated as for an ACS.

Box 50.1 Aortic dissection – alerts

Both the chest X-ray and transthoracic echocardiogram may be normal in acute dissection.

Pulse abnormalities are found in <20% of patients with dissection and may also be caused by other conditions (e.g. arterial stenosis). Asymmetry of blood pressure <20 mmHg may be normal.

Further reading

Mussa FF, Horton JD, Moridzadeh R, Nicholson J, Trimarchi S, Eagle KA (2016) 2016 Acute aortic dissection and intramural hematoma: a systematic review. *JAMA* 316, 754–763.

The Task Force for the diagnosis and treatment of aortic diseases of the European Society of Cardiology (ESC) (2014) 2014 ESC Guidelines on the diagnosis and treatment of aortic diseases. *European Heart Journal* 35, 2873–2926. DOI: 10.1093/eurheartj/ehu281.

CHAPTER 51

Heart valve disease and prosthetic heart valves

JOHN B. CHAMBERS

Significant valve disease occurs in 13% of people aged over 75. The main aetiologies in industrialized countries are calcific aortic stenosis and functional mitral regurgitation. The population prevalence of mitral prolapse is 2% and of bicuspid aortic valve about 1%.

Heart valve disease may present:

- With infective endocarditis (see Chapter 52)
- With arrhythmia, hypotension or pulmonary oedema
- Coincidentally, when it increases the mortality in other acute illnesses including acute coronary syndrome or stroke or after road traffic collisions
- Coincidentally, when detected peri-operatively (e.g. after hip fracture)

Priorities

- Immediate echocardiography (Table 51.1) is indicated for unexplained hypotension or pulmonary oedema. A murmur may be inaudible in the presence of low flow even with severe valve disease.
- If there is a coincidental murmur in a patient presenting with a clear non-valve problem, echocardiography is indicated with an urgency depending on the clinical circumstance. Echocardiography should be performed before non-cardiac surgery unless this is an emergency.
- Refer for immediate advice from a cardiologist if there is:
  - Severe valve disease or
  - Apparently moderate valve disease with prior exertional symptoms or current hypotension, pulmonary oedema or LV impairment on the echocardiogram
- Consider the causes of acute valve disease or deterioration in previously stable valve disease (Table 51.2).

Table 51.1 Echocardiography in valve disease: key information.

- Valve(s) affected and grade of stenosis or regurgitation
- Left ventricular size and function
- If there is acute severe aortic regurgitation, evidence of raised left ventricular end-diastolic pressure (early closure of the mitral valve and E deceleration time <150 ms)
- Evidence for aetiology, for example infective endocarditis (Chapter 52), ruptured cord
- Pulmonary artery pressure and right ventricular function
- Ascending aortic diameter and evidence of abscess or dissection

---

Acute Medicine: A Practical Guide to the Management of Medical Emergencies, Fifth Edition. Edited by David Sprigings and John B. Chambers.
© 2018 John Wiley & Sons Ltd. Published 2018 by John Wiley & Sons Ltd.

Table 51.2 Causes of acute presentation in valve disease.

Acute regurgitation
- Endocarditis
- Deceleration injury
- Ruptured mitral chord (with mitral prolapse)
- Papillary muscle rupture (acute mitral regurgitation)
- Aortic dissection (acute aortic regurgitation)

Acute decompensation of previously stable native or prosthetic valve disease

Valve-related
- Endocarditis
- Progression of native disease
- Prosthetic valve dysfunction
  - Dehiscence
  - Thrombosis
  - Structural degeneration (i.e. valve failure)

Non-valvar
- Decompensation of long-standing LV dysfunction
- Acute myocardial infarction or myocardial ischaemia
- Arrhythmia
- Fluid-load
  - Poor compliance with diuretic therapy
  - Drugs causing fluid retention (e.g. NSAIDs, steroids)
  - Iatrogenic fluid overload
- Intercurrent illness (e.g. pneumonia, anaemia)

Table 51.3 Target (and range) international normalized ratio (INR) for mechanical prostheses.

Prosthesis thrombogenicity	No patient risk factors*	>1 risk factor*
Low	2.5 (2.0–3.0)	3.0 (2.5–3.5)
Medium	3.0 (2.5–3.5)	3.5 (3.0–4.0)
High	3.5 (3.0–4.0	4.0 (3.5–4.5)

Prosthesis thrombogenicity:
Low: Carbomedics, Medtronic Hall, St Jude Medical, On-X**
Medium: other bileaflet valves
High: Lillehei-Kaster, Omniscience, Starr-Edwards, Bjork-Shiley and other tilting-disc valves

*Patient-related risk factors: mitral or tricuspid valve replacement; previous thromboembolism; atrial fibrillation; mitral stenosis of any degree; left ventricular ejection fraction <35%.
** The OnX aortic valve has recently received a licence for an INR target 1.8 and range 1.5–2.0.

Further management

This depends on the valve lesion.

Severe aortic stenosis presenting with heart failure
- Start a loop diuretic.
- If hypotensive start dobutamine (p. 13 Table 2.7).

- The only definitive treatment is valve replacement (or a transcatheter procedure).
- A low left ventricular ejection fraction may be reversible and is not a contraindication to aortic valve replacement.

Severe aortic stenosis noted incidentally

- Symptomatic severe aortic stenosis is a contraindication to all but life-saving non-cardiac surgery.
- Asymptomatic severe aortic stenosis requires a cardiology opinion but usually the original management plan can proceed if the non-cardiac surgery is low or moderate risk. The following precautions are necessary:
  - Invasive monitoring and HDU nursing.
  - Avoid epidural anaesthetics (which may cause vasodilatation).
  - Avoid vasodilators, for example angiotensin-converting enzyme inhibitors, which should only be used under specialist guidance.
  - Avoid drugs with negative inotropic effect.
  - Moderate aortic stenosis may also cause symptoms and be associated with sudden death and should prompt cardiac referral.

Severe aortic regurgitation presenting with heart failure

- Consider infective endocarditis.
- Request an urgent cardiac opinion. This must be immediate if there are echocardiographic signs of a high LV end-diastolic pressure since these patients can deteriorate rapidly.
- Critical aortic regurgitation can lead to vasoconstriction with normalization of the diastolic pressure (usually <70 mmHg and often 30 or 40 mmHg in severe regurgitation).
- Give a loop diuretic.
- If systolic BP <100 mmHg start dobutamine.
- If oxygen saturation <92% despite 60% oxygen and patient tiring, discuss mechanical ventilation.
- Discuss urgent specialist investigation and surgery with a cardiologist.

Severe aortic regurgitation noted incidentally

- Refer for a cardiology opinion especially if there are indications for surgery:
  - Exertional breathlessness
  - LV systolic diameter >50 mm or diastolic diameter >70 mm
  - Significant aortic root dilatation
- Patients with compensated LV function usually tolerate non-cardiac surgery well.

Mitral stenosis presenting with pulmonary oedema

- Give a loop diuretic.
- Left atrial pressure is highly dependent on heart rate. Treat atrial fibrillation with digoxin and if the ventricular rate is >100/min, add verapamil or a beta blocker. If there is sinus tachycardia give a beta blocker, for example metoprolol 25 mg 12-hourly PO.
- Avoid mechanical ventilation unless essential because of the risks of circulatory collapse. Maintain peripheral vascular resistance with noradrenaline.
- Discuss mitral valve replacement or balloon valvotomy with a cardiologist.

Mitral stenosis noted incidentally

- Indications for surgery are:
  - Symptoms
  - High pulmonary artery pressure
  - RV dysfunction

- Patients with severe mitral stenosis tolerate non-cardiac surgery and pregnancy badly even if asymptomatic. Refer for a cardiac opinion for considering urgent balloon valvotomy.

Mitral regurgitation presenting with heart failure

- Start a loop diuretic.
- Start dobutamine if systolic BP <100 mmHg, or noradrenaline if systolic BP <90 mmHg.
- Discuss with a cardiologist the insertion of a balloon pump preparatory to surgery.

Mitral regurgitation noted incidentally

- Refer for a cardiology opinion especially if there are indications for surgery:
  - Exertional breathlessness
  - LV systolic diameter >40 mm (in repairable mitral prolapse)
- Patients with LV compensation usually tolerate non-cardiac surgery well.

Prosthetic heart valve presenting with heart failure

Because of the difficulty of assessing prosthetic failure a cardiac referral should be made even if there is severe LV dysfunction sufficient to cause the presentation.

- Obstruction is recognized by reduced or absent opening of the cusps or mechanical leaflet associated with a high-pressure drop across the valve on echocardiography.
- Regurgitation is obvious if there is a large regurgitant colour jet but may be suspected if there is rocking of the prosthesis or the combination of highly active left ventricle and low cardiac output.

Prosthetic valve as a coincidental observation

The main concern is management of anticoagulation. Avoid giving vitamin K antagonists unless emergency correction is essential.

INR high and no active bleeding (see Chapter 103)

- If INR >5 omit 1-2 doses checking the INR daily and restart at a lower dose.
- If INR >8 give vitamin K 1-5mg orally.

Active bleeding (see Chapter 103)

If there is active bleeding which cannot be controlled by direct pressure (e.g. intracerebral or gastrointestinal):

- Give vitamin K IV (not intramuscularly) in 1 mg aliquots.
- Consider IV prothrombin complex, or if not available then fresh frozen plasma.

If INR low or a surgical procedure is planned (see Chapter 103)

IV heparin gives better control of anticoagulation than s/c:

- If INR is below 2.0 start IV heparin.
- If elective surgery is planned, stop warfarin and start IV heparin when the INR falls below 2.0.

Other complications associated with prosthetic heart valves

Thromboembolism

- The risk of thromboembolism is most closely related to non-prosthetic factors, for example atrial fibrillation, large left atrium, impaired left ventricle.
- Check that there are no signs of prosthetic dysfunction (breathlessness, abnormal murmur, muffled closure sound) or signs of infective endocarditis (Chapter 52).

- Look at the anticoagulation record and check INR, full blood count, C-reactive protein and blood culture (three sets) if white cell count or C-reactive protein raised.
- If INR <2 for a mechanical valve and there is no evidence of endocarditis discuss an increase in warfarin dose with a haematologist. Target INR according to ESC guidelines, (Table 51.3). Arrange an early appointment with the anticoagulation clinic.
- Investigate also for other potential causes. Arrange carotid USS.
- If thromboembolism persists discuss with a cardiologist and consider transoesophageal echocardiography looking for thrombus or pannus formation (endothelial overgrowth which can be a nidus for thrombus formation).

Fever

- Always consider infective endocarditis but do not forget non-cardiac causes.
- Send three sets of blood cultures before starting antibiotic therapy. *Staphylococcus aureus*, and coagulase negative staphylococci are the most common organisms in the first year after surgery and after this, as for native endocarditis, Staphylococcus aureus (including MRSA), Viridans group streptococci (e.g. S. mutans), Streptococcus bovis group, and Enterococci.
- The sensitivity of transthoracic echo for vegetations is much lower than for native valves, and TOE is often necessary to confirm the diagnosis, especially in mechanical valves.
- Surgery is more likely to be necessary in prosthetic than native valve endocarditis

Anaemia

- Investigate as for any anaemia, not forgetting the possibility of infective endocarditis.
- Virtually all mechanical valves produce minor haemolysis (disrupted cells on the film, high LDH and bilirubin, low haptoglobin) caused by normal transprosthetic regurgitation. Usually the haemoglobin remains normal.
- Haemolytic anaemia suggests leakage usually around the valve (paraprosthetic regurgitation), which is often small and only detectable on transoesophageal echocardiography.
- Refer for advice from a cardiologist and haematologist.

Box 51.1 Heart valve disease – alerts.

In severe aortic stenosis with a low cardiac output, the transvalve gradient will fall and the aortic stenosis may be erroneously graded as moderate.

If mitral regurgitation reported as 'mild' or 'moderate' is associated with a hyperdynamic left ventricle in a patient with shock, the likely diagnosis is critical regurgitation. An inexperienced operator can miss severe regurgitation since the jet area may be small as a result of the low pressure difference between left ventricle and left atrium.

In severe valve disease, a murmur may not be obvious if the cardiac output is low and/or breath-sounds loud.

Severe aortic stenosis is frequently associated with systemic hypertension rather than a low pressure and narrow pulse pressure.

Further reading

Nishimura RA, Otto CM, Bonow RO, et al. (2014) AHA/ACC Guideline for the management of patients with valvular heart disease. *J Am Coll Cardiol* 63, e57–e185. DOI: 10.1016/j.jacc.2014.02.536.

The Joint Task Force on the Management of Valvular Heart Disease of the European Society of Cardiology (ESC) and the European Association for Cardio-Thoracic Surgery (EACTS) (2012) Guidelines on the management of valvular heart disease (version 2012). *European Heart Journal* 33, 2451–2496. DOI: 10.1093/eurheartj/ehs109.

CHAPTER 52

Infective endocarditis

John B. Chambers and John L. Klein

Infective endocarditis is uncommon but not rare, and is still under-recognized. It has an average hospital mortality of 20%. Mortality is reduced by early detection, prompt initiation of appropriate antibiotics and timely surgery when indicated. About 40% of patients require surgery as an inpatient and a further 10% in the first two years after discharge.

Patients with prosthetic valves have a 0.3–1.2% incidence per year. Previous infective endocarditis and corrected congenital heart disease also increase susceptibility (Table 52.1). IV drug use greatly increases the risk of left as well as right-sided endocarditis.

Infection of the intra-cardiac leads of implanted cardiac devices (Chapter 58) causes a similar presentation as infection of heart valves. Removal of an infected device is almost always required to achieve cure of infection.

Priorities

1 Think of the diagnosis

Consider if there is fever or raised inflammatory markers and any of:

- High or moderate risk cardiac structural disease (Table 52.1) especially prosthetic heart valve
- Previous episodes of infective endocarditis
- Stroke in a young patient
- Arterial embolism
- IV drug use ('pneumonia' can be caused by septic pulmonary emboli from tricuspid valve endocarditis)
- Tunnelled central venous catheter, including Hickman line or haemodialysis catheter
- Multisystem illness
- Chronic malaise, sweating and weight loss, often for several weeks
- Acute aortic or mitral regurgitation (may present with acute pulmonary oedema)

Box 52.1 Infective endocarditis – alerts

Do not start antibiotics before taking blood cultures.

Care in infective endocarditis should be shared between a cardiologist and an infection specialist.

Seek early advice from a cardiac surgeon if there is severe valve regurgitation, suspected endocarditis of a prosthetic heart valve or fungal endocarditis.

Surgery is usually needed if sepsis is still present after 1–2 weeks of antibiotic therapy.

Acute Medicine: A Practical Guide to the Management of Medical Emergencies, Fifth Edition. Edited by David Sprigings and John B. Chambers.
© 2018 John Wiley & Sons Ltd. Published 2018 by John Wiley & Sons Ltd.

Table 52.1 Conditions predisposing to infective endocarditis.

High risk
Prosthetic heart valve or repair
Previous episode of infective endocarditis
Congenital disease corrected with a valved shunt
Moderate risk
Acquired valve disease
Mitral prolapse
Bicuspid aortic valve
Uncorrected congenital heart disease other than atrial septal defect
Hypertrophic cardiomyopathy
Predisposing conditions
Immunosuppression
Indwelling lines, for example haemodialysis
Intravenous drug use

2 **Send blood cultures**
- If you suspect endocarditis it is essential to send blood cultures before starting antibiotic therapy since prior antibiotic therapy is the most common cause of blood culture-negative endocarditis.
- If the patient is stable, send three cultures taken at 2–4 h intervals.
- If the patient is unstable because of sepsis or severe valve regurgitation take two cultures 30–60 min apart and then start antibiotics.
- Infective endocarditis is often first suspected when a typical organism is grown from the first blood culture (Table 52.2).

3 The clinical assessment is given in Table 52.3 and urgent investigation in Tables 52.4 and 52.5. The diagnosis is aided by the modified Duke criteria (Table 52.6).

4 Emergency surgery may be indicated for heart failure caused by acute mitral or aortic regurgitation, and within 48 h if there are severe valve lesions associated with a stroke or with large residual vegetations. Seek an immediate cardiac opinion.

Table 52.2 Organisms and infective endocarditis.

Organisms characteristically causing infective endocarditis
- Viridans group streptococci are the most common cause in non-IVDU without intracardiac prosthetic material.
- *Streptococcus bovis* group (up to 40% are associated with colorectal tumours, including carcinoma), *Staphylococcus aureus* (the chance of having infective endocarditis is 30% with community-acquired infection and 10% in hospital-acquired infection) or after implantation of a pacemaker or prosthetic valve.
- Coagulase-negative staphylococci are the commonest cause of contaminated blood cultures, but are common causes of endocarditis in patients with prosthetic valves or pacemakers.
- *Enterococcus faecalis* – common in older age groups.

Organisms that rarely cause infective endocarditis
The list is potentially almost endless, but common organisms cultured from blood triggering inappropriate requests for echocardiography are:
Pseudomonas aeruginosa (usually associated with I.V. line infections or pneumonia)
E. coli and other colifoms (usually associated with urinary, biliary or intra-abdominal infections)
Streptococcus milleri group (commonly associated with hepatic and other abdominal abscesses)

Table 52.3 Focused assessment in suspected infective endocarditis.

History
- Major symptoms and time course
- Symptoms of systemic embolism (transient ischaemic attack, stroke, abdominal pain, limb ischaemia) or pulmonary embolism (with right-sided valve endocarditis, typically seen with IV drug use)
- Previous endocarditis or other known high-risk cardiac lesion (Table 52.1)
- Antibiotic history (prior antibiotic therapy may render blood cultures negative)
- Dental history (Regular dental surveillance? Dental extraction within 2–6 weeks)
- IV drug use?

Examination
- Physiological observations and systematic examination
- Careful examination of the skin, nails, conjunctival and oral mucosae and fundi, looking for stigmata of infective endocarditis (petechiae and splinter haemorrhages). Janeway lesions, Osler nodes and Roth spots are rare.
- Search for alternative source of sepsis, for example inflamed venous cannula site, cellulitis, groin infection in IV drug-use.
- Splenomegaly.

Table 52.4 Urgent investigation in suspected infective endocarditis.

- Blood culture (3 sets drawn 2–4 h apart) (unless critically ill in which case take two sets 30–60 min apart)
- Full blood count
- C-reactive protein
- Blood glucose
- Sodium, potassium, creatinine, liver function tests
- Urine stick test, microscopy and culture
- ECG (looking for lengthening of the PR interval as a sign of possible aortic root abscess)
- Chest radiograph
- Consider echocardiography (see Table 52.5)

Table 52.5 Indications for transthoracic echocardiography in suspected infective endocarditis.

Urgent
- Hypotension or pulmonary oedema
- Clinically severe aortic or mitral regurgitation (rapid deterioration may occur)
- Suspicion of an abscess (ill patient, long PR interval, *S. aureus* bacteraemia)

As soon as possible
- Positive blood culture with organism typically associated with endocarditis, for example viridans group streptococci, *Streptococcus bovis* group, community-acquired *S. aureus* or enterococci
- IV drug use
- Prosthetic heart valve
- Central venous catheter-related blood-steam infection persisting for >72 h after antimicrobial therapy
- New regurgitant murmur (endocarditis rarely causes new obstruction)

Not indicated
Low clinical suspicion of endocarditis (e.g. fever with ejection systolic flow murmur) (see Table 52.6)

Table 52.6 Modified Duke criteria for the diagnosis of infective endocarditis.

Type of criterion	Description of criterion
Major	**1** Typical microorganisms from two sets of blood cultures: • Viridans group streptococci, *S. bovis* group, HACEK group or *S. aureus*, or • Community-acquired enterococci with no primary focus, or • Persistently positive with microorganisms consistent with IE (>2 taken more than 12 h apart, or all of three positives or a majority of >4 drawn over a period of 1 h), or • Single positive blood culture for *Coxiella burnetii* or phase I IgG antibody titre>1:800 **2** Imaging positive*: • Vegetations • Local complication (abscess, fistula, pseudoaneurysm) • New prosthetic valve dehiscence • New valve regurgitation or valve destruction
Minor	• Known predisposition to endocarditis (including intravenous drug use) • Temperature >38 °C • Vascular phenomena (e.g. arterial embolus, intracranial haemorrhage) • Immunological features (e.g. glomerulonephritis, Osler's nodes, positive rheumatoid factor) • Positive blood culture but insufficient for major criteria or serological evidence of active infection with an organism consistent with IE

Definite IE: Two major criteria, *or* one major and three minor criteria *or* five minor criteria.
Possible IE: Illness consistent with IE that falls short of *Definite* but is not *Rejected.*
IE rejected: Firm alternative diagnosis; resolution with ≤4 days of antibiotics; no evidence of IE at surgery/autopsy after ≤4 days of antibiotics).
* PET/CT is included in the 2015 ESC guidelines as a major criterion although little high quality data exist on its diagnostic accuracy.

Further management

1 Discuss antibiotic therapy with an infection specialist (clinical microbiologist or infectious diseases physician). Current recommendations are given in Table 52.7.
2 Discuss management with the endocarditis team at your surgical centre. Indications for early transfer are given in Table 52.8.

Table 52.7 Empirical antibiotic therapy in suspected infective endocarditis.

1 Patients with prosthetic heart valves, penicillin allergy, suspected MRSA:
• Vancomycin 1 g 12-hourly IV plus
• Gentamicin 1 mg/kg 8-hourly IV plus
• Consider adding rifampicin 450 mg 12-hourly PO in prosthetic valve infection
2 Acute presentation (ill for <1 week) in patients with native valves (including IVDUs):
• Flucloxacillin 2 g 4–6 hourly IV plus
• Gentamicin 1 mg/kg 8-hourly IV
3 Sub-acute presentation in patients with native heart valves:
• Amoxicillin 2 g 4-hourly IV plus
• Gentamicin 1 mg/kg 8-hourly IV

These are regimens for when therapy has to be started before blood culture results are available. Contact a microbiologist for advice, particularly in patients with penicillin allergy.

Table 52.8 Indications for transfer to a surgical centre.

Prosthetic valve or implantable cardiac electronic device infection
Severe regurgitation even if currently stable haemodynamically
Intracardiac abscess
Invasive organism (e.g. *S. aureus* *)
Organisms that are hard to manage medically (e.g. fungi)
Failure to respond to antibiotics
Stroke (or other embolism) and large residual vegetation
Recurrent emboli
Renal failure[†]

* Some cases of *S. aureus* IE may respond to antibiotic therapy, but IE caused by this organism should trigger discussion with a surgical centre.
[†] Renal failure in IE has many and sometimes multiple origins including glomerulonephritis, renal emboli, aminoglycoside therapy and low cardiac output. It can contribute to the decision for early surgery when associated with severe valve destruction or failure to control sepsis and should therefore trigger a discussion with a surgical centre.

3 Remove infected intravenous cannulae.
4 Consider the appropriate route for antimicrobial delivery (e.g. PICC line).
5 Monitoring is given in Table 52.9.
6 Cardiac surgery is usually needed:
- As an emergency for critical valve destruction causing haemodynamic collapse.
- Within 48h for severe valve disease in the presence of a stroke or large residual vegetation.
- At a time determined by the endocarditis team, usually at 1–2 weeks for: failure to control sepsis; severe valve destruction; emboli despite treatment with the correct antibiotic at the correct dose.
7 Correct anaemia with transfusion if haemoglobin is <80 g/L.
8 If the creatinine rises:
- Consider the possible causes: pre-renal failure; glomerulonephritis related to IE; renal infarct/abscess; vancomycin or gentamicin-nephrotoxicity; interstitial nephritis related to antibiotic; other causes, for example bladder outflow obstruction.
- Check urinalysis and urine microscopy, and arrange ultrasound of the urinary tract.
- Reduce antibiotic doses as necessary.
- Discuss management with a cardiac surgeon if renal failure is due to severe valve regurgitation, uncontrolled sepsis or glomerulonephritis.
- Seek advice from a nephrologist if you suspect glomerulonephritis or interstitial nephritis (casts in urine, large kidneys on ultrasound scan).

Table 52.9 Monitoring in infective endocarditis.

Clinical assessment daily, more frequently if there is a change
Record blood results on a flow chart if electronic systems not in use
Check creatinine and electrolytes, initially daily, then twice weekly as condition improves
Check C-reactive protein and white cell count twice weekly
Check vancomycin/gentamicin levels as directed by microbiology department
With aortic valve endocarditis, record an ECG daily while fever persists (prolongation of PR interval is a sign of abscess formation: arrange transoesophageal echocardiography)
Repeat transthoracic echocardiography if there is a change in clinical status and before discharge (to provide baseline against which to compare grade of regurgitation and size of left ventricle on outpatient studies)

9 Seek further opinions from a:
- Maxillofacial surgeon if endocarditis is due to viridans group streptococci or other oral commensal.
- Gastroenterologist if endocarditis is due to the *Streptococcus bovis* group (up to 40% are associated with colorectal tumours including carcinoma).
- Spinal surgeon if there is back pain (and order MRI of spine).

Problems

Missed infective endocarditis
Some scenarios recur:
- Possible lymphoma in a patient with a prosthetic heart valve.
- Search for source of gastro-intestinal blood or malignancy in a patient with normochromic normocytic anaemia, weight loss and fever/sweats (often subtle and easily missed).
- IV drug use with a chest infection (lung cavitations).

Blood culture-negative endocarditis
Prior antibiotic therapy is the most common cause. Other causes to consider are given in Table 52.10. Ask advice from an infection specialist about:
- Stopping antibiotics and repeating blood cultures if the diagnosis is not secure.
- Sending blood for serology (especially for *Bartonella* and *Coxiella burnetii*).

IV drug use with cavitating lung lesions but normal tricuspid valve
Consider septic thrombophlebitis of the femoral veins and arrange an ultrasound scan of the leg veins.

Should echocardiography be done in all patients with *Staphylococcus aureus* bacteraemia?
All patients with community-acquired *S. aureus* bacteraemia should have echocardiography since the risk of endocarditis is high.

The need in patients with hospital-acquired line-related bacteraemia is less certain and you should be guided by local hospital protocols. Echocardiography is unequivocally indicated if:
- There are suggestive features, for example new regurgitant murmur or splinter haemorrhages.
- The fever fails to settle in 72 h.
- Persistent bacteraemia despite intravenous line removal and antibiotic therapy.

Table 52.10 Causes of blood culture-negative endocarditis.

Prior antibiotic therapy (at least 50%)
Slow-growing organisms (some members of the HACEK* group)
Mould endocarditis (e.g. *Aspergillus* species)
Infective endocarditis due to *Coxiella burnetii* or *Bartonella* species
Thrombotic, non-infected ('marantic') endocarditis (e.g. systemic lupus erythematosus or cancer)

*HACEK is an acronym referring to the following organisms: *Haemophilus* species, *Aggregatibacter* (previously *Actino-bacillus*) species, *Cardiobacterium* hominis, *Eikenella* corrodens, and *Kingella* species. Organisms of the HACEK group are oro-pharyngeal commensals.

Further reading

Cahill TJ, Prendergast B (2016) Infective endocarditis. *Lancet* 387, 882–893.

Chambers J, Sandoe J, Ray S, *et al.* (2014) The infective endocarditis team: recommendations from an international working group. *Heart* 100, 524–527.

The Task Force for the management of infective endocarditis of the European Society of Cardiology (ESC) (2015) 2015 ESC Guidelines for the management of infective endocarditis. http://eurheartj.oxfordjournals .org/content/36/44/3075.

CHAPTER 53

Acute pericarditis

DAVID SPRIGINGS AND JOHN B. CHAMBERS

- Consider acute pericarditis in any patient with pleuritic central chest pain (pericarditis accounts for 5% of patients with acute severe chest pain).
- The typical patient is an otherwise healthy young man with a presumed viral aetiology (male:female ratio 2:1).
- Other causes are given in Table 53.1.
- There is a recurrence rate of 30% by 18 months.

Priorities

1 Review the observations and make a focused clinical assessment (Table 53.2). A pericardial friction rub is heard in less than one-third of cases so its absence does not exclude the diagnosis. If there are clinical signs of cardiac tamponade, arrange urgent echocardiography (see Chapter 54 for further management).

2 Obtain an ECG and other investigations (Table 53.3). The diagnosis of acute pericarditis is based on the clinical features supported by the ECG. The distinction between acute pericarditis, acute coronary syndrome with ST elevation and non-specific chest pain with benign early repolarization can sometimes be difficult: see Table 7.4. A pericardial effusion is common but not invariable in acute pericarditis.

3 Confirmation of the diagnosis of acute pericarditis requires **at least two** of the following **four** features:
- Pericarditic chest pain: central chest pain worse on inspiration and eased by sitting forward
- Pericardial friction rub
- New widespread ST segment elevation or PR depression on ECG
- Pericardial effusion (new or worsening)

4 Relieve pain: an NSAID is usually sufficient (Table 53.4). Severe pain may require morphine.

5 Review the clinical findings and investigation results. Decide on the likely aetiology. Are there any high-risk features?
- Ill patient
- Fever >38°C
- Sub-acute course
- Large pericardial effusion (>20mm thickness on echocardiography)
- Clinical or echocardiographic features of cardiac tamponade (Chapter 54)
- Immunosuppression
- Evidence of myopericarditis
- Pericarditis in the setting of chest trauma
- Oral anticoagulant therapy

Further management

1 **Admit or discharge?**

Admit if there are high-risk features or a specific non-viral cause of pericarditis is suspected.

Low-risk patients with presumed viral pericarditis can be managed as outpatients.

Acute Medicine: A Practical Guide to the Management of Medical Emergencies, Fifth Edition. Edited by David Sprigings and John B. Chambers.
© 2018 John Wiley & Sons Ltd. Published 2018 by John Wiley & Sons Ltd.

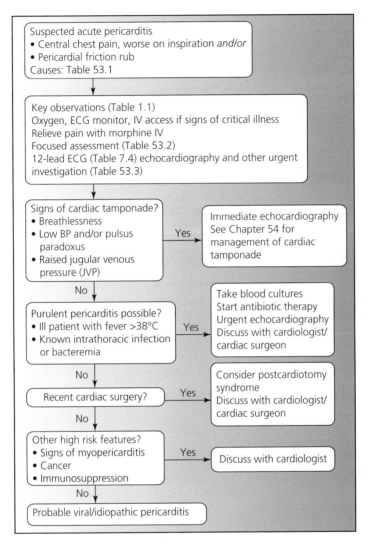

Figure 53.1 Assessment of suspected acute pericarditis.

Table 53.1 Causes of acute pericarditis.

Viruses (Enteroviruses, especially coxsackie and echoviruses; adenoviruses; Parvovirus B19;
Herpes viruses (especially EBV and CMV); HIV
Pyogenic bacteria (e.g. Streptococcus pneumoniae, S. pyogenes, S. aureus, Neisseria meningitidis)
Other bacteria: Mycoplasma pneumoniae, Coxiella burnetii (Q fever agent), Borrelia burgdorferi (Lyme disease agent)
Autoimmune (e.g. SLE, rheumatoid arthritis, scleroderma, ulcerative colitis, chronic active hepatitis)
Neoplasia (e.g. breast, lung, lymphomas)
Metabolic (uraemia)
Drug-related (e.g. dantrolene, doxorubicin, hydralazine, procainamide)
Pericardial injury including cardiothoracic surgery (Dressler's Syndrome)
As a complication of acute myocardial infarction

Table 53.2 Focused clinical assessment in suspected acute pericarditis.

History

Quality of chest pain typically worse on inspiration and in certain postures, for example lying back

Was there a viral prodrome (fever, malaise, sore throat, muscle aching)?

Are there any constitutional symptoms to suggest TB (weight loss, chronic cough)?

Past history of predisposing conditions: SLE, chronic active hepatitis, ulcerative colitis, chronic renal failure

Risk for Dressler syndrome: recent (usually 2–6 weeks; range 1 week to 3 months) cardiac surgery or chest trauma

Country of origin (consider Familial Mediterranean Fever)

Examination

Heart rate

Friction rub?

Signs of tamponade (raised JVP, hypotension, palpable pulsus paradoxus)

Signs of heart failure (basal crepitations) to suggest myocarditis

Table 53.3 Investigation in suspected acute pericarditis.

ECG (see Table 7.4)

Chest X-ray

Echocardiography (urgent if evidence of tamponade or myocarditis)

Plasma troponin

Creatinine, sodium and potassium

Full blood count

C-reactive protein

ESR if Dressler syndrome possible

Blood culture (if suspected bacterial infection)

Autoantibody screen

HIV serology

Table 53.4 Drug therapy in acute pericarditis.

Drug	Comment/Dose
NSAID	Ibuprofen 400 mg 8-hourly PO
Colchicine	Weight >70 kg 500 μgm twice daily PO
	Weight <70 kg 500 μgm once daily PO
	Prednisolone 0.2–0.5 mg/kg/day PO
Prednisolone	If NSAID contraindicated or if there is evidence of auto-immune cause

2 Are there signs of severe sepsis?

Consider purulent pericarditis. This is rare, and is usually due to spread of intrathoracic infection, for example following thoracic trauma or complicating bacterial pneumonia.

Start antibiotic therapy with advice from a microbiologist (e.g. IV vancomycin and ceftriaxone) after taking blood cultures.

Perform pericardiocentesis if there is an effusion large enough to be drained safely (thickness >20 mm), and send fluid for Gram stain and culture.

Consider tuberculous or fungal infection if the effusion is purulent but no organisms are seen on Gram stain. Discuss further management with a cardiologist or cardiothoracic surgeon.

3 Possible Dressler (postpericardiotomy) syndrome

Consider Dressler syndrome if the patient has had recent cardiac surgery (typically 2–4 weeks previously). It is an acute self-limiting illness, with fever, pericarditis and pleuritis.

Investigations show:

- ECG: typical changes of acute pericarditis or only non-specific ST/T abnormalities.
- Chest X-ray: an enlarged cardiac silhouette (due to pericardial effusion), bilateral pleural effusions and transient pulmonary infiltrates.
- ESR: this is typically around 100 mm/h.

If the pain has not settled after 48 h of treatment with NSAID, consider colchicine (Table 53.4).

4 Presumed viral ('idiopathic') acute pericarditis

This is the likely diagnosis in young and otherwise healthy adults. It may be preceded by a flu-like illness and is usually a self-limiting disorder lasting 1–3 weeks.

Give an NSAID with gastroprotection, continued for 1 week after the pain resolves. Colchicine should be co-administered, and continued for 3 months, to reduce the risk of recurrence (Table 53.4).

Patients should be advised to avoid exercise until there is no evidence of active disease (normal inflammatory markers).

5 When are corticosteroids indicated?

Prednisolone should be given in place of NSAIDs when:

- Acute pericarditis complicates autoimmune disease, provided there are no features to suggest bacterial infection
- NSAID are contraindicated in viral pericarditis

Further reading

Imazio M, Gaita F, LeWinter M (2015) Evaluation and treatment of pericarditis: a systematic review *JAMA* 314, 1498–1506.

The Task Force for the diagnosis and management of pericardial diseases of the European Society of Cardiology (ESC) (2015) 2015 ESC Guidelines for the diagnosis and management of pericardial diseases. http://www.escardio.org/static_file/Escardio/Guidelines/Publications/PERICA/2015%20Percardial%20Web%20Addenda-ehv318.pdf.

CHAPTER 54

Cardiac tamponade

JOHN B. CHAMBERS AND DAVID SPRIGINGS

Consider cardiac tamponade if there is hypotension or breathlessness and a raised jugular venous pressure. Have a high index of suspicion in the presence of predisposing conditions (Table 54.1), notably cancer, or after central venous cannulation.

Priorities

1 Give oxygen, attach an ECG monitor and place an IV cannula. Your examination should include an assessment of pulsus paradoxus (Box 10.2). Pulsus paradoxus is an exaggeration of the normal inspiratory fall in systolic blood pressure to >10 mmHg. It may be palpable in the radial artery, with the radial pulse disappearing on inspiration.
2 Obtain an ECG and chest X-ray to exclude other diagnoses, and an urgent echocardiogram (Table 54.2).
3 If a pericardial effusion with clinical and echocardiographic signs of tamponade is confirmed, contact a cardiologist urgently to discuss pericardiocentesis. The technique of pericardial aspiration is described in detail in Chapter 120. If systolic pressure is <90 mmHg and the effusion cannot be drained immediately, treat with IV fluid together with an infusion of noradrenaline (Table 2.7) via a central line.

Further management

This is directed at the underlying cause (Table 54.1).

Consider **purulent pericarditis** if the patient is unwell with signs of sepsis. Start antibiotic therapy with advice from a microbiologist (e.g. IV vancomycin and ceftriaxone) after taking blood cultures.

Patients with **malignant effusions** will usually require further intervention to prevent recurrent tamponade, for example chemotherapy or creation of a pericardial window.

If the patient has pericardial effusion with tamponade complicating **autoimmune disease**, start prednisolone 30–40 mg PO daily, with gastroprotection.

Problems

Signs of tamponade but only small pericardial effusion (echo separation <10 mm)

This can occur with effusive-constrictive pericarditis in malignancy, autoimmune disease and after viral infection. Percutaneous drainage is potentially hazardous and may not relieve the symptoms. Seek urgent advice from a cardiologist.

Acute Medicine: A Practical Guide to the Management of Medical Emergencies, Fifth Edition. Edited by David Sprigings and John B. Chambers.
© 2018 John Wiley & Sons Ltd. Published 2018 by John Wiley & Sons Ltd.

Table 54.1 Causes of cardiac tamponade.

Bleeding into the pericardial space

Penetrating and blunt chest trauma, including external cardiac compression

Bleeding from a cardiac chamber or coronary artery caused by perforation or laceration as a complication of cardiac catheterization, percutaneous coronary intervention, pacemaker insertion, pericardiocentesis or central venous cannulation

Bleeding after cardiac surgery

Cardiac rupture after myocardial infarction

Aortic dissection with retrograde extension into pericardial space

Anticoagulant therapy for atrial fibrillation or other indication in the presence of pericarditis

Thrombolytic therapy given (inappropriately) for pericarditis

Serous or sero-sanguinous pericardial effusion

Neoplastic involvement of the pericardium (most commonly in carcinoma of breast or bronchus, or lymphoma or cardiac angiosarcoma)

Pericarditis complicating connective tissue diseases (e.g. systemic lupus erythematosus, rheumatoid arthritis)

Postcardiotomy syndrome

Tuberculous and viral pericarditis

Uraemic pericarditis

Idiopathic pericarditis (tamponade is a rare complication)

Purulent pericarditis

Pyogenic bacterial infection, usually due to spread of intrathoracic infection, for example following thoracic surgery or trauma, or complicating bacterial pneumonia

Table 54.2 Echocardiography in suspected cardiac tamponade.

Is there a pericardial effusion?

Presence, size and distribution (circumferential or loculated) of pericardial fluid

Be aware that a pleural effusion or dilated right ventricle may be misdiagnosed on echocardiography as a pericardial effusion

Are there echocardiographic signs of cardiac tamponade in a spontaneously breathing subject?

Diastolic collapse of the free wall of the right ventricle

A fall in mitral inflow velocity or aortic velocity by >25% on inspiration

Engorgement of the inferior vena cava with no respiratory variation

Reduction in LV cavity size on inspiration

Is pericardiocentesis feasible and safe? Which approach is preferred? (Chapter 120)

Subcostal drainage (Chapter 120) is safest and there should usually be >20 mm fluid in the subcostal approach.

Drainage may be difficult if the fluid is dense or there are multiple loculations.

Echocardiography can be used to guide pericardiocentesis by confirming the position of the needle tip from the presence of intra-pericardial bubbles on re-injection of the initial fluid sampled, and should be repeated after drainage to assess the size of any residual effusion.

Tamponade early after cardiac surgery

Discuss management with a cardiac surgeon. It may be more appropriate to drain the effusion surgically.

Tamponade with severely impaired left ventricular function

Total pericardiocentesis may lead to further ventricular dilatation. Limit drainage to 1 L. Seek urgent advice from a cardiologist.

Further reading

Ristić AD, Imazio M, Adler Y, *et al.* (2014) Triage strategy for urgent management of cardiac tamponade: a position statement of the European Society of Cardiology Working Group on Myocardial and Pericardial Diseases. *European Heart Journal* 35, 2279–2284. DOI: 10.1093/eurheartj/ehu217.

The Task Force for the diagnosis and management of pericardial diseases of the European Society of Cardiology (ESC) (2015) 2015 ESC Guidelines for the diagnosis and management of pericardial diseases. http://www.escardio.org/static_file/Escardio/Guidelines/Publications/PERICA/2015%20Percardial%20Web%20Addenda-ehv318.pdf.

CHAPTER 55

Severe hypertension

DAVID SPRIGINGS AND JOHN B. CHAMBERS

Severe hypertension is arbitrarily defined as a systolic blood pressure of >180 mmHg, and/or a diastolic blood pressure of >120 mmHg. Acute management is determined by the clinical context and the presence and type of organ damage.

Intravenous therapy has specific indications, but is potentially dangerous, as an abrupt reduction in blood pressure may cause cerebral, myocardial and renal ischaemia.

Priorities

Establish the context and comorbidities by focused clinical assessment and investigation (Tables 55.1 and 55.2).

Management of severe hypertension in specific situations is discussed below. If IV therapy is indicated, transfer the patient to CCU, HDU or ITU for arterial blood pressure monitoring and general care.

Acute aortic dissection

- Make sure adequate analgesia has been given, as pain will contribute to hypertension.
- Put in an arterial line to allow continuous BP monitoring, and a bladder catheter to monitor urine output.
- Start labetalol IV (Table 55.3). Give a bolus of 20 mg over 2 min, followed by an infusion of 1–6 mg/min, increasing the infusion rate every 10 min as needed to achieve target systolic BP.
- Target systolic BP is 100–120 mmHg within 20–30 min, providing urine output remains >30 mL/h, and there is no other clinical evidence of organ ischaemia.
- If target BP is not achieved with labetalol 6 mg/min, add a nitrate infusion (Table 55.3).
- Start or increase oral therapy.
- See Chapter 50 for further management of aortic dissection.

Acute ischaemic stroke

- See Chapter 65 for the assessment of the patient with ischaemic stroke.
- If the patient is a candidate for thrombolysis: start antihypertensive therapy if BP is ≥185/110 mmHg.
- If the patient is not a candidate for thrombolysis, start therapy if BP is ≥220/120 mmHg.
- Give labetalol 10 mg IV bolus over 1 min, followed by an infusion of 1–8 mg/min, increasing the infusion rate every 10 min as needed to achieve target BP.
- Target BP is <185/110 mmHg. If BP is not maintained at or below this target, do not give thrombolysis.
- If target BP is not achieved with labetalol 8 mg/min, add a nicardipine infusion (Table 55.3) at 5 mg/h, and increased the infusion rate by 2.5 mg/h every 10 min to a maximum of 15 mg/h.

Acute Medicine: A Practical Guide to the Management of Medical Emergencies, Fifth Edition. Edited by David Sprigings and John B. Chambers.
© 2018 John Wiley & Sons Ltd. Published 2018 by John Wiley & Sons Ltd.

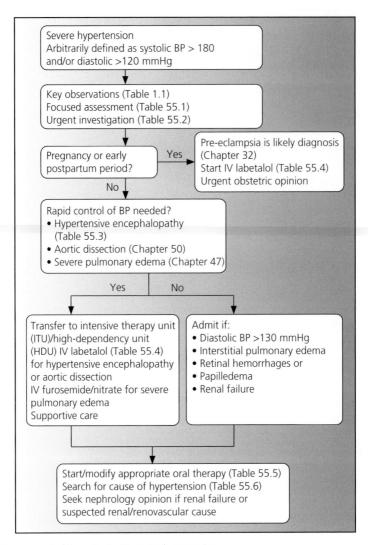

Figure 55.1 Management of the patient with severe hypertension.

- Target BP is <185/110 mmHg. If BP is not maintained at or below this target, do not give thrombolysis.
- Monitor BP every 15 min for 2 hours from the start of thrombolytic therapy, then every 30 minutes for 6 h, and then every hour for 16 h.
- Start or increase oral therapy.

Acute haemorrhagic stroke
- If the patient presents within 6 h of the onset of intracerebral haemorrhage, with systolic BP >150 mmHg, start antihypertensive therapy.
- Target systolic BP is 140 mmHg within 6 h and maintained for at least 7 days.
- Give labetalol or nicardipine by infusion (as for acute ischaemic stroke).
- Start or increase oral therapy.

Table 55.1 Focused assessment in severe hypertension.

History
- Is the patient known to have hypertension? What treatment has been given? What is the compliance with treatment? What investigations have been done to exclude an underlying cause for hypertension? Is there associated cardiac or renal disease?
- Pregnant or within three months of giving birth?
- Drug history? Recent use of drugs that may give hyperadrenergic state (e.g. cocaine, amphetamines, phencyclidine)?
- Any symptoms to suggest stroke or subarachnoid haemorrhage, aortic dissection, acute coronary syndrome, pulmonary oedema?

Examination
- Measure the blood pressure in both arms
- Check for signs of heart failure and aortic regurgitation
- Check the presence and symmetry of the major pulses, and for radio-femoral delay
- Listen for carotid, abdominal and femoral bruits
- Examine the abdomen (palpable kidneys?)
- Examine the fundi: are there retinal haemorrhages, exudates or papilloedema (not due to other causes), which define accelerated-phase or 'malignant' hypertension?
- Assess the conscious level and for focal neurological signs

Table 55.2 Urgent investigation in severe hypertension.

Blood glucose
Sodium, potassium and creatinine (check daily), low Na and K in hyperaldosteronism and renal artery stenosis
Plasma troponin, if acute coronary syndrome suspected
Full blood count
Plasma renin/aldosterone (for later analysis)
Urine stick test and microscopy (renal impairment with minimal proteinuria suggests renal artery stenosis)
Ultrasonography of kidneys and urinary tract
Urinary catecholamine excretion
Urinary free cortisol excretion if suspected Cushing syndrome (Table 55.6)
Chest X-ray
ECG
Computed tomography (CT) or magnetic resonance imaging (MRI) of the brain, if there are neurological symptoms, headache, nausea and vomiting, or retinal haemorrhages, exudates or papilloedema
Contrast enhanced CT of the chest, if aortic dissection is suspected

Table 55.3 Intravenous therapy for severe hypertension with organ damage.

Drug	Properties	Administration
Labetalol	Beta and alpha-adrenergic blocker	IV bolus: 10–20 mg over 1–2 min IV infusion: 1–8 mg/min (see text)
Esmolol	Short-acting beta-adrenergic blocker	IV bolus: 1 mg/kg over 30 s IV infusion: 150–300 µgm/kg/min (see text)
Isosorbide dinitrate	Nitric-oxide-mediated vasodilatation	IV infusion: 2–12 mg/h (see text)
Nicardipine	Dihydropyridine calcium channel blocker	IV infusion: 5–15 mg/h (see text)
Phentolamine	Short-acting, non-selective alpha-adrenergic blocker	IV bolus: 1 mg (response is maximal in 2–3 min and lasts 10–15 min) IV infusion

Subarachnoid haemorrhage
- Make sure adequate analgesia has been given.
- If systolic BP is >160 mmHg, start antihypertensive therapy.
- Target systolic BP is <160 mmHg.
- Give labetalol or nicardipine by infusion (as for acute ischaemic stroke).
- See Chapter 67 for further management of subarachnoid haemorrhage.

Hypertensive encephalopathy
- This is rare. Hypertensive encephalopathy is due to cerebral oedema resulting from hyperperfusion, as a consequence of severe hypertension, with failure of autoregulation of cerebral blood flow. Clinical features are summarized in Table 55.3.
- It may be difficult to distinguish clinically between hypertensive encephalopathy, subarachnoid haemorrhage and stroke. Hypertensive encephalopathy is favoured by the gradual onset of symptoms and the absence (or late appearance) of focal neurological signs. CT should be done to exclude other diagnoses. In hypertensive encephalopathy, neurological status improves with lowering of blood pressure.
- Target BP is 10–20% lower than initial BP after 1 h of therapy, and 25% lower after 24 h.
- Give nicardipine by infusion.
- Start or increase oral therapy.

Acute heart failure
- Treat with a nitrate infusion plus a loop diuretic IV (e.g. furosemide 20–40 mg initially).
- See Chapters 47 and 48 for further management of acute pulmonary oedema and acute heart failure.

Acute coronary syndrome
- Make sure adequate analgesia has been given.
- Treat with a nitrate infusion plus esmolol IV (Table 55.3).
- See Chapters 45 and 46 for further management of acute coronary syndromes.

Phaeochromocytoma hypertensive crisis
- See Chapter 94.
- Treat with phentolamine IV (Table 55.3). Seek expert advice from an endocrinologist.

Table 55.4 Hypertensive encephalopathy.

Early features
- Headache
- Nausea and vomiting
- Delirium
- Retinal haemorrhages, exudates or papilloedema

Late features
- Focal neurological signs
- Fits
- Coma

Suspected pre-eclampsia/eclampsia: pregnancy or within three months of giving birth

- The diagnosis of pre-eclampsia/eclampsia is discussed in Chapter 32.
- Seek urgent advice from an obstetrician.
- Target BP is 130–150/80–100 mmHg.
- Give labetalol 20 mg IV bolus over 2 min, followed by an infusion of 1–2 mg/min.
- If there is pulmonary oedema, add nitrate IV.

Cocaine-induced hypertension

- Sedation with a benzodiazepine is the preferred initial treatment for cocaine-induced hypertension.
- Target diastolic BP is 100–105 mmHg within 2–6 hours.
- Blood pressure will fall as cocaine is metabolized. If treatment in addition to benzodiazepine is needed, use phentolamine IV.

Other patients

1 **Admit for investigation and management if there are any of the following features:**
   - Retinal haemorrhages, exudates or papilloedema
   - Acute kidney injury
   - Interstitial pulmonary oedema
   - Diastolic pressure >130 mmHg

   Recheck the blood pressure after the patient has rested for 30 min in a quiet room.
2 **Start or increase oral therapy. Aim to reduce BP to ≤160/100 mmHg over the first 24 h:**
   - Initial therapy for the patient who is not already receiving anti-hypertensive therapy is given in Table 55.5.
   - Nifedipine MR should be co-administered with amlodipine for the first three days of treatment with amlodipine (as amlodipine has a large volume of distribution, and is therefore of limited efficacy during this period).
   - For patients already on treatment, check compliance, prescribe usual treatment at increased dose if appropriate, or add an agent from another class. If the patient is already taking an ACE-inhibitor or angiotensin-receptor blocker, a calcium channel blocker and a thiazide, consider adding spironolactone 25–50 mg daily.
3 **What is causing severe hypertension?**

   Causes of secondary hypertension, and clues to specific diagnoses, are summarized in Table 55.6.

Table 55.5 Initial oral therapy for severe hypertension in a patient not already receiving anti-hypertensive therapy.

Clinical setting	Drug therapy
Phaeochromocytoma suspected (see Chapter 94)	Labetalol 100–200 mg 12-hourly PO
Renal artery stenosis suspected (see Table 55.6)	Amlodipine* 5–10 mg daily PO plus Bisoprolol 2.5–5 mg daily PO
Heart failure (see Chapter 48)	Amlodipine* 5–10 mg daily PO plus Furosemide 20–40 mg daily PO
Other patients	Patients aged <55: ACE-inhibitor Patients aged ≥55, or Afro-Caribbean origin of any age: calcium-channel blocker or thiazide (if fluid retention present)

*Nifedipine MR should be co-administered with amlodipine for the first three days of treatment with amlodipine (as amlodipine has a large volume of distribution, and is therefore of limited efficacy during this period).

Table 55.6 Causes of secondary hypertension.

Cause	Clues/investigation
Intrinsic renal disease	Family history of heritable renal disease (e.g. polycystic kidney disease)
	Abnormal urine stick test and microscopy Raised creatinine
	Abnormal kidneys on ultrasound Discuss further investigation with nephrologist if intrinsic renal disease suspected
Primary hyperaldosteronism	Low plasma potassium
	High plasma aldosterone with suppressed plasma renin
Cushing syndrome	Truncal obesity, thin skin with purple abdominal striae, proximal myopathy (unable to rise from chair without using arms)
	Increased urinary free cortisol excretion
Pheochromocytoma (see Chapter 94)	Paroxysmal headache, sweating or palpitation
	Hypertensive crisis following anaesthesia or administration of contrast
	Family history of pheochromocytoma Increased urinary catecholamine excretion
Coarctation of aorta	Radiofemoral delay
	Coarctation demonstrated by echocardiography/MRI
Renal artery stenosis	May be due to fibromuscular dysplasia (age <50 with no family history of hypertension) or, more commonly, to atherosclerosis (age >50 with other atherosclerotic arterial disease)
	Refractory hypertension
	Deteriorating blood pressure control in compliant, long-standing hypertensive patients
	Rise in creatinine on treatment with ACE inhibitor
	Renal impairment with minimal proteinuria Low plasma sodium and potassium (due to secondary hyperaldosteronism)
	Difference in kidney size >1.5 cm on ultrasound
Other causes	Many causes including drugs, obstructive sleep apnoea, acromegaly

ACE, angiotensin-converting enzyme.

4 **Seek advice from a nephrologist if there is:**
- Acute kidney injury or chronic kidney disease
- Evidence of acute glomerulonephritis or vasculitis (2+ or more proteinuria and/or red cell casts in the urine)
- Suspected renal artery stenosis
- Suspected scleroderma renal crisis (see Table 25.1)

Further reading

James PA, Oparil S, Carter BL, et al. (2014) 2014 Evidence-Based Guideline for the management of high blood pressure in adults: Report from the panel members appointed to the Eighth Joint National Committee (JNC 8). *JAMA* 311, 507–520. DOI: 10.1001/jama.2013.284427.

Monnet X, Marik PE (2014) What's new with hypertensive crises? *Intensive Care Med* 41, 127–130. DOI: 10.1007/s00134-014-3546-7.

Poulter NR, Prabhakaran D, Caulfield M (2015) Hypertension. *Lancet* 386, 801–812.

CHAPTER 56

Deep vein thrombosis

Charlotte Masterton-Smith and Kevin O'Kane

Consider the diagnosis in any patient presenting with new-onset leg pain or swelling, especially if it is unilateral and if there are risk factors for venous thrombosis (Table 56.1). The assessment and management of suspected deep vein thrombosis is summarized in Figure 56.1.

Priorities

Assess the probability of deep vein thrombosis (DVT), using clinical judgement combined with the Wells score (Table 56.2).

If the clinical probability of DVT is low
Check plasma D-dimer.
- If plasma D-dimer is negative, DVT is effectively excluded. Pursue other diagnoses (Table 56.3).
- If plasma D-dimer is positive, request a duplex scan of proximal leg veins (to be performed within four hours; if this is not possible, give an interim 24-h treatment dose of low-molecular-weight heparin, pending the result of the scan).

If the clinical probability of DVT is intermediate or high
Request a duplex scan of proximal leg veins (to be performed within four hours; if this is not possible, give an interim 24-h treatment dose of low-molecular-weight heparin, pending the result of the scan).
- If the scan is positive for DVT, start anticoagulation.
- If the scan is negative for DVT, check plasma D-dimer. Pursue other diagnoses (Table 56.3). Repeat the duplex scan 6–8 days later in patients with a positive D-dimer test to confirm no DVT.

Further management

Anticoagulation
Anticoagulation is discussed in detail in Chapter 103. Anticoagulation for deep vein thrombosis can be with rivaroxaban, low-molecular-weight heparin or warfarin (preceded by and overlapping with heparin).

Acute Medicine: A Practical Guide to the Management of Medical Emergencies, Fifth Edition. Edited by David Sprigings and John B. Chambers.
© 2018 John Wiley & Sons Ltd. Published 2018 by John Wiley & Sons Ltd.

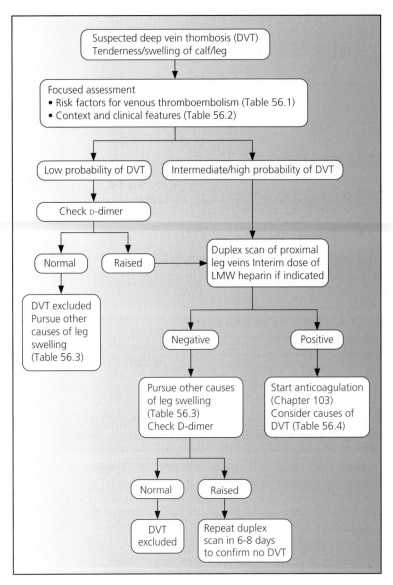

Figure 56.1 Assessment and management of suspected deep vein thrombosis.

Rivaroxaban

Start rivaroxaban 15 mg twice daily PO, unless contraindicated or if creatinine clearance is <15 mL/min. Continue rivaroxaban for 21 days then change to 20 mg daily.

Rivaroxaban is contraindicated in pregnancy, breastfeeding, renal failure, significant liver disease, concomitant use of cytochrome P-450 inhibitors, and is not currently recommended in patients with active cancer.

Low-molecular-weight heparin

Low-molecular-weight heparin (LMWH) is indicated in patients with active cancer (particularly if undergoing chemotherapy) or who are pregnant.

Table 56.1 Risk factors for venous thromboembolism.

Common

Active cancer

Prolonged immobility (long journeys, lower limb fracture)

Recent major surgery

Pregnancy or recent childbirth

Uncommon or rare

Factor V Leiden

Antithrombin III deficiency

Protein C deficiency

Protein S deficiency

Antiphospholipid syndrome

Active inflammatory bowel disease

Myeloproliferative disorders

Oestrogen-containing oral contraceptive (especially when combined with Factor V Leiden)

Nephrotic syndrome

Homocystinuria

Paroxysmal nocturnal haemoglobinuria

Hyperviscosity syndrome

Behcet's disease

Warfarin

Warfarin should be used if rivaroxaban is contraindicated and in the absence of active cancer or pregnancy.

- Warfarin loading is given in Table 103.11.
- It is initially pro-thrombotic, so is co-administered with LMWH or unfractionated heparin. During this period, check both the activated partial thromboplastin time (APTT) and International Normalized Ratio (INR) daily.
- Heparin can be stopped after five days provided the INR is >2.0.
- The target INR is usually 2.0–3.0.

Table 56.2 Estimating the clinical probability of DVT with three-level Wells score.

Clinical feature	Points
History	
Active cancer (treatment ongoing, or within previous 6 months, or palliative)	1
Paralysis, paresis or recent plaster immobilization of the leg	1
Recently bedridden for more than 3 days, or major surgery within 4 weeks	1
Examination	
Localized tenderness along the distribution of the deep venous system	1
Entire leg swollen	1
Calf swelling by >3 cm when compared with asymptomatic leg (measured 10 cm below tibial tuberosity)	1
Pitting oedema (greater in the symptomatic leg)	1
Collateral superficial veins (non-varicose)	1
Alternative diagnosis?	
An alternative diagnosis (Table 56.3) is as likely or more likely than DVT	−2
Clinical probability of DVT	
Score 3 or more: high probability	
Score 1 or 2: intermediate probability	
Score 0 or less: low probability	

Source: Wells PS *et al.* Value of assessment of pretest probability of deep-vein thrombosis in clinical management. *Lancet* 1997; 350: 1795–1798.

Reproduced with permission of Elsevier.

Table 56.3 Causes of leg swelling.

Venous/lymphatic
Deep vein thrombosis
Superficial thrombophlebitis
IVC obstruction (e.g. by a tumour)
Varicose veins with chronic venous hypertension
Post-phlebitic syndrome
Congenital lymphoedema
After vein harvesting for coronary bypass grafting
Dependent oedema (e.g. in a paralysed limb)
Severe obesity with compression of ilio-femoral veins

Musculoskeletal
Calf haematoma
Ruptured Baker's cyst
Muscle tear

Skin
Cellulitis (often presents with tenderness, erythema and induration of the skin)

Systemic (oedema is bilateral, but may be asymmetric)
Heart failure
Liver failure
Acute kidney injury/chronic kidney disease
Nephrotic syndrome
Hypoalbuminaemia
Chronic respiratory failure
Pregnancy
Idiopathic oedema of women
Dihydropyridine calcium antagonists
Drugs causing salt/water retention

Duration of anticoagulation

The duration and dosing of treatment will be monitored by the anticoagulation clinic, which should follow up all patients with a new diagnosis of DVT within a week of diagnosis.

Supportive care

For patients with extensive DVT, bed rest with elevation of the leg for 24–48 h or until swelling is resolving.

Table 56.4 Investigation after unprovoked venous thromboembolism.

Chest X-ray
Full blood count
Biochemical profile
Urinalysis
Prostate-specific antigen (PSA) (in men)
Mammography (in women)
Consider CT of chest, abdomen and pelvis in patients aged >40, to screen for cancer
Consider thrombophilia testing, guided by a haematologist

Why has the patient had a DVT?

Consider the presence of risk factors (Table 56.1). In many patients, the cause of DVT is obvious. Further tests for patients with unprovoked DVT are given in Table 56.4. Patients aged under 50 with unprovoked DVT or with a strong family history of venous thromboembolism should be screened for a thrombophilic disorder: seek advice from a haematologist.

Further reading

Di Nisio M, van Es N, Büller HR. (2016) Deep vein thrombosis and pulmonary embolism. *Lancet.*

Kearon C, Akl EA, Ornelas J, *et al*. (2016) Antithrombotic therapy for VTE disease: CHEST guideline and expert panel report. *Chest* 149, 315–352.

National Institute for Health and Care Excellence (2015) Venous thromboembolic diseases: diagnosis, management and thrombophilia testing Clinical guideline (CG144). https://www.nice.org.uk/guidance/cg144.

CHAPTER 57

Pulmonary embolism

Roshan Navin and Kevin O'Kane

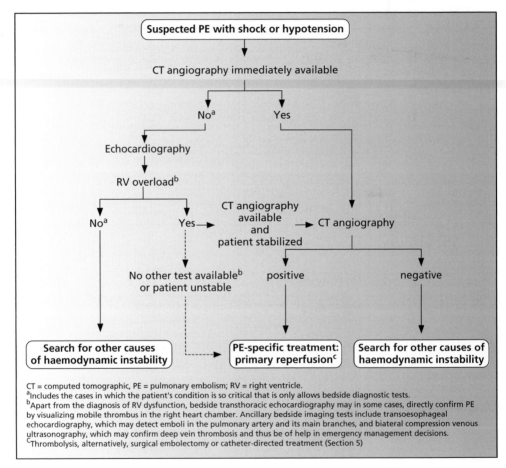

CT = computed tomographic, PE = pulmonary embolism; RV = right ventricle.
[a]Includes the cases in which the patient's condition is so critical that is only allows bedside diagnostic tests.
[b]Apart from the diagnosis of RV dysfunction, bedside transthoracic echocardiography may in some cases, directly confirm PE by visualizing mobile thrombus in the right heart chamber. Ancillary bedside imaging tests include transoesophageal echocardiography, which may detect emboli in the pulmonary artery and its main branches, and biateral compression venous ultrasonography, which may confirm deep vein thrombosis and thus be of help in emergency management decisions.
[c]Thrombolysis, alternatively, surgical embolectomy or catheter-directed treatment (Section 5)

Figure 57.1 Suspected pulmonary embolism with shock or hypotension. Source: Konstantinides SV, Torbicki A, Agnelli G et al. (2014) 2014 ESC Guidelines on the diagnosis and management of acute pulmonary. *Eur Heart J* 35, 3033–3080. Reproduced with permission of Oxford University Press.

Acute Medicine: A Practical Guide to the Management of Medical Emergencies, Fifth Edition. Edited by David Sprigings and John B. Chambers.
© 2018 John Wiley & Sons Ltd. Published 2018 by John Wiley & Sons Ltd.

Consider pulmonary embolism in any patient with:

- Shock or hypotension
- Acute breathlessness, or worsening of chronic breathlessness (e.g. in chronic obstructive pulmonary disease or heart failure)
- Pre-syncope or syncope, with risk factors for venous thromboembolism
- Chest pain (which may be non-pleuritic or pleuritic)
- Haemoptysis

One or more predisposing factors for venous thromboembolism (Table 56.1) are present in most patients, but only 15% have clinical evidence of deep vein thrombosis (DVT).

The clinical classification of the severity of acute pulmonary embolism is based on the clinical status at presentation, with high-risk pulmonary embolism defined by the presence of shock or persistent hypotension: this determines management (Figures 57.1 and 57.2).

Suspected pulmonary embolism with shock or persistent hypotension (Figure 57.1)

Priorities

- If peri-arrest, call the resuscitation team (see Chapter 6 for further management of cardiorespiratory arrest).
- Give high-flow oxygen. Place an IV cannula. Attach ECG and oxygen saturation monitors. Check oxygen saturation. Make a rapid clinical assessment (see Chapters 1 and 2). Clinical judgement supplemented by a prediction rule (Table 57.1) should be used to assess the probability of pulmonary embolism.
- Obtain an ECG, chest X-ray and arterial blood gases. These are principally of value in excluding alternative diagnoses (e.g. myocardial infarction, severe pneumonia, tension pneumothorax).
  - In pulmonary embolism with shock/hypotension, the ECG may show evidence of right ventricular strain (right axis deviation, right bundle branch block, T wave inversion in V1–3).
  - The chest X-ray is often normal, or may show non-specific abnormalities (Table 57.2).
  - A normal ECG and chest X-ray do not exclude pulmonary embolism.
- If pulmonary embolism is the working diagnosis or must be excluded, CT pulmonary angiography (CTPA) should be done if immediately available. If CTPA cannot be done immediately, echocardiography should be performed.

Table 57.1 Clinical prediction rules for pulmonary embolism (PE) probability.

These clinical prediction rules combine elements from the history and examination to determine the probability of PE, stratified either as low/intermediate/high, or as unlikely/likely: this guides further management

Rule	Method	Interpretation	Online calculator
Original Wells (Ann Intern Med 1998; 129: 997-1005)	7 elements scored (including assessment of probability of alternative diagnosis to PE) Total score of 0–12.5 points	<2: low risk of PE 2–6: intermediate risk >6: high risk	https://www.mdcalc.com/wells-criteria-pulmonary-embolism
Modified Wells (Thromb Haemost 2000; 83: 416-420)		≤4: PE unlikely >4: PE likely	https://www.mdcalc.com/wells-criteria-pulmonary-embolism
Revised Geneva (Ann Intern Med 2006; 144: 165-171)	8 elements scored Total score of 0–22 points	0–3: low risk 4–10: intermediate risk ≥11: high risk	https://www.mdcalc.com/geneva-score-revised-pulmonary-embolism

Table 57.2 Chest X-ray findings in pulmonary embolism.

Normal appearances
Elevated hemidiaphragm
Linear atelectasis
Small pleural effusion
Focal shadowing
Regional oligaemia distal to an obstructive embolus (Westermark's sign)
Enlarged right descending central pulmonary artery (Palla's sign)
Local widening of the pulmonary artery by impaction of embolus (Fleischer's sign)
Peripheral pleural-based wedge of airspace opacity with a rounded convex apex implying an area of lung infarction (Hampton's hump)

Table 57.3 Echocardiographic findings in pulmonary embolism with haemodynamic instability.

Right ventricular dilatation and free wall hypokinesis, often with preserved contraction at the apex (McConnell's sign)
D-shaped left ventricle in the parasternal short-axis view
Peak velocity of the jet of tricuspid regurgitation usually <4.0 m/s*
Short time to peak velocity of flow in the pulmonary artery <90 ms*
Inferior vena cava dilated and unreactive
Occasionally thrombus in the pulmonary artery or right-heart*

* Requires a standard echocardiogram.

Source: Adapted from Rimington H, Chambers J (2015) *Echocardiography: Guidelines for Reporting and Interpretation*, 3rd edn. Reproduced with permission of Taylor and Francis.

Table 57.4 Thrombolytic therapy for acute pulmonary embolism with shock or persistent hypotension.

Criteria to be met
- Systolic BP <90 mmHg after standard treatment for 30–60 min
- Pulmonary embolism confirmed on CT pulmonary angiography, or supported by echocardiographic findings (Table 57.3)
- No active bleeding (other contraindications to thrombolysis (Table 45.2) are relative in the context of immediately life-threatening pulmonary embolism)

Regimens
Thrombolytic therapy can be given via a peripheral or central vein

Streptokinase
- 250,000 U IV over 30 min, followed by
- 100,000 U/h IV for 12–72 h

Alteplase
- 10 mg IV over 1–2 min IV, followed by
- 90 mg IV over 2 h (maximum total dose 1.5/kg in patients < 65 kg)
- Check the thrombin time (TT) or activated partial thromboplastin time (APTT) 3–4 h after stopping streptokinase or alteplase. When TT/APTT are less than twice control, restart heparin

- If pulmonary embolism is confirmed by CTPA, or is highly likely on echocardiography (Table 57.3), give systemic thrombolysis if no contraindication (Table 57.4). Surgical embolectomy or local endovascular thrombolysis (with unfractionated heparin infusion as a bridging measure) should be considered if systemic thrombolysis is contraindicated.
- If systolic BP remains <90 mmHg, give dobutamine (2.5–10 µgm/kg/min IV) aiming for systolic BP ≥90 mmHg. Consider adding noradrenaline if a systolic BP ≥90 mmHg (mean arterial pressure >65 mmHg) is still not achieved.
- Transfer the patient to ICU or HDU. Mechanical ventilatory support may be required. Pulmonary vasodilators such as inhaled nitric oxide or nebulized iloprost may have a role (though available data are limited).
- Further management (anticoagulation, investigation for cause of pulmonary embolism) is given below.

Suspected pulmonary embolism without shock or hypotension (Figure 57.2)

Priorities

Review the physiological observations and make a focused clinical assessment. Obtain an ECG and chest X-ray (and arterial blood gases if arterial oxygen saturation is <94% breathing air. In pulmonary embolism without shock or hypotension, the ECG may be normal or show only sinus tachycardia or minor ST/T wave abnormalities. The chest X-ray is often normal or may show non-specific abnormalities (Table 57.2). A normal ECG and chest X-ray do not exclude pulmonary embolism.

Assess the probability of pulmonary embolism, using clinical judgement supplemented by a prediction rule (Table 57.1).

If pulmonary embolism is clinically unlikely

Check the plasma D-dimer. The commonly used assays have high sensitivity (95%) but only low specificity (50%) for venous thromboembolism; the normal range will depend on the assay. Plasma D-dimer levels increase with age. Causes of a raised plasma D-dimer other than venous thromboembolism include renal failure, aortic dissection, infection and malignancy.

- If plasma D-dimer is negative, pulmonary embolism is effectively excluded. A negative D-dimer test in a patient with a modified Wells score of <4 makes PE highly unlikely (0.14–0.5% probability); the negative predictive value of this combination is at least 99.5% and comparable to the most sensitive imaging such as CT pulmonary angiography. Pursue other diagnoses.
- If this is positive, request CT pulmonary angiography or ventilation/perfusion (V/Q) scan (see below). If this is negative for pulmonary embolism, pursue other diagnoses. If positive for pulmonary embolism, start anti-coagulation (see below).

If pulmonary embolism is likely

- Request CT pulmonary angiography (CTPA), or alternative imaging if indicated (see below).
- If imaging is negative for pulmonary embolis/deep vein thrombosis, pursue other diagnoses. If positive for pulmonary embolism, start anticoagulation (see below).
- Thrombolysis may be indicated for some patients with sub-massive pulmonary embolism (defined as acute PE without systemic hypotension (systolic blood pressure >90 mmHg) but with either right ventricular dysfunction or myocardial necrosis): see Problems below.

Alternatives to CT pulmonary angiography

CT pulmonary angiography (CTPA) is the investigation of choice if the chest X-ray is abnormal, or there is underlying respiratory disease (including chronic obstructive pulmonary disease (COPD) and asthma). It also

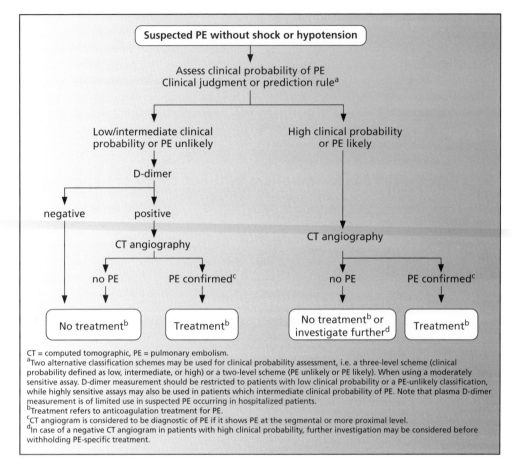

CT = computed tomographic, PE = pulmonary embolism.
[a]Two alternative classification schemes may be used for clinical probability assessment, i.e. a three-level scheme (clinical probability defined as low, intermediate, or high) or a two-level scheme (PE unlikely or PE likely). When using a moderately sensitive assay. D-dimer measurement should be restricted to patients with low clinical probability or a PE-unlikely classification, while highly sensitive assays may also be used in patients which intermediate clinical probability of PE. Note that plasma D-dimer measurement is of limited use in suspected PE occurring in hospitalized patients.
[b]Treatment refers to anticoagulation treatment for PE.
[c]CT angiogram is considered to be diagnostic of PE if it shows PE at the segmental or more proximal level.
[d]In case of a negative CT angiogram in patients with high clinical probability, further investigation may be considered before withholding PE-specific treatment.

Figure 57.2 Suspected pulmonary embolism without shock or hypotension. *Source:* Konstantinides SV, Torbicki A, Agnelli G *et al.* (2014) 2014 ESC Guidelines on the diagnosis and management of acute pulmonary. *Eur Heart J* 35, 3033–3080. Reproduced with permission of Oxford University Press.

gives information on lung parenchyma, aorta, mediastinum, pleural spaces, bones and chest wall, and can reveal alternative diagnoses if PE is excluded. It carries considerably higher radiation exposure than a V/Q scan.

Ventilation/perfusion scan (V/Q scan)

A ventilation/perfusion scan (V/Q scan) is the investigation of choice if the chest X-ray is normal, and there is no underlying respiratory disease such as COPD or asthma. It is also preferable to CTPA in renal failure or previous contrast reaction.

A normal perfusion (Q) scan or ventilation/perfusion (V/Q) scan excludes pulmonary embolism if pulmonary embolism is unlikely on clinical grounds.

A 'high-probability' scan confirms the diagnosis if pulmonary embolism is likely on clinical grounds.

Further diagnostic testing is needed if the scan shows a low or intermediate probability result, or if the scan findings and clinical probability are discordant.

Duplex scan of leg veins

Duplex scan of the leg veins is the first imaging of choice in pregnancy for suspected pulmonary embolism without shock or hypotension, as a positive finding eliminates the need for investigation involving radiation. See Problems below.

Further management

Anticoagulation

Anticoagulation is discussed in detail in Chapter 103. Anticoagulation for pulmonary embolism can be with rivaroxaban, heparin or warfarin (preceded by and overlapping with heparin).

Rivaroxaban

Rivaroxaban (a direct factor Xa inhibitor) is licensed in the UK for the treatment of pulmonary embolism (without the need for adjunctive heparin).

Rivaroxaban is contraindicated in pregnancy, breastfeeding, renal failure, significant liver disease, concomitant use of cytochrome P-450 inhibitors, and is not currently recommended in patients with active cancer.

Low-molecular-weight heparin (LMWH)

LMWH is indicated in patients with active cancer (particularly if undergoing chemotherapy) or who are pregnant.

Unfractionated heparin

Unfractionated heparin by infusion (UFH) should be used if there is:
- Renal failure (eGFR <30 mL/min)
- Increased risk of bleeding
- Peri-operative state
- Peri-partum state

Warfarin

Warfarin should be used if rivaroxaban is contraindicated and in the absence of active cancer or pregnancy.
- Warfarin loading is given in Table 103.11.
- It is initially pro-thrombotic, so is co-administered with LMWH or unfractionated heparin. During this period, check both the activated partial thromboplastin time (APTT) and International Normalized Ratio (INR) daily.
- Heparin can be stopped after five days provided the INR is >2.0.
- The target INR is usually 2.0–3.0.

Duration of anticoagulation

In provoked PE (those with a transient, reversible risk factor), treatment is usually for three months. In unprovoked PE, treatment is usually extended for as long as the underlying risk factor (if identified) is present. If no cause is identified, treatment duration is determined on a case-by-case basis: seek advice from a haematologist.

Ambulatory care, discharge planning and follow-up
- Ambulatory care and outpatient management of patients with low-risk pulmonary embolism is possible. The Pulmonary Embolism Severity Index (PESI) (Table 57.5) score is the most widely validated and used prognostic model for PE, to guide the initial decision to admit to hospital or discharge.
- Serial/repeat PESI scoring can guide the subsequent timing of safe discharge if originally admitted.
- A robust system of communication, support and follow-up is required for the ambulatory care approach to be successful.

Table 57.5 Pulmonary Embolism Severity Index (PESI) score.

Predictors	Points
Age	+1 per year
Male sex	+10
Heart failure	+10
Chronic lung disease	+10
Temperature <36 °C	+20
Arterial oxygen saturation <90%	+20
Respiratory rate >30/min	+20
Pulse rate >110/min	+20
Systolic BP <100 mmHg	+30
Active cancer	+30
Altered mental status	+60

PESI score (total no. of points)	Risk class	30 day mortality rate
≤65	I	0–1.6%
66–85	II	1.7–3.5%
86–105	III	3.2–7.1%
106–125	IV	4.0–11.4%
>125	V	10.0–24.5%

In the stable non-pregnant patient with PESI risk class I or II, ambulatory care may be appropriate, depending on locally-agreed protocols.

Why has the patient had a pulmonary embolism?

- Consider the presence of risk factors (Table 56.1). In many patients, the cause of pulmonary embolism is obvious. Further tests for patients with unprovoked DVT/PE are given in Table 56.3.
- Patients under 50 with unprovoked DVT/PE or with a strong family history of venous thromboembolism should be screened for a thrombophilic disorder: seek advice from a haematologist.

Problems

Sub-massive pulmonary embolism

Sub-massive PE is characterized by:

- Right ventricular (RV) dysfunction (RV dilatation on echo, or raised plasma BNP/NT-pro-BNP)
- Myocardial necrosis (raised plasma troponin)
- Worsening hypoxaemia and respiratory insufficiency
- Extreme tachycardia
- High clot burden

If sub-massive PE suspected, there may be a role for half-dose thrombolysis. Seek expert advice. The incidence of longer-term complications such as chronic thromboembolic pulmonary hypertension (CTEPH) may be reduced by using this strategy.

Currently, the judgement on thrombolysis in sub-massive PE should be individualised and based on local guidelines or specialist advice. It is not generally recommended for those patients with only minor RV dysfunction or myocardial necrosis, and no clinical deterioration. If there are no features of sub-massive PE, proceed with anticoagulation, p. 563.

Suspected pulmonary embolism in pregnancy

- The differential diagnoses of breathlessness, chest pain and shock in pregnancy are discussed in Chapter 32.
- PE is the leading cause of maternal death in the UK, with a mortality rate of 1.56 per 100,000 pregnancies.
- The risk of undiagnosed maternal PE to a mother and her fetus far outweighs any risk from radiation exposure through diagnostic imaging. The commonly used tests are not associated with high levels of radiation.
- D-dimer is negative in up to 50% of pregnant patients up to 20 weeks gestation and should be the first test of choice. If D-dimer is negative, the patient is highly unlikely to have a PE, and alternative diagnoses should be sought.
- If D-dimer is positive, duplex scan of both leg veins should be performed, as confirming the presence of DVT will instigate the same treatment regimen of LMWH as in non-massive PE. If no DVT is found, but there is ongoing suspicion of PE, then a half-dose perfusion (Q) scan, following a (normal) chest X-ray, is the imaging modality of choice and carries a lower maternal radiation exposure than CTPA.
- If the clinical presentation is with shock or hypotension, and echocardiography shows features of massive pulmonary embolism (Table 57.3), CTPA is not necessary.

When to consider placement of an inferior vena cava (IVC) filter

IVC filter use is generally limited to patients in whom anticoagulation is contraindicated, thrombosis has recurred despite adequate anticoagulation, or if temporary cessation of anticoagulation within one month is anticipated, for example in pregnant patients within one month of the expected date of delivery.

Further reading

Kearon C, Akl EA, Ornelas J, *et al.* (2016) Antithrombotic therapy for VTE disease: CHEST guideline and expert panel report. *Chest* 149, 315–352.

Raja AS, Greenberg JO, Qaseem A, *et al.* (2015) Evaluation of patients with suspected acute pulmonary embolism: best practice advice from the Clinical Guidelines Committee of the American College of Physicians. *Ann Intern Med.* 163, 701–711.

The Task Force for the Diagnosis and Management of Acute Pulmonary Embolism of the European Society of Cardiology (ESC) (2014) 2014 ESC Guidelines on the diagnosis and management of acute pulmonary embolism. http://eurheartj.oxfordjournals.org/content/early/2014/08/28/eurheartj.ehu283.

CHAPTER 58

Problems with pacemakers and other cardiac devices

MICHAEL COOKLIN AND DAVID SPRIGINGS

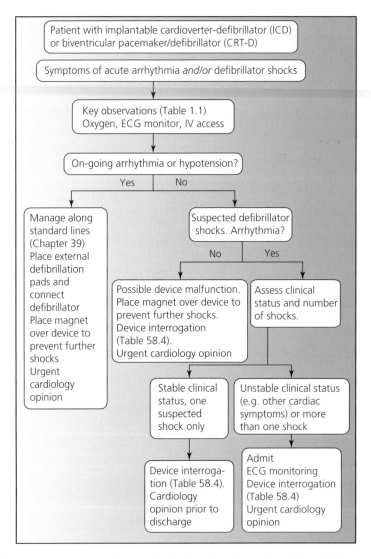

Figure 58.1 Management of acute arrhythmia and/or shocks in the patient with an ICD or CRT-D.

Acute Medicine: A Practical Guide to the Management of Medical Emergencies, Fifth Edition. Edited by David Sprigings and John B. Chambers.
© 2018 John Wiley & Sons Ltd. Published 2018 by John Wiley & Sons Ltd.

Table 58.1 Cardiac device functions.

1. Pacemaker functions		
Pacemaker type/indications	**Pacemaker code**	**Comment**
Single lead atrial pacemaker Indication: sinoatrial disorder (sinus bradycardia/pauses) with normal AV conduction	AAI or AAIR	Pacemaker senses and paces right atrium If no intrinsic activity is sensed within right atrium, the pacemaker paces at its preprogrammed rate AAIR indicates rate-adaptive capability: the pacemaker increases the atrial pacing rate in response to stimuli such as movement
Single lead ventricular pacemaker Indications: AV block with atrial fibrillation, intermittent AV block	VVI or VVIR	Pacemaker senses and paces right ventricle If atrial electrical activity is conducted through the AV node/bundle of His and depolarizes the ventricles, the pacemaker is inhibited If no intrinsic activity is sensed within right ventricle, the pacemaker paces at its preprogrammed rate VVIR indicates rate-adaptive capability: the pacemaker increases the pacing rate in response to stimuli such as movement
Dual lead atrial and ventricular pacemaker Indications: AV block with sinus rhythm, sinoatrial disorder with impaired AV conduction	DDD or DDDR (Figure 58.2)	Pacemaker senses and paces both the right atrium and the right ventricle If no intrinsic activity is sensed in right atrium, the pacemaker paces at its preprogrammed rate; if intrinsic or paced atrial activity is not conducted to the ventricles within a preprogrammed interval, the pacemaker paces the right ventricle DDDR indicates rate-adaptive capability: the pacemaker increases the pacing rate in response to stimuli such as movement
Cardiac resynchronization therapy (CRT) **(biventricular pacing)**	CRT-P or CRT-D	Pacing both right and left ventricle to correct dyssynchronous contraction of the left ventricle and improve ejection CRT may be combined with defibrillation capability (CRT-D) (see below) Pacing leads are placed in the right atrium, right ventricle and in a venous branch over the epicardial free wall of the left ventricle (via the coronary sinus)

2. ICD functions	
ICD function	**Comment**
Sensing **Detection**	Recognition of atrial and ventricular electrogram signals Classification of sensed signals according to programmable heart rate zones
Provision of therapy to terminate ventricular fibrillation (VF) or ventricular tachycardia (VT)	VF is terminated by high energy (up to 30 J) unsynchronized shocks delivered between coil electrode in right ventricle and device casing and/or another electrode VT is managed in one of four ways:

(continued)

Table 58.1 (*Continued*)

2. ICD functions	
ICD function	**Comment**
	• Observation with no action (monitor zone)
	• Antitachycardia pacing (burst pacing at a rate faster than the VT rate)
	• Low energy (<5 J) synchronized shock
	• High energy unsynchronized shock
	Placement of a magnet over the ICD suspends VT/VF detection (but not pacing for bradycardia)
Pacing for bradycardia	As provided by a pacemaker (see above)

AV, atrioventricular.

Table 58.2 Complications of cardiac devices.

At implantation/shortly after implantation
Pneumothorax
Air embolism
Device pocket haematoma
Malposition of lead
Displacement of lead
Perforation of great vessels or myocardium by a lead causing pericardial effusion/tamponade
Diaphragmatic stimulation
Thrombosis of subclavian vein
Later
Lead malfunction (insulation failure, conduction fracture)
Pulse generator/device malfunction
Infection of lead
Infection of device pocket/device
Erosion of device pocket
Thrombosis of subclavian and central veins

Table 58.3 Assessment of suspected pacemaker malfunction.

Check the details of the pacemaker: is it a single or dual chamber system (Table 58.1) and what is the pacing mode?
   Contact the hospital where the system was implanted to obtain further details.
Record a 12-lead ECG, a long rhythm strip and a penetrated chest X- ray for the position of the leads.
Does the ECG show no pacing spikes, spikes without capture or spikes without sensing? Interpretation is given below.
Contact the cardiology department to arrange a check of the pacemaker and discuss management with a cardiologist
   (including need for temporary pacing).

(*continued*)

ECG	Causes
No spikes	Normal sensing
	Malfunction of pulse generator
	Spike buried in QRS complex
	Electromagnetic interference
Spikes without capture (failure to capture)	High threshold:
	• Lead fracture
	• Lead displacement
	• Myocardial fibrosis
	• Myocardial perforation
	Lead not properly connected to pulse generator
	Depletion of battery of pulse generator
	Spike in ventricular refractory period
Spikes without sensing (failure to sense)	Lead displacement
	Low intrinsic P/R wave (i.e. not at sensing threshold)

Table 58.4 Findings and management on interrogation of an implantable cardioverter-defibrillator (ICD) or CRT-D device after the patient reports a shock.

Finding	Action
VT/VF with appropriate termination by shock	Assess potential causes:
	• Myocardial ischaemia
	• Non-compliance with drug therapy
	• Electrolyte disorder
	• Intercurrent illness
	Consider starting/modifying drug therapy to prevent recurrence.
	Refer to a cardiologist
Inappropriate shock due to missensing of SVT/AF	Assess causes and treat (Chapters 42 and 43)
	Refer to a cardiologist
Inappropriate shock due to missensing of electrical noise	Environmental noise: avoid exposure
	Electrical noise from ICD or lead malfunction:
	• Programme VT/VF detection off
	• Admit for further management
	• Refer to a cardiologist
No shock or arrhythmia	Phantom shock, reassure

AF, atrial fibrillation; SVT, supraventricular tachycardia.

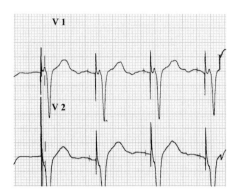

Figure 58.2 ECG showing dual chamber pacing. The small atrial and larger ventricular pacing spikes can be seen, preceding the P waves and QRS complexes, respectively.

Further reading

Report of a joint Working Party project on behalf of the British Society for Antimicrobial Chemotherapy (BSAC, host organization), British Heart Rhythm Society (BHRS), British Cardiovascular Society (BCS), British Heart Valve Society (BHVS) and British Society for Echocardiography (BSE) (2015) Guidelines for the diagnosis, prevention and management of implantable cardiac electronic device infection. *J Antimicrob Chemother* 70, 325–359.

The Task Force on cardiac pacing and resynchronization therapy of the European Society of Cardiology (ESC) (2013) 2013 ESC Guidelines on cardiac pacing and cardiac resynchronization therapy. *European Heart Journal* 34, 2281–2329.

Respiratory

CHAPTER 59

Upper airway obstruction

Matthew Frise

The upper airway runs from the mouth and nose to the carina. Upper airway obstruction (UAO) is a condition where functional or mechanical factors lead to loss of normal airway architecture and patency, compromising ventilation.

- Upper airway obstruction is a life-threatening medical emergency. Precipitous deterioration may occur without warning, so treatment must be swift.
- Causes are given in Appendix 59.1 and Table 59.1. Intervention may need to precede a definitive diagnosis.
- It is important not to make the situation worse by incorrect positioning, for example lying the patient flat, attempting intubation if inexperienced, or giving sedative drugs with an unsecured airway.

Priorities

Don't make the situation worse

- Often simple manoeuvres are all that are required until more experienced help arrives.
- The use of airway adjuncts and attempted intubation in inexperienced hands may worsen the situation and make subsequent attempts at establishing a definitive airway more difficult.
- The conscious patient will often try to assume the position which best relieves obstruction; help the patient to do this. In tracheal compression or laryngeal tumours, lying the patient flat can provoke complete obstruction and respiratory arrest.
- Sedative drugs must be used with extreme caution in patients with possible UAO; sedation before the airway is secured may precipitate respiratory arrest.

Re-establish airway patency to permit adequate ventilation, whilst preventing aspiration

- If the patient is conscious and choking as a result of acute severe airway obstruction by a foreign body, give alternating sequences of five intrascapular back blows and five abdominal thrusts.
- In other conscious patients with suspected UAO:
  - Give high flow supplemental oxygen via non-rebreathe mask whilst making a rapid clinical assessment (Table 59.2). The airway may be lost at any time, leading to hypoxic cardiac arrest, so do not withhold oxygen due to misplaced concerns about toxicity.
  - If there are any features suggestive of anaphylaxis give IM adrenaline 500 µgm immediately and summon help. Treat according to ALS guidelines (see Chapter 38). If there is cardiovascular instability raise the legs rather than lying the patient down and do not instrument the airway unless suitably experienced. If the patient arrests in the meantime, follow ALS guidelines (see Chapter 6).
  - Secure IV access, ideally large bore. If intubation is likely at least two IV access points should be available.

Acute Medicine: A Practical Guide to the Management of Medical Emergencies, Fifth Edition. Edited by David Sprigings and John B. Chambers.
© 2018 John Wiley & Sons Ltd. Published 2018 by John Wiley & Sons Ltd.

Table 59.1 Mechanical causes of upper airway obstruction.

Oedema
Anaphylaxis (Chapter 38)
Angioedema – angiotensin-converting enzyme inhibitors, C1 inhibitor deficiency (Chapter 27)
Post-extubation laryngeal oedema – typically a few hours after extubation

Extrinsic compression
Thyroid masses – benign or malignant
Lymphadenopathy of any cause
Neck haematoma, for example arterial puncture complicating central venous access

Tumours of the airway
Laryngeal carcinoma
Tracheal carcinoma

Infection
Retropharyngeal abscess
Ludwig's angina
Laryngitis and epiglottitis

Vocal cord paralysis
Recurrent laryngeal nerve palsy of any cause
Cricoarytenoid disease in rheumatoid arthritis

Trauma
Acute laryngeal trauma
Facial fractures and associated haemorrhage
Thermal inhalation injury to mucosa
Tracheal stenosis following intubation or tracheostomy

Foreign bodies

- **If the patient is unconscious and has signs of obstruction such as snoring**:
  - Check the airway is clear of debris, suction if necessary and manipulate the airway to see if obstruction can be relieved.
  - Consider an oro- or nasopharyngeal airway (see Chapter 112).
  - If the patient is breathing place in the recovery position with adjuncts and supplemental oxygen in situ.
  - If there is concern about cervical spine injury, use manual in-line stabilization, but the airway takes priority.
  - If there is inadequate or absent respiratory effort despite relief of obstruction, ask for the arrest team to be summoned whilst commencing bag-mask ventilation using 100% oxygen. If this is ineffective, insert a supraglottic airway such as a laryngeal mask airway or an i-gel®. If still ineffective and more experienced help is yet to arrive, attempt endotracheal intubation if appropriately experienced.
  - If at any point cardiac output is lost, follow the ALS algorithm.

Continue your assessment
- If the patient is conscious obtain a brief history (Table 59.2); yes/no answers may be all that is possible.
- Examine the patient. Look closely at the thorax, head and neck for swelling, masses, previous surgical scars (especially from tracheostomy or neck dissection), distended veins or distorted anatomy. **Listen carefully for stridor**.
- If the features suggest mechanical obstruction summon urgent ENT assistance.
- Optimize the patient's position and **stay at the bedside**.

Table 59.2 Clinical features of upper airway obstruction.

Acute partial obstruction

Respiratory distress – dyspnoea, tachypnoea, short sentences, agitation, diaphoresis

Coughing, choking, gagging and altered voice

Grunting and snoring – partial obstruction of pharynx by soft palate or epiglottis

Stridor

Drooling and gurgling

Paradoxical chest wall movements and supraclavicular retraction

Dermal ecchymoses and subcutaneous emphysema – if very forceful respiratory effort

Negative pressure pulmonary oedema – may be misdiagnosed as acute heart failure

Rapid decompensation and progression to complete obstruction

Subacute or chronic partial obstruction

May be almost asymptomatic at rest if develops gradually

Dyspnoea and tachypnoea

Stridor

Voice change

Hypercapnic ventilatory failure

Sudden progression to complete obstruction

Complete obstruction

Inability to breathe and speak

May clasp throat between thumb and index finger to indicate choking

Agitation and panic

Cyanosis

Vigorous respiratory effort becoming feeble as consciousness lost

Respiratory arrest, bradycardia and hypotension followed swiftly by cardiac arrest if not relieved

Further management

Some causes of UAO, such as anaphylaxis, are reasonably quickly reversible and once the patient has recovered from the acute event, extubation can be attempted.

Medical therapies for mechanical upper airway obstruction (UAO)

These are based on relatively little evidence but can be considered (Table 59.3).

Further diagnosis

- Disorders of consciousness that have compromised the airway should be managed as discussed in Chapters 3 and 112.
- For mechanical UAO several approaches to diagnosis are available:
  - **Fibreoptic endoscopy**: allows visualization of the upper airway under local anaesthesia usually via the nose, but may also be performed orally or via an endotracheal tube (ETT) or tracheostomy. It has the advantage of also permitting awake fibreoptic intubation of a patient with UAO who is able to sit up and cooperate, avoiding the risks of a rapid-sequence induction (RSI) in this setting.
  - **Radiographs**: plain films of the thorax and neck may locate a foreign body or tracheal distortion, and can be undertaken in the resuscitation room without the need to move the patient. These may also reveal evidence of complications such as aspiration, negative pressure pulmonary oedema or pneumothorax.
  - **CT**: in a stable patient who is able to lie flat, or otherwise once a definitive airway has been secured, gives excellent cross-sectional imaging of the relevant anatomy and will reveal most pathologies of interest.

Table 59.3 Medical treatments in upper airway obstruction.

Nebulized adrenaline
- This can be used to treat laryngeal oedema in patients with partial UAO who remain conscious and self-ventilating (low grade evidence).
- A typical dose is 1 mL of a 1:1000 solution diluted with saline to 5 mL.
- It is not a substitute for IM adrenaline in anaphylaxis.

Corticosteroids
- Widely used in adults, despite sparse evidence (even in the setting of anaphylaxis). Some studies suggest a reduction in post-extubation laryngeal oedema with prophylactic use.
- Typically used doses are hydrocortisone 100–200 mg IV or dexamethasone 10 mg IV or IM.

Heliox
- This is a mixture of at least 70% helium in oxygen, which reduces the work of breathing by diminishing turbulent flow in the partially obstructed airway.
- Its use may be limited by concomitant lung disease requiring a higher fraction of inspired oxygen. Most research has involved patients with obstructive lung disease, rather than UAO.
- It is only a temporizing measure and does nothing to correct the underlying pathology.

Consider a surgical airway

- This is needed if the cause of UAO is not quickly reversible, for example laryngeal tumour or bilateral vocal cord paralysis.
- Seek advice from an ENT surgeon. Formation of a tracheostomy is increasingly undertaken percutaneously by critical care physicians using the Seldinger technique.
- For the patient with UAO, anatomical considerations may make surgical formation in theatre preferable.

Problems

Transport of the patient with a compromised airway

- If a patient with a compromised airway and/or impaired consciousness requires transfer to another area, such as for diagnostic imaging, careful consideration should be given to intubation beforehand. Doing so in a controlled manner and well-resourced environment of the resuscitation room is far preferable to attempting advanced airway interventions in a CT scanner with limited equipment when the patient has vomited and aspirated.
- If a patient with UAO needs to lie flat (and still) for imaging, intubation may be required in any event.

Aspiration of gastric contents

- Aspiration pneumonitis is a chemical process resulting from lung injury by gastric acid. In the self-ventilating patient, this requires supportive therapy with supplemental oxygen and possibly continuous positive airway pressure (CPAP).
- If true aspiration pneumonia develops as a result of superinfection, antibiotic therapy should be instituted in line with local guidance (see Chapter 63). Evidence is lacking to support the use of empirical antibiotic therapy in all patients with evidence of aspiration.
- Aspiration is the commonest cause of death associated with airway management during anaesthesia.

Negative-pressure pulmonary oedema
- Occasionally the negative pressures generated by a patient's vigorous ventilatory effort in the face of UAO can cause pulmonary oedema.
- Confusingly, this may develop some hours after relief of the obstruction, and misdiagnosis as acute cardiogenic pulmonary oedema or aspiration is possible (Chapter 47).
- Treatment is with supplemental oxygen and CPAP. Depending on volume status, loop diuretics may be helpful.

The patient with a tracheostomy
- Following the national tracheostomy safety project, adult inpatients with a tracheostomy should all have clear guidance at the bedside indicating steps to be taken in the event of an emergency – follow these if called to an acutely ill inpatient with a tracheostomy.
- For patients presenting with signs of airway compromise and a tracheostomy, the priorities are to summon expert help and deliver oxygen by whatever means possible until assistance arrives. General steps are as follows:
  - Give high flow oxygen via the stoma and face.
  - Remove the inner tube and try to pass a suction catheter – if it passes easily, suction and leave the outer tube in place. If respiratory effort is poor or lost, ventilate via the tracheostomy (may need inner tube replaced to attach circuit).
  - If a suction catheter cannot be passed, deflate the tracheostomy cuff and see if this relieves the obstruction. If so leave the cuff down and continue oxygen.
  - If obstruction persists remove the tracheostomy altogether. Occlude the stoma and attempt ventilation from above using BMV with adjuncts or an LMA. If this fails try ventilation via the stoma using a bag and paediatric mask.
- Patients with laryngectomies cannot be ventilated or intubated from above since they do not have an airway above the stoma. Oxygen applied to the face will not be useful for this reason. The default position in the emergency setting where the exact anatomy may not be clear is to apply oxygen to the stoma and the face.

Can't intubate, can't ventilate
- The situation where endotracheal intubation fails and ventilation with bag and mask is impossible is well recognized. Try an LMA or an i-gel® early; if these fail, other options in sick medical patients, for the appropriately experienced, include:
  - **Retrograde intubation**: a guidewire is passed percutaneously across the cricothyroid membrane and up into the retropharynx and the end captured with a pair of forceps; this is then used to guide an ETT into the trachea.
  - **Transtracheal jet ventilation**: a very high pressure oxygen source is used in bursts via a large-bore catheter (IV or specifically-designed) inserted through the cricothyroid membrane. Provides temporary relief of hypoxia but carries serious risks of potentially fatal barotrauma and subcutaneous emphysema. Contra-indicated if complete UAO prevents expiration.
  - **Cricothyroidotomy**: the surgical treatment of choice to re-establish airflow if other interventions fail. A horizontal incision is made through the cricothyroid membrane and a small ETT inserted allowing manual ventilation with 100% oxygen. A formal surgical tracheostomy under local anaesthesia is also an option if available without delay.

Appendix 59.1 Upper airway obstruction

Functional: impairment of consciousness or neurological disease in a patient with an essentially normal airway. Patients with existing obstructive sleep apnoea are at particularly high risk. This is commonly encountered by acute physicians. Simple interventions may be sufficient whilst the underlying problem is identified and treated.

Mechanical: physical obstruction of the airway by a foreign body, tumour or oedema, for example. Anaesthetic or ENT expertise is often required, though temporizing measures are important whilst help is awaited.

Due to a combination of functional and mechanical factors: any functional cause of airway compromise may be complicated by mechanical obstruction, for example aspiration of vomitus in a patient intoxicated with alcohol. Likewise, uncorrected mechanical obstruction eventually results in exhaustion, asphyxia and loss of consciousness.

Obstruction tends to occur at sites of anatomical narrowing and the causes and clinical features differ according the level, though no sign or symptom is pathognomonic. The time course and degree of obstruction are also important. Common mechanical causes of airway obstruction are given in Table 59.1.

Further reading

Al-Qadi MO, Artenstein AW, Braman SS (2013) The 'forgotten zone': acquired disorders of the trachea in adults. *Respir Med* 107, 1301–1313. DOI: 10.1016/j.rmed.2013.03.017.

Patel A, Pearce A (2011) Progress in management of the obstructed airway. *Anaesthesia* 66, Suppl 2, 93–100. DOI: 10.1111/j.1365-2044.2011.06938.x.

CHAPTER 60

Acute asthma

Swapna Mandal

- Asthma (Box 60.1) is one of the commonest causes of breathlessness and wheeze, but other causes should be considered, especially if the response to initial treatment is slow (Table 60.1).
- The severity of an attack is easily underestimated (Table 60.2).
- It is important to establish the severity of the exacerbation to monitor progress and determine if early involvement of the intensive care team is required.

Box 60.1 Asthma.

- Asthma is characterized by variable airways obstruction, and defined by the presence of one or more of the following symptoms: breathlessness, wheeze, chest tightness or cough, with reversible airways obstruction shown by diurnal variation in peak expiratory flow >25%.
- The National Review of Asthma Deaths has shown that the UK has one of the highest death rates for asthma in Europe, with 195 deaths attributable to an acute exacerbation between 2012 and 2013.
- Acute asthma is diagnosed by worsening symptoms with associated signs and a reduction in the patient's usual peak expiratory flow (PEF).

Priorities

Is this acute asthma? If so, how severe?

Many other diseases can mimic acute asthma (Table 60.1). Important diagnoses to consider include:

An **exacerbation of chronic obstructive pulmonary disease** (Chapter 61). The patient tends to be older, with a smoking history.

Upper airway obstruction (Chapter 59). PEF is disproportionately lower than the FEV_1.

Vocal cord dysfunction. Symptoms can be similar to asthma, but usually the periods of breathlessness are short, with difficulty in inspiration (as opposed to expiration in asthma).

Anaphylaxis may also present with wheeze and breathlessness, but typically there are additional features such as urticarial rash and hypotension (Chapter 38).

The severity of acute asthma can be judged by the clinical features and PEF (Table 60.2).

Immediate management (Figure 60.1)

All patients presenting with an acute exacerbation of asthma should receive **oxygen** therapy to maintain an arterial oxygen saturation between 94–98%.

Acute Medicine: A Practical Guide to the Management of Medical Emergencies, Fifth Edition. Edited by David Sprigings and John B. Chambers.
© 2018 John Wiley & Sons Ltd. Published 2018 by John Wiley & Sons Ltd.

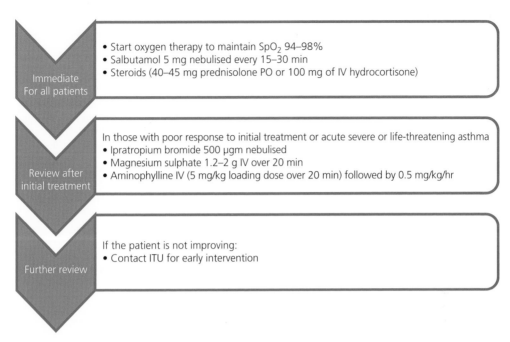

Figure 60.1 Management of acute asthma. Adapted from BTS/SIGN guidelines.

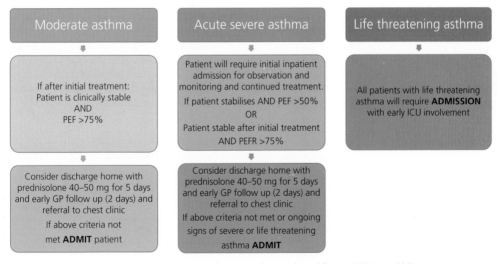

Figure 60.2 Discharge planning of the patient with acute asthma. Adapted from BTS/SIGN guidelines.

High-dose nebulized **β-agonists** (5 mg **salbutamol**) should be given as quickly as possible (the nebulizer should preferably be driven by oxygen); doses can be repeated every 15–30 min.

Ipratropium bromide (500 μgm 6-hourly) can be given to those with acute severe or life-threatening asthma, or in those who have a poor initial response to salbutamol.

Table 60.1 Differential diagnosis of acute asthma.

Disorder	Comment
Acute exacerbation of chronic obstructive pulmonary disease	A relevant smoking history will assist in differentiating between an exacerbation of asthma and an exacerbation of COPD.
Upper airway obstruction	These individuals may have a more chronic course; however, they may present acutely, for example inhalation of a foreign body or acute anaphylaxis. The key in determining the differences will be in the history. In a more chronic setting, flow-volume loops are very helpful.
Vocal cord dysfunction	Acutely VCD can present in a similar manner to acute asthma. It can be difficult to differentiate VCD from asthma as some patients with VCD may also have asthma and respond to acute treatment. Arterial blood gases will be normal in VCD and often patients with VCD find inspiration more difficult than expiration.
Anaphylaxis	Individuals with anaphylaxis can have wheeze and allergy is common in those with asthma. The key to determining the difference will be the history, that is, an acute trigger in those with analphylaxis and other signs such as an urticarial rash and angioedema. Treatment for both will include bronchodilators and steroids. Individuals with anaphylaxis will also require adrenaline.

In patients presenting with atypical histories, signs or symptoms, other important diagnoses to consider are:

Disorder	Comment
Gastro-oesophageal reflux	This often presents more chronically as a cough; however, gastro-oesophageal reflux can exacerbate symptoms of asthma.
Cystic fibrosis	This is an inherited disorder resulting in deficiency of the cystic fibrosis transmembrane receptor. These individuals often have bronchiectasis and can also develop cystic fibrosis related asthma and can therefore present with wheeze and cough. Often these patients will also have thick sputum that can be difficult to expectorate, this would be an unusual finding in those with asthma that is not related to CF.
Heart failure	Heart failure can also present with breathlessness and wheeze. The history is key, the symptoms are often progressive over a period of time, heart failure tends to occur in the older population and those with a significant history of cardiac disease. These individuals will respond well to diuresis.
Foreign body aspiration	There will often be a very acute history involving a feeling of 'choking' whilst having eaten something. If the foreign body is lodged within the upper airway and there is complete obstruction, respiratory arrest may occur. Partial obstruction of the upper airway may cause stridor. If the foreign body passes below the carina a more chronic course of symptoms will occur, such as cough, wheeze and recurrent infection.
Eosinophillic lung disease	Eosinophilic pneumonias are a group of disorders characterized by peripheral blood eosinophilia and evidence of eosinophilia within the airways. Causes of eosinophilic pneumonia include: helminth and tropical infections; medication such as NSAIDs and antibiotics; Churg-Strauss syndrome (eosinophilic granulomatosis with polyangitis); ABPA and idiopathic eosinophilic pneumonias. The history and searching for a trigger, for example medication or travel to endemic areas will assist in the diagnosis. These individuals tend to present with a chronic course of symptoms and blood tests, and often bronchoscopy/lung biopsy may be necessary to clinch the diagnosis. Many of these conditions will respond to steroid treatment
Carcinoid tumour	These are neuroendocrine tumours that can occur in the digestive tract and sometimes the lung. Carcinoid syndrome encompasses the following signs and symptoms: flushing, diarrhoea, telangiectasia, hepatomegaly, heart disease and wheeze caused by bronchospasm. These additional signs and symptoms should alert a

Table 60.1 (*Continued*)

Disorder	Comment
	clinician to a diagnosis other than lone asthma. Diagnosis will be made through imaging and hormone profile; a bronchoscopy may be necessary to determine if there is carcinoid tumour present in the airway.
Interstitial lung disease	ILD often causes cough and breathlessness; wheeze can occur although it is more unusual. Presentation of ILD is often later in life and examination will elicit other findings such as crackles and evidence of an underlying connective tissue disorder.
Churg-Strauss syndrome	Often now called eosinophilic granulomatosis with polyangitis, CSS is a vasculitis of small to medium-sized vessels that is characterized by asthma, peripheral eosinophilia, pulmonary infiltrates, polyneuropathy and allergic rhinitis. The ANCA (predominantly p-ANCA) will often be positive in these individuals. Churg-Strauss syndrome is a multisystem disorder and therefore the presence of other system involvement should suggest a diagnosis of CSS rather than asthma alone.

Corticosteroids should be administered immediately. Either 40–50 mg of oral prednisolone daily or hydrocortisone 100 mg 6-hourly IV or IM should be given. Corticosteroids should be given for a minimum of 5 days.

In those with acute severe asthma with poor response to initial therapy or life-threatening asthma, a single dose of **magnesium sulphate** (1.2–2 g IV over 20 min) can be given.

Aminophylline may be considered in those with life-threatening asthma. A loading dose of 5 mg/kg should be given parenterally over 20 minutes (omit if the patient is on oral aminophylline) followed by an infusion of 0.5 mg/kg/h.

Consider referral to ITU if: hypoxia worsens, hypercapnia or acidaemia is evident, the patient is exhausting, GCS is deteriorating or PEF is deteriorating.

Non-invasive ventilation (NIV) is **not** recommended for asthma and should not be given outside the intensive care environment.

Table 60.2 Assessment of severity of acute asthma.

	Moderate exacerbation of asthma	Acute severe asthma	Life-threatening asthma
Symptoms	Worsening chest tightness, breathlessness, wheeze, cough	Worsening chest tightness, breathlessness, wheeze, cough	
PEF	50–75% of best/predicted	33–50% of best/predicted	<33% of best/predicted
Physiological variable		RR $\geq$25 breaths/min HR $\geq$110 breaths/min	SaO_2 <92% PaO_2 <8 kPa $PaCO_2$ 4.6–6.0 kPa
Other signs		Unable to complete sentences in one breath	Reduced GCS Exhaustion Silent chest Cyanosis Poor respiratory effort Arrhythmia Hypotension

Adapted from BTS/SIGN guidelines.

Table 60.3 Monitoring of the patient with acute asthma.

Regular monitoring	To be monitored as required
Peak expiratory flow rate	ABG (initially if SpO_2 <92% and repeat after treatment)
SaO_2	Serum theophylline concentrations
Respiratory rate	Serum electrolytes
Heart rate	

Other treatments

- Antibiotics may be considered in those with signs of infection but should not be routinely used in the management of acute asthma.
- Patients who are dehydrated may require IV fluids.

Investigations and monitoring (Table 60.3)

Whilst treating these patients, investigations can be initiated, these include:
- PEF (once the patient is stabilized PEF should continue to be monitored)
- Arterial blood gas (ABG)
- Serum electrolytes (as patients will be receiving salbutamol they may become hypokalaemic)
- Chest X-ray to rule out exacerbating factors including pneumothorax or pneumonia

Further management

All patients with life-threatening asthma must be admitted. Those with moderate or acute severe asthma may be considered for discharge home (Figure 60.2). Pitfalls to avoid are summarized in Box 60.2.

Box 60.2 Pitfalls in the management of acute asthma.

- Be vigilant for pneumothoraces; small ones may be difficult to detect.
- Beware of the tiring patient. Escalate treatment and involve the ICU team if:
  - Wheeze disappears: this is a silent chest not an improvement in symptoms
  - $PaCO_2$ normalizes
- If you are giving a one-off stat dose of IV hydrocortisone, ensure you give a dose of oral prednisolone also.
- Ensure at discharge that:
  - Inhaled corticosteroid is started in addition to a course of oral steroids
  - Inhaler technique is checked
  - Smoking cessation advice given if necessary
  - A peak flow meter is given to continue monitoring
  - Specialist follow-up is arranged (urgently for those with an acute, severe or life-threatening episode)

Asthma in pregnancy

Asthma control can deteriorate in pregnancy. Pregnant women with acute asthma should be treated in exactly the same manner as those who are not pregnant. In addition, there should be continuous foetal monitoring and involvement of the obstetric team.

Further reading

British Thoracic Society and Scottish Intercollegiate Guidelines Network (2016) British guideline on the management of asthma: A national clinical guideline. https://www.brit-thoracic.org.uk/document-library/clinical-information/asthma/btssign-asthma-guideline-2016/.

CHAPTER 61

Exacerbation of chronic obstructive pulmonary disease (COPD)

Eui-Sik Suh

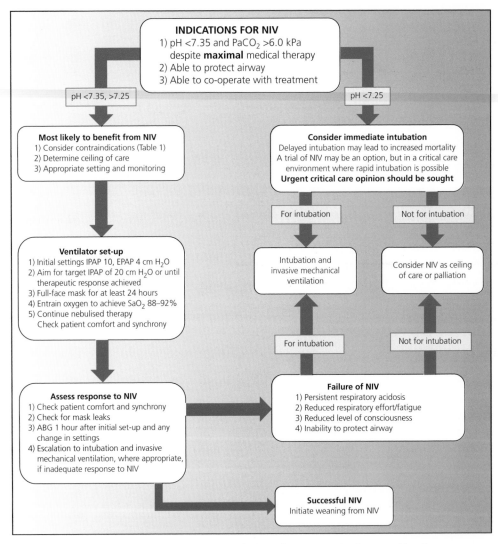

Figure 61.1 Algorithm for the use of NIV in acute exacerbations of COPD. IPAP: inspiratory positive airway pressure; EPAP: expiratory positive airway pressure.

Acute Medicine: A Practical Guide to the Management of Medical Emergencies, Fifth Edition. Edited by David Sprigings and John B. Chambers.
© 2018 John Wiley & Sons Ltd. Published 2018 by John Wiley & Sons Ltd.

- Among hospitalized patients with an exacerbation of COPD, 90-day mortality is 14%, and one-third of patients are readmitted over this period.
- Exacerbations of COPD are associated with a decline in lung function and quality of life, and therefore impose a significant burden on patients and their carers.
- Left ventricular failure and pulmonary embolism may be misdiagnosed as, or be associated with, an acute exacerbation of COPD.
- COPD may be associated with coronary disease. Angina or myocardial infarction may complicate an acute exacerbation of COPD.

Priorities

The working diagnosis is made in a patient with chronic obstructive pulmonary disease (COPD) by an acute change in dyspnoea, cough and/or sputum production, beyond normal day-to-day variation.

Consider pneumonia (Chapter 62), heart failure (Chapter 48) and pulmonary embolism (Chapter 57) in the differential diagnoses; these may coexist with an exacerbation of COPD.

Oxygen

- Give 28% via a Venturi mask.
- Aim initially for arterial oxygen saturation (SaO_2) 88–92% until an arterial blood gas (ABG) sample is obtained.
- If $PaCO_2$ is normal, aim for SaO_2 94–98% unless there is a history of previous hypercapnic (type 2) respiratory failure requiring ventilatory support, but repeat ABG in 1 hour.
- Monitor closely for decreases in respiratory rate and conscious level, as this may indicate oxygen-induced hypercapnic encephalopathy. Repeat ABG if this occurs.
- If the patient is hypercapnic and PaO_2 >8 kPa, consider reducing FiO_2 and repeat ABG.
- If PaO_2 <8 kPa and the patient has a respiratory acidosis, consider NIV (Figure 61.1 and Chapter 113).

Bronchodilators
- Give nebulized salbutamol 2.5–5 mg 4 hourly, although continuous ('back-to-back') salbutamol nebulization may be required in severely breathless patients.
- Ipratropium 0.5 mg up to 4-hourly. Stop long-acting anti-muscarinic agents (e.g. tiotropium) for the duration of ipratropium therapy.

Corticosteroid
- Give prednisolone 30 mg daily for 7–10 days.
- Hydrocortisone (100–200 mg IV 6-hourly) may be given if the patient is unable to swallow tablets.
- In the presence of radiographic consolidation, patient should be treated as having pneumonia; while a substantial proportion of COPD patients with community-acquired pneumonia will be commenced on steroid therapy, there are currently no strong data to support the use of steroids in the routine treatment of severe pneumonia.

Antibiotic therapy
- Indicated if there is a history of increased sputum purulence or radiographic evidence of pneumonia.
- Amoxicillin, doxycycline or macrolides may be appropriate according to local policy.

Table 61.1 Focused clinical assessment in suspected acute exacerbation of COPD.

History

Known COPD? Severity?
- Mild COPD: post-bronchodilator FEV1/forced vital capacity (FVC) ratio <0.7, FEV1 ≥60% predicted
- Moderate COPD: post-bronchodilator FEV1/FVC ratio <0.7, 30%, ≤FEV1 <60% predicted
- Severe COPD: post-bronchodilator FEV1/FVC ratio <0.7, FEV1 <30% predicted

Symptoms
- Breathlessness
- Wheeze
- Increased sputum volume and/or purulence
- Increased use of bronchodilators

Functional limitation
- Reduced exercise tolerance
- Impaired ability to perform activities of daily living

Pre-hospital treatment
- Rescue pack use
- Antibiotics and/or steroids

Disease severity prior to acute episode
- Usual MRC dyspnoea scale score:

Grade	Description of breathlessness
0	Breathless with strenuous exercise
1	Breathless when hurrying on level ground or walking up a slight hill
2	On level ground, walks slower than people of the same age because of breathlessness, or has to stop for breath when walking at own pace
3	Has to stop for breath after walking about 100 yards or after a few minutes on level ground
4	Too breathless to leave the house or breathless when dressing

Previous lung function
Comorbidities, for example cardiac, other respiratory pathology
Exacerbation frequency (e.g. in the previous 12 months)
Previous mechanical ventilation (invasive or non-invasive)

Examination
Conscious level (Glasgow Coma Scale)
Observations (respiratory rate, SaO_2, heart rate, blood pressure, temperature)
Accessory muscle use
Hyperinflated chest
Abdominal paradox
Added lung sounds
Reduced breath sounds
Evidence of cor pulmonale – plethora, oedema
Evidence of hypercapnia – asterixis, bounding pulse

Source: Fletcher CM, Elmes PC, Fairbairn MB, *et al.* (1959) The significance of respiratory symptoms and the diagnosis of chronic bronchitis in a working population. *BMJ* 2, 257. Reproduced with permission of BMJ Publishing Ltd.

Table 61.2 Investigation in suspected acute exacerbation of COPD.

Investigation	Comment
Arterial blood gases and pH	State FiO_2. Note the bicarbonate level to determine whether any respiratory acidosis is acute or acute-on-chronic.
Chest X-ray	Look for pneumothorax, consolidation, other pathologies, for example pulmonary oedema, interstitial lung disease, lung cancer.
ECG	Atrial fibrillation is common in acute exacerbation of COPD. Cardiac ischaemia P Pulmonale
Full blood count	
C-reactive protein	
Electrolytes and creatinine	
Troponin	A stable raised troponin level is associated with a relatively reduced long-term prognosis. A rise, then fall in troponin level suggests associated coronary disease.
BNP or NTproBNP	High BNP levels suggest heart failure and should trigger echocardiography.
Sputum culture	
Swabs for respiratory viruses	
Echocardiography	Warranted if there is a suspicion of left ventricular dysfunction as a cause of breathlessness and wheeze. There is also a high prevalence (at least 31%) of left ventricular dysfunction in patients with severe exacerbations of COPD requiring ICU admission.
CT pulmonary angiography	Indicated in patients who fail to respond to standard therapy or in whom there is a high index of suspicion for pulmonary embolism. Wheeze may be a presenting symptom of pulmonary embolism. In hospitalized patients with exacerbation of COPD, 20% may have pulmonary embolism according to a recent systematic review.

- Intravenous therapy may be indicated in severely unwell patients.
- Adjust antibiotic therapy when sputum or blood cultures become available.

Aminophylline
- Consider giving under expert guidance when conventional bronchodilator therapy has failed.
- There is a narrow therapeutic index and a risk of arrhythmia.
- Cardiac monitoring.
- 250–500 mg (5 mg/kg) IV over 20 minutes unless the patient is already on a theophylline.
- Then 0.5 mg/kg/hour IV infusion.
- Check aminophylline levels within 24 hours of commencing, then as clinically indicated.

Non-invasive ventilation
- In acute hypercapnic respiratory failure complicating an exacerbation of COPD, NIV improves survival, reduces intubation rates and reduces length of ICU stay.
- The use of NIV is summarized in Figure 61.1 and detailed in Chapter 113.

Establishing the ceiling of care
- Predicting survival in COPD patients who require admission to the ICU is difficult: clinicians' estimates of mortality are variable, inaccurate and generally pessimistic.
- Any decision to limit the escalation of care should be made by a senior physician, taking into account the patient's wishes expressed during or before hospital admission. A ruling by the Court of Appeal in England and

Wales in 2014 now places a legal obligation on physicians to consult with patients before making do-not-attempt-resuscitation (DNAR) orders.
- Age, arterial blood pH and reduced conscious level are predictive of mortality. Functional status, body mass index, requirement for supplemental oxygen when stable, comorbidities and previous admissions to the ICU should also be considered when assessing whether invasive mechanical ventilation is appropriate.

Further management

Supportive care
- Ensure a fluid intake of 2–3 L/day.
- Check electrolytes the day after admission. Salbutamol and steroids may result in significant hypokalaemia. Give potassium supplement if the plasma level is <3.5 mmol/L.
- Physiotherapy is of little value unless sputum is copious (>25 mL/day) or there is mucus plugging with lobar atelectasis.
- DVT prophylaxis with stockings/LMW heparin. Assess/treat comorbidities, for example atrial fibrillation, congestive heart failure.

If the patient is not improving, consider:
- Wrong diagnosis: reconsider pneumonia, heart failure and pulmonary embolism. Other causes of respiratory failure with raised $PaCO_2$ are given in Table 23.4. Echocardiography is indicated to exclude left ventricular dysfunction.
- Missed pneumothorax.
- Inadequately treated infection. Consider changing to cefuroxime or cefotaxime IV and adding a macrolide.
- Inadequate bronchodilator therapy. Check that nebulizers are being run at the correct flow rate. Nebulized salbutamol and ipratropium can be given 2-hourly if necessary, or salbutamol can be given by IV infusion 5–30 mg/min (see xxx).
- Cor pulmonale. Fluid retention with peripheral oedema may occur in patients with COPD complicated by acute or chronic respiratory failure even without right ventricular dysfunction. The diagnosis of cor pulmonale is made from a raised JVP, enlarged cardiac silhouette on the chest X-ray, and ECG evidence of right ventricular hypertrophy (not an invariable feature). Obtain an echocardiogram to confirm right ventricular dysfunction, estimate pulmonary artery pressures and exclude left ventricular or aortic/mitral valve disease. Treat fluid retention with a diuretic. There is no definite evidence for the use of digoxin (unless indicated for rate control in atrial fibrillation) or ACE inhibitors in cor pulmonale. Resistant cor pulmonale raises the suspicion of obstructive sleep apnoea.

Arrhythmias
- Supraventricular arrhythmias are common in acute exacerbations of COPD. Check plasma potassium: salbutamol and steroids may result in significant hypokalaemia. Give potassium replacement if plasma potassium is <3.5 mmol/L.
- Treat atrial fibrillation/flutter with digoxin, combined if needed with verapamil or diltiazem. Treat multifocal atrial tachycardia with verapamil if the ventricular rate is >110/min. DC cardioversion is ineffective.

Chest pain
- Chest pain from coronary disease occurs in acute exacerbations of COPD and may be caused by hypoxia, sepsis or tachycardia. A rise and fall in troponin T may also occur without chest pain or acute ECG changes
- Ask for advice from a cardiologist. There is evidence that a beta blocker, aspirin and a statin improve outcome.
- Further cardiac investigation with a functional test may be indicated in individual cases.

Enuring safe discharge

- Patients should be off intravenous therapy for >24 hours before discharge and established on discharge medication.
- Refer for early post-exacerbation pulmonary rehabilitation, and arrange supported discharge package or social support as appropriate.
- Check functional status in the context of the patients' home circumstances.
- Check inhaler technique.
- Prescribe a rescue pack of oral corticosteroids and antibiotics for patients with frequent exacerbations and educate them on recognizing an exacerbation.
- Record spirometry at discharge.
- Give smoking cessation counselling if required.
- Arrange primary care review within 1 week and chest clinic review within 4–6 weeks.

Further reading

Aleva FE, Voets LWLM, Simons SO, et al. (2016) Prevalence and localization of pulmonary embolism in unexplained acute exacerbations of COPD: A systematic review and meta-analysis. *Chest* 151, 544–554.

Davidson AC, Banham S, Elliott M, et al. (2016) British Thoracic Society/Intensive Care Society Acute Hypercapnic Respiratory Failure Guideline Development Group. BTS/ICS Guidelines for the ventilatory management of acute hypercapnic respiratory failure in adults. *Thorax* 71, ii1–ii35. https://www.brit-thoracic.org.uk/document-library/clinical-information/acute-hypercapnic-respiratory-failure/ bts-guidelines-for-ventilatory-management-of-ahrf/. Global Initiative for Chronic Obstructive Lung Disease website: http://goldcopd.org/

MacDonald MI, Shafuddin E, King PT, Chang CL, Bardin PG, Hancox R.J. (2016) Cardiac dysfunction during exacerbations of chronic obstructive pulmonary disease. *Lancet Respir Med* 4, 138–148.

Vanfleteren LEGW, Spruit MA, Wouters EFM, Franssen F.M.E. (2016) Management of chronic obstructive pulmonary disease beyond the lungs. *Lancet Respir Med* 4, 911–924.

CHAPTER 62

Community-acquired pneumonia

AHMED YOUSUF

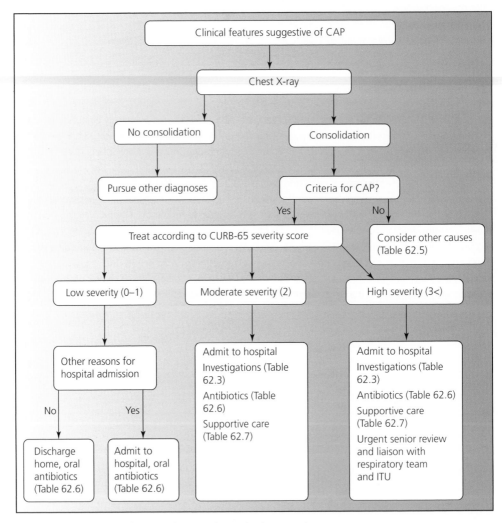

Figure 62.1 Management of suspected community-acquired pneumonia.

Acute Medicine: A Practical Guide to the Management of Medical Emergencies, Fifth Edition. Edited by David Springings and John B. Chambers.
© 2018 John Wiley & Sons Ltd. Published 2018 by John Wiley & Sons Ltd.

Box 62.1 Definitions.

Community-acquired pneumonia: pneumonia acquired outside hospital (including residency in a care home or nursing home), or which appears within 48 h of admission to hospital.

Hospital-acquired pneumonia: pneumonia that develops 48 h or longer after hospital admission, and was not subclinical on admission.

Lower respiratory tract infection: an acute illness with cough and at least one other lower respiratory tract symptom, presumed to be due to infection. The definition includes pneumonia, acute bronchitis and infective exacerbation of chronic obstructive pulmonary disease.

Community-acquired pneumonia (CAP) (see Box 62.1 for definition) usually presents with acute respiratory symptoms, but should always be considered in patients with unexplained sepsis or delirium. Examination of the chest may be normal and, if you suspect pneumonia, a chest X-ray is need to make the diagnosis.

A broad range of pathogens can cause CAP. *Streptococcus pneumoniae* (pneumococcus) is the most common bacterial pathogen, accounting for up to 50% of cases. Other common pathogens are *Staph. aureus, Legionella pneumophila* and influenza.

Priorities

Is this pneumonia? How severe is it?
- Suspect pneumonia in the presence of one or more of the following clinical features:
  - Fever
  - Cough
  - Purulent sputum
  - Pleuritic chest pain
  - Focal lung crackles or bronchial breathing
- Consider the differential diagnosis (Table 62.1). A chest X-ray showing new focal shadowing is essential for the diagnosis (Table 62.2). Other investigations needed are given in Table 62.3. For low severity (CURB-65 = 0–1) urine antigen or serological investigations may be considered during outbreaks (e.g. Legionnaires' disease) or epidemic mycoplasma years, or when there is a particular clinical or epidemiological reason.
- The severity of CAP can be assessed by the CURB-65 score (Table 62.4).

Choice of initial antibiotic therapy for CAP
- Your initial therapy depends on the clinical setting, severity of pneumonia and local antimicrobial policy (Table 62.5).
- Start antibiotic therapy as soon as diagnosis of CAP is suspected. Antibiotics should not be withheld if there is a delay in taking blood for culture.

Further management

Oxygen
Humidified O_2 should be continued to keep arterial PaO_2 >8.0 kPa, oxygen saturation >92% (>88% in patients with chronic obstructive pulmonary disease).

Table 62.1 Differential diagnosis of suspected pneumonia.

Disorder	Comment
Cardiovascular disorders	
Pulmonary embolism	Risk factor(s) for venous thromboembolism
	Sudden-onset shortness of breath
	See Chapter 57.
Tricuspid valve endocarditis	IVDU or indwelling venous cannula e.g. for haemodialysis in blood cultures.
Neoplastic disorders	
Bronchial carcinoma	Weight loss, chronic cough, abnormal CXR (nodule or mass, mediastinal lymphadenopathy)
Alveolar cell carcinoma	Similar CXR appearance to pneumonia. If there is no leucocytosis or fever or if the patient doesn't respond to antibiotics.
Immune-mediated disorders	
Wegener granulomatosis	Haematuria, haemoptysis, epistaxis, scleritis, uveitis
Diffuse alveolar haemorrhage in pulmonary-renal syndromes	Haematuria, haemoptysis, positive anti-GBM, ANCA antibodies
Systemic lupus erythematosus	Skin rash, sensitivity to sunlight, positive ANA
Acute interstitial pneumonia	Ground glass changes and traction bronchiectasis on HRCT
Eosinophilic pneumonia syndromes	Peripheral blood eosinophilia, peripheral infiltrate within the outer two-thirds of the lung fields on X-ray, responds to steroids
Bronchiolitis obliterans – organizing pneumonia	Acute to subacute onset of symptoms, migratory patchy infiltrates on X-ray, responds to steroids
Other disorders	
Drug toxicity (e.g. amiodarone pneumonitis)	Restrictive spirometry, decreased gas transfer, responds to steroids and stopping offending drug(s)
Radiation pneumonitis	History of recent radiotherapy, responds to steroids

Table 62.2 Chest X-ray findings in pneumonia.

Element	Comment
Focal shadowing	Required to make the diagnosis of pneumonia.
	Lobar pneumonia is the result of disease that starts in the periphery and spreads from one alveolus to another. As the disease reaches a fissure, this will result in a sharp delineation, since consolidation will not cross a fissure. The alveoli that surround the bronchi become denser and the bronchi become more visible, resulting in an air-bronchogram.
	Bronchopneumonia starts in the airways as acute bronchitis. It will lead to multifocal ill-defined densities. When it progresses it can produce diffuse consolidation.
Pleural effusion	If present, arrange for ultrasound-guided aspiration of effusion and send samples for Gram stain and culture, pH and biochemistry (LDH, protein, glucose).
Cavitation	Associated with tuberculosis and *Staphylococcus aureus* infection, but may also occur in Gram-negative and anaerobic infections.
Lung abscess	Chest X-ray typically demonstrates an air-fluid level, but chest CT is more sensitive and can confirm the diagnosis in difficult cases. Most patients with lung abscess do well with conservative management and a prolonged course of antibiotics.
Pneumothorax	May occur in cavitating pneumonia and is particularly associated with *Pneumocystis jiroveci* pneumonia (Chapter 34).

Table 62.3 Urgent investigations in suspected community acquired pneumonia.

Test	Comment
Chest X-ray	See Table 62.2.
Full blood count	Leucocytosis or leucopenia are markers of sepsis and severe infection.
Electrolytes, urea and creatinine	To assess renal function and disease severity (urea >7.0).
C-reactive protein	As biomarker of treatment response.
Liver function tests	The identification of underlying or associated hepatic disease.
Arterial blood gases (ABG)	If oxygen saturations <92% on air, or in patients with COPD to assess for type 2 respiratory failure.
Urine for Legionella antigen	In those with severe CAP or during an outbreak.
Blood culture	Identification of pathogens and antibiotic sensitivity patterns allows selection of optimal antibiotic regimens. Blood for culture must be taken prior to starting antibiotics.
'Atypical' serology	For patients with severe CAP or unresponsive to beta lactam antibiotics. 'Atypical' pathogens that cause pneumonia are *Mycoplasma pneumoniae*, *Chlamydia pneumoniae*, *Chlamydia psittaci* and *Coxiella burnetii*.
Sputum culture	For patients with CAP who are able to expectorate sputum. Sputum samples should be sent for Gram stain, culture and sensitivity tests.
HIV test	HIV testing should be offered to all adult patients with community-acquired pneumonia.

Fluid balance

- Insensible losses are greater than normal due to fever (allow 500 mL/day/°C fever) and tachypnoea.
- Patients with severe pneumonia should receive IV fluids (2–3 L/day), with daily assessment of fluid status and measurement of renal function. Adequate hydration also helps with expectoration of sputum.

Antibiotic therapy

- Review this after 48 h. If there has been clinical improvement, with a fall in C-reactive protein level, switch to oral therapy in those patients initially given IV therapy.
- Management of patients who fail to improve after 48 h antibiotic therapy is discussed below (see Problems).

Venous thromboembolism prophylaxis

Give prophylaxis with anti-embolism stockings and low-molecular-weight heparin.

Table 62.4 CURB-65 Score.

Score 1 point each for:

- New **C**onfusion (abbreviated mental test score 8 or less, or new disorientation)
- Blood **U**rea >7.0 mmol/L
- **R**espiratory rate >30 breaths/min
- Low **B**lood pressure (systolic BP <90 mmHg or diastolic BP <60 mmHg)
- Age ≥**65** years).

Score 0–1: low severity (mortality <3%): manage as outpatient.
Score 2: moderate severity (mortality 9%): admit to general or respiratory ward.
Score 3 or more: high severity (mortality of 15–40%): admit to HDU or ICU.

Table 62.5 Initial empirical treatment regimens for community-acquired pneumonia in adults (source: adapted from British Thoracic Society guidelines).

Severity	Site	Preferred treatment	Penicillin allergy
Low (CURB-65 = 0–1, mortality <3%)	Home	Amoxicillin 500 mg TDS orally for 5 days.	Doxycycline 200 mg loading dose then 100 mg orally *or* clarithromycin 500 mg bd orally for 5 days.
Low severity (CURB-65 = 0–1, mortality <3%) but admission indicated for reasons other than pneumonia severity (e.g. social reasons)	Hospital	Amoxicillin 500 mg tds orally. If oral administration not possible: amoxicillin 500 mg tds IV for 5 days.	Doxycycline 200 mg loading dose then 100 mg od orally *or* clarithromycin 500 mg bd orally for 5 days.
Moderate severity (CURB-65 = 2, 9% mortality)	Hospital	Amoxicillin 500 mg –1.0 g tds orally *plus* clarithromycin 500 mg bd orally. If oral administration not possible: amoxicillin 500 mg tds IV *plus* clarithromycin 500 mg bd IV.	Doxycycline 200 mg loading dose then 100 mg orally *or* levofloxacin 500 mg od orally *or* moxifloxacin 400 mg od orally.
High severity (CURB-65 = 3–5, 15–40% mortality)	Hospital	Co-amoxiclav 1.2 g tds IV plus clarithromycin 500 mg bd IV.	Vancomycin 1.g bd IV plus clarithromycin 500.mg bd IV or Lower case 500 mg bd IV or Cefuroxime 1.5 g tds IV or cefotaxime 1 g tds IV or ceftriaxone 2 g od IV, plus clarithromycin 500 mg bd IV

Pain relief

Relieve pleuritic chest pain with paracetamol and/or NSAIDs, to facilitate sputum expectoration.

Chest physiotherapy

- Chest physiotherapy is helpful if the patient is producing sputum but having difficulty expectorating it, and in bronchiectasis.
- Nebulized hypertonic saline may be helpful when sputum is thick and difficult to expectorate, but tends to cause a greater degree of bronchoconstriction than normal saline. Give bronchodilator therapy before nebulized hypertonic saline.

Bronchodilator therapy

Nebulized salbutamol or ipratropium should be prescribed to patients with asthma or COPD if there is wheeze.

Checklist before discharge

Clinically stable for >24 h:
- Normal mental state (or at baseline)
- Temperature <37.5 °C
- Respiratory rate <24/min
- Arterial oxygen saturation breathing air >92% (>88% if COPD)
- Heart rate <100/min
- Systolic BP >90 mmHg

- Able to eat without assistance (or at baseline)
- Able to walk at least short distances unaided (or close to preadmission functional status)
- Social support at home organized if needed
- Advice on smoking cessation given if needed
- General practitioner follow-up arranged within one week
- Follow-up appointment in chest clinic at six weeks, with chest X-ray taken before visit

Problems

Failure to improve after 48 h antibiotic therapy

Address the following points:
- Review the clinical, microbiological and radiological findings.
  - Are you confident the diagnosis is pneumonia (consider the diagnoses in Table 62.1), and that the patient's current antibiotic therapy is appropriate for the possible pathogens?
  - Consider broadening your antibiotic therapy, in case the organism is unusual or resistant: ask advice from a microbiologist.
- Re-examine the patient, and check for signs of metastatic infection, such as septic arthritis, pericarditis or infective endocarditis.
- Repeat the chest X-ray. Are there any new findings such as cavitation or pleural effusion? If pleural fluid is now present, this should be aspirated and sent for Gram stain and culture. If the fluid is cloudy rather than mildly turbid, drain completely and treat as empyema (discuss with a chest physician). A pH <7.20 also favours empyema rather than a parapneumonic effusion.
- In an IV drug user or a patient with an indwelling venous cannula consider tricuspid valve endocarditis with septic pulmonary emboli.
- Consider underlying airways or lung disease, such as chronic obstructive pulmonary disease, bronchiectasis, bronchial carcinoma and inhaled foreign body.
- Consider pulmonary tuberculosis in patients with risk factors for TB. Send sputum for Ziehl-Neelsen stain. If no sputum is being produced, consider fibreoptic bronchoscopy. A Mantoux skin test (0.1 mL or 1 in 10,000 intradermally) may be performed, but interpretation can be difficult – a strongly positive test is good evidence of active infection, but a negative reaction can occur in the presence of active infection.
- Consider HIV/AIDS. Test for HIV if this has not already been done.
- Ask advice from a chest physician. CT or fibreoptic bronchoscopy may be indicated to clarify the diagnosis.

Further reading

National Institute for Health and Care Excellence (2014) Pneumonia in adults: diagnosis and management. Clinical guideline (CG191). https://www.nice.org.uk/guidance/cg191

Prina E, Ranzani OT, Torres A. (2015) Community-acquired pneumonia. *Lancet* 386, 1097–1108.

CHAPTER 63

Hospital-acquired pneumonia

AHMED YOUSUF

Hospital-acquired (or nosocomial) pneumonia (HAP) (Box 63.1) is defined as a lower respiratory **tract** infection occurring 48 h or more after admission which was not incubating at the time of admission.

Consider hospital-acquired pneumonia in a patient with:

- New cough productive of purulent sputum or purulent tracheal secretions
- Acute breathlessness (Chapter 10)
- Increased oxygen requirement/respiratory failure (Chapter 11)
- New delirium
- Core temperature >38 or <36 °C

Priorities

Make a rapid but systematic assessment using the ABCDE approach (Chapter 1).

Airway: ensure a clear airway (Chapters 59 and 112). If the airway is compromised, seek urgent help from an anaesthetist.

Box 63.1 Hospital-acquired pneumonia.

Hospital-acquired pneumonia (HAP) affects 0.5–1.0% of inpatients and is the commonest healthcare-associated infection contributing to death.

The mortality rate of HAP is between 30–70%. It increases hospital stay by 7–9 days.

In immunocompetent patients, HAP is typically caused by bacteria (e.g. *Pseudomonas aeruginosa*, *Escherichia coli*, *Klebsiella pneumoniae*, *Staphylococcus aureus*) and rarely by viral or fungal pathogens.

Risk factors for hospital-acquired pneumonia are:

- Age >70
- Chronic lung disease
- Diabetes
- Reduced level of consciousness
- Recent chest or abdominal surgery
- Mechanical ventilation
- Nasogastric feeding
- Immunosuppression (e.g. long-term corticosteroid use, chemotherapy)

Acute Medicine: A Practical Guide to the Management of Medical Emergencies, Fifth Edition. Edited by David Sprigings and John B. Chambers.
© 2018 John Wiley & Sons Ltd. Published 2018 by John Wiley & Sons Ltd.

Table 63.1 Initial antibiotic therapy of hospital-acquired pneumonia (HAP).

| Severity of HAP | Initial antibiotic therapy | |
	No penicillin allergy	Penicillin allergy
Non-severe	Co-amoxiclav 1.2 g 8-hourly IV for 5–10 days[*]	Clarithroymycin 500 mg 12-hourly IV/PO for 5–10 days
Severe[†]	Tazocin 4.5 g 8-hourly IV + gentamicin for 5–10 days or Ceftazidime 1 g 8-hourly IV + gentamicin (+ vancomycin if MRSA is suspected)	Meropenem 0.5–1 g 8-hourly IV + gentamicin or Levofloxacin 500 mg 12-hourly IV

[*] Consider switching to oral therapy after 48 h if there is clinical improvement and plasma C-reactive protein level is falling.
[†] Treat as severe HAP if any of the following are present: rapidly progressive consolidation on chest X-ray; respiratory rate >30, PaO_2 <8 kPa, high oxygen requirement; shock (systolic BP <90 mmHg or diastolic BP <60 mmHg); admitted to high dependency unit or intubated and ventilated.

Breathing: maintain adequate oxygenation. Give supplemental oxygen as needed to maintain oxygen saturation at 94–96% (88–92% if known chronic obstructive pulmonary disease and at risk of CO_2 retention).

Circulation: maintain adequate cardiac output/systemic blood pressure:

- Volume-replacement with IV crystalloid if dehydrated.
- Correct major arrhythmia (Chapter 39). Rate-control if fast atrial fibrillation (Chapter 43).

  While doing this, collect information about the patient, the current problem, the context and comorbidities. Establish what has been decided regarding the ceiling of care and resuscitation status of the patient.

Check arterial blood gases, arrange a chest X-ray and record an ECG

See Chapter 11 for management of respiratory failure. Compare the chest X-ray with previous chest X-rays if available. Focal shadowing (Table 62.2) is required to make the diagnosis of pneumonia. Consider the differential diagnosis (Table 62.1). CT chest may be needed in patients with abnormal chest X-ray.

If the working diagnosis is hospital-acquired pneumonia, start antibiotic therapy (Table 63.1)

The choice of antibiotic therapy is governed by local hospital policy (which takes into account knowledge of local microbial pathogens). Seek advice from a microbiologist on antibiotic therapy for patients with severe hospital-acquired pneumonia. Treat as severe HAP if any of the following are present:

- Rapidly progressive consolidation on CXR
- Respiratory rate >30, PaO_2 <8 kPa, high oxygen requirement
- Shock (systolic BP <90 mmHg or diastolic BP <60 mmHg)
- Admitted to high dependency unit or patient is intubated and ventilated.

  Consider switching to oral therapy after 48 h if there is clinical improvement and plasma C-reactive protein level is falling.

  If aspiration pneumonia is suspected (Appendix 63.1; Table 63.2), discuss further management and whether bronchoscopy is indicated with a chest physician or intensivist.

Appendix 63.1 Aspiration pneumonia syndromes

- Aspiration is the misdirection of oropharyngeal or gastric contents into the larynx and lower respiratory tract. Around 45% of healthy people aspirate during sleep. Aspiration is more common in hospital patients,

Table 63.2 Aspiration pneumonia syndromes.

Inoculum	Effects on airway and lungs	Clinical features	Management
Acid	Chemical pneumonitis	Acute dyspnoea, tachypnoea, possible cyanosis, bronchospasm, fever, pink frothy sputum, infiltrates in one or both lower lobes, hypoxaemia	Positive-pressure breathing, IV fluids, tracheal suction
Oropharyngeal bacteria	Bacterial infection	Usually insidious onset; cough, fever, purulent sputum, infiltrate involving dependent pulmonary segment or lobe, with or without cavitation	Antibiotic therapy (Table 63.1)
Inert fluids	Mechanical obstruction, reflex airway closure	Acute dyspnoea, cyanosis, pulmonary oedema	Tracheal suction, intermittent positive-pressure breathing with oxygen, bronchodilator
Particulate matter	Mechanical obstruction	Dependent on level of obstruction, ranging from acute apnoea to chronic cough with or without recurrent infections	Extraction of particulate matter, antibiotic therapy (Table 63.1)

particularly after a stroke or with a reduced conscious level, when the upper airway becomes colonized with Gram-negative bacteria.

- Conditions that predispose to aspiration pneumonia include:
  - Reduced consciousness, resulting in a compromise of the cough reflex and glottic closure
  - Dysphasia from neurologic deficits
  - Disorders of the upper gastrointestinal tract including oesophageal disease, surgery involving the upper airways or oesophagus, and gastric reflux
  - Mechanical disruption of the glottic closure due to tracheostomy, endotracheal intubation, bronchoscopy, upper GI endoscopy, and nasogastric feeding
  - Protracted vomiting
  - Large volume NG tube feedings
  - Feeding gastrostomy
- Aspiration pneumonia syndromes and management is summarized in Table 63.2.

Further reading

Infectious Diseases Society of America and the American Thoracic Society (2016) Management of adults with hospital-acquired and ventilator-associated pneumonia: 2016 Clinical Practice Guidelines by the Infectious Diseases Society of America and the American Thoracic Society. *Clinical Infectious Diseases* 63, e61–e111. http://cid.oxfordjournals.org/content/63/5/e61.long.

CHAPTER 64

Pneumothorax

ROB HALLIFAX

Consider pneumothorax (Table 64.1) in any patient with:

- Sudden breathlessness or chest pain, particularly in young, otherwise fit adults or following invasive procedures, for example subclavian vein cannulation, lung biopsy, chest aspiration.
- Exacerbation of chronic obstructive pulmonary disease (or rarely asthma): pneumothorax may be painless and contribute to respiratory failure.
- Hypoxia, an increase in inflation pressure or unexplained hypotension in the mechanically ventilated patient: asymmetry of chest expansion is a useful clue.

Management of suspected pneumothorax is summarized in Figure 64.1.

Box 64.1 The chest X-ray in suspected pneumothorax.

Pneumothorax is diagnosed by the presence of a white visceral pleural line on the chest X-ray, with no pulmonary vessels visible beyond this.

Look carefully at the lung parenchyma for evidence of underlying disease.

Contralateral shift of the trachea and mediastinum with depression of the hemi-diaphragm are typical features of tension pneumothorax although may not always be evident.

Do not mistake an emphysematous bulla for a small pneumothorax. Points in favour of a bulla are:

- Adhesions between the lung and the parietal pleura
- A scallop-shaped edge to the cavity
- Faint markings over the lucency caused by the lung enfolding the bulla
- The presence of other bullae

If you suspect a pneumothorax, but the chest X-ray appears normal, recheck the lung apices and the right border of the heart. In the supine patient look for:

- Unusually sharp appearance of the cardiac border or diaphragm, with increased transradiancy of the adjacent parts of the thorax and abdomen
- A vertical line parallel to the chest wall (caused by retraction of the middle lobe from the chest wall)
- A diagonal line from the heart to the costophrenic angle

Acute Medicine: A Practical Guide to the Management of Medical Emergencies, Fifth Edition. Edited by David Sprigings and John B. Chambers.
© 2018 John Wiley & Sons Ltd. Published 2018 by John Wiley & Sons Ltd.

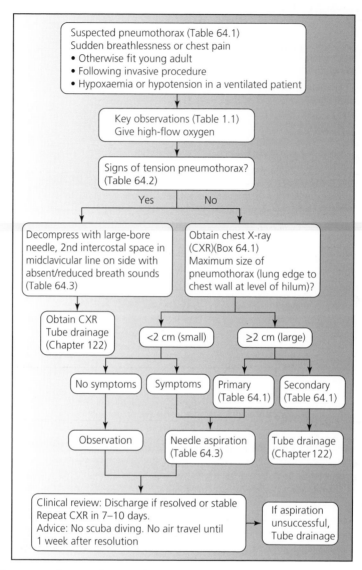

Figure 64.1 Management of suspected pneumothorax.

Table 64.1 Classification and causes of pneumothorax.

Spontaneous pneumothorax

Primary (PSP)
- No clinical lung disease
- Typically occurs in tall thin males aged 15–30 years
- Association with tobacco and cannabis smoking
- Rare in patients aged over 40

Secondary (SSP)
- Airways disease (COPD, cystic fibrosis, acute severe asthma)
- Infectious lung disease (*Pneumocystis carinii* (*jiroveci*) pneumonia; necrotizing pneumonia caused by anaerobic, Gram-negative bacteria or *Staphylococcus aureus*)

- Interstitial lung disease (e.g. sarcoidosis)
- Connective tissue disease (e.g. rheumatoid arthritis, Marfan syndrome)
- Malignancy (bronchial carcinoma or sarcoma)
- Thoracic endometriosis ('catamenial' pneumothorax)

Traumatic pneumothorax (due to penetrating or blunt chest trauma) should be managed by surgical team

Iatrogenic pneumothorax
- Transthoracic needle aspiration
- Subclavian vein puncture
- Thoracentesis and lung biopsy
- Pericardiocentesis
- Barotrauma related to mechanical ventilation

COPD, chronic obstructive pulmonary disease.

Table 64.2 Signs of tension pneumothorax.

- Respiratory distress (dyspnoea, tachypnoea, ability to speak only in short sentences or single words, agitation, sweating)
- Falling arterial oxygen saturation
- Ipsilateral hyperexpansion, hypomobility, hyperresonance with decreased breath sounds
- Tachycardia
- Hypotension (late sign)
- Tracheal deviation (inconsistent sign)
- Elevated jugular venous pressure (inconsistent sign)

Table 64.3 Needle aspiration of pneumothorax.

1 Identify the 2nd or 3rd intercostal space in the mid-clavicular line.
2 Infiltrate with lidocaine down to and around the pleura.
3 Connect a 21 G (green) needle to a three-way tap and a 60 mL syringe.
4 With the patient semi-recumbent, insert the needle into the pleural space. Withdraw air and expel it via the three-way tap.
5 Aspirate up to a maximum of 2.5 L.
6 Obtain a chest X-ray to assess resolution of the pneumothorax.
7 If aspiration fails to sufficiently re-inflate the lung, insert small bore (<14F) chest drain (Chapter 122).

Further reading

Bintcliff AJ, Hallifax RJ, Edey A, *et al.* (2015) Spontaneous pneumothorax: time to rethink management? *Lancet Respir Med* 3, 578–88.

Pasquier M, Hugli O, Carron PN. (2013) Videos in clinical medicine. Needle aspiration of primary spontaneous pneumothorax. *N Engl J Med* 368, e24. http://www.nejm.org/doi/full/10.1056/NEJMvcm1111468.

Tschopp J-M, Bintcliffe O, Astoul P, *et al.* (2015) European Respiratory Society task force statement: diagnosis and treatment of primary spontaneous pneumothorax. *Eur Respir J* 46, 321–335. http://erj.ersjournals.com/content/erj/46/2/321.full.pdf.

Neurological

CHAPTER 65

Stroke

Tony Rudd and Ajay Bhalla

Stroke typically causes rapidly-developing neurological symptoms or coma. About 85% of strokes are due to cerebral infarction (Appendix 65.1), for which thrombolysis should be considered. Headache, vomiting and coma at onset are more common in haemorrhagic stroke, but accurate differentiation requires computed tomography (CT), which should be done immediately in suspected stroke. Management is summarized in Figure 65.1.

Priorities

1 **If the patient is unconscious**, initial resuscitation is as for coma from any cause (Chapter 3). Check blood glucose to exclude hyper- or hypoglycaemia.
2 **Is this a stroke and not another disease mimicking stroke?**
   - The clinical assessment of the patient with suspected stroke is summarized in Tables 65.1 and 65.2, and investigations needed urgently in Table 65.3.
   - Differentiation of stroke from stroke-like presentations of other diseases can sometimes be difficult. The acute onset (or presence on waking from sleep) of asymmetric face, arm or leg weakness, speech disturbance or visual field defect support a diagnosis of stroke. Fever at presentation, prominent headache, or neck stiffness should make you consider alternative diagnoses. Syncope or seizure activity suggest against the diagnosis.
   - The disorders which are most commonly misdiagnosed as stroke are summarized in Table 65.4, and atypical presentations of stroke in Table 65.5.
3 **If the working diagnosis is stroke due to cerebral infarction, is thrombolysis or thrombectomy indicated?**

Thrombolysis
- This should only be considered when the patient is in a hospital with a well-organized stroke service, which has trained staff, immediate access to neuroimaging, protocols in place to manage complications, and systems to audit outcomes. Indications for thrombolysis are:
  - Any patient, regardless of age or stroke severity, where treatment can be started within 3 h of known symptom onset and who has been shown not to have an intracerebral haemorrhage or other contra-indications (Table 65.6).
  - Between 3 and 4.5 h of known symptom onset, patients under 80 years who have been shown not to have an intracerebral haemorrhage or other contraindication.
  - Between 4.5 and 6 h of known symptom onset, patients should be considered on an individual basis, recognizing that the benefits to treatment are likely to be smaller but that the risks of a worse outcome, including death, will not be increased.
- Table 65.7 summarizes how to administer alteplase for thrombolysis.

Acute Medicine: A Practical Guide to the Management of Medical Emergencies, Fifth Edition. Edited by David Sprigings and John B. Chambers.
© 2018 John Wiley & Sons Ltd. Published 2018 by John Wiley & Sons Ltd.

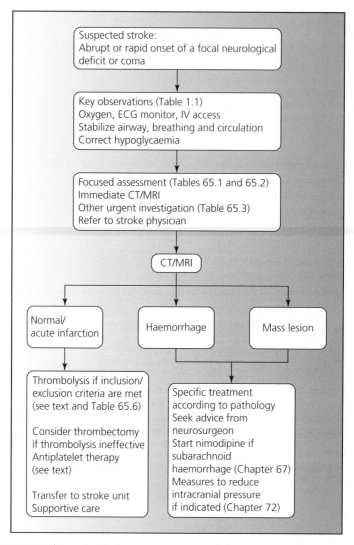

Figure 65.1 Management of suspected stroke.

Thrombectomy

- Clot retrieval for selected patients with proximal anterior and middle cerebral artery occlusion is beneficial, and while few centres currently offer this service, it should be considered if thrombolysis is ineffective.
- Thrombectomy is time-critical and should be undertaken in centres with the relevant expertise within a maximum of 6 h of the onset of symptoms.

Anti-platelet therapy

- Aspirin 300 mg once daily for 14 days should be started 24 h after thrombolysis, or as soon as possible within 48 h of the onset of symptoms in patients who do not receive thrombolysis.
- Patients with aspirin hypersensitivity, or those intolerant of aspirin despite co-administration of a proton pump inhibitor, should receive clopidogrel 75 mg once daily.

Table 65.1 Focused assessment of the patient with suspected stroke.

History

Pattern of onset
Time of onset or when last known to be well
Medication and compliance (particularly anticoagulants)
Previous level of function and comorbidities

Examination
General – hydration, temperature
Cardiovascular – blood pressure, heart rate and rhythm, peripheral circulation, carotid bruits
Respiratory – oxygenation, evidence of infection
Alimentary – swallowing
Skin – pressure areas
Urological – bladder, continence
Neurological: see Table 65.2

Table 65.2 National Institute of Health Stroke Score (NIHSS). This should be completed on all patients with stroke to ensure that the stroke deficits are collected in a systematic way and the less obvious signs of stroke are not missed.

Level of consciousness	Alert	0
	Not alert, but arousable with minor stimuli	1
	Not alert, needs repeated stimuli	2
	Coma	3
Level of consciousness questions	Answers both correctly	0
	Answers one correctly	1
	Answers both incorrectly	2
Level of consciousness commands	Performs both correctly	0
	Performs one correctly	1
	Performs neither correctly	2
Best gaze	Normal	0
	Partial gaze palsy	1
	Forced deviation	2
Visual field testing	No visual loss	0
	Partial hemianopia	1
	Complete hemianopia	2
	Bilateral hemianopia	3
Facial paresis	Normal facial movements	0
	Minor paralysis	1
	Partial paralysis	2
	Complete paralysis of one or both sides	3
Right arm motor function	No drift	0
	Drift	1
	Some effort against gravity	2
	No effort against gravity	3
	No movement	4
Left arm motor function	No drift	0
	Drift	1
	Some effort against gravity	2
	No effort against gravity	3
	No movement	4

(*continued*)

Table 65.2 (*Continued*)

Right leg motor function	No drift	0
	Drift	1
	Some effort against gravity	2
	No effort against gravity	3
	No movement	4
Left leg motor function	No drift	0
	Drift	1
	Some effort against gravity	2
	No effort against gravity	3
	No movement	4
Limb ataxia	Absent	0
	Present one limb	1
	Present two limbs	2
Sensory	Normal	0
	Mild to moderate loss	1
	Severe to total	2
Best language	Normal	0
	Mild to moderate aphasia	1
	Severe aphasia	2
	Mute	3
Dysarthria	Normal	0
	Mild to moderate	1
	Severe/mute/anarthric	2
Extinction/inattention	No abnormality	0
	Visual, tactile, auditory or personal inattention	1
	Profound hemi inattention of extinction to more than one modality	2

Further management

All stroke patients should be managed on a stroke unit unless other conditions requiring specialist care dominate (e.g. need for intensive care).
- Specialist interdisciplinary care is the most significant intervention that is available for the management of stroke patients.
- All stroke patients should have access to inpatient stroke-specific rehabilitation facilities, followed by early supported discharge to community stroke teams and longer-term rehabilitation.

Table 65.3 Urgent investigation in suspected stroke.

Blood glucose
Full blood count
Coagulation screen if on anticoagulants or suspicion of bleeding disorder
Haemoglobin electrophoresis if possible sickle cell disease or thalassaemia
Creatinine and electrolytes
Lipids
Blood culture if febrile at presentation
ECG
Chest X-ray
CT head

Table 65.4 Diseases which may mimic stroke.

Disease	Comment
Subdural haematoma	May present with focal neurological deficits. Often no history of trauma. May have headache, fluctuating symptoms and signs. Diagnosis on brain imaging.
Subarachnoid haemorrhage	Classically presents with sudden onset headache with or without focal neurological signs. Diagnosis on brain imaging and lumbar puncture.
Brain tumour	Often progressive symptoms with or without symptoms of raised intracranial pressure. Diagnosis with contrast enhanced brain imaging.
Encephalitis	More often global signs such as clouding of consciousness, confusion, headache together with symptoms and signs of sepsis. Can have focal neurology. Diagnosis on lumbar puncture.
Hypertensive encephalopathy and posterior reversible encephalopathy syndrome (PRES)	Usually generalized rather than focal symptoms such as headache, vomiting, clouding consciousness and seizures. May present with cortical blindness and other visual disturbance. Diagnosis on brain imaging and clinical picture. Patients often make good recovery with reversal of radiological abnormalities.
Cerebral vasculitis	Presents with focal neurological signs, sometimes in patients with known systemic vasculitis. Fluctuating course. Diagnosis on brain imaging, inflammatory and autoimmune markers and may need brain biopsy.

- Cognitive and mood disturbance after stroke are common and psychological support may be needed.
- The underlying cause of the stroke needs to be established and appropriate secondary prevention provided.

Supportive care

- Rehabilitation should start early, although intensive mobilization within the first few hours of the stroke should be avoided.
- Maintain close observation and management of normal homeostasis, for example hydration, electrolytes, nutrition, oxygenation, temperature.

Table 65.5 Some atypical presentations of stroke.

Site of stroke	Clinical features
Brainstem	Isolated cranial nerve disorders, vertigo, crossed motor and sensory signs, ataxia
Frontal lobe	Change in behaviour/personality without focal neurological signs
Localized language area	Mobile aphasic patient often initially diagnosed as delirium/dementia
Bilateral thalamic infarction	Confusion
Pons	Locked in syndrome
Cortical lesions	Focal seizures
Basal ganglia	Abnormal movements, for example asterixis, hemifacial spasms
Visual cortex	Isolated visual symptoms, for example Anton's syndrome, Balint's syndrome
Frontal or posterolateral parietal lobe	Alien hand syndrome

Table 65.6 Contraindications to thrombolysis for cerebral infarction.

Evidence of intracerebral haemorrhage or previous intracerebral haemorrhage
Time of onset 6 h or more before treatment or evidence on the scan of established recent infarction
Uncontrolled hypertension (above 185/110 mmHg)
Witnessed seizure at stroke onset
Taking warfarin with INR >1.7, or a direct-acting oral anticoagulant
Bleeding diathesis
Severe previous neurological disability
Arterial puncture or bleeding at non-compressible site within last 7 days
Within 14 days of major surgery
Rapidly improving symptoms

- Patients with primary intracerebral haemorrhage presenting within the first 6 h of the onset and with a systolic blood pressure of over 150 mmHg should have their blood pressure lowered to 140 mmHg for at least 7 days unless there is any contraindication. Patients with ischaemic stroke should have their blood pressure kept below 185/110 mmHg.
- Screen for swallowing abnormalities before any food or fluid is given and certainly within 4 h of admission. This should be done using a standardized screening protocol such as one that first checks the ability of the patient to cough and then goes on to test the ability to swallow teaspoons of water, followed by a glass of water. If a patient is unable to swallow safely, start feeding with a nasogastric tube within 24 h of admission. If intravenous fluids are required (and enteral hydration is preferred) then avoid the use of glucose solutions as hyperglycaemia may worsen outcomes.
- Venous thrombo-embolism is common. Do not use anticoagulants even in low dose for prophylaxis. Evidence shows that intermittent pneumatic compression devices are safe and effective at preventing DVT in patients with hemiparetic legs. TED stockings (both short and long) should not be used. At best they are useless, uncomfortable and expensive, at worst harmful.
- Patients should be carefully monitored for infection, which should be treated early. This requires monitoring of temperature, pulse, blood pressure and oxygen saturation, at least daily examination of the chest, and monitoring for urinary tract infection. There is no evidence to support the use of prophylactic antibiotics after stroke.
- Depression is very common after stroke and can be difficult to identify, particularly in dysphasic patients. All patients should be screened for depression. Cognitive behavioural therapy is usually the treatment of first choice.

Table 65.7 Thrombolysis with alteplase for ischaemic stroke.

Explain risks and benefits (2–5% symptomatic haemorrhage rate; it will not affect mortality rate overall, improved chance of surviving with less disability. NNT of 7 treating within 3 h of symptom onset and NNT of 14 when treating within 4.5 h).
Give alteplase 0.9 mg/kg to a maximum of 90 mg with 10% of the bolus over 2 min intravenously and the remainder by an infusion over 60 min.
Check neurological signs and general observations:
- Every 15 min for 2 h
- Every 30 min for 6 h
- Every 60 min for 16 h
Repeat brain imaging after 24 h.
Keep blood pressure at or below 180/105 mmHg for first 24 h.
Do not give aspirin until 24 h after thrombolysis.

- All patients should be screened for cognitive impairment using a validated score after stroke.
- Urinary catheterization should be avoided. It is rarely indicated for the management of incontinence.
- Constipation is common in immobile patients. Manage initially by early mobilization, good hydration, a diet rich in complex polysaccharides, and the use of commodes or toilets rather than bedpans.

Establishing the cause of the stroke

Investigations needed are summarized in Table 65.8.

Preventing another stroke (secondary prevention)
All patients

- Give advice and support for smoking cessation if indicated.
- Give advice on diet and exercise.
- Blood pressure management. Probably the lower the blood pressure the better, so most patients will benefit from antihypertensive treatment.
- Patients should be started on a statin if fasting total cholesterol is >3.5 mmol/L.

Following cerebral infarction due to arterial atherothromboembolism

- Give aspirin 300 mg daily for 2 weeks, followed by clopidogrel 75 mg thereafter.
- If the patient cannot tolerate clopidogrel, give the combination of aspirin 75 mg daily and dipyridamole MR 200 mg 12-hourly.
- Patients should be considered for carotid endarterectomy if they have between 50 and 99% carotid stenosis (measured using the NASCET method) on the symptomatic side. The earlier the surgery is performed after TIA or minor stroke the better, as the risk of recurrence is highest in the first few days. There is rarely an indication for operating on asymptomatic stenosis.

Table 65.8 Further investigation to determine the cause of stroke.

Cerebral infarction
Cervical artery imaging: (duplex, CT angiography or MR angiography), to identify significant carotid stenosis (where surgery might be considered) or cervical artery dissection or vasculitis, for example Takayasu arteritis.

Echocardiography:
- Transthoracic echocardiography (TTE) where a cardio-embolic cause for stroke is being considered. If the patient is in known atrial fibrillation, then may not need echocardiography as patient will be anticoagulated anyway. Use to look for endocarditis, aortic dissection, atrial myxoma or where there is an undiagnosed cardiac murmur or abnormal ECG.
- Use transthoracic echocardiography with bubble injection where patent foramen ovale is suspected.
- Consider transoesophageal echocardiography (TOE) for patients with possible endocarditis and a normal TTE, mechanical heart valve prosthesis and for unexplained stroke in patients <50 years.

Ambulatory ECG monitoring: do a 24-h recording if atrial fibrillation is suspected and the standard ECG shows sinus rhythm. If 24-h recording is normal consider an 8-day recording.

Intracerebral haemorrhage
Intracranial arteriography: if suspected vasculitis, aneurysm, arteriovenous malformation, cavernoma

Subarachnoid haemorrhage
See Chapter 67.

Cerebral venous sinus thrombosis and venous infarction
Need to consider the diagnosis from the history (headache, vomiting, seizures, focal neurological deficits) and then specifically ask for CT venography or MR venography to confirm.

Following cerebral infarction related to atrial fibrillation

- Give aspirin 300 mg daily for 2 weeks, followed by anticoagulation with warfarin or a direct-acting anticoagulant (Chapter 103).
- If the stroke is small and the patient is being discharged from hospital, then earlier commencement of anticoagulation is appropriate as the risk of haemorrhagic transformation of the infarct is low.

Appendix 65.1 Classification of stroke

Arterial ischaemic

Cardioembolic

- Atrial fibrillation (thrombus in left atrium)
- Left ventricular mural thrombus
- Paradoxical embolism through a patent foramen ovale
- Embolism from infective endocarditis
- Atrial myxoma

Atherothromboembolic

- Carotid atheroma
- Vertebral atheroma
- Cerebral artery occlusion (may complicate aortic dissection)
- Cervical artery dissection

Small vessel disease

- Hypertensive arterial disease
- Diabetic vasculopathy
- Cerebral vasculitis

Others

- CADASIL syndrome (cerebral autosomal dominary arteriopathy with subcortical infarcts and leukoencephalopathy
- MELAS syndrome (mitochondrial myopathy, encephalopathy, lactic acidosis and stroke-like episodes)

Haemorrhage

Subarachnoid haemorrhage (see Chapter 67)

- Aneurysm
- Arteriovenous malformation

Parenchymal haemorrhage

- Hypertensive arterial disease
- Amyloid angiopathy
- Arteriovenous malformation
- Bleeding disorder (see Chapter 102)
- Haemorrhagic transformation of cerebral infarction (commonly seen in infarction due to cerebral venous thrombosis)
- Reperfusion after carotid endarterectomy/angioplasty
- Mycotic aneurysm complicating infective endocarditis

Venous stroke

Cerebral venous thrombosis (risk factors as for deep vein thrombosis (Table 56.1), plus local infection and trauma.

Further reading

Fernandes PM, Whiteley WN, Hart SR, Salman RA-S. (2013) Stroke: mimics and chameleons. *Pract Neurol* 13, 21–28.

Hankey GJ. (2017) Stroke. *Lancet* 389, 641–654.

Intercollegiate Stroke Working Party (2016) National clinical guideline for stroke 5th edn. http://guideline.ssnap.org/2016StrokeGuideline/index.html.

CHAPTER 66

Transient ischaemic attack

AJAY BHALLA AND TONY RUDD

Transient ischaemic attack (TIA) is defined as a transient episode of neurological dysfunction caused by focal brain, spinal cord, or retinal ischaemia, without evidence of acute infarction on brain imaging. The symptoms of confirmed TIA typically last only minutes. Rapid and accurate diagnosis of TIA is crucial as without appropriate treatment, the patient is at high risk of subsequent stroke. The risk of stroke is 10% within the first two weeks after a TIA, and higher in patients who have two or more TIAs within one week (crescendo TIA), or who have a severe internal carotid artery stenosis or are in atrial fibrillation.

Priorities

Clinical assessment and investigation are directed at answering these questions:

1 **Was it a TIA?**

Establish if the symptoms were:

- Focal neurological or monocular rather than global (Tables 66.1, 66.2).
- Of sudden onset.
- Maximum at the onset, rather than spreading or stuttering (spreading of sensory symptoms over several seconds tends to indicate seizure activity, whereas spreading of sensory symptoms over several minutes indicates migraine).
- Negative (loss of function, e.g. weakness or numbness) rather than positive (e.g. jerking as a result of seizure or parathesiae due to seizure or migraine).

If the answer is 'yes' to all four questions, then a diagnosis of TIA is highly likely. Other causes of transient neurological or visual symptoms to be considered when the diagnosis of TIA is less likely are given in Table 66.3.

2 **Which arterial territory?**

Carotid and vertebrobasilar territory TIAs give rise to differing patterns of symptoms (Table 66.4). Establishing which territory was involved (or if TIAs have occurred in both territories) is important in the interpretation of the carotid duplex scan and further management.

Acute Medicine: A Practical Guide to the Management of Medical Emergencies, Fifth Edition. Edited by David Sprigings and John B. Chambers.
© 2018 John Wiley & Sons Ltd. Published 2018 by John Wiley & Sons Ltd.

Table 66.1 Focal neurological symptoms: attributable to a focal area of the brain and therefore more likely to represent TIA.

Weakness (hemiparesis) or uncoordination of one side of body
Dysphagia
Ataxia

Dysphasia (receptive or expressive)
Dysarthria
Dyslexia
Dysgraphia
Dyscalculia

Hemisensory disturbance
Transient monocular blindness
Hemianopia or quadrantinopia
Bilateral blindness
Diplopia

Vertigo (only in association with other brain stem focal symptoms, unusual for vertigo as an isolated symptom to represent a TIA)

Dyspraxia
Visual spatial dysfunction (visual neglect)
Amnesia (as an isolated symptom does not indicate TIA)

Note: if multiple stereotypical focal events over a period of time with the same symptoms then a diagnosis of TIA is very unlikely: consider seizure activity.

Table 66.2 Non-focal (global) neurological symptoms: not attributable to a focal area of the brain and therefore very unlikely to represent TIA.

Generalized weakness
Generalized sensory disturbance
Faints or light-headedness
Blackouts or drop attacks (syncope)
Faecal or urinary incontinence
Confusion

If isolated symptom, in the absence of other focal neurological symptoms:
• Vertigo
• Tinnitus
• Dysarthria
• Dysphagia
• Diplopia
• Ataxia

Table 66.3 Causes of transient neurological or monocular visual symptoms.

Cause	Comment
Migraine aura (with or without headache)	Stereotypical positive symptoms such tingling and visual symptoms, spreading over several minutes and typically resolving within 60 min. Often positive family history for migraine.
Partial epileptic seizure	Positive symptoms (jerking or tingling, marching over several seconds). May have impaired awareness (partial complex seizure).
Transient global amnesia	Loss of anterograde memory usually accompanied by repetitive questioning. Resolves usually within 6 h. No language deficit. Able to recognize surroundings and familiar individuals.
Metabolic	Hypoglycaemia: consider if recurrent events associated with low blood glucose. See Chapter 81.
Structural lesion	For example brain tumour, chronic subdural haematoma. See Chapter 72.
Demyelination	Subacute onset in young adults. MRI clarifies diagnosis.
Mononeuropathy	Look for lower motor neuron signs.
Myasthenia gravis	Check for fatigability.
Monocular visual symptoms	Ocular or optic nerve disease. See Chapter 19.

3 Does the TIA have a potentially treatable cause (Box 66.1)?

This is determined by clinical assessment and investigation (Table 66.5).

Always consider:

- Atherosclerotic carotid artery disease. A carotid bruit is not a sensitive or specific sign of severe carotid stenosis. Carotid duplex scan is indicated in patients who have had a carotid territory TIA (Table 66.4) and would be candidates for endarterectomy.

Table 66.4 TIA: Which vascular territory was involved?

Symptom	Carotid territory	Vertebrobasilar territory
Dysphasia	Yes	No
Monocular visual loss	Yes	No
Unilateral weakness	Yes	Yes
Unilateral sensory loss	Yes	Yes
Dysarthria	Yes	Yes
Homonymous hemianopia	Yes	Yes
Ataxia/unsteadiness	Yes	Yes
Dysphagia	Yes	Yes
Diplopia	No	Yes
Vertigo	No	Yes

Box 66.1 Causes of transient ischaemic attack.

Large arterial atherothromboembolism (45%)

Atherosclerotic disease of the aorta or extracranial carotid and vertebral arteries

Embolism from the heart (20%)
Atrial fibrillation (left atrial thrombus)
Infective endocarditis (see Chapter 52)
Prosthetic heart valve (see Chapter 51)
Recent myocardial infarction (left ventricular thrombus)
Dilated cardiomyopathy (left ventricular thrombus)
Rheumatic mitral stenosis (left atrial appendage thrombus may be present even if in sinus rhythm at presentation)
(see Chapter 51)
Have a high index of suspicion of a cardiac embolic source if the clinical presentation of TIA suggests involvement
of multiple cerebral arterial territories

Small artery microatheroma (25%)

Carotid or vertebral dissection (5%)
Consider diagnosis if focal neurological symptoms preceded by headache (either frontal headache over the eye in
carotid dissection of neck pain in vertebral dissection); look for Horner's syndrome in carotid dissection.

Others (5%)
Arteritis (consider if associated headache or systemic symptoms, raised C-reactive protein/ESR, headache; see
Chapter 99)
Haematological (hyperviscosity syndrome, sickle cell disease)

ESR, erythrocyte sedimentation rate.

Table 66.5 Investigation after TIA.

All patients
Full blood count
ESR or C-reactive protein (if raised, consider vasculitis, infective endocarditis, cardiac myxoma or systemic infection)
INR (if taking warfarin)
Sickle cell test (if sickle cell disease considered)
Electrolytes and creatinine
Lipid profile
Blood glucose (exclude hypoglycaemia and diabetes mellitus)
Blood culture if febrile or infective endocarditis suspected (e.g. prosthetic heart valve)
ECG (atrial fibrillation, previous myocardial infarction, left ventricular hypertrophy)
Chest X-ray (exclude lung neoplasm, assess heart size)

Selected patients
Neuroimaging
MRI is indicated for the following in the first instance unless the patient cannot tolerate this, in which case CT should be
done:
• Diagnosis is unclear
• Exclude structural intracranial lesion such as meningioma, subdural haematoma
• When vascular territory is unclear (diffusion-weighted MRI)

(*continued*)

Table 66.5 (*Continued*)

* When duration of focal neurological symptoms was >1 h (diffusion-weighted MRI)
* If the patient may be suitable for carotid endarterectomy and need to be certain whether anterior or posterior circulation

Arterial imaging
* Carotid duplex scan, following carotid territory TIA or transient monocular visual loss
* CT or MR angiography if carotid dissection or large-vessel vasculitis is suspected

Echocardiography
When cardiac embolic source is suspected or must be excluded:
* Transthoracic echocardiography (TTE) where a cardio-embolic cause for stroke is being considered. Use to look for endocarditis, aortic dissection, atrial myxoma or where there is an undiagnosed cardiac murmur or abnormal ECG.
* Use transthoracic echocardiography with bubble injection where patent foramen ovale is suspected.
* Consider transoesophageal echocardiography (TOE) for patients with possible endocarditis and a normal TTE, mechanical heart valve prosthesis and for unexplained stroke in patients <50 years.

Ambulatory ECG monitoring
* Ambulatory monitoring for 24 h if paroxysmal atrial fibrillation (AF) is suspected
* If ECG monitoring for 24 h does not reveal paroxysmal AF, but clinical suspicion is high, consider 7-day recording

* Embolism from the heart (e.g. atrial fibrillation, mechanical heart valve replacement with INR <2).
* Arteritis, suggested by headache or systemic symptoms, with elevated ESR and C-reactive protein.
* Haematological disease (e.g. erythrocytosis, thrombocythaemia (Chapter 100)).

Further management

Patients with suspected TIA should have:
* Assessment and investigation by stroke specialist within 24 h of onset (same-day neurovascular clinic assessment or hospital admission)
* Antiplatelet therapy (300 mg aspirin, followed by 75 mg clopidogrel)
* Statin therapy (e.g. simvastatin 40 mg)
* BP maintained <140/80 mmHg
* Carotid endarterectomy within one week of onset, if carotid duplex imaging demonstrates a stenosis between 50–99% (and surgery is not contraindicated)

Patients with crescendo TIA (two or more TIAs in one week) should be treated as being at high risk of stroke. Consider dual antiplatelet therapy short term for at least seven days (aspirin and clopidogrel).

Patients in atrial fibrillation should be anticoagulated with rapid-onset anticoagulants (Chapter 103) once brain imaging has excluded intracerebral haemorrhage and there are no contraindications to anticoagulation.

All patients with TIA should be informed that they must not drive for one month following onset.

Further reading

Li L, Yiin GS, Geraghty OC, *et al.* on behalf of the Oxford Vascular Study (2015) Incidence, outcome, risk factors, and long-term prognosis of cryptogenic transient ischaemic attack and ischaemic stroke: a population-based study. *Lancet Neurol* 14, 903–913.

Nadarajan V, Perry RJ, Johnson J, Werring DJ. (2014) Transient ischaemic attacks: mimics and chameleons. *Pract Neurol* 14, 23–31.

CHAPTER 67

Subarachnoid haemorrhage

Michael Canty

Consider subarachnoid haemorrhage (SAH) (Box 67.1) in any patient with:
- A clear history of sudden onset, severe headache
- Headache with reduced conscious level, neurological deficit, or seizure
- Any sudden, unexplained collapse with presentation in coma

Most patients with SAH will complain of nausea and vomiting, photophobia, and eventually neck stiffness. Some will present in an acute confusional state and a collateral history is essential.

In the conscious patient, examination is often normal. In others, there may be objective neck stiffness, mild disorientation, or subtle deficits such as dysphasia or pronator drift. Uncommonly, the presence of subhyaloid or vitreous haemorrhage is detected on fundoscopy; in the context of a suggestive history these findings are usually pathognomonic.

Box 67.1 Subarachnoid haemorrhage (SAH).

SAH is bleeding beneath the arachnoid layer of the dura. All bleeding into cerebrospinal fluid (e.g. basal cisterns, cerebral ventricles) is subarachnoid haemorrhage.

Rupture of an intracranial aneurysm accounts for 85% of cases. Identification and obliteration of such aneurysms is needed to reduce the risk of rebleeding. Of the remainder, 10% have no identifiable cause, and are labelled non-aneurysmal SAH.

Rarer causes account for the last 5% of cases, including arterial dissection, rupture of an arteriovenous malformation, and posterior reversible encephalopathy syndrome (PRES). Subarachnoid haemorrhage is often seen in trauma, but is a completely different clinical entity and is not considered here.

Accounts for approximately 3% of all strokes, and occurs with an incidence of 10.5 per 100,000 person-years. It occurs more commonly in women, and is strikingly more common in Finland and Japan. Family history is an important risk factor, and having a first-degree relative with SAH increases the relative risk three to seven-fold. Three main modifiable risk factors have been identified: smoking, hypertension and heavy alcohol consumption.

SAH is a potentially devastating condition. Approximately half of all patients with SAH will die. Of the remainder, one-third will not recover functional independence.

Acute Medicine: A Practical Guide to the Management of Medical Emergencies, Fifth Edition. Edited by David Sprigings and John B. Chambers.
© 2018 John Wiley & Sons Ltd. Published 2018 by John Wiley & Sons Ltd.

Priorities

1 If you suspect SAH

- Assess the airway, breathing and circulation, and correct abnormal physiology.
- Assess the conscious level: seek an urgent anaesthetic/intensive care opinion for patients flexing to painful stimuli or worse.
- Nurse the patient 30° head-up to optimize cerebral venous drainage; provide oxygen if arterial oxygen saturation is <94%; establish IV access; make nil by mouth; start IV 0.9% saline, usually at 125 mL/h.
- Check full blood count, coagulation screen, blood glucose, urea, creatinine and electrolytes.
- Record an ECG to assess for myocardial ischaemia or 'stunning' secondary to SAH.
- Provide analgesia – opioid if required. Stop antiplatelet therapy and reverse anticoagulation (Chapter 103).

2 Arrange brain CT

- The primary investigation in suspected SAH is non-contrast CT scanning of the brain, from vertex to foramen magnum. As a general rule, this should be performed as an emergency including when out of hours. Many UK units will defer imaging to daylight hours in fully conscious patients without neurological deficit; this decision should be made by a senior clinician in the context of each individual case.
- It is helpful to think of CT as a screening investigation to decide whether or not a lumbar puncture (LP) is necessary. In the presence of a 'positive' CT scan demonstrating SAH, a lumbar puncture is not required and a referral should be made immediately to neurosurgery. If, however the CT does not demonstrate SAH or an alternative diagnosis, LP should be considered mandatory to confirm or exclude SAH.
- In a conscious patient with a severe headache, the presence of a unilaterally dilated pupil, often accompanied by a significant ptosis of the same eye, usually indicates an expanding aneurysm of the ipsilateral posterior communicating artery. Refer urgently to neurosurgery, even if the CT scan is normal: a so-called 'painful third nerve palsy' often heralds an imminent aneurysm rupture.

3 If CT is normal, perform lumbar puncture (LP)

- LP should be performed >12 h after the onset of symptoms; earlier LP may be falsely negative. See Chapter 123 for the technique of LP.
- Ideally performed by an experienced clinician to reduce the risk of a 'traumatic tap', which often makes a definite diagnosis impossible.
- Measure opening pressure; send CSF for microscopy, cell count and culture, and spectrophotometry to assess for the presence of CSF bilirubin. Samples should be analysed immediately on receipt; if analysis is delayed, false positives may occur.
- All positive or equivocal results should be referred to neurosurgery. A negative result excludes SAH (but see Box 67.2).

Further management

1 If SAH is confirmed by CT/LP, refer immediately to neurosurgery

- CT or MR angiography is occasionally requested following advice from the regional neurosurgical unit in specific cases. This should only be requested with the agreement of local radiology. Regional neuroradiology consultation may be required to offer a specialist opinion on such imaging.
- Consider starting nimodipine 60 mg orally/NG 4-hourly (to reduce the incidence of delayed ischaemic neurological deficit) after discussion with neurosurgery. In severe hypertension, active pharmacological blood pressure control (Chapter 55) may be required: discuss with neurosurgery.
- Most patients with SAH will be transferred to the regional neurosurgical unit for further assessment and management. Specialist management usually involves further investigation with CT angiography, which identifies causative aneurysms or arteriovenous malformations with high sensitivity. If CT angiography is normal, most patients will proceed to digital-subtraction catheter angiography.

Box 67.2 Pitfalls in the diagnosis of subarachnoid haemorrhage.

Clinical

The history in SAH is crucial. The onset of the headache must be specifically enquired about. The majority of haemorrhages occur with a severe headache, usually the worst of the patient's life, and are maximal within seconds.

Patients presenting in an acute confusional state may give no history of headache and careful witness accounts must be sought.

In patients with gradual onset, retro-orbital headache, always examine the pupils and eyelids carefully – a partial or complete III nerve palsy mandates that an expanding posterior communicating artery aneurysm is excluded. Discuss with neurosurgery, even if a plain CT scan is normal.

Some patients with SAH will present as physiologically unstable, with abnormal cardiac rhythms, such as atrial fibrillation, or with signs of myocardial ischaemia. It is important to separate the cardiac sequelae from the neurological presentation, as these events usually require no specific treatment, and antiplatelet or anticoagulant therapy may be disastrous.

CT

Recent North American literature has suggested that in selected patients, a normal CT scan within 6 h of symptom onset is sufficiently specific to exclude SAH without the requirement for lumbar puncture. This is not yet widely accepted, and usual UK neurosurgical practice would be to advise lumbar puncture in all patients in whom SAH is suspected, if CT is normal.

LP

The obtaining, measurement, and interpretation of CSF bilirubin is prone to error and care must be taken. Samples should be obtained after 12 h and analysed as soon as possible. The 'three tube' technique to assess for falling red blood cell counts as a method to distinguish traumatic tap from SAH is notoriously unreliable. If spectrophotometry is unavailable (e.g. overnight), lumbar puncture should be delayed until the biochemistry lab can perform the analysis. The presence of bilirubin indicates red cell breakdown products in the CSF. In a rapidly-analysed sample, this indicates blood in the CSF present prior to the lumbar puncture, that is, SAH. Spectrophotometry has replaced the visual inspection of CSF supernatant for xanthochromia.

A 'traumatic tap', where inadvertent venous contamination causes the CSF to be overly bloody, often results in an equivocal biochemistry analysis, as the large spectrophotometric peak produced by oxy-haemoglobin 'masks' any bilirubin peak which may be present. One option is to immediately repeat a lumbar puncture, if this can be done less than 6 h since the first attempt; otherwise such patients should be discussed with neurosurgery.

- If systolic BP is > 160 mmHg, start antihypertensive therapy aiming for a target < 160 mmHg. We would not normally expect referring clinicans to institute vasoactive blood pressure management of SAH; doing so and inadvertently dropping BP precipitously is potentially dangerous.
- Consider giving labetalol or nicardipine by infusion (as for acute ischaemic stroke): see Chapter 55. However be cautious about excessive lowering of blood pressure.

2 **Management of culprit intracranial aneurysm**

- Definitive treatment of responsible aneurysms has markedly changed since the publication of the International Subarachnoid Aneurysm Trial (ISAT) in 2005. This trial demonstrated the superiority of endovascular 'coiling' of aneurysms versus the traditional method of surgical 'clipping' via craniotomy.

- Clipping is now carried out almost exclusively by subspecialist vascular neurosurgeons, usually for complex aneurysms not easily treated by coiling, or in the presence of an intracerebral haematoma requiring evacuation.

3 **Management of other complications of SAH**

Delayed ischaemic neurological deficit (DIND)

- Incidence peaks at 4–14 days post-ictus.
- Presents with new focal neurological deficit, severe headache, or reduced conscious level.
- Managed with aggressive fluid administration, induced hypertension (assuming a secured aneurysm), and occasionally endovascular intervention such as balloon angioplasty and intra-arterial administration of nimodipine or nicardipine.

Hydrocephalus

- Often occurs very early in SAH, but may also present weeks or months post-ictus.
- Typically presents with features of raised intracranial pressure, with headache, vomiting, lethargy, confusion, incontinence or deterioration in mobility. CT imaging of the brain usually confirms the diagnosis.
- Acute presentation with hydrocephalus requires an urgent neurosurgical opinion. Most of these patients will require surgical CSF diversion (e.g. insertion of an external ventricular drain). Hydrocephalus presenting in a delayed fashion is often picked up once the patient is in the rehabilitation phase, and may simply present with a plateau or regression in rehab progress. Most of these patients will benefit from permanent CSF diversion, usually a ventriculoperitoneal shunt, and this should be discussed with neurosurgery.

Hyponatraemia

- Common post-SAH and may by itself cause neurological deterioration.
- The usual differential diagnosis is syndrome of inappropriate ADH secretion (SIADH) and cerebral salt wasting (CSW). Differentiating between the two is difficult, but crucial as treatment varies markedly (although perhaps less so in SAH – see below).
- Cerebral salt wasting manifests as salt loss in a dehydrated patient. The patient may be clinically dry; have biochemical features such as a high haemoglobin/haematocrit, high urea, or high serum urate. Urine output is relatively high; urinary sodium levels are elevated; plasma osmolality is low (due to salt loss).
- SIADH manifests as inappropriate free water retention in a euvolaemic patient. Similarly to CSW, urinary sodium levels are high, while plasma osmolality is low; however, urine output is relatively low, and the patient is not dehydrated.
- CSW is treated by increasing intravascular volume with fluids; depending on the degree of hyponatraemia they may also require salt, usually in the form of hypertonic saline. SIADH is classically treated with fluid restriction; however, in acute subarachnoid haemorrhage this is usually contraindicated as it may contribute towards the development of DIND. Most SIADH is mild and resolves spontaneously; if sodium drops precipitously then hypertonic saline may be required.

Further reading

Macdonald RL, Schweizer TA. (2016) Spontaneous subarachnoid haemorrhage. *Lancet* 389, 655–666.

CHAPTER 68

Bacterial meningitis

DAVID SPRIGINGS AND JOHN L. KLEIN

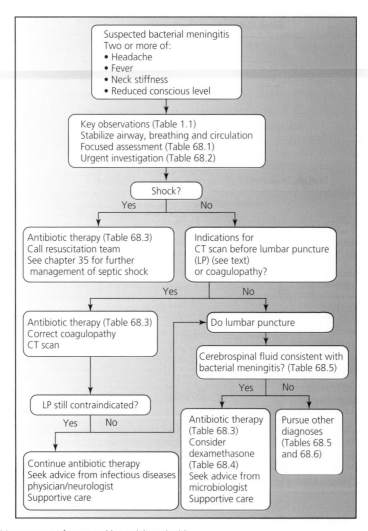

Figure 68.1 Management of suspected bacterial meningitis.

Acute Medicine: A Practical Guide to the Management of Medical Emergencies, Fifth Edition. Edited by David Sprigings and John B. Chambers.
© 2018 John Wiley & Sons Ltd. Published 2018 by John Wiley & Sons Ltd.

Consider bacterial meningitis in any patient with fever, headache, neck stiffness or a reduced conscious level: 95% of patients with bacterial meningitis will have at least two of these four features. Bacterial meningitis can also present as septic shock. Management of suspected bacterial meningitis is summarized in Figure 68.1.

Most cases in the developed world are caused by *Neisseria meningitidis* or *Streptococcus pneumoniae*. In the context of immunosuppression, alcohol-use disorder or age >60 years, *Listeria monocytogenes* should also be considered. In resource-poor settings, *M. tuberculosis* may predominate (Appendix 68.1).

Disorders which can mimic meningitis include subarachnoid haemorrhage (Chapter 67), viral encephalitis (Chapter 69), brain abscess, subdural empyema and cerebral malaria.

Priorities

1 Review the physiological observations, make a focused clinical assessment (Table 68.1) and arrange urgent investigations (Table 68.2).
2 If the clinical picture is consistent with bacterial meningitis, and the patient has shock, a reduced conscious level or a petechial/purpuric rash (suggesting meningococcal infection), take blood for culture and immediately start antibiotic therapy (Table 68.3), plus adjunctive dexamethasone (Table 68.4), if indicated.
3 In patients with suspected meningitis without signs of shock or severe sepsis, lumbar puncture (LP) should be performed within 1 h of arrival at hospital, provided there is no contraindication to LP. Antibiotic therapy (Table 68.3) should be started immediately after LP, and within the first hour.

   If LP cannot be done within 1 h (e.g. because of the need for CT or the presence of a coagulopathy), take blood for culture and immediately start antibiotic therapy (Table 68.3).
4 CT should be done before LP if there are risk factors for an intracranial mass lesion, or signs of raised intracranial pressure:
   - Immunosuppression (e.g. HIV/AIDS, immunosuppressive therapy)
   - History of brain tumour or focal infection
   - Major seizures within one week of presentation
   - Papilloedema
   - Reduced conscious level (Glasgow Coma Scale score <13)
   - Focal neurological signs (not including cranial nerve palsies)
5 If the patient is taking antiplatelet or anticoagulant therapy, or has thrombocytopenia or a coagulopathy, discuss management with a haematologist before LP. See also Chapters 102 and 103.
6 The technique of LP is described in detail in Chapter 122.
   - Measure and record the opening pressure. If the opening pressure is >40 cm CSF, indicating severe cerebral oedema, give mannitol 0.5 g/kg IV over 10 min plus dexamethasone 12 mg IV. Discuss further management with a neurologist.
   - Send CSF for cell count, protein concentration, glucose (fluoride tube), Gram stain and culture. PCR for meningococcus and pneumococcus should be undertaken if blood/CSF cultures are negative. Consider requesting microscopy and culture for acid-fast bacilli if tuberculosis is suspected (Appendix 68.1); in immunosuppressed patients (especially those with HIV infection), request an India ink stain and a cryptococcal antigen test (Appendix 68.2).
7 Patients with suspected bacterial meningitis should be isolated (contact precautions) until at least 24 h into treatment.
8 Blood-stained CSF may be due to a traumatic tap or subarachnoid haemorrhage. The presence of bilirubin in the CSF (detected by spectrophotometry) indicates red cell breakdown products and confirms subarachnoid haemorrhage (Chapter 67).

Table 68.1 Clinical findings in bacterial meningitis.

Prodromal illness for 1–2 days

Fever

Purpuric/petechial rash (especially meningococcal infection)

Signs of meningeal irritation: headache, neck stiffness, vomiting, photophobia

Reduced conscious level

Seizures

Cranial nerve palsies

Focal neurological signs (if bacterial meningitis is complicated by cerebral venous sinus thrombosis or arteritis)

General examination may show signs of predisposing disorders:

- Ear infection
- Sinusitis
- Pneumonia

Table 68.2 Urgent investigation in suspected meningitis.

Blood culture (x2)

Lumbar puncture (if not contraindicated: see text)

Throat swab (request culture for meningococci)

Full blood count

EDTA sample for PCR (for meningococci and pneumococci) – especially if blood cultures drawn after antibiotic therapy

Coagulation screen if there is petechial or purpuric rash or low platelet count

C-reactive protein

Blood glucose (for comparison with CSF glucose)

Creatinine and electrolytes

Arterial blood gases, pH and lactate

Chest X-ray (pneumonia or lung abscess?)

Skull X-ray if suspected sinus infection (nasal discharge, sinus tenderness) or skull fracture

CT if suspected intracranial mass lesion or skull X-ray abnormal

Table 68.3 Initial antibiotic therapy for suspected bacterial meningitis in adults.

Setting	No penicillin allergy	Penicillin allergy
Adult aged under 60	Cefotaxime 2 g qds or ceftriaxone 2 g bd	Minor allergy: cefotaxime 2 g qds or ceftriaxone 2 g bd Severe allergy: chloramphenicol 25 mg/kg qds
Age over 60, Immunocompromised or chronic alcohol abuse **In regions with a high prevalence of penicillin-resistant pneumococci**	Cefotaxime 2 g qds or ceftriaxone 2 g bd + amoxicillin 2 g 4 hourly Add vancomycin 15–20 mg/kg bd	Minor allergy: cefotaxime 2 g qds or ceftriaxone 2 g bd Severe allergy: chloramphenicol 25 mg/kg qds + co-trimoxazole 15 mg/kg (trimethoprim component) tds

Table 68.4 Adjunctive dexamethasone in suspected bacterial meningitis.

Indications
Strong clinical suspicion of bacterial meningitis, especially if CSF is turbid

Situations where dexamethasone not advised
Antibiotic therapy already begun (although consider using up to 12 h after antibiotics in pneumococcal meningitis)
Septic shock
Suspected meningococcal disease (petechial/purpuric rash)
Immunosuppressed patient

Regimen
Give dexamethasone 10 mg IV before or with the first dose of antibiotic therapy (Table 68.3)
Continue dexamethasone 10 mg 6-hourly IV for 4 days if CSF shows Gram-positive diplococci, or if blood/CSF cultures are positive for *Streptococcus pneumoniae*

Further management

1 If organisms are seen on Gram stain of the CSF, bacterial meningitis is confirmed. The cell count will usually be high, with a polymorphonuclear leucocytosis, but may be low in overwhelming infection or immuno-suppression. Modify or start antibiotic therapy (Table 68.3). Ask advice from a microbiologist or infectious diseases physician on the best antibiotic regimen and duration of treatment.

2 If no organisms are seen on Gram stain, management is directed by the clinical picture and CSF formula (Table 68.5):

Normal cell count: that is, bacterial meningitis highly unlikely. Consider other infectious diseases which may give rise to meningism (e.g. bacterial tonsillitis).

High polymorph count: this is typical of pyogenic bacterial meningitis, although may occur early in the course of viral meningitis. Modify or start antibiotic therapy (Table 68.3). Ask advice from a microbiologist or infectious diseases physician on the best antibiotic regimen and duration of treatment.

High lymphocyte count: this may be seen in many diseases (Table 68.6). Distinguishing between viral and partially treated pyogenic bacterial meningitis can be difficult. If in doubt, start antibiotic therapy, awaiting the results of culture of blood and CSF. If tuberculous or cryptococcal meningitis is possible on clinical grounds (see

Table 68.5 CSF formulae in meningitis and encephalitis.

Element	Pyogenic meningitis	Viral meningitis	Tuberculous meningitis	Cryptococcal meningitis	Viral encephalitis
White cell count/mm³	>1000	<500	<500	<150	<250
Predominant cell type	Polymorphs	Lymphocytes	Lymphocytes	Lymphocytes	Lymphocytes
Protein concentration (g/L)	>1.5	0.5–1.0	1.0–5.0	0.5–1.0	0.5–1.0
CSF: blood glucose	<50%	>50%	<50%	<50%	>50%

- The values given are typical, but many exceptions occur.
- Red cells may be seen in the CSF in herpes encephalitis, reflecting cerebral necrosis.
- Antibiotic therapy substantially changes the CSF formula in pyogenic bacterial meningitis, leading to a fall in cell count, increased proportion of lymphocytes and fall in protein level. However, the low CSF glucose level usually persists.

Table 68.6 Causes of meningitis with a high CSF lymphocyte count.*

Viral meningitis
Partially treated pyogenic bacterial meningitis
Other bacterial infections – tuberculosis (Appendix 68.1), leptospirosis, brucellosis, syphilis, listeriosis
Fungal (cryptococcal) infection (Appendix 68.2)
Parameningeal infection – brain abscess or subdural empyema
Neoplastic infiltration

*Viral encephalitis (Chapter 69) may give a similar CSF picture.

Appendices 68.1 and 68.2), or on the results of CSF examination, ask for microscopy and culture for acid-fast bacilli and an India ink stain/cryptococcal antigen test.

3 Supportive care of the patient with bacterial meningitis includes:
- Analgesia as required (e.g. paracetamol, NSAID or codeine).
- Control of seizures (See chapter 16).
- Attention to fluid balance. Losses are increased due to fever. Aim for an intake of 2–3 L/day, supplementing oral intake with IV normal saline/5% glucose if needed. Check creatinine and electrolytes initially daily. Hyponatraemia may occur due to inappropriate ADH secretion.

4 Contacts of patients with confirmed or suspected meningococcal meningitis should be identified. Ciprofloxacin (500 mg stat PO for adults) should be offered to household contacts and other close contacts (e.g. sexual partners). Rifampicin (600 mg twice daily PO in adults for two days) is an alternative.

5 The district community medicine specialist should be informed promptly about confirmed cases of meningitis.

Appendix 68.1 Tuberculous meningitis

Element	Comment
At risk	Birth in a region with a high incidence of tuberculosis (TB) (e.g. India, Pakistan and Africa)
	Recent contact with TB
	Previous pulmonary TB
	Alcohol- or substance-use disorder
	Immunosuppression (organ transplant, lymphoma, steroid therapy, anti-TNF therapy, HIV/AIDS)
Suggestive clinical features	Subacute onset
	Cranial nerve palsies
	Retinal tubercles (pathognomonic but rarely seen)
	Evidence of extra-meningeal TB (e.g. miliary change on CXR)
	Hyponatraemia
CSF findings	Raised opening pressure
	High lymphocyte count
	High protein level
	Rare for acid-fast bacilli to be seen on microscopy, but PCR for *M. tuberculosis* DNA has a higher sensitivity
CT brain	Hydrocephalus common
	Cerebral infarction due to arteritis may be seen
	Tuberculomas may be seen
Treatment	Combination chemotherapy with isoniazid (plus pyridoxine to avoid neuropathy), rifampicin, pyrazinamide and ethambutol
	Consider adjunctive dexamethasone (seek expert advice)

Appendix 68.2 Cryptococcal meningitis

Element	Comment
At risk	Immunosuppression (organ transplant, lymphoma, steroid therapy, HIV/AIDS)
Suggestive clinical features	Insidious onset
	Neck stiffness absent or mild
	Papular or nodular skin lesions
CSF findings	Raised opening pressure
	High lymphocyte count (20–200/mm^3)
	Protein and glucose levels usually only mildly abnormal
	Cryptococci may be seen on Gram stain
	India ink preparation positive in 60%
	CSF culture positive
	Cryptococcal antigen test positive (highly sensitive)
CT brain	Usually normal
	May show hydrocephalus
	May show mass lesions (~10%)
Treatment	Amphotericin B plus flucytosine: seek expert advice

Further reading

Brouwer MC, Tunkel AR, McKhann II GM, van de Beek D (2014) Brain abscess. *N Engl J Med* 371, 447–456.

Jarrin I, Sellier P, Lopes A (2016) Etiologies and management of aseptic meningitis in patients admitted to an internal medicine department. *Medicine* 95, e2372. Open access.

McGill F, Heyderman RS, Michael BD, *et al.* (2016) The UK joint specialist societies guideline on the diagnosis and management of acute meningitis and meningococcal sepsis in immunocompetent adults. *Journal of Infection* 72, 405–438. Open access. http://www.journalofinfection.com/article/S0163-4453(16)00024-4/pdf.

CHAPTER 69

Encephalitis

DAVID SPRIGINGS

Consider encephalitis in any febrile patient with headache, abnormal behaviour or reduced conscious level. These clinical features have a broad differential diagnosis (Table 69.1), which must be considered. As prompt treatment of herpes simplex encephalitis (Appendix 69.1) can minimize brain injury and improve outcomes, aciclovir should be given to all patients with possible encephalitis, until the results of diagnostic tests are known.

- Empirical antibiotic therapy for bacterial meningitis (Chapter 68) should also be given if the patient has features of both meningitis and encephalitis.
- Tuberculous and cryptococcal meningitis should considered in at-risk groups (see Appendices 68.1 and 68.2). Meningism may be absent or mild in these diseases.
- Infectious diseases acquired abroad (e.g. malaria, typhoid) should be considered in patients with the relevant travel history (Chapter 33).

Table 69.1 Causes of fever with headache, abnormal behaviour or reduced conscious level.

Intracranial infection

Viral encephalitis
Other infectious causes of encephalitis
Bacterial meningitis (Chapter 68)
Tuberculous meningitis (Appendix 68.1)
Cryptococcal meningitis (Appendix 68.2)
Subdural empyema
Brain abscess

Systemic infection

Septic encephalopathy
Infective endocarditis
Mycoplasma and Legionella infection
Syphilis, Lyme disease, leptospirosis
Cerebral malaria

Non-infectious

Poisoning (e.g. with amphetamine or cocaine)
Alcohol withdrawal syndrome (Chapter 106)
Cerebral vasculitis
Cerebral venous thrombosis
Acute disseminated encephalomyelitis (seen in young adults; usually follows infection)
Auto-immune encephalitis (fever seen in ~50% cases)
Neuroleptic malignant syndrome (Appendix 69.2)
Acute intermittent porphyria
Heatstroke

Acute Medicine: A Practical Guide to the Management of Medical Emergencies, Fifth Edition. Edited by David Sprigings and John B. Chambers.
© 2018 John Wiley & Sons Ltd. Published 2018 by John Wiley & Sons Ltd.

Table 69.2 Focused assessment in suspected encephalitis.

Current major symptoms and their time course (confirm with family or friends)

Recent foreign travel (Chapter 33)

Insect or animal exposure (occupational/recreational)

Contact with infectious disease

Sexual history

Immunization history

Immunosuppression? Consider immunosuppressive therapy, HIV-AIDS, active cancer, advanced chronic kidney disease, liver failure, diabetes, malnutrition, splenectomy, IV drug use

Drug history (if treated with neuroleptic in preceding two weeks, consider neuroleptic malignant syndrome (Appendix 69.2))

Alcohol/substance use

Priorities

1 Review the physiological observations and make a focused clinical assessment (Table 69.2).

2 If you suspect encephalitis, start aciclovir 10 mg/kg 8-hourly IV. If meningism is present, or there are other reasons to suspect bacterial meningitis, take blood cultures and start appropriate antibiotic therapy (Chapter 68).

3 Arrange CT, LP and other urgent investigations (Table 69.3). In high-resource countries, the ready availability of CT makes it reasonable to do CT before LP in every case. CT should definitely be done before LP if there are risk factors for an intracranial mass lesion, or signs of raised intracranial pressure:
   - Immunosuppression (e.g. HIV-AIDS, immunosuppressive therapy)
   - History of brain tumour or focal infection
   - Major seizures within one week of presentation
   - Papilloedema
   - Reduced conscious level (Glasgow Coma Scale score <13)
   - Focal neurological signs (not including cranial nerve palsies)

Table 69.3 Urgent investigation in suspected encephalitis.

Blood culture (×2)

CT

LP if not contraindicated (send CSF for PCR for HSV-1 in addition to other tests) (Chapter 123)

Throat swab

Full blood count and film

Blood film for malaria if indicated

Coagulation screen

C-reactive protein

Blood glucose

Sodium, potassium, urea and creatinine

Liver function tests

Creatine kinase

Urinalysis

Toxicology screen if poisoning is possible (send serum (10 mL) + urine (50 mL))

Arterial blood gases and pH

Chest X-ray

Serological testing (if indicated) for other infectious diseases

Immunological tests if suspected autoimmune encephalitis

Further management

1 Management is directed by the clinical picture, neuroimaging and CSF formula (see Tables 68.5 and 68.6).
2 If viral encephalitis is probable or cannot be excluded, continue aciclovir and seek advice from an infectious diseases physician and neurologist.
3 Supportive treatment of viral encephalitis includes:
  • Analgesia as required (e.g. paracetamol, NSAID or codeine).
  • Control of seizures (see Chapter 16).
  • Attention to fluid balance. Losses are increased due to fever. Aim for an intake of 2–3 L/day, supplementing oral with IV normal saline if needed. Check electrolytes and creatinine, initially daily. Hyponatraemia may occur due to inappropriate ADH secretion.

Further reading

Graus F, Titulaer MJ, Balu R (2016) A clinical approach to diagnosis of autoimmune encephalitis. *Lancet Neurol* 4, 391–404.
Solomon T, Michael BD, Smith PE, *et al.* (2012) Management of suspected viral encephalitis in adults: The Association of British Neurologists and British Infection Association National guidelines.
  J Infect 64, 347–373. Open access. http://www.journalofinfection.com/article/S0163-4453(11)00563-9/pdf.

Appendix 69.1 Herpes simplex encephalitis

Element	Comment
Clinical features	Acute onset (symptoms usually <1 week)
	Fever
	Headache
	Personality change/abnormal behaviour
	Alteration in conscious level
	Seizures
	Focal neurological abnormalities (cranial nerve palsies, dysphasia, hemiparesis, ataxia)
CT brain	May be normal
	May show generalized brain swelling with loss of cortical sulci and small ventricles
	May show areas of low attenuation in the temporal and/or frontal lobes
CSF findings	High lymphocyte count (50–500/mm^3), with predominance of polymorphs in early phase, and red cells often present
	Protein concentration increased, up to 2.5 g/L
	Glucose is usually normal but may be low
	Herpes simplex DNA may be detected in CSF by PCR
Electroencephalography	Abnormal in two-thirds of cases, with a spike and slow wave pattern localized to the area of brain involved.
Management	Aciclovir 10 mg/kg 8-hourly IV
	Seek expert advice from an infectious diseases physician and neurologist

Appendix 69.2 Neuroleptic malignant syndrome

Element	Comment
Clinical features	Preceding use of neuroleptic (usually develops within two weeks of starting medication)
	Agitated delirium progressing to stupor and coma
	Generalized 'lead-pipe' muscular rigidity, often accompanied by tremor
	Temperature >38 °C (may be >40 °C)
	Autonomic instability: tachycardia, labile or high blood pressure, tachypnoea, sweating
CT brain	Typically normal
CSF findings	Typically normal
	May show raised protein
Electroencephalography	Generalized slow wave activity
Blood tests	High creatine kinase (typically >1000 units/L, and proportionate to rigidity)
	High white cell count (10–40×10^9/L)
	Electrolyte derangements and raised creatinine common
	Low serum iron level
Management	Stop neuroleptic
	Supportive care
	Use benzodiazepine if needed to control agitation
	Consider use of dantrolene, bromocriptine or amantadine
	Seek expert advice from a neurologist

CHAPTER 70

Spinal cord compression

Michael Canty

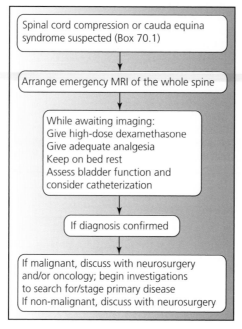

Figure 70.1 Management of suspected spinal cord compression or cauda equina syndrome.

Malignant spinal cord compression

- The spine is the most common site of bony metastases in patients with cancer. Malignant spinal cord or cauda equina compression will occur in 5–10% of patients with a malignancy. The thoracic region (70%) is the most common site of compression, followed by the lumbar (20%) and cervical (10%) spine.
- The most common primaries leading to spinal metastases are cancers of the lung, breast, and prostate, accounting for 70% of cases; however, cord or cauda equina compression may also occur secondary to myeloma, lymphoma, melanoma, renal, and gastrointestinal cancer.
- Metastases spread to the spine either directly, or haematogenously, via arterial supply or venous drainage (e.g. prostate malignancy spreads from the pelvis via the valveless veins of Batson's plexus).

Acute Medicine: A Practical Guide to the Management of Medical Emergencies, Fifth Edition. Edited by David Sprigings and John B. Chambers.
© 2018 John Wiley & Sons Ltd. Published 2018 by John Wiley & Sons Ltd.

- Treatment rarely prolongs survival but can reduce pain and improve quality of life, especially in crucial areas such as mobility and continence.

Other types of cord and cauda equina compression

- Degenerative disease, such as spondylosis and intervertebral disc disease, can cause an insidious onset of myelopathy in a variety of demographics and age groups. With the exception of cauda equina syndrome secondary to acute lumbar disc prolapse, definitive management of this subgroup is rarely as urgent as in malignant disease, but investigation and referral should still occur promptly.
- Spinal extradural abscess is a rare entity, usually presenting with severe spinal pain and systemic upset. In the presence of neurological signs and symptoms, investigation and management must be rapid.
- Spinal extradural haematoma is a very rare condition, usually a complication of anticoagulation. It tends to present suddenly with dramatic progressive deterioration.

Priorities

1 **Clinical assessment**
   Examine the spine and perform a full neurological examination, including assessment of perineal and perianal sensation, and anal tone (Box 70.1).
2 **If the clinical features indicate spinal cord compression or cauda equina syndrome, arrange emergency MRI imaging of the entire spine**
   - If MRI imaging is unavailable, discuss with neurosurgery or oncology whether referral for imaging elsewhere is indicated. Consider CT scanning of the spine.
   - Plain X-rays may confirm the diagnosis while waiting for MRI. Look for bone loss, pedicle destruction (the 'winking owl' sign), collapse or deformity.
   - Arrange baseline blood tests and a chest X-ray.
3 **If malignancy is thought likely, give high dose dexamethasone**
   Typically 8–16 mg IV as a loading dose. Always co-prescribe a proton pump inhibitor or ranitidine.

Further management

Confirmed malignant spinal cord or cauda equina compression
- Refer urgently to neurosurgery and oncology for consideration of surgery and/or radiotherapy, and to get advice on further management.
- Patients able to walk, but with a recent motor or sphincter deterioration, non-radiosensitive tumours, single-site compression, and with a prognosis of >6 months, are good candidates for surgery. Surgery may also be required for tissue diagnosis in an unknown primary where CT-guided biopsy is not possible or unavailable.
- Patients with minimal deficit, or complete, established weakness, may be better managed by radiotherapy. Radiotherapy confers excellent pain relief.
- Surgery may also be indicated in patients with actual or impending instability, and good performance status. These patients should be maintained on strict bed rest. Seek advice from neurosurgery, or a spinal surgeon
- Surgery is also considered in radio-resistant tumours, such as melanoma, renal, or gastrointestinal carcinoma, or in patients that have progressed despite radiotherapy. However, infection and impaired tissue healing is a major concern in the latter group.

Box 70.1 Clinical features of spinal cord compression and cauda equina syndrome.

Clinical feature	Comment
Spinal pain	Almost all patients with cord compression due to malignant disease will have spinal pain, and pain is typically the first symptom. May be focal, radicular or referred.
Site of compression	Around 70% of cases occur in the thoracic spine. The vast majority (>90%) are extradural; intramedullary (within the spinal cord) metastases are very rare.
	Thoracic pain following mild trauma may distract from the underlying diagnosis: trauma can precipitate a pathological fracture in pre-existing disease.
	Around 75% of patients have limb weakness at the time of diagnosis
	Spasticity and hyperreflexia take time to develop, and may be absent in the acute setting.

Motor system	Site of compression	Type of weakness
	Above C5	Spastic quadraparesis: upper motor neuron (UMN) distribution with spasticity and brisk reflexes in all four limbs and extensor plantars
	Between C5 and T1	Lower motor neuron (LMN) weakness at the level of the lesion (e.g. in the hands) and UMN weakness below
	Between T1 and L1	Spastic paraparesis: UMN weakness in the lower limbs; upper limbs unaffected
	Below L1	LMN weakness in the lower limbs

Sensory system See Figure 18.2 Sensory innervation of the skin	Site of compression	Sensory level
	Above C5	Neck
	Between C5 and T1	Upper limbs
	Between T1 and T6	Thorax
	Between T7 and T12	Abdomen
	Below L1	Lower limbs

Sphincter disturbance	Abnormalities of bladder function almost always precede those of bowel function. **Lesions at or above the conus medullaris** (the termination of the spinal cord) lead to a reflex neurogenic, or 'automatic' bladder, with overactivity, urgency and incomplete emptying; this is an UMN lesion, best thought of as bladder spasticity. Bowel abnormalities present as constipation.
	Lesions compressing the cauda equina cause overflow urinary incontinence due to a loss of bladder motor function, so that the bladder passively fills; this is a LMN lesion, best thought of as bladder flaccidity. Bowel abnormalities present as loss of anal sphincter tone and faecal incontinence. There is perineal sensory loss – the classic 'saddle anaesthesia'.

Box 70.2 Spinal cord compression – alert.

All patients requiring emergency MRI or CT scan may have a surgical diagnosis (e.g. cord compression, unstable spinal deformity) and should be kept nil by mouth pending their definitive imaging and discussion with a spinal surgeon.

Keep the patient on bed rest; prescribe adequate analgesia. If there is significant sphincter involvement, particularly if in urinary retention, insert a bladder catheter.

- Arrange further investigations to seek a primary tumour, if none is known; or to re-stage known disease, depending on specialist advice. This is usually in the form of a CT scan of the chest, abdomen and pelvis; a myeloma screen; tumour markers; and a bone scan.

Confirmed non-malignant spinal cord or cauda equina compression

Stop steroids. Seek advice on further investigation and management from neurosurgery.

Further reading

Al-Qurainy R, Collis E (2016) Metastatic spinal cord compression: diagnosis and management. *BMJ* 353, i2539. DOI: 10.1136/bmj.i2539

Fehlings M, Nater A, Tetreault L, *et al.* Survival and clinical outcomes in patients with metastatic epidural spinal cord compression: results from the AOSpine prospective multi-centre study of 142 patients. *Global Spine J* 2016; 06-GO223. DOI: 10.1055/s-0036-1582880.

CHAPTER 71

Guillain-Barré syndrome

Simon Rinaldi

Consider Guillain-Barré syndrome (GBS) (Appendix 71.1) in the patient with progressive symmetrical limb or facial weakness. Management of the patient with suspected GBS is summarized in Figure 71.1.

Priorities

The priorities are to establish the diagnosis in a timely manner (Tables 71.1 and 71.2; Box 71.1), exclude potential mimics (Table 71.3), and institute appropriate monitoring and therapy to manage or prevent potential complications. The most feared of these are life-threatening – neuromuscular respiratory failure, cardiovascular autonomic disturbance and pulmonary embolism.

Immediate management
- Involve ICU promptly if there is respiratory compromise or autonomic dysfunction.
- Continue to monitor cardiorespiratory function, including regular spirometry, in progressive phase.
- Measurement of vital capacity with bedside spirometry is an absolute requirement in the safe management of patients with GBS. Frequent monitoring is required during the progressive phase of the illness.
  - An adult vital capacity of <1.5 L/<20 mL/kg is of immediate concern and warrants discussion with ICU as a minimum.
  - At <1 L/<15 mL/kg, or with a fall of 50% from baseline on serial testing, prompt ICU involvement is required, and intubation may be necessary.

Box 71.1 Pitfalls in the diagnosis of Guillain-Barré syndrome

The more common diagnostic pitfalls relate to distinguishing GBS from spinal cord or cauda equina syndromes. Acute (radiculo-) neuropathies related to nutritional deficiency, critical illness, haematological malignancy, infection or vasculitis are also occasional mimics.

Confusion also sometimes surrounds the concept of ascending weakness. As GBS is most often demyelinating, proximal weakness is usually found in an affected limb, and the typical progression is from legs to arms to cranial nerves and respiratory muscles – not from distal to proximal in individual limbs. Exceptions exist, but descending weakness (starting with the cranial musculature) should prompt thoughts of botulism, not GBS.

Acute Medicine: A Practical Guide to the Management of Medical Emergencies, Fifth Edition. Edited by David Sprigings and John B. Chambers.
© 2018 John Wiley & Sons Ltd. Published 2018 by John Wiley & Sons Ltd.

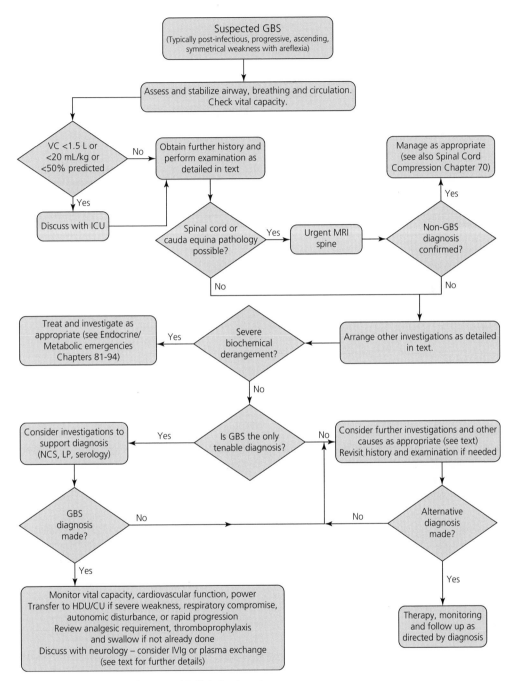

Figure 71.1 Management of suspected Guillain-Barré syndrome.

- Peak expiratory flow or arterial blood gas measurements are inadequate for assessing neuromuscular respiratory compromise.
- Treat pain. Paracetamol and opioids can be used, but neuropathic pain agents (e.g. gabapentin, pregabalin, amitriptyline) are often required.

Table 71.1 Clinical assessment.

History

Prodromal illness? Other potential trigger?

Backpain? Weakness? Sensory disturbance? Autonomic symptoms? Sphincter disturbance? Ataxia? Diplopia? Dysphagia? Dysarthria?

Onset? Progression? Fever? Rash? Ongoing systemic upset?

Prior episodes? Past history/comorbidities? HIV? Haematological malignancy? Tick bite? Alcohol excess? Poor diet?

Travel? Toxin/heavy metal exposure? Drugs?

Red flags for **alternative** diagnosis?

> Hyperacute onset? Marked fluctuation/fatigability? Sphincter disturbance at onset? Persistent bowel/bladder dysfunction? Progression greater than four weeks from onset? Neurological dysfunction developing concurrently with systemic upset?

Examination

Supportive findings:

- Largely symmetrical, proximal *and* distal flaccid limb weakness.
- Areflexia: bilateral facial palsy +/− other cranial nerve palsies; autonomic dysfunction.

Examination red flags for **alternative** diagnosis: marked asymmetry; upper motor neuron signs; sensory level; rash; fever; fatigable weakness.

- Prevent complications: thromboprophylaxis, pressure area care, assess swallow and place nil by mouth (with feeding by nasogastric tube) if compromised.
- Consider disease modifying treatment: IV immunoglobulin (IVIg) (0.4 g/kg × 5 days) or plasma exchange (PLEx), in discussion with a neurologist.

Monitoring

- Close monitoring of cardiorespiratory function is required initially. As a minimum, two sets of observations an hour apart, including measurement of vital capacity, are suggested following initial presentation. In the rapidly deteriorating patient, even more frequent assessment may be appropriate.
- Transient arrhythmias (supraventricular tachycardia or bradycardia) without haemodynamic compromise require no treatment. Severe prolonged bradycardia can occur, requiring temporary pacing. Sustained severe hypertension (diastolic BP >120 mmHg) should be treated with labetalol by infusion (p. 349). If hypotension does not respond to IV fluids (guided by measurement of CVP), treat with dopamine or noradrenaline infusion (p. 13).
- Regular assessment of power can also help to identify whether the disease is in a progressive, plateau or recovery phase.
- With progressive deterioration, frequent monitoring will need to be maintained, and ICU involved in the event of respiratory compromise, as detailed above. On the other hand, if serial assessments show stability, the frequency of monitoring can be relaxed.
- In spinal cord pathology, upper motor neuron signs can subsequently develop from what was initially a flaccid paralysis, revealing the true location of the lesion.

Selection of patients for ambulatory care, hospital admission and HDU/ICU admission

- All patients in the progressive phase of the disease will require admission for monitoring as a minimum.
- Non-ambulant patients and those with cardiovascular autonomic involvement should usually be monitored in a high dependency setting at least.

Table 71.2 Investigation in suspected Guillain-Barré syndrome.

Test	Comment
CSF analysis	CSF protein is usually elevated, but may be normal, especially early in the disease course. CSF lymphocyte count >10/mm^3 is unusual, and counts >50/mm^3 are 'never' seen in GBS, such that alternative diagnoses (haematological malignancy, HIV, Borrelia) must be strongly considered in this setting.
MRI spine	Mandatory if spinal cord/cauda equina compression is in the differential (see Figure 71.1).
Nerve conduction studies/ electromyography (NCS/EMG)	Can support the diagnosis by demonstrating an acute neuropathy, and may classify into demyelinating (slowing, temporal dispersion, conduction block) or axonal (reduced amplitudes) subtypes. Electrophysiological studies do not make or break the diagnosis in isolation, however. Interpretation in the context of the clinical presentation, with expert opinion where required, is recommended.
Blood tests	**All patients** Blood glucose. Creatinine and electrolytes (including calcium, phosphate and magnesium) (severe electrolyte disturbance may cause flaccid weakness). Liver function tests. Serum protein electrophoresis and immunoglobulin levels (to detect paraproteins and exclude IgA deficiency). Creatine kinase (to exclude rhabdomyolysis). Full blood count. Erythrocyte sedimentation rate and C-reactive protein (usually elevated in vasculitic mononeuritis multiplex, which can mimic GBS). Thyroid function tests. **In selected patients** Anti-ganglioside antibodies (anti-GQ1b antibodies have 90–95% sensitivity for Miller Fisher syndrome (MFS), anti-GM1 or GD1a may support diagnosis of acute motor axonal neuropathy (AMAN)). Serological tests for prodromal infections (*C.jejuni*, EBV, CMV, hepatitis E, Mycoplasma pneumonia (before IVIg is given)). ANA/ENA (vasculitis?). Anti-acetylcholine receptor antibodies (myasthenia gravis?). Anti-voltage gated calcium channel antibodies (Lambert-Eaton?). Thiamine/red cell transketolase (dry beriberi?).
Stool	Culture for *Campylobacter jejuni*.
Urine	Porphyrins/porphobilogen. Myoglobin.

- With evidence of neuromuscular respiratory compromise and/or pronounced cardiovascular autonomic instability involvement of ICU is recommended.

Risk-assessment models
- Risk of mechanical ventilation in first week can be assessed by the Erasmus GBS Respiratory Insufficiency Score (EGRIS, measured at time of admission). Overall, around one in four patients with GBS will require intubation.
- Long-term prognosis (the probability of being unable to walk independently at four weeks, three months and six months) can be calculated by the modified Erasmus GBS Outcome Score (mEGOS).
  Both are available via https://gbsstudies.erasmusmc.nl/tools

Table 71.3 Causes of acute weakness (see also Table 17.1).

Site	Causes
Brain	Stroke
	Mass lesion with brainstem compression
	Encephalitis
	Central pontine myelinolysis
	Sedative drugs
Spinal cord	Spinal cord/cauda equina/root compression (see Chapter 70)
	Transverse myelitis
	Anterior spinal artery occlusion
	Haematomyelia
	Poliomyelitis
	Rabies
Peripheral nerve	Guillain-Barré syndrome
	Critical illness neuropathy
	Toxins (heavy metals, biological toxins or drug intoxication)
	Acute intermittent porphyria
	Vasculitis (with mononeuritis multiplex)
	Lymphomatous neuropathy
	Diphtheria
Neuromuscular junction	Myasthenia gravis
	Lambert-Eaton syndrome
	Botulism
	Biological or industrial toxins
Muscle	Hypokalaemia
	Hypophosphataemia
	Hypomagnesaemia
	Inflammatory myopathy
	Critical illness myopathy
	Acute rhabdomyolysis (see Appendix 25.1)
	Trichinosis
	Periodic paralyses

Further management

Patients who fail to improve, or continue to deteriorate, after initial treatment with IVIg or PLEx may require a repeat or alternative treatment. There is little evidence to support this decision and discussion with a neurologist is recommended.

For patients in the plateau or recovery phase of their disease, pain management, pressure area care and thromboprophylaxis remain important. Fatigue and low mood are also common problems which may require treatment. Input from physiotherapy is extremely valuable in maintaining and then improving mobility and functional ability. With the aid of occupational therapy, discharge home might be considered at this time, with or without an intermediate period spent in a specialist rehabilitation setting as appropriate.

Patient support groups

http://www.gaincharity.org.uk/
http://www.gbs-cidp.org/

Appendix 71.1 Guillain-Barré syndrome

Guillain-Barré syndrome (GBS) is an acute, inflammatory neuropathy. Typical cases are characterized by largely symmetric, post-infectious, ascending weakness with arreflexia. Cranial nerve palsy (especially facial), pain and sensory symptoms are common, sensory signs less so.

By definition, progression of weakness ceases within four weeks of onset. Nadir is reached earlier than this in most cases.

GBS has become the most common cause of acquired neuromuscular paralysis. GBS follows infection in approximately two-thirds of cases. Most often the infection is of upper respiratory tract, although *Campylobacter jejuni* (causing gastroenteritis) is the most frequently identified prodromal agent. In the Western world, the resulting neuropathy is of a demyelinating type (Acute Inflammatory Demyelinating Polyradiculoneuropathy, AIDP) in the majority of cases. Axonal subtypes are also seen (such as Acute Motor Axonal Neuropathy, AMAN).

Miller Fisher syndrome (MFS), characterized by a triad of ophthalmoplegia, ataxia and areflexia, is usually considered a regional variant of GBS, but is significantly less common. Other regional and overlap syndromes are also described.

The recovery phase in GBS can be extremely long, and at least 20% of patients fail to return to their premorbid baseline. Nevertheless, continuing improvement is possible even at two years from the initial presentation.

The risk of recurrent GBS is small but significant, at around 5%. Occasionally a further deterioration after initial improvement can represent a fluctuation related to the acute treatment 'wearing off' or indicate a diagnosis of chronic inflammatory demyelinating polyradiculoneuropathy (CIDP).

Further reading

Wilson HJ, Jacobs BC, van Doorn PA (2016) Guillain-Barré syndrome. *Lancet* 388, 717–727.

CHAPTER 72

Raised intracranial pressure

Michael Canty

Owing to its diverse causes (Table 72.1), raised intracranial pressure (ICP) can affect all ages and demographics. It can often present in an insidious manner with symptoms that may be difficult to differentiate from more benign pathologies. Recognition of raised ICP and urgent identification of the cause is crucial: because of the intracranial pressure-volume relationship (Box 72.1), even seemingly well, stable patients can deteriorate rapidly and without warning.

The importance of regular and reliable neurological observations should be emphasized to the nursing staff. In certain conditions, such as malignant MCA syndrome secondary to ischaemic stroke, even subtle changes to conscious level may be of critical importance and trigger urgent intervention.

Priorities

1 **If you suspect raised intracranial pressure (Table 72.2):**
- Assess the airway, breathing and circulation, and correct abnormal physiology.
- Assess the conscious level: seek an urgent anaesthetic/intensive care opinion for patients flexing to painful stimuli or worse.

Box 72.1 Intracranial pressure-volume relationship

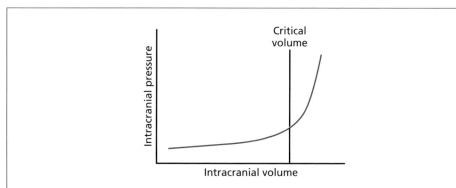

The relationship between intracranial pressure and volume is explained by the pressure-volume curve. The Monro-Kellie hypothesis states that in the rigid container of the skull, the volume of the intracranial constituents is constant (i.e. brain, blood and CSF). An increase in any component, or the addition of a component (i.e. a brain tumour), must be offset by a decrease in one or more of the others if intracranial pressure is to remain constant. Once this compensatory reserve is exhausted, ICP rises precipitously.

Acute Medicine: A Practical Guide to the Management of Medical Emergencies, Fifth Edition. Edited by David Sprigings and John B. Chambers.
© 2018 John Wiley & Sons Ltd. Published 2018 by John Wiley & Sons Ltd.

Table 72.1 Causes of raised intracranial pressure.

Mechanism	Pathologies	Comment
Vascular	Haemorrhagic stroke Subarachnoid haemorrhage Cerebral venous sinus thrombosis Ischaemic stroke with mass effect ('malignant MCA (middle cerebral artery) syndrome')	Vascular causes typically present suddenly, with headache, vomiting and neurological deficit. Patients with raised ICP secondary to ischaemic stroke present with pressure symptoms usually over 24 h following the infarct, with severe headache and progressive reduction in conscious level.
Disorders of CSF hydrodynamics	Obstructive hydrocephalus Communicating hydrocephalus Idiopathic intracranial hypertension	Obstructive hydrocephalus due to a mass lesion such as a tumour presents subacutely, but conscious level may deteriorate very rapidly. Such patients, particularly if young, may lose the ability to look upwards, due to dorsal midbrain compression. Communicating hydrocephalus usually occurs due to disruption of CSF reabsorption, such as following subarachnoid haemorrhage, or meningitis. Idiopathic intracranial hypertension (previously known as benign intracranial hypertension) occurs almost exclusively in young, obese females. It is characterized by headache, papilloedema, and markedly raised CSF pressures on lumbar puncture.
Infection	Brain abscess Subdural empyema Meningitis Encephalitis	Brain abscess and empyema present with headache, confusion and seizures. There is usually a source such as sinusitis, dental abscess or infective endocarditis. Meningitis and encephalitis cause raised intracranial pressure secondary to cerebral inflammation, venous congestion and thrombosis, and secondary hydrocephalus.
Trauma	Severe head injury with traumatic haematoma (e.g. subdural or extradural haematoma) Chronic subdural haematoma	Acutely raised intracranial pressure secondary to trauma presents with a clear history in a usually comatose patient. Chronic subdural haematoma is a common presentation to medicine, usually in elderly patients with a great variety of presentations. Most commonly it presents with deterioration in mobility, headache, confusion, and occasionally focal deficit.
Neoplasia	Primary brain tumour Brain metastasis Extra-axial tumour (e.g. meningioma)	Brain tumours present subacutely with headache, nausea and vomiting, and focal deficits. There may be a history of previous cancer in patients presenting with brain metastasis. A small number of patients, usually with cerebellar metastasis, present in extremis with obstructive hydrocephalus.
Metabolic disorder	Acute liver failure Diabetic ketoacidosis Hypoxic-ischaemic brain injury Severe hyponatraemia Acute mountain sickness	Metabolic presentations of raised ICP are varied, and the diagnosis is often suspected by the systemic condition of the patient, for example cerebral oedema in a young patient with diabetic ketoacidosis following fluid administration.

Table 72.2 Clinical features of raised intracranial pressure.

Feature	Comment
Headache	Classically wakes the patient from sleep in the early hours of the morning, due to recumbency and the vasodilating effect of hypercapnia while asleep. Also exacerbated by lying down or bending over, coughing, sneezing or laughing.
Vomiting	Vomiting is a late feature of raised ICP. It typically occurs after waking, and is associated with morning headache.
Visual symptoms	These include a deterioration in visual acuity, field loss, blurring of vision and visual obscurations with episodic darkening of vision.
Reduced conscious level	As ICP increases, there is a progressive fall in conscious level (which should be assessed by the Glasgow coma scale score) due to caudal displacement of the diencephalon and midbrain.
Seizures	Seizures are extremely deleterious in raised ICP and should be treated aggressively. Prophylaxis is often appropriate, especially in intracranial infection – seek specialist advice.
Papilloedema	Optic nerve head swelling suggests relatively long-standing raised ICP, as well as a threat to vision, and mandates urgent investigation. Retinal haemorrhages may also be present.
Focal neurological deficits	These include extraocular muscle palsy, facial nerve palsy, limb weakness or numbness, upper motor neuron signs such as extensor plantar response, ataxia, dysphasia, dysarthria. An abnormal neurological examination in the context of a suggestive history requires urgent investigation.

- Arrange brain CT. Emergent or urgent CT is required in almost all cases to determine the cause of raised ICP.
- Seek urgent advice on management from neurology or neurosurgery. Lumbar puncture may be indicated, but should only be done on specialist advice (Box 72.2).

2 **Prevent secondary brain injury**

- The cornerstone of preventing secondary brain injury is maintenance of normal physiology. Arterial oxygen and carbon dioxide tensions should be kept within normal limits. Hypo- and hypertension should be avoided. Treat fever aggressively. Maintain normal blood glucose and treat electrolyte abnormalities.
- Nurse the patient 30° head-up to optimize cerebral venous drainage.
- Seizures are extremely deleterious in raised ICP and should be treated aggressively. Prophylaxis is often appropriate, especially in intracranial infection – seek specialist advice.

Box 72.2 Cautions before lumbar puncture

Lumbar puncture is often an important investigation in certain suspected diagnoses, such as sub-arachnoid haemorrhage, meningitis and idiopathic intracranial hypertension. However, it has absolute and relative contraindications, many of which are encountered in raised ICP.

No patient should have a lumbar puncture without a CT scan of the brain. Decreased conscious level is a relative contraindication, and if there are concerns about the safety of lumbar puncture, specialist advice should be sought before proceeding. In the absence of an obvious mass lesion, CT or MR imaging of the brain are poor at identifying raised intracranial pressure, and should not be relied on for this purpose.

3 **Consider therapy to reduce intracranial pressure**
- Give **dexamethasone** 4 mg 6-hourly IV/PO to treat tumour-related vasogenic cerebral oedema. Steroids are contraindicated in trauma. They may be used sparingly in intracranial abscess or empyema if significant mass effect is present, but only on neurosurgical advice. Always co-prescribe a proton pump inhibitor or ranitidine to prevent steroid-induced gastritis and ulceration.
- Consider **mannitol** 20% 0.5–1 g/kg IV to treat severely raised ICP secondary to cerebral oedema, and/or to buy time prior to neurosurgical intervention in life-threatening situations. Seek specialist advice. Mannitol must not be used in systemic hypotension. Check plasma osmolality; further doses may be given until osmolality reaches 320 mosmol/kg. Beyond this, mannitol may cause rebound intracranial hypertension.

Further management

Further management is determined by the cause of raised ICP:
- Most cases of haemorrhagic or ischaemic stroke will be managed by stroke teams; only a small number will proceed to neurosurgical intervention.
- In general, hydrocephalus, raised ICP due to trauma and primary brain tumours will be managed by neurosurgical units, depending on the age and comorbidities of the patient. Patients with a new diagnosis of an intracranial tumour should be discussed with a neurosurgeon, but if stable generally require further investigation such as staging CT examination of the chest, abdomen and pelvis, and MRI of the brain.
- Patients with metabolic causes of raised ICP will often be managed by non-neuroscience clinical teams; however, advice on management should always be obtained.

Further reading

Bradley D, Rees J (2013) Brain tumour: mimics and chameleons. *Pract Neurol* 13, 359–371.
Piper RJ, Kalyvas AV, Young AMH, Hughes MA, Jamjoom AAB, Fouyas IP (2015) Interventions for idiopathic intracranial hypertension. *Cochrane Database of Systematic Reviews 2015*, Issue 8. Art. No.: CD003434. DOI: 10.1002/14651858.CD003434.pub3. www.cochranelibrary.com.

Abdominal

CHAPTER 73

Acute upper gastrointestinal bleeding

SIMON ANDERSON AND UDI SHMUELI

- This usually presents with haematemesis or melaena (Box 73.1), but should be considered in any patient with unexplained hypotension or syncope, or decompensated chronic liver disease.
- Causes of upper gastrointestinal (GI) bleeding are given in Table 73.1. About 90% of non-variceal bleeds and 50% of variceal bleeds stop spontaneously. Mortality is around 7–10% in patients with non-variceal bleeds, and 30% in those with variceal bleeds. Almost all deaths occur in patients >65 years and those with major comorbidities, most often from multi-organ failure secondary to hypovolaemia/hypotension.
- In patients with severe upper GI bleeding, a good outcome requires vigorous resuscitation, and close collaboration with medical, endoscopic, radiological and surgical teams: it is important to involve these specialists as early as possible to discuss the management plan.

Priorities

1 **Make a rapid clinical assessment**, to include an estimate of the volume of blood lost (Table 73.2). Put in a large-bore IV cannula (e.g. green or grey Venflon), and take 20 mL of blood for urgent investigations (Table 73.3). Initial fluid resuscitation should be with IV crystalloid. Give blood when available if the patient is shocked, or actively bleeding with a haemoglobin of <90 g/L.

Box 73.1 Manifestations of acute upper GI bleeding

Haematemesis is the vomiting of red blood, and indicates moderate or severe acute upper GI bleeding.

Coffee-ground vomiting is the vomiting of dark brown vomitus that resembles coffee grounds. It results from the oxidation of haem to haematin by gastric acid, and indicates minor upper GI bleeding that has slowed or stopped.

Melaena is black, tarry stool and typically indicates upper GI bleeding. Small intestinal or right colon bleeding can also cause melaena. (see Chapter 74, Table 74.1). Upper GI bleeding of >50–100 mL is required to cause melaena, which may persist for several days after bleeding has ceased. Black stool that is not melaena may result from ingestion of iron or some foods.

Haematochezia is the passage of liquid blood or clots per rectum, and usually indicates lower GI bleeding (see Chapter 74, Table 74.2), but sometimes can result from severe upper GI bleeding with rapid transit of blood through the gut.

Acute Medicine: A Practical Guide to the Management of Medical Emergencies, Fifth Edition. Edited by David Sprigings and John B. Chambers.
© 2018 John Wiley & Sons Ltd. Published 2018 by John Wiley & Sons Ltd.

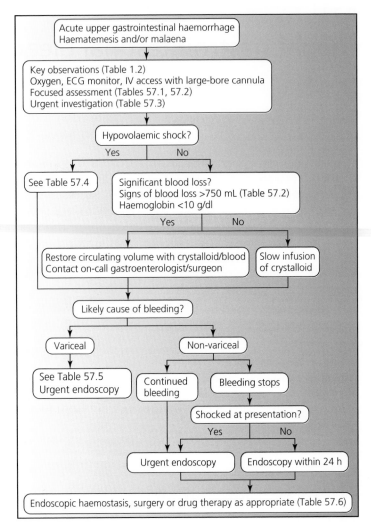

Figure 73.1 Management of acute upper gastrointestinal bleeding.

The Blatchford score (Table 73.4) is a screening tool to assess the probability that endoscopic intervention or blood transfusion will be needed, and is helpful when discussing the patient's management with colleagues.

2 If there is hypovolaemic shock (systolic blood pressure ≤90 mmHg, pulse ≥100/min, cold extremities):
- Give oxygen 60–100% and attach an ECG monitor.
- Obtain help:
  - Inform gastroenterology/surgical colleagues, and contact the on-call endoscopy service, to arrange urgent endoscopy.
  - Put out a major haemorrhage call.
  - Call the on-call anaesthetist for endotracheal intubation if there is respiratory failure or a reduced level of consciousness (e.g. Glasgow coma scale score <9).
- Transfuse blood products within the pre-assembled packs. If systolic blood pressure remains <100 mmHg, use uncrossmatched O Rhesus negative blood (Rhesus positive blood is acceptable for males and

Table 73.1 Causes of upper gastrointestinal haemorrhage.

Common

Gastric or duodenal peptic ulcer

Oesophageal or gastric varices

Erosive oesophagitis, gastritis or duodenitis

No lesion identified (10–15% cases; usually because the lesion is obscured by blood, difficult to identify, such as Dieulafoy's lesion, or healed by the time of the gastroscopy)

Less common or rare

Portal hypertensive gastropathy

Angiodysplasia

Gastric antral vascular ectasia (GAVE), (long red stripes arising from the pylorus, also known as 'watermelon' stomach)

Mass lesions (polyp or cancer)

Mallory-Weiss syndrome (see Chapter 75)

Dieulafoy's lesion (an abnormally large submucosal vessel that erodes the gastric epithelium bleeding intermittently; there is no primary ulcer and so in the absence of bleeding it is difficult to see)

Haemobilia (bleeding from the bile duct)

Haemosuccus pancreaticus (bleeding from the pancreatic duct)

Aorto-enteric fistula (fistula between aneurysmal aorta or aortic graft and the gut, most often duodenum; endoscopy is primarily to exclude bleeding from other causes; the fistula may not be visualized)

Cameron lesions (linear ulcers within the sac of a hiatus hernia at the diaphragmatic impression)

Table 73.2 Focused assessment in acute upper GI bleeding.

History

Has there been haematemesis, melaena or both? Did vomiting precede the first haematemesis (suggesting Mallory-Weiss tear, although this history is absent in 50% of cases)? Was bleeding associated with syncope?

Has there been previous upper gastrointestinal bleeding? What was the cause?

Current and recent drug therapy: ask specifically about non-steroidal anti-inflammatory drugs (NSAIDs), aspirin, clopidogrel, warfarin and direct-acting oral anticoagulants (fondaparinux, rivaroxaban, apixaban, dabigatran)

Usual and recent alcohol intake

Known chronic liver disease

Other medical problems, for example heart disease, chronic kidney disease, haematological conditions.

Examination

Estimate the volume of blood loss from the physiological observations:

Major bleed (>1500 mL; >30% of blood volume)	Minor bleed (≤750 mL; <15% of blood volume)
Pulse ≥120/min	Pulse <100/min
Systolic BP <120 mmHg (note this is influenced by age and usual blood pressure)	Systolic BP ≥120 mmHg, with postural fall <20 from lying to sitting
Cool or cold extremities	Normal perfusion of extremities
Tachypnoea (respiratory rate >20/min)	Normal respiratory rate
Abnormal mental state: agitation, confusion, reduced conscious level	Normal mental state

Signs of chronic liver disease?

Abdominal tenderness or masses?

Hepatomegaly, splenomegaly or ascites?

Table 73.3 Urgent investigation in acute upper GI bleeding.

Full blood count
Group and screen serum: crossmatch at least 4 units of whole blood if there is shock, significant blood loss or initial haemoglobin <100 g/L
Coagulation screen
Sodium, potassium, urea and creatinine
Liver function tests
ECG if age ≥50 or known cardiac disease
Chest X-ray

post-menopausal females). Start transfusing crossmatched blood as soon as it is available, via a second IV cannula. Use a blood warmer if infusing at >50 mL/kg/hour.
- Correct clotting abnormalities (see below).
- Insert a urinary catheter to monitor the urine output (aim for urine output of 0.5 mL/kg/hour).

3 Correct clotting abnormalities
- If the fibrinogen level is <1.5 g/L, or the prothrombin time (or international normalized ratio, INR) is >1.5 × control, give 2 units of fresh frozen plasma.
- If the patient is taking warfarin and is actively bleeding, give vitamin K, 5–10 mg by slow IV injection, and consider giving prothrombin complex concentrate: discuss with a haematologist (see Chapter 103).

Table 73.4 Blatchford score.

Add the scores for each risk marker. If no value applies for a particular marker, score 0. A total score can range from 0 to 23. A score above zero indicates the need for admission and inpatient endoscopy.

Risk marker on admission	Score
Blood urea (mmol/L)	
≥6.5 <8.0	2
≥8.0 <10.0	3
≥10.0 <25	4
≥25	6
Haemoglobin (g/L) for men	
≥120 <130	1
≥100 <120	3
<100	6
Haemoglobin (g/L) for women	
≥100 <120	1
<100	6
Systolic blood pressure (mmHg)	
100–109	1
90–99	2
<90	3
Other markers	
Pulse ≥100/min	1
Presentation with malaena	1
Presentation with syncope	2
Hepatic disease	2
Heart failure	2

- If the patient is taking a direct-acting oral anticoagulant (e.g. dabigatran, rivaroxaban), discuss management with a haematologist (see Chapter 103).
- If the platelet count is $<50 \times 10^9$/L, and the patient is actively bleeding, give platelet concentrate: discuss with a haematologist.

4 If you suspect bleeding oesophageal or gastric varices (because of a past history of variceal bleeding or chronic liver disease):

- Give terlipressin 2 mg IV followed by 1–2 mg 4–6 hourly until bleeding is controlled, for up to 5 days.
- Give IV antibiotic (e.g. coamoxiclav 1.2 g 8-hourly IV or tazocin 4.5 g 8-hourly IV), to prevent bacterial infection (including spontaneous bacterial peritonitis, Chapter 24), which is a common complication.
- Contact the endoscopy service for urgent endoscopy, to define the source of bleeding and for therapeutic endoscopy (banding of bleeding varices).
- If bleeding continues, or there is any impairment in conscious level, contact an anaesthetist to discuss endotracheal intubation.
- If there is continued variceal bleeding (and the airway is protected by endotracheal intubation), a Sengstaken-Blakemore tube (Chapter 125) can be inserted by an experienced operator.
- Other supportive measures for patients with decompensated chronic liver disease are discussed in Chapter 77.

5 In patients without shock but with evidence of significant blood loss (e.g. syncope in association with bleeding; clinical signs of blood loss >750 mL) or haemoglobin <100 g/L:

- Start an infusion of crystalloid to maintain systolic blood pressure >100 mmHg.
- Transfuse blood if the initial haemoglobin is <70 g/L.
- Correct clotting abnormalities (see above).
- Contact the on-call endoscopy service to arrange endoscopy within 24 hours.

Further management

Blood transfusion

Once the volume deficit has been corrected, recheck the haemoglobin and transfuse blood if this is 70 g/L or below.

Endoscopy

- Urgent endoscopy is needed for patients with shock on admission (but not before adequate resuscitation), with known varices or signs of chronic liver disease, or evidence of continued bleeding.
- Other patients should have endoscopy within 24 hours of admission (with the exception of those with a Blatchford score of zero, who can be considered for discharge with outpatient endoscopy). They can be allowed to eat, but must be nil by mouth for >4 hours prior to endoscopy.

Drug therapy

- Stop nonsteroidal anti-inflammatory drugs (NSAIDs).
- Anticoagulant and antiplatelet therapy should be stopped/reversed, if the benefits of doing so outweigh the risks: for patients with a mechanical prosthetic heart valve, recent acute coronary syndrome or coronary stents, discuss this with a cardiologist. See Chapter 103.
- There is no evidence that starting a proton pump inhibitor (PPI) before endoscopy alters outcome. Treatment with a PPI makes testing for *Helicobacter pylori* unreliable.
- There is no firm evidence to support antifibrinolytic therapy (tranexamic acid) before or after endoscopy.
- The HALT-IT trial is assessing whether early administration of tranexamic acid can reduce the in-hospital mortality of upper GI bleeding, and improve outcomes. The trial aims to complete recruitment in 2017.

Table 73.5 Rockall score post-endoscopy.

Add the scores at the top of each column for each of the variables to derive a total risk score. The total score can range from 0 to 11.

	Score			
	0	**1**	**2**	**3**
Age	<60	60–79	≥80	
Shock on admission?	No shock (systolic blood pressure ≥100, pulse <100)	Tachycardia (systolic BP ≥100, pulse ≥100)	Hypotension (systolic BP <100)	
Comorbidity	None		Heart failure, ischaemic heart disease, any other comorbidity	Renal failure, liver failure, disseminated malignancy
Diagnosis at endoscopy	Mallory-Weiss tear, no lesion seen, no signs of recent bleeding	All other diagnosis	Malignancy of upper GI tract	
Major stigmata of recent bleeding at endoscopy	None or dark spot only		Blood in upper GI tract, adherent clot, visible or spurting vessel	

Management after endoscopy
- Calculate the Rockall score (Table 73.5). Those with a score ≤2 can be discharged (predicted mortality <1%). Those with a score ≥3 should remain in hospital for close observation.
- Further management is determined by the endoscopic diagnosis, and should be discussed with a gastroenterologist.

Peptic ulcer
- Patients with low-risk peptic ulcer bleeding based on clinical and endoscopic criteria (e.g. clean ulcer base) can be discharged on the same day as endoscopy.
- Most patients with high-risk peptic ulcer bleeding based on clinical and endoscopic criteria (e.g. stigmata of recent haemorrhage) should remain hospitalized for at least 72 h.
- Start a proton pump inhibitor (PPI). If the patient is stable and able to tolerate oral medication, this can be administered by mouth (e.g. omeprazole 40 mg PO 12-hourly). If the patient is at high risk of further bleeding (high Rockall score) or unable to tolerate oral medication, give a bolus of omeprazole (or pantoprazole) 80 mg IV followed by an infusion of 8 mg/hour for 72 h.
- Rebleeding after an initial endoscopy requires either a repeat endoscopy or referral to interventional radiology, depending on the initial findings at endoscopy. If interventional radiology is not promptly available, refer for surgery.
- Full dose PPIs should be given for at least four weeks.
- Most patients with gastric ulcers should have a repeat endoscopy at 6–8 weeks to confirm healing and exclude malignancy.
- If *Helicobacter pylori* positive, start eradication treatment according to local protocols. Most ulcers not due to NSAIDs or aspirin are associated with *H. pylori* infection. As the Clotest taken at endoscopy may be falsely negative when taken at the time of an acute bleed, a high index of suspicion should be kept and a urease

breath test (off PPIs) should be ordered after the acute event when appropriate. Gastric biopsies taken for histology at the time of the initial endoscopy, can also improve the detection rate.

- Anticoagulant and antiplatelet therapy: NSAIDs should be stopped; low-dose aspirin, if needed for secondary prevention of vascular events or coronary stent thrombosis, can be continued with concomitant PPI therapy. Other antiplatelet agents (e.g. clopidogrel) should be stopped temporarily and timing of restarting discussed with the appropriate specialist (cardiologist or stroke physician).

Erosive gastritis

There are two groups of patients:

- Previously well patients in whom erosive gastritis is related to aspirin, NSAIDs or alcohol. Bleeding usually stops when these agents are withdrawn and no specific treatment is needed. A short course of a PPI can be given to limit concomitant damage from acid exposure. *H. pylori* should be treated if present.
- In critically ill patients with stress ulceration, in whom the mortality is high, correct clotting abnormalities and give a PPI. Sucralfate is also an option.

Oesophagitis and oesophageal ulcer

Give a PPI for 4 weeks, followed by a further 4–8 weeks treatment if not fully healed.

Oesophageal and gastric varices

- Variceal bleeding stops spontaneously in 50% of patients. The risk of further bleeding can be substantially reduced by follow-up endoscopic therapy to obliterate residual varices, and administration of a non-selective beta blocker (e.g. propranolol or carvedilol).
- Discuss management of the varices and the underlying cause of portal hypertension with a gastroenterologist or hepatologist.

Mallory-Weiss tear

- Bleeding usually stops spontaneously and rebleeding is rare.
- If bleeding continues, the options are repeat endoscopy with a view to endotherapy (argon-plasma coagulation, application of haemostasis clip), tamponade using a Sengstaken-Blakemore tube, or interventional radiology for embolization.

Negative endoscopy

- In 15–20% of patients, the first endoscopy does not reveal a source of bleeding. Discuss repeating the endoscopy, especially if blood or food obscured the views obtained, or the patient has chronic liver disease (as varices which have recently bled may not be visible).
- Patients who presented with melaena alone, should be investigated for a small bowel or proximal colonic source of bleeding (Chapter 74, Table 74.1). A normal blood urea suggests a colonic cause of melaena, except in patients with chronic liver disease (in whom urea levels are often low).
- CT angiography can be useful after two negative endoscopies, but only if performed when the patient is actively bleeding.

Further reading

Gerson LB, Fidler JL, Cave DR, *et al.* (2015) American College of Gastroenterology Clinical Guideline: Diagnosis and management of small bowel bleeding. *Am J Gastroenterol* 110, 1265–1287.

National Institute for Health and Care Excellence (2015) *Blood transfusion*. NICE guideline (NG24). https://www.nice.org.uk/guidance/ng24.

National Institute for Health and Care Excellence (2016) *Acute upper gastrointestinal bleeding in over 16s: management.* Clinical guideline (CG141). https://www.nice.org.uk/guidance/cg141?unlid=122385053201610212730.

Tripathi DJ, Stanley AJ, Hayes PC (2015) UK guidelines on the management of variceal haemorrhage in cirrhotic patients. *Gut* 1–25. DOI: 10.1136/gutjnl-2015-309262.

CHAPTER 74

Acute lower gastrointestinal bleeding

Sophia Savva and Andrew Dixon

Acute lower gastrointestinal bleeding can present with melaena or haematochezia (the passage of liquid blood or clots per rectum). Causes are given in Tables 74.1 and 74.2.

An upper gastrointestinal source must always be excluded in patients with evidence of severe bleeding, and these patients should be managed accordingly (see Chapter 73). Haematochezia usually originates from the left side of the colon or rectum, and bleeding stops without intervention in most cases.

Priorities

1 **Consider (and exclude by urgent endoscopy) an upper gastrointestinal source of bleeding in patients with severe bleeding**
   - Look for clinical clues (Table 73.2): is there a history of liver disease, excess alcohol consumption, known varices, haematemesis, upper abdominal pain or NSAID use? Are there signs of major blood loss? Is the blood urea raised (Table 73.3), suggesting an upper GI source?
   - If there is reason to suspect severe upper GI bleeding, management hinges on vigorous resuscitation, followed by upper GI endoscopy as soon as the patient is stabilized. Please refer to Chapter 73 for detailed advice on the management of upper GI bleeding.
   - Focused assessment of the patient with acute lower GI bleeding is summarized in Table 74.3, and investigation needed urgently in Table 74.4.
2 **Involve the surgical team promptly if there is acute lower GI bleeding with haemodynamic compromise or major blood loss**
   Although 85% of lower GI bleeding is self-limiting, surgery can be life-saving if bleeding is severe and persistent.
3 **Consider correction of clotting abnormalities**
   - Consider stopping or reversing antiplatelet and anticoagulant drugs at presentation (Chapter 103). In cases of minor self-limiting rectal bleeding, this may not be necessary. If there is more severe or persistent bleeding, the decision may be difficult, and the risk of further bleeding has to be balanced against the risk of stopping these medications, for example in the patient with recent coronary stent placement.
   - Correction of clotting abnormalities is described on in Chapters 102 and 103. Seek advice from a haematologist.
4 **Blood transfusion**
   Blood transfusion is rarely necessary in cases of lower GI bleeding. As with other causes of blood loss, the transfusion threshold should be a haemoglobin <80 g/L, or haemoglobin <100 g/L if there is ongoing bleeding. This is a guideline only and the decision should include careful clinical assessment of the patient.

Acute Medicine: A Practical Guide to the Management of Medical Emergencies, Fifth Edition. Edited by David Sprigings and John B. Chambers.
© 2018 John Wiley & Sons Ltd. Published 2018 by John Wiley & Sons Ltd.

Table 74.1 Small bowel and proximal colonic sources of melaena.

Arteriovenous malformation, including angiodysplasia (a common cause of bleeding in the elderly).
Meckel's diverticulum (usually causes acute lower GI bleeding in children but can present in young adults).
Right colon diverticulosis (more common in non-Western countries, where the diverticula are predominantly left sided).
Inflammatory bowel disease (Crohn's disease).
Haemobilia (bleeding from the biliary tree usually occurs after instrumentation (e.g. ERCP), surgery (cholecystectomy) or trauma. It may be associated with jaundice and biliary colic).
Haemosuccus pancreaticus (bleeding from the pancreatic duct).
Aorto-enteric fistula (fistula between aneurysmal aorta or aortic graft and the gut, most often duodenum).
Ectopic varices (usually but not invariable associated with upper GI tract varices; ectopic varices can be difficult to detect especially if not considered to be a cause of bleeding).

5 Admit or discharge?
- Patients with minor lower GI bleeding that stops spontaneously can be investigated by early outpatient sigmoidoscopy and clinic review.
- Admit patients with moderate or severe bleeding, persistent bleeding, or significant comorbidities.

Further management

Once clotting abnormalities have been corrected, 85% of lower GI bleeding stops without intervention.

Flexible sigmoidoscopy
Once the patient is stabilized, the source of bleeding must be identified. In most cases flexible sigmoidoscopy is a reasonable first investigation; the earlier it is undertaken, the higher the diagnostic yield. Blood in the GI tract acts as a laxative, so often flexible sigmoidoscopy can be undertaken without bowel preparation by means of an enema.

Lower GI bleeding with negative sigmoidoscopy
- If bleeding continues and its cause cannot be determined by flexible sigmoidoscopy, a full colonoscopy and/or CT angiogram is needed. If these do not reveal a cause, mesenteric angiography and technetium-labelled RBC scanning may localize the source of bleeding.

Table 74.2 Causes of haematochezia.

Severe upper gastrointestinal bleeding (the patient will usually be shocked and, in contrast to a lower GI bleed, plasma urea will be disproportionately raised).
Diverticular disease (the commonest cause particularly in the elderly, usually with no pre-existing symptoms).
Ulcerative colitis (almost invariably associated with diarrhoea and a pre-existing history; inflammatory markers may be normal in left-sided disease).
Left-sided colonic cancer (usually low-grade but recurrent bleeding; should always be actively excluded as a cause).
Post-polypectomy bleeding (delayed bleeding occurs on average 5–7 days post-procedure; risk factors include: polyps >10 mm, age >65, cardiovascular or renal disease, use of anti-coagulant or antiplatelet agents).
Ischaemic colitis (older adult with risk factors for arterial thromboembolism (atherosclerosis or vasculitis) or acute hypotension, e.g. post cardiac arrest; there is usually associated abdominal pain).
Angiodysplasia (venous bleeding and therefore less severe).
Radiation colitis (often following radiotherapy for cancer of prostate; can cause acute bleeding shortly after treatment and also delayed bleeding, typically within two years).
Rectal varices (these are relatively common in all cases of portal hypertension but seldom cause significant bleeding; they should be distinguished from haemorrhoids).
Haemorrhoids (will still require endoscopic evaluation to exclude a more serious cause).

Table 74.3 Focused assessment in acute lower GI bleeding.

See also Table 73.2 Focused assessment in acute upper GI bleeding

History
Ask about prior episodes and pre-existing conditions such diverticulosis, colitis or recent colonoscopy.
Take careful drug history for anti-inflammatory drugs antiplatelet drugs and anticoagulants.
Explore preceding symptoms such as weight loss and change in bowel habit, which may suggest malignancy.
Check for significant comorbidities such as cardiac disease or renal impairment.

Examination
Estimate the volume of blood loss from the physiological observations:

Major bleed (>1500 mL; >30% of blood volume)	Minor bleed (≤750 mL; <15% of blood volume)
Pulse ≥120/min	Pulse <100/min
Systolic BP <120 mmHg (note this is influenced by age and usual blood pressure)	Systolic BP ≥120 mmHg, with postural fall <20 from lying to sitting
Cool or cold extremities	Normal perfusion of extremities
Tachypnoea (respiratory rate >20/min)	Normal respiratory rate
Abnormal mental state: agitation, confusion, reduced conscious level	Normal mental state

Examine for signs of chronic liver disease/cirrhosis.
Look for cachexia or obvious weight loss that may indicate an underlying malignancy.
Rectal examination is essential to assess the stool and for rectal masses. This should always be performed in a sensitive manner with an appropriate chaperone. Unless the patient requests their presence, friends and family with the patient should be asked to leave the room when you perform this examination.

- For mesenteric angiography to be diagnostic, bleeding has to be ongoing at a rate of >0.5 mL/minute to be diagnostic. Trans-catheter embolization can follow angiography to stop the bleeding.
- If the bleeding stops and its cause cannot be determined by flexible sigmoidoscopy, a full colonoscopy should be performed as an urgent outpatient procedure.
- On the rare occasions where there is ongoing bleeding and the above investigations have failed to identify the source, upper GI endoscopy, push enteroscopy or capsule endoscopy may be considered.

Endoscopic haemostasis

- Bleeding points, for example post-polypectomy or from a bleeding diverticulum, can be treated endoscopically by the application of endoclips or heater probe.
- Angiodysplasia or radiation proctitis can be treated using argon plasma coagulation.

Table 74.4 Urgent investigation in acute lower GI bleeding.

Full blood count
Group and screen serum: crossmatch at least four units of whole blood if there is shock, significant blood loss or initial haemoglobin <100 g/L
Coagulation screen
Sodium, potassium, urea and creatinine
Liver function tests
ECG if age ≥50 or known cardiac disease
Chest X-ray

- Bleeding tumours are often harder to treat endoscopically as there may not be a single bleeding point; haemostasis is sometimes achieved using the above methods.

Emergency surgery

- If there is persistent severe bleeding despite supportive measures and attempts at endoscopic haemostasis, emergency surgery may be needed,
- Efforts should be directed at identifying the source of bleeding prior to surgery as this improves outcomes. Pre-operative localization of the source of bleeding (i.e small bowel, right or left colon) is important to minimize the duration of the operation and minimize the length of bowel needed to be resected.

Bleeding from inflammatory bowel disease

- See Chapter 76. Patients with a flare of ulcerative colitis typically have bloody diarrhoea. The bleeding usually settles with medical management but a colectomy may be needed to treat the colitis itself. Crohn's disease can present with a large lower GI bleed with minimal pre-existing symptoms. Ulceration in the ileo-caecal region is the usual cause. The diagnosis is usually clear from the history, but in a new presentation differentiation from infective colitis or ischaemic colits can be difficult and treatment may be started empirically.
- LMWH prophylaxis for venous thromboembolism should be given as these patients are at high risk.
- Blood transfusion may be needed to maintain a haemoglobin of about 100 g/L.

Further reading

Cirocchi R, Grassi V, Cavaliere D, *et al*. (2015) New trends in acute management of colonic diverticular bleeding: a systematic review. *Medicine* 94, e1710.

Strate LL, Gralnek IM (2016) American College of Gastroenterology Clinical Guideline: Management of patients with acute lower gastrointestinal bleeding. *Am J Gastroenterol* 111, 459–474.

CHAPTER 75

Acute oesophageal disorders

Sophia Savva and Andrew Dixon

Causes of oesophageal perforation and rupture are given in Table 75.1.

History

Typical presentation is vomiting followed by severe lower retrosternal chest pain in a middle-aged male, often with a background of heavy alcohol intake. Oesophageal rupture may occur without vomiting, and may follow straining (e.g. in labour or with weight-lifting), coughing or hiccoughing. Often there is an underlying diagnosis of eosinophilic oesophagitis or Barrett's oesophagus.

Examination

Pneumomediastinum may result in subcutaneous emphysema (found in ~25% patients) and crackling sounds on auscultation of the heart. There may be signs of pleural effusion/pneumothorax. Signs of septic shock (from mediastinitis) may dominate the clinical picture and are seen in ~25% of patients at presentation.

Differential diagnosis

Includes myocardial infarction, aortic dissection, pulmonary embolism, pericarditis, pneumonia, spontaneous pneumothorax, perforated peptic ulcer, acute pancreatitis. Misdiagnosis of spontaneous oesophageal rupture is common.

Investigation (Table 75.2)
Initial management

- Urgent surgical opinion
- Admit to high-dependency unit (HDU)/intensive care unit (ICU)
- Nil by mouth
- Opioid analgesia and antiemetic

Acute Medicine: A Practical Guide to the Management of Medical Emergencies, Fifth Edition. Edited by David Sprigings and John B. Chambers.
© 2018 John Wiley & Sons Ltd. Published 2018 by John Wiley & Sons Ltd.

Table 75.1 Causes of oesophageal perforation and rupture

Spontaneous oesophageal rupture, typically associated with vomiting (Boerhaave syndrome; Table 75.2) (usually occurs in the left posterolateral wall of the lower third of the oesophagus, with leak into the left pleural cavity).
Blunt trauma to the chest.
Instrumentation of the oesophagus (risk with diagnostic endoscopy very low; risk increased with procedures such as dilatation of stricture or sclerotherapy of varices).
Surgery to the oesophagus or adjacent structures.
Left atrial radiofrequency ablation for atrial fibrillation (causing atrioesophageal fistula)
Ingestion of a corrosive substance.

- IV fluids
- Antibiotic therapy to cover anaerobic and Gram-positive/Gram-negative aerobic bacteria: for example piperacillin/tazobactam + metronidazole + gentamicin
- IV proton pump inhibitor
- Management of septic shock if present (chapter 35)

Mallory-Weiss tear

- Small tears at the gastro-oesophageal junction.
- Accounts for 5–10% of acute upper gastrointestinal bleeding (chapter 73).
- A history of retching is only elicited in around 30% of cases.
- Around 80% stop bleeding spontaneously and rebleeding is uncommon outside of the context of coagulopathy.
- Rarely need endoscopic therapy except if high-risk stigmata are present, for example visible vessel.

Table 75.2 Urgent investigation in suspected Boerhaave syndrome.

Test	Comment
Chest X-ray	Almost always abnormal in Boerhaave syndrome although changes may be subtle at presentation.
	Abnormalities seen include pneumomediastinum, mediastinal widening, subcutaneous emphysema, pleural effusion (usually on left), pneumothorax, free peritoneal gas.
CT chest	Indicated if chest X-ray is non-diagnostic and other diagnoses such as aortic dissection or pulmonary embolism are more likely.
	In Boerhaave syndrome, CT may show extra-oesophageal gas, peri-oesophageal fluid, mediastinal widening, and gas and fluid in pleural spaces, retroperitoneum and lesser sac.
Water-soluble (Gastrografin) contrast swallow	Definitive test. Reveals location and extent of extravasation of contrast medium.
	If negative despite high clinical index of suspicion, barium swallow should be done.
Aspiration of pleural effusion if present	Exudative pleural effusion with low pH, high amylase level, purulent; may contain undigested food.
Tests to exclude other diagnoses and needed in management	ECG, arterial blood gases and pH, full blood count, group and screen, biochemistry, blood culture.

Food bolus obstruction

Usually caused by large pieces of meat or small chicken or fish bones.

Patients present with sudden onset dysphagia and a sensation of a blockage.

Chest pain due to muscle spasm is common and can mimic angina.

AP and lateral chest X-rays are useful to asses for mediastinal free air.

Most pass spontaneously, but due to the potential for localized ischaemia within the oesophagus, endoscopy should be performed within 12 hours.

Underlying oesophageal pathology has been reported in 80%, including benign and malignant strictures, dysmotility and eosinophilic oesophagitis (diagnosed on biopsy).

Once the obstruction has been cleared hospitalization is rarely necessary, although repeat outpatient endoscopy is sometimes indicated (e.g. for stricture dilatation).

Further reading

Furuta GT, Katzka DA (2015) Eosinophilic esophagitis. *N Engl J Med* 373, 1640–1648.

Kim HS (2015) Endoscopic management of Mallory-Weiss tearing. *Clin Endosc* 48, 102–105. http://www.e-ce. org/upload/pdf/ce-48-102.pdf.

Markar SR, Mackenzie H, Wiggins T, *et al.* (2015) Management and outcomes of oesophageal perforation: a national study of 2,564 patients in England. *Am J Gastroenterol* 110, 1559–1566. DOI: 10.1038/ ajg.2015.304.

Nirula R. Esophageal perforation (2014) *Surg Clin North Am* 94, 35–41.

CHAPTER 76

Inflammatory bowel disease flare

SOPHIA SAVVA AND ANDREW DIXON

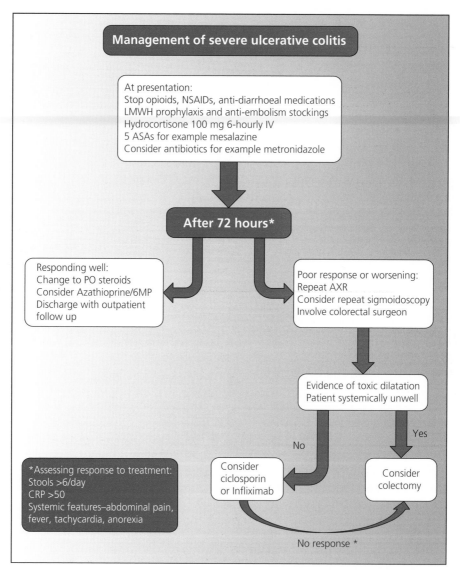

Figure 76.1 Management of severe ulcerative colitis.

Acute Medicine: A Practical Guide to the Management of Medical Emergencies, Fifth Edition. Edited by
David Sprigings and John B. Chambers.
© 2018 John Wiley & Sons Ltd. Published 2018 by John Wiley & Sons Ltd.

Consider a flare of inflammatory bowel disease (IBD) (Appendix 76.1) in patients presenting with:

- Diarrhoea, especially bloody diarrhoea (Chapter 22)
- Abdominal pain (Chapter 21)
- Acute lower gastrointestinal bleeding (Chapter 74)

Assessment and management of the patient presenting with undifferentiated acute diarrhoea are given in Chapter 22.

Priorities

Establish the diagnosis by clinical assessment (Table 76.1) and urgent investigation (Table 76.2).

Key differentials to consider are:

Infective diarrhoea. Missing this diagnosis in someone with colitis can result in serious harm if they are subsequently immunosuppressed.

Colorectal cancer in a patient with long-standing colitis. This can occur even in young patients.

Ischaemic colitis, particularly in patients who are over 50 and known arteriopaths or have a history of atrial fibrillation.

Diverticular disease.

Radiation colitis (following radiotherapy).

Where there is any diagnostic doubt, request colonoscopy. Limited examinations can often be performed without bowel preparation. Biopsies are often key to establishing the diagnosis and differentiating between Crohn's colitis and ulcerative colitis, and can reveal the presence of cytomegalovirus and other infections. Other pathologies such as colorectal cancer and ischaemic colitis can also be identified.

Immediate management of a flare of IBD

- Establish a stool chart. This is essential for assessing progress. A sudden reduction in stool production should be followed up with an abdominal film to rule out toxic megacolon.
- Prescribe low-molecular-weight heparin thromboprophylaxis and anti-embolism stockings. This should be done even in patients with rectal bleeding as long as they are not anaemic or haemodynamically compromised. Active inflammatory bowel disease confers a very high thromboembolic risk.
- Prescribe hydrocortisone 100 mg 6-hourly IV.
- Prescribe a 5-ASA for colitis, which can be given rectally in limited left-sided disease. These are not effective drugs for use in small-bowel Crohn's disease.
- Advise a low residue diet.
- If proximal constipation is seen on the abdominal film, prescribe laxatives.
- Discontinue opioids, NSAIDs and anti-diarrhoeal agents, as these can precipitate toxic megacolon.
- Involve the gastroenterology team and the inflammatory bowel disease nurse.
- Well patients with no high-risk features can be managed as outpatients, with oral steroids in the form of prednisolone or budesonide.
- Treat any underlying or suspected infection.
- Patients with signs of peritonitis, toxic dilatation, fistulating or obstructing disease should be referred urgently to the surgical team.

Table 76.1 Focused assessment in suspected inflammatory bowel disease flare.

History

Mode of onset (abrupt, sub-acute or gradual) and duration of symptoms
Stool frequency, volume, consistency; watery or containing blood or mucus
Nocturnal diarrhoea?
Associated abdominal pain? Relation to defaecation
Upper GI symptoms? (nausea and vomiting may be due to stricturing small bowel disease in Crohn's)
Past history
Drug history

Examination
Physiological observations
Nutritional status
Extra-intestinal manifestations of IBD (erythema nodosum, iritis, arthritis)
Abdomen (scars, masses)
Perianal and rectal examination

Further management

Ulcerative colitis

This is summarized in Figure 76.1.

Imaging
Abdominal X-ray should be done to rule out toxic dilatation and proximal constipation. It can also often give an idea as to the extent of the disease.

Table 76.2 Investigations in a flare of inflammatory bowel disease.

Element	Comment
Full blood count	Patients on immunomodulators can become neutropenic, and therefore susceptible to infections. A full blood count may also reveal anaemia or a raised white cell count indicating infection or steroid use.
C-reactive protein (CRP)	Ten percent of patients with inflammatory bowel disease do not develop a raised CRP even during active disease. In these patients it is often useful to look at the platelet count as a marker of inflammation.
Electrolytes, urea and creatinine	Dehydration is unusual in flare-ups of inflammatory bowel disease unless there is underlying obstruction or the patient has presented late.
Amylase	In patients with abdominal pain pancreatitis is an important differential. Both steroids and azathioprine can cause pancreatitis.
Plain radiographs	Plain abdominal films may show loops of inflamed bowel, proximal constipation, obstruction or toxic dilatation of the colon. Chest X-ray may show concurrent chest infection or air under the diaphragm suggesting perforation.
Stool culture	Always send at least three stool cultures were possible. Even in patients with known colitis infection can trigger an exacerbation. In patients with previous hospital admissions or recent antibiotic use always consider Clostridium infection. CMV colitis can also occur in immunosuppressed patients.

Other forms of imaging are rarely necessary. Occasionally a CT abdomen may be indicated if complications are suspected, but as IBD patients have a high lifetime exposure to ionizing radiation, this should be avoided wherever possible.

Nutrition

Maintenance of caloric intake is essential to promote bowel microbiome health and prevent weight loss, but during periods of active disease, a low-residue diet should be given to prevent further disease exacerbation.

Drug therapy

The initial treatment of an acute flare is with corticosteroid. In a severe flare, oral steroid is not adequately absorbed by inflamed mucosa, so parenteral treatment should be given initially. If the response is good, oral steroid (e.g. prednisolone 40–60 mg daily, with gastric and bone protection) can be substituted after 72 hours, and can be given from the outset in mild-moderate flares.

If a severe flare does not respond to parenteral corticosteroid, ciclosporin or infliximab may be used. This must always be under the supervision of a gastroenterologist.

Surgery

Colectomy remains the most effective treatment for ulcerative colitis. However, it should be reserved for the patient in whom medical treatment has failed. Of vital importance is the firm establishment of the diagnosis of ulcerative colitis (UC) as opposed to Crohn's colitis, as colectomy is curative in the former but not in the latter. Surgical intervention in UC carries a much better prognosis when performed as a planned procedure rather than as an emergency. This is why it is important to involve the surgical team early, and also why sometimes certain drugs such as ciclosporin can be given as a bridge to surgery.

Crohn's disease

Imaging

In small bowel Crohn's disease, further imaging may be warranted. Consider small-bowel ultrasound scanning, MRI enterocleisis or CT of the abdomen to look for collections, obstructions, perforations or fistulas.

When requesting imaging in Crohn's disease remember that these patients are often young, with a lifelong illness, and their exposure to radiation is often significant over the years. Consider imaging techniques that do not involve exposure to ionizing radiation where available.

Capsule endoscopy

Crohn's disease can often present in an occult fashion with iron-deficiency anaemia, non-specific abdominal pain, nausea and vomiting, or weight loss. In these cases, capsule endoscopy may be useful to image the small bowel, but this is usually performed on an outpatient basis.

Nutrition

Nutritional assessment is an essential part of management, particularly if there is a history of weight loss or multiple surgeries resulting in a short gut. Elemental diets have been shown to be useful in treating complicated Crohn's disease, especially in the presence of strictures, but compliance is low. In severe cases supplementary NG feeding or even parenteral feeding may become necessary, but this should always be instigated on the advice of a nutrition consultant.

Drug therapy

The initial treatment of an acute flare is with corticosteroid. In a severe flare, oral steroid is not adequately absorbed by inflamed mucosa, so parenteral treatment should be given initially. If the response is good, oral steroid (e.g. prednisolone 40–60 mg daily, with gastric and bone protection) can be substituted after 72 hours, and can be given from the outset in mild-moderate flares.

If a severe flare does not respond to parenteral corticosteroid, ciclosporin or infliximab may be used. This must always be under the supervision of a gastroenterologist.

Surgery

The place of surgery in the management of Crohn's disease is less clear cut than in UC. Endoscopic recurrence of the disease post-surgery is around 80% after the first year, and for this reason surgery is reserved for complications of Crohn's disease or disease refractive to medical management. In general, surgery focuses on removing as little of the bowel as possible, as over many years these patients can end up with a short gut and the complications that follow.

Appendix 76.1 Inflammatory bowel disease

Crohn's disease

Affects about one in every 650 people in the UK and is increasing in incidence.

Inflammation can affect any area of the GI tract from the mouth to the perianal area. Upper GI Crohn's disease is more common in children, affecting around 10% of patients, but much rarer in adults (thought to be about 1%).

Inflammation can be transmural and skip lesions can be present. Crohn's can be further complicated by fistulating or stricturing disease.

Perianal disease, small-bowel disease or fistulas are features of Crohn's and not seen in ulcerative colitis.

Ulcerative colitis (UC)

Inflammation is limited to the rectum and colon and occasionally the terminal ileum, and confined to the mucosa.

Inflammation is always continuous from the rectum (unless partially treated).

Bloody diarrhoea is more common in UC.

UC may be difficult to distinguish from infective causes of diarrhoea, but often a history of chronicity will help to differentiate the two.

Abdominal pain is not a common presenting feature of UC.

Further reading

National Institute for Health and Care Excellence (2012) Crohn's disease: management. Clinical guideline (CG152). https://www.nice.org.uk/guidance/cg152?unlid=5300026042016102323343.

National Institute for Health and Care Excellence (2013) Ulcerative colitis: management. Clinical guideline (CG166). https://www.nice.org.uk/guidance/cg166.

Seah D, De Cruz P (2016) Review article: the practical management of acute severe ulcerative colitis. *Aliment Pharmacol Ther* 43, 482–513.

CHAPTER 77

Acute liver failure and decompensated chronic liver disease

B EN W ARNER AND M ARK W ILKINSON

Acute liver failure

- Consider acute liver failure (ALF) in any patient with jaundice, reduced consciousness or coagulopathy. Decompensated chronic liver disease is a more frequent occurrence, distinguished from ALF in that the patient has pre-existing cirrhosis with either progression or a superimposed insult. Particular aetiologies favour ALF (e.g. paracetamol toxicity or Budd-Chiari syndrome). Common causes for ALF are shown in Table 77.1.
- The prognosis of ALF is related to the time taken for encephalopathy to develop and the aetiology. Hyperacute liver failure (the development of encephalopathy <7 days after jaundice) is associated with a better prognosis than acute liver failure (jaundice to encephalopathy between 8 and 28 days) and sub-acute liver failure (jaundice to encephalopathy in 4–12 weeks). Aetiologies with the worst prognosis include non-A, non-B causes for ALF, while paracetamol toxicity and pregnancy-related syndromes have the most favorable outcomes.

Priorities

If you suspect ALF:

1 Check the blood glucose, as hypoglycaemia is a common complication.
- If <4.0 mmol/L, give 100 mL of 20% glucose or 200 mL of 10% glucose over 15–30 min IV. Recheck blood glucose after 10 min, if still <4.0 mmol/L, repeat the above IV glucose treatment.

Box 77.1 Liver failure

The term liver failure is applied to two distinct syndromes: acute liver failure and decompensated chronic liver disease. Management of suspected liver failure is summarized in Figure 77.1.

Acute liver failure (ALF) is defined as severe acute liver injury with encephalopathy and impaired liver synthetic function (prothrombin time/international normalized ratio ≥ 1.5) in the absence of pre-existing liver disease; an illness duration of <26 weeks distinguishes acute from chronic liver failure. ALF has an annual incidence of around 5 per million in the UK. Causes are given in Table 77.1.

Decompensated chronic liver disease (acute on chronic liver failure) is defined as a syndrome in patients with chronic liver disease, with or without previously diagnosed cirrhosis, characterized by acute hepatic decompensation resulting in liver failure (jaundice and prolongation of the prothrombin time/ international normalized ratio), and one or more extrahepatic organ failures. Management is focused on identification and treatment of the precipitant(s) (Table 77.6) while providing supportive care.

Acute Medicine: A Practical Guide to the Management of Medical Emergencies, Fifth Edition. Edited by David Sprigings and John B. Chambers.
© 2018 John Wiley & Sons Ltd. Published 2018 by John Wiley & Sons Ltd.

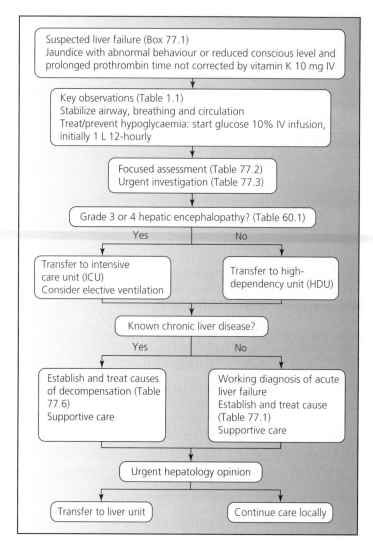

Figure 77.1 Management of suspected acute liver failure.

- Start an IV infusion of 10% glucose, initially 1 L/12 h, to prevent hypoglycaemia; use a large peripheral vein as it can cause thrombophlebitis.

2 Make a focused clinical assessment (Table 77.2), including a detailed drug history (including any herbal and over-the-counter medications) from the patient or family members, and arrange urgent investigations (Table 77.3).

- If there is any suspicion that ALF is due to paracetamol poisoning, then give N-acetylcysteine (NAC) without delay using the standard regimen (Table 36.9), as this improves outcomes even when given up to 48 h after ingestion.

3 If there is grade 3 or 4 encephalopathy, transfer the patient to an ICU for elective intubation and ventilation. Other patients with ALF should be nursed in a high-dependency unit.

4 Obtain advice on management from a hepatologist or your regional liver unit, with the investigation results to hand when you make the phone call.

Table 77.1 Causes of acute liver failure (fulminant hepatic failure).

Cause	Comment
Drug-related	Paracetamol poisoning is the commonest cause of ALF in the UK; AST/ALT are typically >3500 units/L
	Idiosyncratic reaction (usually occurs within six months of starting drug); many drugs implicated, for example coamoxiclav
Viral hepatitis	Hepatitis A, B, C, D or E virus
	Herpes simplex virus (a rare cause; usually seen in patients taking immunosuppressive therapy or in third trimester of pregnancy)
Ischaemic hepatitis ('shock liver')	May occur after cardiac arrest or prolonged hypotension, or in severe heart failure, and therefore often associated with acute kidney injury
	Markedly raised AST/ALT
Acute Budd-Chiari syndrome	Due to acute hepatic vein thrombosis
	Typically occurs in women aged 20–40 years, with underlying haematological disorder (e.g. polycythemia rubra vera, paroxysmal nocturnal haemoglobinuria) or other cause of thrombophilia (P. 567 Table 100.6)
	Presents with right upper quadrant pain, hepatomegaly and ascites (Chapter 24)
	Diagnosed by duplex ultrasonography of hepatic veins and IVC
Acute fatty liver of pregnancy	Occurs in last trimester of pregnancy
	Often associated with pre-eclampsia
	See Chapter 32
Autoimmune hepatitis	Consider if there are other autoimmune disorders (e.g. haemolytic anaemia, idiopathic thrombocytopenic purpura, type 1 diabetes, thyroiditis, coeliac disease)
	Autoantibodies (antinuclear antibodies, anti-smooth muscle antibodies) and hypergammaglobulinaemia usually present
***Amanita phalloides* poisoning**	Suspect if the patient has eaten wild mushrooms
	Usually associated with severe gastrointestinal poisoning symptoms (nausea, vomiting, diarrhoea, abdominal pain), which develop within hours to one day of ingestion
Wilson disease	Suspect in a patient age <30 with liver failure and haemolytic anaemia (giving markedly elevated bilirubin)
	Kayser-Fleischer rings are present in ~50%
	Serum ceruloplasmin is typically low (but may be normal in ~15% and is often reduced in other forms of ALF) and serum/urinary copper levels high
	Alkaline phosphatase and urate are low
Malignant infiltration	May occur in breast cancer, small cell lung cancer, lymphoma and melanoma
	Associated with hepatomegaly
	Diagnosis made by imaging and biopsy
Cause unclear	Retake the drug history
	Consider transjugular liver biopsy

ALF, acute liver failure; ALT, alanine aminotransferase; AST, aspartate aminotransferase; IVC, inferior vena cava.

Determining the cause of ALF (Table 77.1)

- In the UK, paracetamol poisoning causes around 50% of ALF, and viral hepatitis around 40%. The mortality of patients with paracetamol poisoning who reach medical attention is 0.4%. Where ALF occurs due to viral hepatitis, mortality is around 40% and 60% due to non-A, non-B viral hepatitis.
- Consider mushroom (*Amanita phalloides*) poisoning in patients with a compatible history; severe nausea, vomiting, diarrhoea and abdominal pain develop within hours to one day of ingestion. Penicillin G 300,000 units/kg/day and milk thistle (silibinin) 30–40 mg/kg/day PO or IV are recognized treatments.

Table 77.2 Focused assessment of the patient with possible acute liver failure.

History

Duration and time course of jaundice and other symptoms (e.g. fever, abdominal pain)

Known liver or biliary tract disease?

Full drug history: including all non-prescription drugs, herbal remedies, dietary supplements, mushroom ingestion or khat, taken over the past year

Risk factors for viral hepatitis (foreign travel, IV drug use, men who have sex with men, multiple sexual partners, body piercing and tattoos, blood transfusion and blood products, needle-stick injury in health-care worker)?

Pregnancy?

Usual and recent alcohol intake?

Other medical problems (e.g. cardiovascular disease, transplant recipient, cancer, HIV/AIDS, haematological disease)?

Family history of jaundice/liver disease?

Examination

Physiological observations and systematic examination

Conscious level and mental state; grade of encephalopathy if present:

Grading of hepatic encephalopathy	
Grade	**Clinical features**
Subclinical	Impaired work, personality change, sleep disturbance
	Abnormal findings on psychomotor testing
Grade 1	Mild confusion, agitation, apathy, oriented in time and place
	Fine tremor, asterixis
Grade 2	Drowsiness, lethargy, disoriented in time
	Asterixis, dysarthria
Grade 3	Sleepy but rousable, disoriented in time and place
	Hyperreflexia, hyperventilation
Grade 4	Responsive only to painful stimuli or unresponsive

Asterixis? Ask the patient to hold the arms outstretched with the wrists extended and fingers spread apart, and eyes closed, for 30 seconds or longer. The sign is positive if after a brief latent period, there is a sudden lapse of maintenance of the posture.

Hepatic foetor?

Signs of chronic liver disease?

Right upper quadrant tenderness?

Liver enlargement (seen in early viral hepatitis, alcoholic hepatitis, malignant infiltration, congestive heart failure, acute Budd-Chiari syndrome)?

Splenomegaly?

Ascites (Chapter 24)?

- Wilson's disease and autoimmune hepatitis, although both forms of chronic liver disease, can be treated as if they are ALF. Wilson's classically presents with a Coombs-negative haemolytic anaemia and a high bilirubin to ALP ratio. The diagnosis is confirmed by high urinary copper levels. Treatment aims to lower serum copper levels via haemofiltration. Penicillamine is not recommended acutely. Autoimmune hepatitis should be treated with 40–60 mg prednisolone PO per day.
- The presence of a nodular liver on imaging in a patient suspected of having ALF does not necessarily indicate that the patient has pre-existing cirrhosis. Nodularity can occur with benign conditions. As the severity of

Table 77.3 Urgent investigation in suspected acute liver failure.

Needed urgently

Prothrombin time (PT)/international normalized ratio (INR) and activated partial thromboplastin time (APTT)

Full blood count and reticulocyte count

Blood glucose

Sodium, potassium, urea and creatinine (urea may be low because of reduced hepatic synthesis; if markedly elevated with a normal creatinine, suspect upper gastrointestinal bleeding)

Liver function tests: bilirubin, aspartate transaminase, alanine transaminase, gamma-glutamyl transpeptidase, alkaline phosphatase, albumin

Amylase and lipase

Paracetamol level if unexplained acute liver failure or paracetamol poisoning is suspected

Arterial blood gases, pH, lactate and ammonia

Blood culture

Urine stick test, microscopy and culture

Microscopy and culture of ascites if present (aspirate 10 mL for cell count (use EDTA tube) and culture (inoculate blood culture bottles) (see Chapter 24)

Chest X-ray

Ultrasound of liver, biliary tract and hepatic/portal veins

Pregnancy test in women of childbearing age

For later analysis

Markers of viral hepatitis (anti-HAV IgM, HBsAg, anti-HBc IgM, anti-HCV, anti-HDV, anti-HEV, anti-HSV, anti-VZV)

HIV test

Autoimmune profile (antinuclear antibodies, antismooth muscle antibodies, immunoglobulins)

Plasma ceruloplasmin in patients aged <50 (to exclude Wilson's disease)

Serum (10 mL) and urine (50 mL) for toxicological analysis if needed

Blood group and screen

EDTA, ethylene diaminetetra-acetic acid; HAV, hepatitis A virus; HBc, hepatitis B core; HBsAG, hepatitis B surface antigen; HCV, hepatitis C virus; HDV, hepatitis D virus; HEV, hepatitis E virus; HSV, herpes simplex virus; VZV, varicella zoster virus; IgM, immunoglobulin M.

fibrosis increases, so, too, does the diagnostic accuracy of ultrasound at detecting cirrhosis. The gold standard for diagnosing cirrhosis is liver biopsy, or non-invasively by a Fibroscan.

- ALF in women in the third trimester of pregnancy is most commonly due to HELLP syndrome (coexistent hypertension and proteinuria) or acute fatty liver of pregnancy (AFLP) (see Chapter 32). AFLP can be confirmed by hepatic steatosis on imaging. Other causes of ALF, however, also occur in pregnancy. Treatment is alongside maternity staff and commonly involves prompt delivery of the foetus.

Further management of acute liver failure before transfer to a Liver Unit

General care and monitoring

- Nurse the patient with 20 head-up tilt in a quiet area of an ICU or high-dependency unit, avoiding unnecessary disturbance.
- Monitor the conscious level, pulse, blood pressure, temperature and plasma glucose 1–4-hourly. Monitor oxygen saturation by pulse oximeter and give oxygen by mask to maintain SaO_2 >90%.
- Give platelet concentrate before placing central venous and arterial lines if the platelet count is <50 × 10^9/L. Avoid giving fresh frozen plasma (FFP) unless there is active bleeding, as this affects coagulation tests – the best

prognostic marker – for several days, and can precipitate fluid overload. If correction of coagulopathy is needed, discuss with your local haematologist: typically FFP is given in combination with recombinant activated factor VIIa.

- If encephalopathy is grade 2 or more, or if systolic BP is <90 mmHg, central venous pressure monitoring and a urinary catheter will be required. Other causes of reduced consciousness need excluding by clinical assessment and CT head. Fluid resuscitation should be with 4.5% human albumin solution or normal saline unless the blood glucose levels are low.
- If encephalopathy progresses to grade 3 or 4, arrange elective intubation and ventilation.
- If there is any evidence of sepsis, then commence antibiotics and antifungals after a full septic screen.
- Give lactulose to assist in ammonia excretion and prevent worsening encephalopathy. Avoid any potentially nephrotoxic agents.
- Put in a nasogastric tube for gastric drainage if the patient is vomiting or is ventilated. Start enteral feeding early or parenteral feeding if required. Replace potassium, magnesium and phosphate as needed (Chapters 86, 88 and 89).

Management of complications

Complications of ALF and management of complications are summarized in Table 77.4.

Table 77.4 Major complications of acute liver failure and their management.

Complication	Management
Cerebral oedema	See text
Hypotension	Correct hypovolaemia with blood or 4.5% human albumin solution
	Use epinephrine, norepinephrine or dopamine infusion (P. 13 Table 2.7) to maintain mean arterial pressure >60 mmHg
Acute kidney injury	Correct hypovolemia
	Avoid high-dose furosemide
	See Appendix 77.1 Hepatorenal syndrome
	Start renal replacement therapy if anuric or oliguric with plasma creatinine >400 µmol/L
Hypoglycaemia	Give glucose 10% IV 1 L 12-hourly to prevent hypoglycaemia
	Check blood glucose 1–4 hourly
	If blood glucose is <4.0 mmol/L, give 100 mL of 20% glucose or 200 mL of 10% glucose over 15–30 min IV; recheck blood glucose after 10 min, if still <4.0 mmol/L, repeat
Coagulopathy	Give vitamin K 10 mg IV daily
	Give platelet transfusion if count <50 × 10⁹/L Give fresh frozen plasma only if there is active bleeding
Gastric stress ulceration	Prophylaxis with proton pump inhibitor, ranitidine or sucralfate
Hypoxaemia	Many possible causes: inhalation, infection, pulmonary oedema, atelectasis, intrapulmonary haemorrhage.
	Increase inspired oxygen
	Ventilate with positive end-expiratory pressure if SaO₂ remains <92%
Sepsis	Daily culture of blood, sputum and urine
	Early treatment of presumed infection with broad-spectrum antibiotic therapy: discuss with microbiologist
	Consider antifungal therapy if fever with negative blood cultures

Cerebral oedema occurs in 75–80% of patients with grade 4 encephalopathy and is often fatal. It may result in paroxysmal hypertension, dilated pupils, sustained ankle clonus and sometimes decerebrate posturing (papilloedema is usually absent). Intracranial pressure (ICP) should be maintained below 25 mmHg. To avoid raised ICP:

- Give mannitol 20% 100–200 mL (0.5–1.0 g/kg) IV over 10 min alongside maintenance of mean arterial pressure (MAP) at >75 mmHg using vasopressors, with a cerebral perfusion pressure of 60–80 mmHg.
- Increase plasma sodium to 145–155 mmol/L with hypertonic normal saline (Chapter 85).
- Avoid seizures by using phenytoin alongside short-acting benzodiazepines.
- Consider therapeutic hypothermia 32–34 °C as a bridge to transplantation.

Criteria for liver transplantation
These are summarized in Table 77.5.

Table 77.5 Criteria for transplantation in acute liver failure (ALF) (King's College Hospital)*.

ALF due to paracetamol poisoning
- Arterial pH <7.3 after volume resuscitation
- International normalized ratio (INR) >6.5
- Creatinine >300 micromol/L
- Grade 3 or 4 encephalopathy

ALF due to other cause
- INR >6.5
  Or any three of the following features:
- Non-A, non-B viral hepatitis, drug-induced, Wilson's or indeterminate aetiology of ALF
- Time from jaundice to encephalopathy >7 days
- Age <10 or >40
- INR >3.5
- Serum bilirubin >200 micromol/L

Absolute contraindication to transplantation
- AIDS
- Extrahepatic malignancy
- Advanced cardiopulmonary disease
- Cholangiocarcinoma

Relative contraindications to transplantation
- HIV positivity
- Age >70
- HBV DNA positivity
- Active alcohol/substance misuse
- Severe psychiatric disorder
- Portal vein thrombosis
- Pulmonary hypertension

Table 77.6 Precipitants of decompensated chronic liver disease.

Intercurrent infection, especially spontaneous bacterial peritonitis (Appendix 24.1)
Acute gastrointestinal bleeding (variceal and non-variceal) (Chapter 73)
Drugs: diuretics, hypnotics, sedatives and opioid analgesics
Alcoholic hepatitis
Viral hepatitis
Major surgery and anaesthesia
Liver ischaemia secondary to hypotension
Acute portal vein thrombosis
Hypokalaemia and hypoglycaemia
Constipation
Development of hepatocellular carcinoma
No cause apparent (in up to 40% of patients)

Decompensated chronic liver disease

Priorities

Search for and treat precipitants (Tables 77.6).

- Spontaneous bacterial peritonitis (SBP) is common and may not be accompanied by abdominal tenderness. If there is ascites, aspirate 10 mL for microscopy and culture (inoculate blood culture bottles). Assume peritonitis is present if ascitic fluid shows >250 white blood cells/mm^3, of which >75% are polymorphs, and treat with third-generation cephalosporin, for example cefotaxime 2 g 8-hourly IV for 5 days, followed by a quinolone PO for 5 days. See Appendix 24.1 for further discussion of SBP.
- A rectal examination must be performed to exclude melaena. Evaluation and management of acute upper and lower gastrointestinal bleeding is described in Chapters 73 and 74.

  Start a liver failure regimen.

Reduce the intestinal nitrogenous load: start lactulose 30 mL 3-hourly PO until diarrhoea begins, then reduce to 30 mL 12-hourly, adjusted to achieve passage of two soft stools/day.

Enteral nutrition should be started early to prevent a hypercatabolic state.

Reduce the risk of gastric stress ulceration: give prophylaxis with omeprazole, ranitidine or sucralfate.

Maintain blood glucose >4.0 mmol/L. Give dextrose 10% IV infusion initially 1 L 12-hourly. Check blood glucose 1–4-hourly and immediately if conscious level deteriorates.

Fluid and electrolyte balance: the diet should be low in sodium. Give potassium supplements to maintain a plasma level >3.5 mmol/L. If IV fluid is needed, use 4.5% human albumin solution or glucose 5% or 10%. Avoid normal saline. In the absence of renal impairment, treat ascites with spironolactone combined with a loop diuretic if necessary, aiming for weight loss of 0.5 kg/day. If ascites is refractory to diuretic therapy, use paracentesis with IV infusion of 100 mL of 20% human albumin solution. See Chapter 24 for further management of ascites.

Thromboprophylaxis: as patients remain at high risk of venous thromboembolism even when prothrombin time is prolonged, prescribe low-molecular-weight heparin prophylaxis unless there is active bleeding or the platelet count is <50 × 10^9/L.

Drugs: give vitamin K 10 mg IV (not intramuscularly) and folic acid 15 mg PO once daily. Avoid sedatives and opioids. Other drugs that are contraindicated are listed in the *British National Formulary*.

  Seek advice on further management from a hepatologist or gastroenterologist.

Appendix 77.1 Hepatorenal syndrome

Definition
Acute kidney injury (AKI) in a patient with acute or chronic liver disease complicated by severe liver failure and portal hypertension, when other causes of AKI have been excluded (see Chapter 25).

Background
Hepatorenal syndrome occurs in around 20–25% of patients with acute liver failure and decompensated chronic liver disease. Spontaneous bacterial peritonitis (Appendix 24.1) is complicated by AKI in 30–40% of cases, and is a common precipitant of hepatorenal syndrome.

Diagnosis
Acute kidney injury (see Chapter 25 for definition and staging)

Exclusion of other causes of acute kidney injury (Chapter 25)

No or minimal proteinuria

Normal or near-normal urine microscopy

Urine sodium concentration <10mmol/L (if not taking diuretic); urine osmolality greater than plasma osmolality

Failure of renal function to improve after withdrawal of diuretics and with volume expansion with human albumin solution 1 g/kg (up to 100 g) IV daily for two days.

Management
Seek advice from a hepatologist

Treat the underlying liver disease

Exclude/treat spontaneous bacterial peritonitis (Appendix 24.1)

General management of acute kidney injury (Chapter 25)

Consider treatment with terlipressin (0.5–2.0 mg IV every 4–12 h) for 5–15 days plus human albumin solution, 1 g/kg (up to 100 g) IV on days 1 and 2, followed by 20–40 g daily, for 5–15 days

Further reading

Baekdal M, Ytting H, Larsen FS. (2016) Acute liver failure. *J Hepatol Gastroint Dis* 2, 3 (open access).

Bernal W, Wendon J. (2013) Acute liver failure. *N Engl J Med* 369, 2525–2534.

Bernal W, Jalan R, Quaglia A, *et al*. (2015) Acute on chronic liver failure. *Lancet* 386, 1576–1587.

National Institute for Health and Care Excellence (2016) Cirrhosis in over 16s: assessment and management NICE guideline (NG50). https://www.nice.org.uk/guidance/ng50.

Wijdicks EFM. (2016) Hepatic encephalopathy. *N Engl J Med* 375, 1660–1670.

CHAPTER 78

Alcoholic hepatitis

BEN WARNER AND MARK WILKINSON

Alcoholic hepatitis is distinguished from other causes of acute hepatitis by:
- A history of heavy alcohol use (Chapter 106)
- An AST: ALT ratio of ≥2, which is rarely seen in other forms of liver disease

Severe acute alcoholic hepatitis is a life-threatening disease. Treatment with corticosteroid can improve survival, but mortality remains high, with 35% of patients dying within six months.

Seek urgent advice from a hepatologist or gastroenterologist if you suspect alcoholic hepatitis.

Table 78.1 Alcoholic hepatitis: diagnosis.

Clinical features and blood results
- Jaundice
- Prolonged history of alcohol excess
- Stigmata of chronic liver disease may be present
- Fever
- Tender hepatomegaly and a hepatic bruit
- Ascites
- Raised white cell count (may be $>20 \times 10^9$/L) and C-reactive protein
- Prothrombin time prolonged >5 s over control
- Mildly raised AST and ALT (typically 2–3 times level of normal, AST: ALT ratio of ≥2; increases of >10 times suggests viral hepatitis or drug toxicity)
- Raised gamma-glutamyl transpeptidase and serum IgA
- Raised bilirubin
- Raised ferritin (often >1000 μgm/L)
- Low sodium, low potassium, low urea, variable creatinine, low haemoglobin, high MCV, low platelet count

Identification of clinically severe alcoholic hepatitis
- An index of severity ('discriminant function', DF) can be calculated: DF = ([patient's prothrombin time – control] × 4.6) + (bilirubin (μmol/L) ÷ 17.1)
- A DF of >32 identifies patients with severe alcoholic hepatitis (mortality ~50%) who may need intensive care and who may benefit from corticosteroids in the absence of sepsis or other contraindications to steroids.

ALT, alanine aminotransferase; AST, aspartate aminotransferase; IgA, immunoglobulin A; MCV, mean corpuscular volume.

Acute Medicine: A Practical Guide to the Management of Medical Emergencies, Fifth Edition. Edited by David Sprigings and John B. Chambers.
© 2018 John Wiley & Sons Ltd. Published 2018 by John Wiley & Sons Ltd.

Table 78.2 Alcoholic hepatitis: management.

- Seek advice from a gastroenterologist/hepatologist
- Avoid diuretics and ensure adequate volume replacement (use 4.5% human albumin solution and/or salt-poor albumin; avoid normal saline)
- Supportive management of alcohol withdrawal (Chapter 106)
- Start nasogastric feeding early aiming for 2000 calories/day
- Give oral/IV thiamine
- Start broad-spectrum antibiotics after taking cultures of blood, urine and ascites
- Check renal function and prothrombin time daily until there is a consistent improvement
- A full liver screen must be done to exclude other causes of hepatitis (Chapter 23)
- Consider early transjugular liver biopsy
- Consider corticosteroid therapy in patients with DF >32 (prednisolone 40 mg daily for 28 days, with gastroprotection and bone protection)

DF, discriminant function (see Table 78.1).

Further reading

Thursz M, Morgan TR. (2016) Treatment of severe alcoholic hepatitis. *Gastroenterology* 150, 1823–1834.

CHAPTER 79

Biliary tract disorders and acute pancreatitis

Ben Warner and Mark Wilkinson

Table 79.1 Biliary tract disorders: clinical features and management.

Disorder	Clinical features and blood results	Management
Biliary colic	Severe pain, typically in right upper quadrant or epigastrium, but may be retrosternal, lasts 20 min to 6 h Nausea and vomiting	Analgesia (e.g. pethidine) Elective ultrasound of biliary tract
Acute cholecystitis due to gallstones	Severe pain, typically in right upper quadrant, lasts >12 h Often previous biliary colic, nausea and vomiting Often afebrile at presentation or only low grade fever Right upper quadrant tenderness Raised white cell count (usually 12–15 × 10^9/L) in ~60% Liver function tests and amylase normal or only mildly raised; ALT rises before alkaline phosphatase	Analgesia (e.g. pethidine) Nil by mouth Nasogastric drainage if there is vomiting Fluid replacement Antibiotic therapy (e.g. third-generation cephalosporin or quinolone; in severe case, add metronidazole) Surgical opinion Urgent ultrasound of biliary tract
Acute cholangitis	Pain, typically in right upper quadrant, may be mild May follow ERCP Jaundice (in ~60%) Fever with rigors Raised white cell count Abnormal liver function tests and raised amylase Positive blood culture (in ~30%)	Analgesia (e.g. pethidine) Nil by mouth Nasogastric drainage if there is vomiting Fluid replacement Antibiotic therapy (e.g. third-generation cephalosporin or quinolone + metronidazole; if recent ERCP, give piperacillin/tazobactam (or ciprofloxacin if penicillin allergy) + metronidazole + gentamicin) Surgical opinion Urgent ultrasound of biliary tract Biliary drainage by ERCP

ALT, alanine aminotransferase; ERCP, endoscopic retrograde cholangiopancreatography.

Acute Medicine: A Practical Guide to the Management of Medical Emergencies, Fifth Edition. Edited by David Sprigings and John B. Chambers.
© 2018 John Wiley & Sons Ltd. Published 2018 by John Wiley & Sons Ltd.

Table 79.2 Acute pancreatitis (AP): clinical features and management.

Element	Comment
Common causes	Gallstones
	Alcohol
Less common causes	Complication of ERCP Hyperlipidaemia Drugs (e.g. thiopurines, sodium valproate) Hypercalcaemia Pancreas divisum
	Abdominal trauma
	HIV infection
Clinical features and blood results	Epigastric pain, typically sudden in onset when due to gallstones, may increase in severity over a few hours in other causes, may last for several days
	Nausea and vomiting
	Abdominal tenderness/guarding
	Fever at presentation may reflect cytokine-mediated systemic inflammation or acute cholangitis
	Shock, respiratory failure, renal failure and multiorgan failure may occur
	Raised amylase and lipase
	Raised white cell count and C-reactive protein Abnormal liver function tests (elevated ALT more than three times the upper limit of normal is highly predictive of gallstone pancreatitis if alcohol is excluded)
	Hypoglycaemia, hypocalcaemia, hypomagnesaemia and disseminated intravascular coagulation may occur
Identification of severe (10–15%) AP	APACHE II score of 8 or more
	Persistent organ failure (shock, respiratory failure, renal failure) and of SIRS
Genetic predispositions to acute pancreatitis	Mutations in SPINK1 may predispose patients to pancreatitis and to a more severe course

AP, acute pancreatitis; SIRS, systemic inflammatory response; ALT, alanine aminotransferase; APACHE II, severity of illness scoring system based on acute physiology and chronic health evaluation; ERCP, endoscopic retrograde cholangiopancreatography.

Table 79.3 Management of AP

Early fluid resuscitation with 250–500 mL/HR (with careful monitoring of fluid status) of Ringer's lactate or Hartmann's solution aiming to maintain low urea and haematocrit levels.

ICU referral for patients with organ failure.

Urgent abdominal ultrasound to confirm the diagnosis. CT/MRCP for those who fail to improve or deteriorate at 48–72 h. In the absence of gallstones and alcohol excess measure triglyceride levels (>1000 mg/dl suggests primary or secondary hypertriglyceridaemia as the cause).

Consider pancreatic tumours in patients over the age of 40.

Analgesia with opioid and anti-emetics.

Antibiotic therapy with meropenem indicated only for patients with evidence of infected necrosis or extrapancreatic sepsis, for example chest or urinary sepsis.

ERCP within 24 hours for patients with gallstone pancreatitis in whom biliary obstruction is suspected on the basis of raised bilirubin and clinical cholangitis.

Nutritional support: in mild AP, oral feeding with low fat solid food is sufficient.

In severe AP a nasogastric tube may be required in the context of vomiting with the patient fed upright to avoid aspiration.

Parenteral feeding should be avoided.

Infected necrosis is considered in cases where SIRS persists beyond 7–10 days of hospitalization and is confirmed by CT.

Antibiotics are recommended as first line in the stable patient followed by endoscopic/surgical/radiographical intervention if required but not before 4 weeks.

If SIRS fails to improve then CT FNA is needed to confirm antibiotic choice.

The unstable patient requires earlier intervention.

Further reading

Lankisch PG, Apte M, Banks PA. (2015) Acute pancreatitis. *Lancet* 386, 85–96.

National Institute for Health and Care Excellence (2014) Gallstone disease: diagnosis and management. Clinical guideline (CG188). https://www.nice.org.uk/guidance/cg188?unlid=78410445201622195914.

Updated Tokyo Guidelines for acute cholangitis and acute cholecystitis (2013) (open access). http://link.springer.com/journal/534/20/1/page/1.

CHAPTER 80

Urinary tract infection

CAROLYN HEMSLEY AND CLAIRE VAN NISPEN TOT PANNERDEN

Consider urinary tract infection when the patient has symptoms directly referable to the urinary tract:
- Dysuria, frequency, sensation of incomplete voiding
- Haematuria
- Lower abdominal, suprapubic or loin pain
- Abdominal pain and/or fever in pregnancy

In the differential diagnosis of non-specific presentations:
- Unwell after urological intervention or catheterization
- General malaise or fever in patients with long-term urinary catheter
- Delirium or vomiting, with or without fever (especially in children or the elderly)
- Septic shock, without localizing signs (Chapter 35).

Point-of-care urinary testing by urinary dipstick in those with symptoms suggestive of UTI, assessing for pyuria, is sensitive and specific in the non-immunosuppressed population, and can support or exclude the diagnosis at the patient's bedside.

Priorities

1 Determine whether the infection is uncomplicated or complicated (Table 80.1) by clinical assessment (Table 80.2), review of previous microbiology results and investigation (Tables 80.3 and 80.4). This will guide the need for further investigation, the choice of empirical antibiotic therapy, the length of treatment, and the requirement for follow-up.

It is not always apparent at the time of acute presentation whether the infection is complicated or not, but this may become obvious later in the course of treatment.
- Uncomplicated – simple lower urinary tract infection in an otherwise healthy, non-pregnant woman.
- Complicated – UTI in the presence of an underlying condition that increases the risk of infection or the chance of failing therapy (Table 80.1).

Box 80.1 Definitions.

> A urinary tract infection (UTI) is defined by the presence of $\geq 10^3$–10^4 organisms per mL urine, associated with clinical symptoms. Causative organisms are given in Appendix 80.1.
>
> UTI encompasses simple lower urinary tract infection (cystitis), upper urinary tract infection (pyelonephritis, pyonephritis) and infection resulting in bacteraemia and septic shock.

Acute Medicine: A Practical Guide to the Management of Medical Emergencies, Fifth Edition. Edited by David Sprigings and John B. Chambers.
© 2018 John Wiley & Sons Ltd. Published 2018 by John Wiley & Sons Ltd.

Table 80.1 Factors suggestive of complicated urinary tract infection.

Patient demographics
  Very young or advanced age
  Pregnancy
  Male sex
Comorbidities
  Diabetes mellitus
  Immunosuppression
  Renal transplant
  Chronic kidney disease
Anatomical abnormalities
  Urinary tract instrumentation, including urethral catheter, ureteric stent, nephrostomy
  Prostatic pathology
  Urethral stricture
  Renal or bladder stones
Other factors
  Health-care-associated infection
  Failure of recent antimicrobial therapy

Table 80.2 Focused assessment of the patient with suspected urinary tract infection.

History
- Major symptoms and time course – differentiate between lower urinary tract symptoms, upper tract symptoms and systemic features
- Previous history of urinary tract infections
- Antibiotic history
- Presence/absence of urinary catheter, recent catheterization, blocked catheter, catheter change
- History of recent urinary tract intervention or urological intervention
- Previous history of renal tract pathology such as chronic kidney disease, renal stones, single kidney, structural abnormality
- Pregnancy?
- Diabetes?
- Sexual history
- If primarily urethritis or penile discharge, consider sexually transmitted infections (*Neiserria gonorrhoea*, *Chlamydia trachomatis*, *Herpes simplex*, *Trichomonas vaginalis*)
- Symptoms of sexually transmitted infections and epididymo-orchitis?
- Review any recent GP or hospital microbiology results
- Consider points relevant to differential diagnosis – gastrointestinal symptoms

Examination
- Vital signs and key observations if critically ill and resuscitate as appropriate
- Assessment of presence/absence of loin tenderness
- Presence or absence of catheter and quality of catheter urine
- Consider alternative source of sepsis

Note: Gram-negative sepsis secondary to a urinary focus can masquerade as suspected acute respiratory tract infection in the elderly and is often misdiagnosed as such at the time of acute admission.

Table 80.3 Urgent investigations in suspected urinary tract infection.

Suspected simple uncomplicated UTI
- Urine for dipstick as a point-of-care test to detect presence/absence of nitrites and leucocyte esterase
- Urine dipstick for glucose
- Send urine for microscopy, culture and sensitivities – before antibiotics are started (may not be needed if first presentation of lower urinary tract infection in a woman)

Suspected complicated UTI
- Urine dipstick and culture as above
- Full blood count
- C-reactive protein
- Electrolytes, urea and creatinine
- Liver function tests
- Blood glucose
- Pregnancy test in women of childbearing age with lower abdominal symptoms
- CT KUB – if history of renal stones or features of renal colic
- Renal/urinary tract ultrasonography – urgent in the setting of acute kidney injury

Table 80.4 Indications for renal/urinary tract imaging.

Urgent

Features of renal colic or suspicion of renal stones +/− renal tract obstruction (plain X-ray and CT KUB)

As soon as possible (renal ultrasound is the usual initial investigation):
- Acute kidney injury
- Pyelonephritis in men or children
- Recurrent episode of pyelonephritis in women
- History of renal pathology
- Persistent fever despite 48–72 h of appropriate antibiotic
- Uncertain diagnosis, for example considering genitourinary pathology or appendicitis

Referral for renal tract imaging post treatment of acute infection
- Urinary infection in boys and men with no known risk factors for UTI
- Recurrent urinary tract infections (>3/year)
- Haematuria

Not indicated
- Uncomplicated lower tract infection in women
- First episode of pyelonephritis in women with no AKI and rapid treatment response (within defervescence within 48–72 h)

2 If the patient is febrile or has significant systemic upset send peripheral blood as well as urine for culture before starting appropriate empirical antibiotics (Tables 80.5 and 80.6).
- The choice of agent depends on local epidemiology and resistance rates of common urinary pathogens and is usually indicated by local guidelines.
- Consider recent antibiotic history, especially if considering treatment failure.
- Consider recent microbiological culture results if available.
- Mode of delivery of the antibiotic (intravenous versus oral) will depend on the acuity of the illness and ability of patient to tolerate oral antibiotics.
- Review antibiotic choice in pregnancy.

Table 80.5 Empirical antibiotic therapy in suspected urinary tract infection.

Always refer to any local guidelines as resistance rates vary depending on geography, and consider community versus health-care associated infection (HAI). HAIs are commonly more resistant than community acquired UTIs. Examples of standard recommendations are given below.

Simple community-acquired lower urinary tract infection
Trimethoprim 50 mg 6-hourly PO or nitrofurantoin 100 mg 12-hourly PO

Women 3 days   Men 7 days
(Nitrofurantoin is not appropriate if upper renal tract or prostatitis is possible as it does not achieve reliable prostatic or renal parenchymal tissue concentrations. Nitrofurantoin is also not appropriate if eGFR is <45 mL/min.)

Simple health-care-associated acquired lower urinary tract infection
Cephalexin 500 mg 8-hourly PO or co-amoxiclav 625 mg 8-hourly PO

Women 3 days   Men 7 days

Suspected pyelonephritis
Aminoglycoside (e.g. gentamicin 5 mg/kg) IV **plus** IV co-amoxiclav
or
Aminoglycoside (e.g. gentamicin 5 mg/kg) IV **plus** a second-generation cephalosporin IV (e.g. cefuroxime)
or
Oral quinolone (e.g. ciprofloxacin) if mild pyelonephritis in a patient in whom the likelihood of quinolone resistance is <10% (based on local epidemiology) and there has been no quinolone exposure in the last 3–6 months.
Course length 10–14 days. Seven days of ciprofloxacin has shown to be equivalent to 14 days.
In all cases, subsequent antibiotic therapy post 48 h should be tailored to an appropriate single agent on receipt of susceptibility data and consider IV to oral switch depending on defervescence and clinical improvement.

Table 80.6 Common antimicrobials in the treatment of urinary tract infection.

Drug	Absorption (bioavailability following oral admin)	Amount excreted unchanged in urine	Dosing in renal impairment
Amoxicillin	89%	60%	Oral – high dose amoxicillin reduce dose if eGFR <10 mL/min IV – high dose amoxicillin reduce dose if eGFR <30 mL/min (risk of crystalluria with high doses)
Co-amoxiclav	75%	60% amoxicillin 40% clavulanic acid	Oral – no dose adjustment required IV – reduce dose if eGFRI <30 mL/min
Cefalexin	>90%	>90%	Reduce dose if eGFR <50 mL/min
Ciprofloxacin	70–80%	40–70%	Oral – reduce dose if eGFR <20 mL/min IV – reduce dose if eGFR <20 mL/min
Trimethoprim	>90%	40–60%	Reduce dose if eGFR <30 mL/min
Nitrofurantoin	94% (lower if administered without food)	30–40%	**Contraindicated** if eGFR <45 mL/min
Fosfomycin	40%	>70%	Avoid if eGFR <10 mL/min
Gentamicin	N/A	95%	Reduce dose if eGFR <20 mL/min
Amikacin	N/A	95%	Reduce dose if eGFR <20 mL/min

Table 80.7 Indications for referral to urology.

Urgent

Septic shock with associated ureteric obstruction/hydronephrosis with suspicion or pyonephrosis

Fever and features of renal colic

As soon as possible

Hydronephrosis/ureteric obstruction on imaging +/- AKI OR persisting fever after 72 h on appropriate antibiotic therapy

Renal abscess detected on renal tract imaging

Emphysematous cystitis or pyelonephritis detected on imaging

Non-obstructing stones found on imaging

Acute on chronic retention requiring catheterization

Routine follow-up through clinic

Unexplained recurrent urinary tract infection

Recurrent urinary tract infections in children

3 If suspected uncomplicated urinary tract infection (i.e. only lower urinary tract symptoms in a young woman with no features of systemic upset and no previous antimicrobial therapy) then treatment with empirical antibiotic without the need for urine culture is appropriate (Table 80.5). The patient should be advised to return if treatment fails to resolve symptoms, at which point urinary culture is indicated to guide further correct antimicrobial selection. Uncomplicated UTI or pyelonephritis in a young woman with complete symptom resolution does not need follow-up.

4 Relieve acute urinary retention. UTI is a common precipitant for acute on chronic retention in older men with prostatic enlargement and partial bladder outflow obstruction.
   - Catheterize if in acute urinary retention.
   - Unblock or replace blocked urinary catheters with appropriate antibiotic cover if long-term catheter in situ.

5 If there is an associated acute kidney injury, manage this along standard lines (Chapter 25).
   - Ensure appropriate fluid management including input/output chart.
   - Arrange ultrasonography of the kidneys and urinary tract to exclude obstruction requiring intervention.

6 Consider the need for urinary tract imaging (Table 80.4).

Further management

1 Review urinary culture results and change antimicrobial therapy as guided by susceptibility data. Urine culture results will be available at 24–48 h. Antibiotic course length depends on the clinical picture and whether it is uncomplicated or complicated UTI (Tables 80.1, 80.5 and 80.6).

2 If persisting fever at 72 h or ongoing symptoms or sepsis despite antimicrobial therapy:
   - Consider if wrong diagnosis. If dysuria, consider perineal candidiasis, vaginitis, urethritis or sexually transmitted infection.
   - If suprapubic or abdominal discomfort, review the need for abdominal imaging to exclude an alternative diagnosis, for example salpingitis, diverticulitis, appendicitis. Is the patient on the appropriate antimicrobial therapy?
   - Review microbiology results and discuss antibiotic therapy with microbiologist or infection specialist.
   - Has renal tract imaging been performed (Table 80.4)? Consider the presence of underlying complete or partial upper renal tract obstruction needing decompression. Consider the presence of a collection requiring drainage (radiologically guided or surgical).

3 Decide if you should refer to a urologist, either acutely or for follow-up (Table 80.7):
   - Decompression of upper renal tract if ureteric obstruction is present, for example by nephrostomy.

- Drainage of perinephric collections or renal abscess.
- Men with recurrent cystitis should be evaluated for prostatitis.

4 Change long-term urinary catheters. In catheter-associated urinary tract infections (CAUTIs), urinary catheter colonization with bacteria is inevitable and hard to eradicate. Replacement of urinary catheters whilst on antibiotic treatment is advisable.

5 Presentation with recurrent symptoms within a few weeks of treatment should have further evaluation for complicated UTI:

- Have they had renal/urinary tract imaging?
- Repeat a urine culture for resistant bacteria.
- Consider performing urodynamics. Is there bladder dysfunction or incomplete emptying?
- Consider referral to urologist for cystoscopy.

Appendix 80.1 Causative agents of urinary tract infection (UTI) and urethritis

Organism	Comment
Typical	
Escherischia coli	Responsible for >80% of urinary tract infections. Increasing resistance amongst urinary isolates both in hospital acquired UTI and community settings since 2000.
Klebsiella sa	Intrinsically resistant to amoxicillin. As with *E coli* increasingly resistant isolates seen in UTI.
Proteus sa	Often associated with stone formation and therefore indication for renal tract imaging.
	Intrinsically resistant to nitrofurantoin.
Staphylococcus saphrophyticus	Common cause of UTI in young women.
Less common	
Other enterobacteriacae (*Enterobacter* sa, *Serratia* sa, *Citrobacter* sa)	More common in health-care associated infection. Typically more resistant to standard antibiotics. Often harbour ESBLs (extended spectrum beta lactamases) conferring resistance to penicillins and third-generation cephalosporins.
Enterococcus sa	
Unusual	
Pseudomonas aeruginosa	Unusual community pathogen. More commonly seen in CAUTIs, history of renal tract intervention, renal stones or health-care exposure.
Candida	When seen in culture often reflects perineal organisms or genital mucosal candidiasis as a cause of dysuria as opposed to true UTI. However, can (rarely) be isolated as a genuine urinary pathogen, and isolation in true UTI would be an indication for renal tract imaging to exclude micro-abscesses or candida balls.
Staphylococcus aureus	Atypical urinary pathogen outside the setting of urinary tract instrumentation. Bacteriuria can be seen in the setting of *Staph aureus* bacteraemia from a non-urinary focus and UTI should not automatically be attributed as primary focus.

Further reading

Hooton TM (2012) Uncomplicated urinary tract infection. *N Engl J Med* 366, 1028–1037.
Shaeffer AJ, Nicolle LE (2016) Urinary tract infections in older men. *N Engl J Med* 374, 562–571.

Metabolic

CHAPTER 81

Hypoglycaemia

Vimal Venugopal, Vito Carone and Manohara Kenchaiah

In hospital inpatients with diabetes, hypoglycaemia is defined as a blood glucose <4.0 mmol/L and it should be corrected.

In a person without diabetes, the diagnosis of hypoglycaemia is based on Whipple's triad:

- Symptoms of hypoglycaemia (Table 81.1)
- Simultaneous demonstration of low blood glucose (<4.0 mmol/L)
- Resolution of symptoms with correction of low blood glucose

Hypoglycaemia must be excluded in any patient with seizures, abnormal behaviour, delirium, reduced conscious level or abnormal neurological signs. Hypoglycaemia is most often due to the treatment of diabetes mellitus, but other causes should be considered (Table 81.2).

Priorities

- If hypoglycaemia is suspected, check a bedside capillary blood glucose and if this is <5 mmol/L, send a venous sample for laboratory testing. Capillary blood glucose maybe falsely low in patients with reduced perfusion of the extremities.
- If hypoglycaemia is confirmed, it should be treated without delay.

Asymptomatic (incidental) or mildly symptomatic hypoglycaemia

Give 20 g of oral glucose (as a sugary drink, snack (e.g. five soft sweets) or glucose gel).

If the patient is drowsy or fitting (this may sometimes occur with mild hypoglycaemia, especially in young patients with diabetes):

- Give 100 mL of 20% glucose or 200 mL of 10% glucose over 15–30 min IV, or glucagon 1 mg IV/IM/SC.
- Recheck blood glucose after 10 min, if still below 4.0 mmol/L, repeat the above IV glucose treatment.
- In patients with malnourishment or alcohol-use disorder, there is a remote risk of precipitating Wernicke encephalopathy by a glucose load: prevent this by giving thiamine 100 mg IV before or shortly after glucose administration.

When the patient is alert and able to swallow, and blood glucose is >4 mmol/L, give a long-acting carbohydrate of the patient's choice, for example two biscuits, one slice of bread/toast or a 200–300 mL glass of milk.

If hypoglycaemia recurs or is likely to recur (e.g. liver disease, sepsis, excess sulphonylurea):

- Give 20 g of oral long-acting carbohydrate if able to eat.
- If unable to eat, start an IV infusion of glucose 10% at 100mL/h via a central or large peripheral vein. Adjust the rate to keep the blood glucose level at 5–10 mmol/L.

Acute Medicine: A Practical Guide to the Management of Medical Emergencies, Fifth Edition. Edited by David Sprigings and John B. Chambers.
© 2018 John Wiley & Sons Ltd. Published 2018 by John Wiley & Sons Ltd.

Table 81.1 Manifestations of hypoglycaemia.

Autonomic	Neuroglycopaenic
Dizziness	Irritability
Sweating	Confusion
Palpitations	Transient loss of consciousness
Tremor	Seizures
Blurred vision	Coma
Anxiety	Focal neurological abnormalities
Hunger	
Paraesthesia	

Table 81.2 Causes of hypoglycaemia.

In patients with diabetes mellitus

Excess insulin

Incorrect insulin injection technique

Increased exercise (relative to usual)

Gastroparesis and malabsorption

Excess insulin secretagogues (e.g. sulphonylureas)

Development of renal failure (with reduced clearance of insulin and sulphonylurea)

Development of other endocrine disorders (adrenal insufficiency, hypothyroidism, hypopituitarism)

Early pregnancy and breast-feeding

In patients with or without diabetes mellitus

Alcohol binge (inhibits hepatic gluconeogenesis)

Starvation

Severe liver disease (Chapter 77)

Sepsis (Chapter 35)

Salicylate poisoning

Adrenal insufficiency (Chapter 90)

Hypopituitarism (Chapter 93)

Other drugs known to cause hypoglycaemia (e.g. propranolol, salicylates and disopyramide)

Falciparum malaria (Chapter 33)

Insulinoma

Nesidioblastosis (acquired hyperinsulinism due to beta cell hyperplasia)

Insulin autoimmune hypoglycaemia

Accidental or non-prescribed use of insulin or insulin secretagogues

Factitious hypoglycaemia

After excess sulphonylurea therapy, maintain the glucose infusion for 24–36 h as the risk of hypoglycaemia may persist for up to 24–36 h following the last dose, especially if there is concurrent renal impairment.

If hypoglycaemia is only partially responsive to glucose 10% infusion:

- Give glucose 20% 100 mL/h IV via a central vein.
- If the cause is intentional insulin overdose, consider local excision of the injection site.

Prevent further or recurrent hypoglycaemia
- This is a fundamental step in all patients with DM, and a crucial one in those with hypoglycaemia unawareness.
- Implicated drugs should be discontinued or amended; specific conditions (e.g. insulinoma, cortisol deficiency) should be directly addressed wherever possible, but this will require specialist input.

Further management

- Identify and treat the cause (Table 81.2).
- In patients without diabetes presenting with blood glucose levels below 3.0 mmol/L with symptoms and no obvious cause, check simultaneous insulin and C-peptide levels. Elevated insulin and C-peptide levels indicate endogenous hyperinsulinaemia, whereas low C-peptide levels in the presence of elevated insulin levels suggest exogenous insulin as the cause of hypoglycaemia.
- Full blood count, renal and liver function tests should be checked in all patients. Additional testing will be directed by the clinical picture and differential diagnosis.
- Give advice to the patient about driving (consult Driver and Vehicle Licensing Authority guidance). Patients with diabetes treated with insulin or oral therapy can continue to drive a car, provided they have adequate awareness of hypoglycaemia, and have had no more than one episode of severe hypoglycaemia (requiring assistance from another person) in the preceding 12 months.

Further reading

Joint British Diabetes Societies Inpatient Care Group (2013) The hospital management of hypoglycaemia in adults with diabetes mellitus. https://www.diabetes.org.uk/Documents/About%20Us/Our%20views/Care%20recs/JBDS%20hypoglycaemia%20position%20(2013).pdf.

CHAPTER 82

Hyperglycaemic states

Vimal Venugopal, Vito Carone and Manohara Kenchaiah

Urine should be tested for glucose in all hospital patients. Blood glucose must be tested in any patient with glycosuria, any ill patient with diabetes and any patient with a clinical state in which derangements of blood glucose are common or must be excluded (Table 82.1). Hyperglycaemia is defined as plasma glucose concentration >11 mmol/L.

Plasma blood glucose >11 mmol/L

- Assess the conscious level and state of hydration, and establish if the patient is taking treatment for diabetes.
- Check urine or plasma for ketones. If there is ketonuria 2+ or greater, or ketonaemia, and the patient is unwell, check venous plasma bicarbonate concentration.
- The patient can now be placed in one of three groups (Table 82.2):
  - Diabetic ketoacidosis: see Chapter 83
  - Hyperosmolar hyperglycaemic state: see Chapter 84
  - Newly-diagnosed or poorly-controlled insulin-treated diabetes: see below

Further management of newly-diagnosed or poorly-controlled diabetes

- If the patient is already on treatment for diabetes, consider increasing the doses of current medication: seek specialist advice.
- If blood glucose is persistently >20 mmol/L, give 4–6 units of rapid-acting insulin SC, repeated every 6 hours, until blood glucose is <11 mmol/L. Check blood glucose 1–2 hourly.
- Use a variable-rate insulin infusion (VRII; 'sliding scale') (Table 82.3) if the patient:
  - Is critically unwell
  - Is vomiting
  - Is unable to eat and drink (e.g. in perioperative period)
  - Has acute coronary syndrome (DIGAMI regimen; Table 82.4)
  - Has a complication of pregnancy

Acute Medicine: A Practical Guide to the Management of Medical Emergencies, Fifth Edition. Edited by David Sprigings and John B. Chambers.
© 2018 John Wiley & Sons Ltd. Published 2018 by John Wiley & Sons Ltd.

Table 82.1 Clinical states in which derangements of blood glucose must be excluded.

Coma or reduced conscious level
Transient loss of consciousness
Seizures
Delirium/acute behavioural disturbance
Suspected stroke/TIA
Poisoning
Metabolic acidosis
Severe hyponatraemia
Liver failure
Hypothermia
Parenteral nutrition
Corticosteroid therapy
Acute coronary syndrome

- If the patient is normally on long-acting insulin, this should be continued while the VRII is being administered. The VRII should be continued no longer than 24 h, (exceptionally 48 h).

Switching from variable-rate insulin infusion to a subcutaneous insulin regimen

- Estimate the daily insulin requirement from the total dose given by infusion over the previous 24 h. Give one-third as long-acting background insulin subcutaneously (SC) at 2200 h. Divide the remaining two-thirds into three and give as short-acting insulin SC before meals.
- Monitor plasma glucose pre-prandially and at 2200 h, and adjust doses of insulin as needed.
- Ask advice from a diabetologist on long-term management. In general:
  - Insulin treated DM, with good control (HbA1c <7.5%): return to usual regime.
  - Insulin treated DM, with poor control (HbA1c >7.5%): review regimen.
  - Oral therapy with good control (HbA1c <7.5%): return to usual therapy.
  - Oral therapy with poor control (HbA1c >7.5%): transfer to insulin.
  - Newly-diagnosed DM: individualized treatment.

Table 82.2 Categorization of the patient with blood glucose >11 mmol/L.

	Blood glucose (mmol/L)	Ketonaemia/ Ketonuria	Venous bicarbonate (mmol/L)	Dehydration	Drowsiness
DKA	>11	3+	<15	++	+/++
HHS	>30	1+	>15	++++	+++
Diabetes[*]	>11	− to 2+	>15	−/+	−

DKA, diabetic ketoacidosis; HHS, hyperosmolar hyperglycaemic state.
[*] Either newly-diagnosed or poorly-controlled.

Table 82.3 Variable-rate insulin infusion ('sliding scale').

Regimens must be individualized.

If the patient is already receiving a long-acting insulin analogue, this should be continued.

Obese patients require more insulin per hour because of insulin resistance.Capillary blood glucose (CBG) measurement should be used to determine the initial insulin infusion rate, and checked hourly to ensure that the infusion rate is appropriate.

1 Make 50 units of soluble insulin up to 50 mL with normal saline (i.e. 1 unit/mL). Flush 10 mL of the solution through the line before connecting to the patient (as some insulin will be adsorbed onto the plastic).

2 Check blood glucose and start the insulin infusion at the appropriate rate (see below).

3 Administer 1 L of 0.45% saline with 5% glucose at 125 mL/h IV (83 mL/h if heart or renal failure).

4 Co-administer potassium chloride IV at an appropriate rate if plasma potassium is <5.5 mmol/L.

5 Check capillary blood glucose (CBG) hourly. Adjust the insulin infusion rate as needed, aiming to keep blood glucose between 6 to 10 mmol/L.

- If CBG is within the target range or falling towards it, continue same rate of insulin infusion.
- If CBG remains over >12 mmol/L for 3 consecutive readings and is not dropping by 3 mmol/L/hr or more the rate of insulin infusion should be increased.
- If CBG drops to below 4.0 mmol/L, the insulin infusion should be stopped and hypoglycaemia should be treated irrespective of whether the patient has symptoms. Insulin infusion should be restarted at a stepped-down rate once CBG is >4.0 mmol/L.

Capillary blood glucose (mmol/L)	Insulin infusion rate (1 unit/mL)		
	Insulin-sensitive	Standard	Insulin-resistant
<4.0	Stop infusion and treat for hypoglycaemia if indicated (Chapter 81). When CBG is >4.0 mmol/L, restart infusion at lower rate.		
4.1–8.0	0.5	1	2
8.1–12.0	1	2	4
12.1–16.0	2	4	6
16.1–20.0	3	5	7
20.1–24.0	4	6	8
>24.0	6	8	10

Table 82.4 Management of hyperglycemia after acute coronary syndrome (DIGAMI regimen).

New diagnosis of DM or known DM with plasma glucose >10 mmol/L:[*]

- Confirm initial capillary blood glucose levels with laboratory measurement; check also plasma potassium and HbA1c.
- Start a variable-rate insulin infusion (Table 82.3).
- Continue the variable-rate insulin infusion until there is stability of plasma glucose (target 4–10 mmol/L) and cardiovascular system, and the patient is able to eat and drink normally. At this point, change to SC insulin (see text).
- While the patient is receiving IV insulin infusion, give glucose 5% IV at a rate of 500 mL 12-hourly. Add 40 mmol KCL to this solution, unless plasma potassium is >5.3 mmol/L.

Known DM and plasma glucose <10 mmol/L

Continue usual treatment and monitor plasma glucose pre-prandially and at 2200 h. If plasma glucose rises >10 mmol/L, manage as above.

[*] Current ESC guidance is to treat if the plasma glucose is >10 mmol/L although the DIGAMI trial used the threshold >11 mmol/L

Further reading

American Diabetes Association (2016) Classification and diagnosis of diabetes. *Diabetes Care* 39 (Suppl. 1), S13–S22. DOI: 10.2337/dc16-S005.

Palmer BF, Clegg DJ (2015) Electrolyte and acid-base disturbances in patients with diabetes mellitus. *N Engl J Med* 373, 548–559.

CHAPTER 83

Diabetic ketoacidosis

VIMAL VENUGOPAL, VITO CARONE, AND MANOHARA KENCHAIAH

Consider diabetic ketoacidosis (DKA) in any ill patient with diabetes, especially if nausea, vomiting or abdominal pain are prominent. DKA typically occurs in patients with type 1 diabetes, but may also be seen in those with type 2 diabetes (ketosis-prone type 2 diabetes).

Priorities

1 Is this DKA?
- Clinical assessment and investigation of the patient with suspected DKA are summarized in Tables 83.1 and 83.2.
- Examination typically shows signs of volume depletion (average deficit 6 L) and tachypnoea from the metabolic acidosis. There may also be features of an associated disorder that has precipitated DKA.
- DKA is confirmed by a blood glucose >11 mmol/L, serum ketones >3 mmol/L and venous blood pH <7.3 or bicarbonate <15 mmol/L.
- Venous blood gases are preferred to arterial blood gases as venous sampling is easier and less painful for the patient. The differences in venous and arterial pH and bicarbonate levels are not significant enough to affect management. Capillary blood glucose and capillary blood ketones are sufficiently accurate for monitoring.

2 If DKA is confirmed, start treatment immediately
- The treatment of DKA (Tables 83.3, 83.4, 83.5) involves fluid replacement to restore the circulating volume, replacement of lost potassium and the use of fixed-rate intravenous insulin infusion to correct the ketonaemia and acidosis.
- If the patient is taking a long-acting insulin, this should be continued, as this allows earlier weaning from the infusion.
- If the patient has a continuous subcutaneous insulin infusion pump, this should be disconnected unless you are instructed not to do so by a specialist diabetes team.

3 Identify and treat the precipitant of DKA
- Infection is a common precipitant (~30% cases) and complication of DKA and may not cause fever. Check carefully for a focus of infection, including examination of the feet and perineum.
- Seek a surgical opinion if abdominal pain or abnormal signs do not resolve with correction of acidosis.
- Other causes of DKA are an inappropriate reduction in, or poor compliance with, insulin therapy (~20% cases), errors in insulin prescription or administration, surgery, acute coronary syndrome, alcohol or substance use and emotional stress (~25% cases).
- DKA may also be the first presentation of type 1 (and, less commonly, type 2) diabetes (~25% cases).

Acute Medicine: A Practical Guide to the Management of Medical Emergencies, Fifth Edition. Edited by David Sprigings and John B. Chambers.
© 2018 John Wiley & Sons Ltd. Published 2018 by John Wiley & Sons Ltd.

Table 83.1 Focused assessment in suspected diabetic ketoacidosis.

History

Diabetes history (duration, treatment, complications)

Polydipsia, polyuria, weight loss?

Nausea, vomiting, abdominal pain?

Possible precipitant of DKA? Consider:

- Inappropriate reduction in, or poor compliance with, insulin therapy
- Error in insulin prescription or administration
- Alcohol or substance use
- Emotional stress
- Infection
- Acute coronary syndrome

Comorbidities

Pregnancy?

Examination

Physiological observations

Focus of infection? Check feet and perineum

Abdominal signs?

4 Consider admission to ICU/HDU if the patient

- Is aged 18–25 years (as higher risk of cerebral oedema) or >70 years (as higher risk of fluid overload)
- Has a reduced conscious level or hypotension which is not corrected by fluid replacement
- Has cardiac or renal failure
- Is pregnant
- At presentation has one or more of the following features:
  - Plasma ketones >6.0 mmol/L
  - Venous bicarbonate <5 mmol/L
  - Venous pH <7.0
  - Plasma potassium <3.5 mmol/L
  - Anion gap >16 mOsmol/kg (calculated as [(plasma sodium+potassium)-(plasma chloride+bicarbonate)]

Table 83.2 Urgent investigation in suspected diabetic ketoacidosis.

Capillary blood glucose

Venous plasma glucose

Capillary blood or urinary ketones

Venous plasma bicarbonate

Sodium, potassium, urea and creatinine

Plasma osmolality, measured directly or calculated from the formula: plasma osmolality = [2 (plasma Na) + glucose + urea]

Venous blood gases

Full blood count

C-reactive protein

Two blood cultures

Urine dipstick, microscopy and culture

Chest X-ray

ECG

Table 83.3 Fluid replacement in diabetic ketoacidosis.

This must take account of:
- The likely fluid deficit (typically 100 mL/kg body weight)
- The blood pressure, central venous pressure and urine output
- Coexisting cardiac or renal disease

1. Give normal saline 1 L IV over 30–60 min (give the faster rate if systolic BP is <90 mmHg), followed by 1 L over 1 h, without added potassium. Consider placement of a central line to monitor central venous pressure (CVP) in patients with cardiac or renal failure.
2. Give further normal saline (with potassium added according to the plasma level, see Table 83.4). As a general guideline, for an adult with DKA (average fluid deficit 6 L) and systolic BP >90 mmHg, the following regimen can be used:
   - 1 L normal saline over 1 h
   - 1 L normal saline (with added potassium) over the following 2 h
   - 1 L normal saline (with added potassium) over the following 2 h
   - 1 L normal saline (with added potassium) over the following 4 h
   - 1 L normal saline (with added potassium) over the following 4 h
   - 1 L normal saline (with added potassium) over the following 6 h
3. Once blood glucose level falls <14 mmol/L, glucose 10% should be given at a rate of 125 mL/h alongside the saline infusion, at the rate required to correct fully the fluid deficit.

Table 83.4 Potassium replacement in diabetic ketoacidosis*.

Plasma potassium (mmol/L)	Potassium added (mmol/L)
<3.5	Regimen needs review[†]
3.5–5.5	40
>5.5	None

* Check plasma potassium on admission, 60 min, 120 min, and then 2-hourly from then on.
[†] Can increase the rate of the overall fluid infusion if fluid balance permits, infusion rates of up to 20 mmol/h of potassium can be given peripherally. If there is persistent hypokalaemia, rates of up to 40 mmol/h can be given via a central venous catheter, with monitoring in a high dependency unit.

Table 83.5 Fixed rate insulin infusion in diabetic ketoacidosis.

Continue basal insulin in patients on basal bolus insulin regimen.
Switch off continuous subcutaneous insulin pump if the patient has one.

1. Make 50 units of soluble insulin up to 50 mL with normal saline (i.e. insulin 1 unit/mL). Flush 10 mL of the solution through the line before connecting to the patient (as some insulin will be adsorbed onto the plastic).
2. Start the infusion at 0.1 units/kg/hr. Check hourly capillary blood glucose and ketones, send venous glucose if capillary blood glucose meter reads 'high'.
3. Aim for blood ketones to fall by 0.5 mmol/L/h. If blood ketones do not fall, increase insulin infusion in 1 unit/h increments until blood ketones fall by at least 0.5 mmol/L/h. If there is no fall in blood ketones or glucose, confirm that the pump is working and the IV line is connected properly. Consult diabetes specialist team if blood ketone levels are still not falling.

Table 83.6 Switching from IV to SC insulin after resolution of diabetic ketoacidosis.

1. Resolution of DKA requires a venous pH >7.3 and blood ketones <0.6 mmol/L.
2. In patients already on basal bolus regime, the basal dose should have been continued throughout the DKA treatment.
3. In patients newly diagnosed with diabetes, start a long-acting insulin 0.25 units/kg and request diabetes specialist team input.
4. Half of the total daily dose should be as long-acting insulin SC at evening. Divide the remaining half into three to calculate the dose of short-acting (soluble) insulin SC before meals.
5. Once DKA has resolved and patient is able to eat, give the fast-acting insulin with a meal and stop the intravenous fixed rate insulin one hour later.
6. Check blood glucose before meals and at 2200 h, and adjust doses of insulin as needed, aiming for levels 4–7 mmol/L.
7. Refer to diabetes team for advice on further management.

Further management

Supportive care
- Place a nasogastric tube if the patient is too drowsy to answer questions or there is a gastric succussion splash. Aspirate the stomach and leave on continuous drainage. Inhalation of vomit is a potentially fatal complication of DKA.
- Use graduated compression stockings and prophylactic low-molecular-weight heparin to reduce the risk of deep vein thrombosis.

Monitoring
- Continuous display of ECG and oxygen saturation
- Check hourly:
  - Conscious level (e.g. by AVPU or Glasgow Coma Scale score) until fully conscious
  - Respiratory rate until stable and then 4-hourly
  - Blood pressure until stable and then 4-hourly
  - Fluid balance
  - Capillary blood glucose and plasma ketones
  - Venous blood glucose by laboratory measurement until capillary blood glucose is <20 mmol/L
- Check venous pH, bicarbonate and potassium on admission, at 60 min, 120 min and then 2-hourly on a blood gas analyser
- Put in a bladder catheter if no urine has been passed after 1 h, or if the patient is incontinent, but not otherwise

Insulin infusion
- The blood glucose should fall with the administration of IV insulin. However, as long as ketoacidosis persists, the fixed rate insulin infusion must be continued even if the blood glucose enters the normal range. When blood glucose is <14 mmol/L, start an infusion of 10% glucose to prevent hypoglycaemia (the commonest complication of treatment of DKA)
- Once the exit criteria for DKA are met, and the patient is eating and drinking, the IV insulin infusion can be weaned off (Table 83.6).

Further reading

Joint British Diabetes Societies Inpatient Care Group (2013) *The management of diabetic ketoacidosis in adults,* 2nd edition. https://www.diabetes.org.uk/Documents/About%20Us/What%20we%20say/Management-of-DKA-241013.pdf.

CHAPTER 84

Hyperosmolar hyperglycaemic state

Vimal Venugopal, Vito Carone, and Manohara Kenchaiah

Consider hyperosmolar hyperglycaemic state (HHS) in any ill patient with diabetes, especially if volume depletion and drowsiness are prominent.

- HHS typically occurs in patients with type 2 diabetes, but can also occur in type 1 diabetes. Any illness that leads to a reduced fluid intake can precipitate HHS, which may be the first presentation of diabetes.
- The onset of HHS is usually over a number of days, and slower compared to DKA. However, an overlap syndrome with features of both HHS and DKA may be seen.
- Mortality of patients with HHS is high (up to 50%), with the major causes of death being the precipitating illness, thromboembolism and aspiration pneumonia.

Hyperosmolar hyperglycaemic state is differentiated from diabetic ketoacidosis (Chapter 83) by:

- Blood glucose >30 mmol/L, but no ketoacidosis (plasma ketones <3 mmol/L, venous bicarbonate >15 mmol/L) and
- Plasma osmolality >350 mOsmol/kg (normal range 285–295 mOsmol/kg); this can be measured directly or calculated from the formula: plasma osmolality = [2 (plasma Na) + glucose + urea].

Management

Clinical assessment, investigation and management are as for DKA (Chapter 83), with the differences noted below. Identify and treat any precipitating illness.

- Use normal saline to correct the fluid deficit. Switch to 0.45% sodium chloride solution if plasma osmolality is not falling despite adequate fluid replacement. Plasma sodium may rise initially but this is not an indication to use 0.45% sodium chloride solution.
- The rate of fall of plasma sodium should not exceed 10 mmol/L in 24 h.
- The fall in blood glucose should be no more than 5 mmol/L/h. Low dose IV insulin (0.05 units/kg/h) should only be administered if there is significant ketonaemia/ketonuria (plasma ketones >1 mmol/L or urine ketones greater than 2+), or if blood glucose is not falling despite correction of the fluid deficit.
- Aim for a positive fluid balance of 3–6 L by 12 h and the remaining replacement of estimated fluid losses within next 12 h (average deficit in HHS is 10 L). Encourage the patient to drink when conscious level allows safe swallowing.
- The risk of foot ulceration is high, particularly if the patient has a reduced conscious level. The heels should be protected and the feet checked daily.

Acute Medicine: A Practical Guide to the Management of Medical Emergencies, Fifth Edition. Edited by David Sprigings and John B. Chambers.
© 2018 John Wiley & Sons Ltd. Published 2018 by John Wiley & Sons Ltd.

- The risk of thromboembolism is high. Unless contraindicated (e.g. recent stroke), give full-dose low-molecular-weight heparin or unfractionated heparin by IV infusion (Chapter 103) until mobile.

  Continue insulin unless the total daily requirement falls below 20 units, when an oral hypoglycaemic can be tried. Most patients can subsequently be maintained on oral hypoglycaemic therapy (or even managed by diet alone), although recovery of endogenous insulin production may be delayed. Ask advice from the diabetes team on an appropriate regimen before discharge.

Further reading

Joint British Diabetes Societies Inpatient Care Group (2012) The management of the hyperosmolar hyperglycaemic state (HHS) in adults with diabetes. https://www.diabetes.org.uk/Documents/Position%20statements/JBDS-IP-HHS-Adults.pdf.

CHAPTER 85

Disorders of plasma sodium concentration

James Crane, Paul Carroll, and Martin Crook

Disorders of plasma sodium concentration (Box 85.1) are usually due to deranged water handling by the kidney. Defective concentration of the urine, without an adequate intake of water, results in hypernatraemia, whilst defective dilution of the urine (often due to non-osmotic release of antidiuretic hormone, ADH) results in hyponatraemia. Hyponatraemia is almost always accompanied by a reduced plasma osmolality (<280 mOsmol/kg), but if an excess of other osmolytes exists, the osmotic drag of water into the extracellular space can result in hyponatraemia (as seen with hyperglycaemic states (Chapter 82).

Hypernatraemia

Principles of management

Treat the underlying disorder: causes of hypernatraemia are given in Table 85.1, and management summarized in Figure 85.1.

Assess the volume status of the patient (Box 85.2) and review fluid balance charts. Is there polyuria (>3 L/day)? In diabetes insipidus, the serum osmolality is usually >300 mOsmol/kg in the presence of an inappropriately dilute urine, that is, urine osmolality is less than serum osmolality.

Box 85.1 Disorders of plasma sodium concentration.

Plasma sodium concentration (mmol/L)	Classification	Clinical features
>155	Severe hypernatraemia	Delirium, reduced conscious level, coma
150–155	Moderate hypernatraemia	Muscle weakness, delirium
143–150	Mild hypernatraemia	Typically asymptomatic
138–143	**Normal range**	
130–138	Mild hyponatraemia	Typically asymptomatic
125–130	Moderate hyponatraemia	Headache, nausea, vomiting, muscle weakness, lethargy, delirium
<125	Severe hyponatraemia	Delirium, ataxia, reduced conscious level, respiratory failure and seizures (reflecting cerebral oedema), especially when hyponatraemia has developed within 48 h.

Acute Medicine: A Practical Guide to the Management of Medical Emergencies, Fifth Edition. Edited by David Sprigings and John B. Chambers.
© 2018 John Wiley & Sons Ltd. Published 2018 by John Wiley & Sons Ltd.

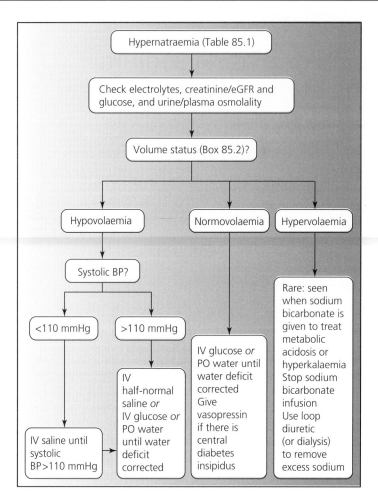

Figure 85.1 Management of hypernatraemia.

Box 85.2 Assessment of volume status.

Volume status	Reliable physical signs
Hypervolaemia	Elevated jugular venous pressure
	Oedema without hypotension
Euvolaemia	Absence of reliable signs of hypervolaemia or hypovolaemia
Hypovolaemia	Postural fall in systolic BP >20 mmHg (with BP measured after >2 min resting in the supine position, and then 1 min after standing)
	Postural increase in pulse rate >30/min (with pulse taken after >2 min resting in the supine position, and then 1 min after standing; count the pulse for 30 s and double the result)

Adapted from: McGee S, Abernethy WB, Simel DL (1999) The rational clinical examination: Is this patient hypovolemic? JAMA 281, 1022–1029.

Table 85.1 Causes of hypernatraemia.

Artefactual hypernatraemia
Blood sample contaminated with sodium citrate or pseudohypernatraemia

Hypovolaemic hypernatraemia
- Poor water intake (may be seen in advanced dementia, with diminished thirst)
- Osmotic diuretics
- Vomiting
- Diarrhoea
- Fistulas
- Major burns
- Hyperosmolar hyperglycaemic state (HHS)

Euvolaemic hypernatraemia
- Increased insensible water loss, for example hyperventilation
- Osmotic diuresis such as glycosuria
- Diabetes insipidus (cranial or nephrogenic causes)

Hypervolaemic hypernatraemia
- Excessive sodium intake, for example hypertonic saline, or drugs containing sodium such as carbenicillin or sodium bicarbonate, salt poisoning
- Mineralocorticoid excess, for example Conn's syndrome or Cushing's syndrome

Check serum sodium, potassium, urea, creatinine, eGFR, calcium and plasma glucose, and serum and urine osmolality.

The choice of fluid and the route and rate of administration depend on the volume status of the patient and the chronicity of the hypernatraemia. Too rapid correction or overcorrection of hypernatraemia may result in brain damage. In mild to moderate hypernatraemia, treating the cause such as hyperglycaemia, or stopping diuretics may be sufficient to correct the derangement.

If the hypernatraemia is chronic (duration >24 h or unknown), aim for a rate of decrease of plasma sodium of no more than 0.5 mmol/L/h, and no more than 10 mmol/L/day, with a target plasma sodium of 145 mmol/L.

If the hypernatraemia has occurred rapidly over a few hours, then prompt correction decreases the risk of osmotic demyelination and improves prognosis without risk of cerebral oedema. Here it is usually appropriate to try to reduce the serum sodium concentration to about 145 mmol/L within 24 h.

Hypovolaemic hypernatraemia

If the patient has hypotension with signs of low cardiac output, give normal saline IV until systolic BP is >110 mmHg.

Then give half-normal (0.45%) saline or 5% glucose IV, or water PO, until the water deficit is corrected.

See Chapter 84 for management of hyperosmolar hyperglycaemic state.

Normovolaemic hypernatraemia

Correct the water deficit with 5% glucose IV or water PO. If the patient has central diabetes insipidus, give vasopressin; if nephrogenic diabetes insipidus, ask advice from a nephrologist.

Hypervolaemic hypernatraemia

This is rare. It may be seen when hypertonic sodium bicarbonate is given for the treatment of metabolic acidosis or hyperkalaemia, or following inappropriate administration of hypertonic saline, or the ingestion of salt. Hyperaldosteronism can cause mild hypervolaemic hypernatraemia.

If related to a hypertonic infusion, discontinue the infusion. Use a loop diuretic (or dialysis) to remove excess sodium.

Hyponatraemia

Principles of management

Treat the underlying disorder: causes of hyponatraemia are given in Table 85.2, and management summarized in Figure 85.2.

Assess the volume status of the patient (Box 85.2) and review fluid balance charts. Check serum sodium, potassium, urea, creatinine, calcium and plasma glucose, with serum and urine osmolality and also check TSH and serum cortisol. Exclude pseudo-hyponatraemia, for example due to lipaemia or severe hyperproteinaemia. In normo-osmolar hyponatraemia consider also hyperglycaemia and sick cell syndrome.

In most cases, hyponatraemia is accompanied by low plasma osmolality (<280 mOsmol/kg) (hypo-osmolar hyponatraemia) and results from an excess of free water, almost always due to the activity of ADH at the renal collecting ducts. This is usually due to appropriate physiological stimuli of ADH secretion from the posterior pituitary, but occasionally to disordered regulation of ADH secretion, the syndrome of inappropriate antidiuretic

Table 85.2 Causes of hypo-osmolar hyponatraemia.

Category	Cause		Mechanism
Hypovolaemic	Gastrointestinal losses	Vomiting Diarrhoea	Sodium loss outstrips water loss, non-osmotic (baroreceptor) stimulation of ADH secretion
	Third space disease, for example ileus		
	Renal losses	Diuretics Salt-losing nephropathy Mineralocorticoid insufficiency/adrenal insufficiency Cerebral salt-wasting	Sodium loss outstrips water loss, non-osmotic (baroreceptor) secretion of ADH secretion
Euvolaemic	Glucocorticoid insufficiency		ACTH stimulation and non-osmotic (baroreceptor) stimulation of ADH secretion,
	Severe hypothyroidism		Non-osmotic (baroreceptor) stimulation of ADH secretion
	Psychogenic polydipsia/water intoxication		Water intake exceeds renal capacity for excretion (typical threshold >15 L daily if renal function and solute intake normal)
	Very low solute intake (e.g. 'beer potomania')		Maximally dilute urine is 50 mOsmol/Kg. Reduced daily solute limits water excretion capacity, e.g. if 50 mOsmol/day, maximal urine volume is 1 L
	Excess hypotonic fluid, for example 5% dextrose post-operatively		Oncotic pressure overcomes impermeability of collecting duct to water which is retained in excess of sodium
Hypervolaemic	Cardiac failure		Non-osmotic (baroreceptor) stimulation of ADH secretion
	Renal failure		Reduced water excreting capacity
	Liver failure, cirrhosis/ascites		Splanchnic vasodilatation, isotonic third space fluid loss (ascites), non-osmotic (baroreceptor) stimulation of ADH secretion
	Hypoalbuminaemia, for example nephrotic syndrome		Isotonic loss of fluid to interstitial space, non-osmotic (baroreceptor) stimulation of ADH secretion

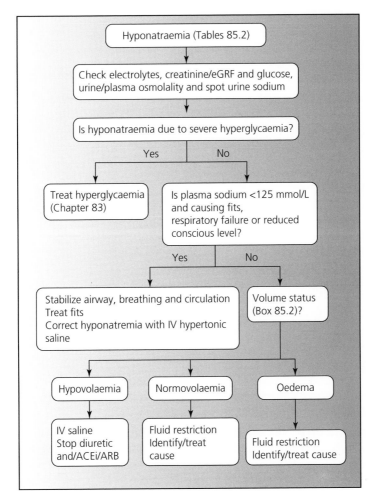

Figure 85.2 Management of hyponatraemia.

hormone, SIADH (Table 85.3). SIADH is overdiagnosed. It is only SIADH if no appropriate stimulus for ADH exists. Hypothyroidism and adrenal insufficiency must be excluded before SIADH can be diagnosed. If SIADH is confirmed, arrange CT head/chest/abdomen and pelvis, to investigate for the cause.

Hypo-osmolar hyponatraemia can be categorized into three clinical groups: hypervolaemic, euvolaemic and hypovolaemic.

Rapid correction of hypo-osmolar hyponatraemia is only indicated if this is the cause of severe neurological abnormalities (reduced conscious level, coma, major seizures); it may result in osmotic demyelination of pontine neurons, especially if the brain has adapted to hyponatraemia. The risk of osmotic demyelination is increased in patients with liver failure, malnutrition and potassium depletion, and elderly women taking thiazide diuretics.

Accurate fluid balance assessment is difficult but critical to the correct management of hyponatraemia. Re-evaluate this if serum sodium is not correcting as expected.

Over-rapid correction of hyponatraemia can lead to catastrophic neurological consequences. Frequent evaluation of serum sodium concentration during treatment is essential to avoid doing harm.

Table 85.3 Syndrome of inappropriate ADH secretion (SIADH).

Criteria for diagnosis of SIADH
- Hyponatraemia and reduced plasma osmolality
- Urine sodium concentration >20 mmol/L and urine osmolality greater than plasma osmolality or not maximally dilute
- No oedema or signs of hypovolaemia
- Normal renal, thyroid and adrenal function
- The patient is not taking diuretics or purgatives

Causes of SIADH
Malignant disease
Small cell carcinoma of bronchus, thymoma, lymphoma, sarcoma, mesothelioma, carcinoma of pancreas and duodenum

Chest disorders
Pneumonia, tuberculosis, empyema, asthma, pneumothorax, positive-pressure ventilation

Neurological disorders
Meningitis, encephalitis, head injury, brain tumour, cerebral abscess, subarachnoid haemorrhage, Guillain–Barré syndrome, acute intermittent porphyria

Drugs
Antidepressants, carbamazepine, cytotoxics, MDMA ('ecstasy'), NSAIDs, opioids, oxytocin, phenothiazines, thiazides, vincristine

Others
Post-operative state
HIV infection
Idiopathic
Reset osmostat

Hyponatraemia with severe neurological abnormalities
Assess airway, breathing and circulation and take appropriate resuscitative action where necessary.

Check baseline investigations as above. Place a bladder catheter and send urine for sodium concentration and osmolality. Consider a central line for venous pressure monitoring.

Administer hypertonic saline. Infuse 150 mL 3% saline over 20 minutes. Recheck serum sodium after the infusion. Administer repeated 150 mL infusions of 3% saline. Aim to raise serum sodium by a maximum of 5 mmol/L in the first hour. Continue hypertonic saline infusions until either a) symptoms improve, or b) the serum sodium reaches 125 mmol/L. Aim to raise serum sodium by a maximum of 10 mmol/L in the first 24 hours and 8mmol/L in subsequent 24 hour periods.

Use of selective vasopressin (V2) antagonists may be considered under expert guidance.

Hyponatraemia without severe neurological symptoms
If the patient has no symptoms attributable to hyponatraemia or is only mildly symptomatic (e.g. headache, nausea, lethargy), hypertonic saline should not be given.

Management depends principally on the patient's fluid status.
- **Hypovolaemic hyponatraemia** is managed with isotonic intravenous fluid, for example 0.9% saline, aiming for a correction rate of no greater than 12 mmol/L/day.
- **Euvolaemic and hypervolaemic hyponatraemia** are managed with fluid restriction. In euvolaemic hyponatraemia, oral sodium supplementation may be added if total body sodium is suspected to be deficient. This should be avoided in hypervolaemic hyponatraemia due to cardiac failure and cirrhosis. The selective vasopressin (V2) antagonists such as conivaptan and talvaptan may have a place here, but seek expert advice.

Hyponatraemia associated with glucocorticoid, mineralocorticoid or thyroid hormone deficiencies should correct on replacement.

Drugs associated with hyponatraemia should be stopped.

- Thiazide diuretics. Act via SIADH as well as via their effect on the Na^+/Cl^- symporter of the distal convoluted tubule.
- Loop diuretics. Less able to cause hyponatraemia than thiazides since their action diminishes the medullary concentration gradient and limits the ability of the kidney to resorb free water as a result of ADH activity.
- Angiotensin-converting-enzyme inhibitors and angiotensin receptor blockers. They usually cause only mild hyponatraemia but limit the ability of the kidney to retain sodium to correct hyponatraemia.
- Antidepressants (tricyclic and SSRI), phenothiazine antipsychotics, quinolone antibiotics, non-steroidal anti-inflammatory drugs and protonpump inhibitors increase ADH secretion or potency.

Further reading

Society for Endocrinology: Endocrine Emergency Guidance. Emergency management of severe symptomatic hyponatraemia in adult patients. http://www.endocrineconnections.com/content/5/5/G4.

Spasovski G, Vanholder R, Allolio B, *et al.* on behalf of the Hyponatraemia Guideline Development Group (2014) Clinical practice guideline on diagnosis and treatment of hyponatraemia. *European Journal of Endocrinology* 170, G1–G47.

Sterns RH. (2015) Disorders of plasma sodium — causes, consequences, and correction. *N Engl J Med* 372, 55–65.

CHAPTER 86

Disorders of plasma potassium concentration

Martin Crook

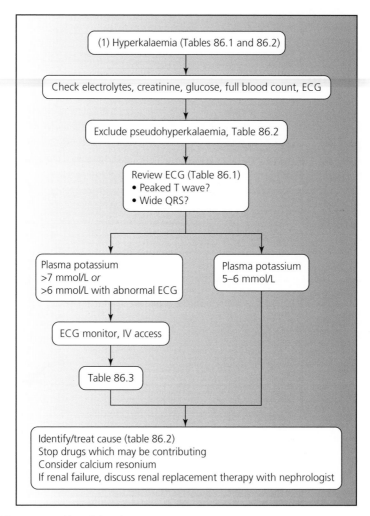

Figure 86.1 Management of hyperkalaemia.

Acute Medicine: A Practical Guide to the Management of Medical Emergencies, Fifth Edition. Edited by David Sprigings and John B. Chambers.
© 2018 John Wiley & Sons Ltd. Published 2018 by John Wiley & Sons Ltd.

Disorders of plasma potassium concentration (Box 86.1) may be an acute effect of drugs, or result from disordered renal plasma potassium handling, release of potassium from damaged cells or excessive gut loss of potassium.

Hyperkalaemia

Hyperkalaemia must be excluded in any patient with acute kidney injury (AKI) or advanced chronic kidney disease (CKD). Severe hyperkalaemia may be asymptomatic until it results in cardiac arrest.

   If the plasma potassium is discordant with the clinical picture, consider pseudohyperkalaemia, for example haemolysis, potassium-EDTA contaminated sample, old sample, sample kept in fridge or severe thrombocytosis/leukocytosis.

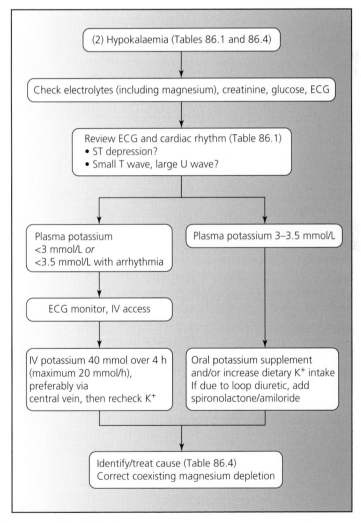

Figure 86.2 Management of hypokalaemia.

Box 86.1 Disorders of plasma potassium concentration.

Plasma potassium concentration (mmol/L)	Classification	Clinical and ECG features
>6.5	Severe hyperkalaemia	Often asymptomatic. Muscle weakness may occur. ECG: tall peaked T wave with shortened QT interval → Progressive lengthening of the PR interval and QRS duration → Sine wave QRS pattern → Ventricular standstill or fibrillation.
5.5–6.5	Moderate hyperkalaemia	May be asymptomatic.
5.0–5.5	Mild hyperkalaemia	May be asymptomatic.
3.5–5.0	**Normal range**	
3.0–3.5	Mild hypokalaemia	May be asymptomatic.
2.5–3.0	Moderate hypokalaemia	ECG: arrhythmias may occur, especially in patients with underlying cardiac disorders or taking antiarrhythmic drugs.
<2.5	Severe hypokalaemia	Muscle necrosis may occur. Below 2 mmol/L there may be ascending paralysis, resembling Guillain-Barré syndrome. Ileus. ECG: ST depression, reduced T wave amplitude, increased U wave amplitude. Arrhythmias commonly occur: extrasystoles, atrial fibrillation, atrioventricular block, ventricular tachycardiac and fibrillation.

Principles of management (Figure 86.1)

Treat the underlying disorder: causes of hyperkalaemia are given in Table 86.1.

Check renal function and address any reversible causes of renal impairment.

Review acid-base status, as hyperkalaemia can be associated with metabolic acidosis.

If the patient is taking digoxin, check plasma digoxin drug level.

Stop drugs which may be contributing to hyperkalaemia, and reduce the dietary intake of potassium.

To increase excretion of potassium, the options are to improve renal function, start renal replacement therapy, or use an ion-exchange resin such as calcium resonium to bind potassium in the gut.

Severe hyperkalaemia with ECG abnormalities

If the plasma potassium is >7 mmol/L or the ECG has abnormalities associated with hyperkalaemia (widening of the QRS complex, loss of the P wave, peaking of the T wave or a sine wave pattern) then:

1 Give 10 mL of calcium chloride 10% IV over 5–10 min to stabilize cardiac muscle. This can be repeated every 5 min up to a total dose of 50 mL. Calcium chloride is more toxic to veins than calcium gluconate, but provides more calcium per ampoule (272 mg of calcium in 10 mL of calcium chloride 10%; 94 mg of calcium in 10 mL of calcium gluconate 10%). The ECG may change within a couple of minutes.

2 Consider 10–20 mg nebulized salbutamol (contraindicated if unstable angina or acute MI); this may reduce potassium by about 0.5–1.0 mmol/L in 15–30 min and lasts for a couple of hours.

3 Give insulin and glucose IV: add 10 units of Actrapid® to 50 mL of glucose 50% and infuse over 30 min. Avoid hypoglycaemia by monitoring blood glucose. The plasma potassium should decrease by about 0.6–1.0 mmol/L

Table 86.1 Causes of hyperkalaemia.

Pseudohyperkalaemia (see text)

Predominantly renal causes

Acute kidney injury or chronic kidney disease

Mineralocorticoid deficiency:

- Adrenal insufficiency
- Hyporeninaemic hypoaldosteronism
- Renal tubular acidosis type 4

Drugs, for example angiotensin-conventing-enzyme inhibitors, angiotensin receptor blockers, potassium-sparing diuretics, spironolactone

Predominantly non-renal causes

Oral or intravenous potassium input excess

Severe tissue damage:

- Rhabdomyolysis
- Tumour-lysis syndrome

Acidosis or hypoxia

Digoxin toxicity

Familial hyperkalaemic periodic paralysis (rare)

---

in 15 min and the reduction lasts for about an hour. Recheck plasma potassium 30 min afterwards and monitor plasma electrolytes and renal function 1–2 h later.

4 The use of intravenous sodium bicarbonate in severe hyperkalaemia in the face of severe acidosis is controversial and expert opinion should be consulted.

5 Stop potassium supplements or any drugs (e.g. ACE inhibitors, angiotensin receptor blockers, potassium-retaining diuretics, spironolactone), which may be contributing to hyperkalaemia. Start calcium resonium (15 g 8-hourly PO or 30 g by retention enema).

6 Recheck plasma potassium after 2 h. If hyperkalaemia is due to AKI or CKD, renal replacement therapy may need to be started to prevent a recurrence: discuss this with a nephrologist.

Mild or moderate hyperkalaemia

Stop potassium supplements or any drugs which may be contributing to hyperkalaemia, and reduce the dietary intake of potassium.

Start calcium resonium (15 g 8-hourly PO or 30 g daily by retention enema) in patients with hyperkalaemia complicating renal failure.

Hypokalaemia

Hypokalaemia may result in muscle weakness and arrhythmias. When plasma potassium falls below 2.5 mmol/L, muscle necrosis may occur; below 2 mmol/L, there may be ascending paralysis. Cardiac arrhythmias may occur when plasma potassium is <3 mmol/L, especially in patients with underlying cardiac disorders or taking anti-arrhythmic drugs. The ECG may show flattened T waves, ST depression and prominent U waves. In patients with cardiac arrhythmias, target plasma potassium is 4–4.5 mmol/L.

Principles of management (Figure 86.2)

Treat the underlying disorder: causes of hypokalaemia are given in Table 86.2.

Table **86.2** Causes of hypokalaemia.

Predominantly renal causes

Mineralocorticoid excess:
- Conn's syndrome
- Cushing's syndrome
- Bartter/Gitelman syndrome
- Liquorice excess
- Glucocorticoid therapy

Fanconi syndrome

Hypomagnesaemia

Drugs, for example loop diuretics, thiazides, carbonate dehydratase inhibitors

Renal tubular acidosis type 1 and 2

Predominantly non-renal causes

Redistribution:
- Alkalosis
- Catecholamines
- Vitamin B12 therapy
- Insulin
- Rapidly growing tumours

Gastro-intestinal loss:
- Prolonged diarrhea or vomiting
- Intestinal fistula
- Purgative abuse

Poor intake of potassium

Familial hypokalaemic periodic paralysis (rare)

A spot urine potassium concentration may help distinguish between predominately non-renal versus renal causes: a urine potassium >20 mmol/L in a patient with hypokalaemia suggests renal potassium loss. Each 0.3 mmol/L reduction in plasma potassium concentration reflects 100 mmol/L deficit in body potassium stores.

Hypokalaemia is most often due to diuretic therapy or gut loss of potassium, and replacement of sodium and water may also be needed. Magnesium depletion commonly coexists with potassium depletion: check plasma magnesium (normal range 0.70–1.20 mmol/L) in patients with hypokalaemia, and correct hypomagnesaemia (Chapter 88) with IV or oral supplements.

Review acid-base status as hypokalaemia can be associated with metabolic alkalosis.

Severe hypokalaemia or hypokalaemia associated with cardiac arrhythmias

Attach an ECG monitor.

Give potassium by IV infusion, initally 40 mmol over 4 h, and then recheck potassium. Give further potassium as needed, up to 200 mmol over 24 h. The maximum rate of infusion should not exceed 20 mmol/h. Potassium given via a peripheral vein may cause pain at the infusion site and tissue necrosis if there is extravasation: administration via a central vein is preferable.

Mild or moderate hypokalaemia without cardiac arrhythmias

Give oral potassium, for example Sando-K 2 tablets (12 mmol per tablet) 8-hourly PO for 3–7 days, and increase the dietary intake of potassium; beware of gastric irritation particularly with Slow-K preparations.

If hypokalaemia is due to the use of a loop diuretic, consider adding a potassium-retaining diuretic (e.g. amiloride or spironolactone), but avoid in patients with renal impairment.

Further reading

McDonald TJ, Oral RA, Vaidya B. (2015) Investigating hyperkalaemia in adults. *BMJ* 351, h4762. DOI: 10.1136/bmj.h4762

UK Renal Association Clinical Practice Guidelines (2014) Treatment of acute hyperkalaemia in adults 2014. http://www.renal.org/docs/default-source/guidelines-resources/joint-guidelines/treatment-of-acute-hyperkalaemia-in-adults/hyperkalaemia-guideline—march-2014.pdf?sfvrsn=2.

CHAPTER 87

Disorders of plasma calcium concentration

Martin Crook

Disorders of plasma calcium concentration (Box 87.1) usually result from deranged handling of calcium by the gut, kidneys or bone. Calcium exists in the extracellular fluid in three forms: the physiologically important ionized fraction (50%), the protein-bound fraction (40%) and a small fraction (10%) complexed to anions. Most laboratories measure total calcium, which should be corrected for the plasma albumin concentration (a major determinant of the ionized calcium fraction):

$$\text{Plasma corrected calcium (mmol/L)} =$$
$$\text{Measured plasma calcium} + (40\text{-plasma albumin concentration g/l}) \times 0.02 \text{ mmol/L}$$

Box 87.1 Disorders of plasma calcium concentration.

Plasma total calcium concentration (mmol/L)	Classification	Clinical and ECG features
>3.5	Severe hypercalcaemia	Delirium and coma ECG: QT interval shortening
3.0–3.5	Moderate hypercalcaemia	Polyuria (from hypercalciuria-induced nephrogenic diabetes insipidus), vomiting, constipation, abdominal pain, renal calculi, joint pain
2.6–3.0	Mild hypercalcaemia	Usually asymptomatic
2.2–2.6	**Normal range**	
1.9–2.2	Mild hypocalcaemia	Usually asymptomatic
1.5–1.9	Moderate hypocalcaemia	Paraesthesiae, muscle cramps, positive Chvostek and Trousseau signs
<1.5	Severe hypocalcaemia	Tetany, carpopedal spasm, seizures, laryngospasm ECG: QT prolongation which may progress to ventricular fibrillation or heart block

Acute Medicine: A Practical Guide to the Management of Medical Emergencies, Fifth Edition. Edited by David Springings and John B. Chambers.
© 2018 John Wiley & Sons Ltd. Published 2018 by John Wiley & Sons Ltd.

Table 87.1 Causes of hypercalcaemia.

Common

Cancer involving bone (carcinoma of breast, bronchus, renal, thyroid, and prostate); haematological cancer, for example myeloma and lymphoma. Mechanisms: secretion of parathyroid-hormone-related protein; bone metastases; increased production of 1,25-dihydroxy vitamin D; ectopic parathyroid hormone production.

Primary hyperparathyroidism.

Chronic kidney disease with tertiary hyperparathyroidism and treatment with calcium and vitamin D metabolites.

Uncommon

Sarcoidosis and other granulomatous diseases such as tuberculosis

Other cancers with humoural effects (see above)

Thyrotoxicosis

Vitamin D excess

Milk-alkali syndrome

Adrenal insufficiency

Paget's disease with immobilization

Acromegaly

HIV infection

Vitamin A toxicity

Drugs, for example thiazides, lithium therapy

Hypocalciuric hypercalcaemia

Hypercalcaemia

Although primary hyperparathyroidism is the commonest cause of hypercalcaemia, cancer is most often the cause of severe hypercalcaemia requiring inpatient management. Typically this occurs in a patient known to have a cancer involving bone (e.g. carcinoma of the breast, bronchus, renal, thyroid or prostate) or a haematological cancer such as myeloma or lymphoma, but may sometimes be the presenting complaint. Hypercalcaemia in patients with cancer is related to osteolytic metastases in 20% cases and to secretion of parathyroid-hormone-related protein (PTHrP) in 80% cases. A small percentage is due to increased production of 1,25-dihydroxy vitamin D (associated with lymphoma) and ectopic PTH secretion.

Principles of management

Treat the underlying disorder: causes of hypercalcaemia are listed in Table 87.1.

Investigation of the patient with hypercalcaemia is given in Table 87.2.

Correct hypovolaemia and increase the renal excretion of calcium.

Inhibit accelerated bone resorption.

Avoid thiazides and lithium carbonate, which contribute to hypercalcaemia and also patient immobilization.

Moderate or severe hypercalcaemia (total calcium >3 mmol/L)

1 The first-line treatment is rehydration. In patients with mild symptoms, oral rehydration (a fluid intake of at least 2–3 L/day) may be sufficient. Patients with more severe symptoms should receive normal saline 1 L 6–8-hourly IV. The use of furosemide is no longer recommended in the management of hypercalcaemia.

2 If plasma calcium remains >3 mmol/L despite rehydration, drug therapy to inhibit osteoclast-mediated bone resorption is indicated. The most commonly used agents are given in Table 87.3.

3 Specific treatment will be needed to prevent a recurrence of hypercalcaemia (e.g. chemotherapy for malignancies, surgery for primary hyperparathyroidism).

4 For severe refractory hypercalcaemia, haemodialysis may be needed: seek advice from a nephrologist.

Table 87.2 Investigation in hypercalcaemia.

Full blood count
Plasma sodium, potassium, urea and creatinine with eGFR
Uncuffed sample for plasma calcium, phosphate, magnesium, total protein, albumin, alkaline phosphatase
Chest X-ray
ECG
If the cause of hypercalcaemia is not known:
Serum and urine protein electrophoresis
Parathyroid hormone (PTH)
Parathyroid hormone related protein (PTH related hormone is very rarely required and is offered by few laboratories)
C-reactive protein and ESR
Thyroid function tests
Vitamin D (25-hydroxy vitamin D)
Urine calcium concentration

Table 87.3 Drug therapy in moderate or severe hypercalcaemia.

Class of drug	Indication
Bisphosphonate (e.g. pamidronate, zolendronic acid)	First choice in hypercalcaemia usually due to non-haematological malignancy or primary hyperparathyroidism
Calcitonin	Failure to respond to bisphosphonate
Glucocorticoid	Hypercalcaemia due to myeloma, lymphoma, vitamin D toxicity and sarcoidosis

Hypocalcaemia

Causes of hypocalcaemia are given in Table 87.4. Acute severe hypocalcaemia (with tetany) is most commonly seen in patients with chronic kidney disease after elective subtotal parathyroidectomy or total thyroidectomy.

Be aware that hyperventilation may also cause carpopedal spasm due to reduced ionized calcium, resulting from a respiratory alkalosis.

Table 87.4 Causes of hypocalcaemia.

Following parathyroidectomy or total thyroidectomy
Hypoparathyroidism, for example autoimmune, infiltration, Di George syndrome
Acute pancreatitis
Severe hypomagnesaemia
Vitamin D deficiency, for example poor intake, malabsorption
Chronic kidney disease
Cancer (either involving bone, with increased osteoblastic activity, or in response to chemotherapy, with phosphate released from tumour cells forming complexes with plasma calcium)
Multiple citrated blood transfusions
Rhabdomyolysis
Septic shock
Pseudohypoparathyroidism
Hypercalciuric hypocalcaemia
Drugs, for example loop diuretics, phenytoin
Ethylene glycol poisoning

Acute severe hypocalcaemia, for example with tetany

Give 10 mL of calcium gluconate 10% (2.25 mmol) IV over 5 min, followed by a continuous infusion of calcium gluconate. This can be repeated and, if indicated, followed with infusion of calcium gluconate 10% infusion 40 mL (9 mmol) over 24 h.

It is essential to monitor serum calcium concentrations regularly and also exclude and manage concomitant hypomagnesaemia.

If hypocalcaemia is likely to continue, give oral vitamin D with patient follow-up.

Seek expert advice on further management.

Further reading

Goldner W. (2016) Cancer-related hypercalcemia. *J Oncol Pract* 12, 426–432. DOI: 10.1200/JOP.2016.011155.

Society for Endocrinology: Endocrine Emergency Guidance. Emergency management of acute hypercalcaemia in adult patients. http://www.endocrineconnections.com/content/5/5/G9.

Society for Endocrinology: Endocrine Emergency Guidance. Emergency management of acute hypocalcaemia in adult patients. http://www.endocrineconnections.com/content/5/5/G7.

CHAPTER 88

Disorders of plasma magnesium concentration

MARTIN CROOK

Magnesium is a predominately intracellular divalent cation, which is an essential cofactor to many enzyme systems. It is also important in cell membrane function and can antagonize calcium in cellular responses.

Classification of plasma magnesium concentration is given in Box 88.1.

Hypermagnesaemia

Causes of hypermagnesaemia are given in Table 88.1.

Hypercalcaemia and hyperkalaemia are associated with hypermagnesaemia, and plasma levels of these ions should be checked, as well as renal function, including eGFR and phosphate.

In resistant hypermagnesaemia, exclude hypothyroidism and adrenal insufficiency.

Box 88.1 Classification of plasma magnesium concentration

Plasma magnesium concentration (mmol/L)	Classification	Clinical and ECG features
>2.50	Severe hypermagnesaemia	Seizures, respiratory depression, hypotension Atrioventricular block, cardiac arrest
1.50–2.50	Moderate hypermagnesaemia	Nausea, hyporeflexia
1.20–1.50	Mild hypermagnesaemia	Usually asymptomatic
0.70–1.20	**Normal range**	
0.60–0.70	Mild hypomagnesaemia	Usually asymptomatic
0.50–0.60	Moderate hypomagnesaemia	Nausea, abdominal pain Paraesthesiae, muscle cramps
<0.50	Severe hypomagnesaemia	Tetany, seizures, muscle weakness, ataxia ECG: PR prolongation, widened QRS, ST depression, torsade de pointes

Acute Medicine: A Practical Guide to the Management of Medical Emergencies, Fifth Edition. Edited by David Sprigings and John B. Chambers.
© 2018 John Wiley & Sons Ltd. Published 2018 by John Wiley & Sons Ltd.

Table 88.1 Causes of hypermagnesaemia.

Increased intake of magnesium

Certain antacids

Milk-alkali syndrome

Magnesium-containing purgatives

Inappropriate magnesium infusion

Reduced renal excretion of magnesium

Acute kidney injury

Chronic kidney disease

Others

Familial hypocalciuric hypercalcaemia

Lithium treatment

Hypothyroidism

Adrenal insufficiency

Symptomatic severe hypermagnesaemia

Treat the underlying cause.

Give 5–10 mL of 10% calcium gluconate slowly IV over 30 s with ECG monitoring.

Insulin and glucose infusion can be used in severe hypermagnesaemia, as for severe hyperkalaemia.

If renal function is normal, urinary magnesium loss can be increased by forced saline diuresis.

If there is impaired renal function, seek advice from a nephrologist: haemodialysis may be indicated, particularly if plasma magnesium concentration is >4 mmol/L.

Hypomagnesaemia

Causes of hypomagnesaemia are given in Table 88.2. The manifestations of hypomagnesaemia are very similar to those of hypocalcaemia (Chapter 87).

Hypocalcaemia, hypophosphataemia and hypokalaemia are associated with hypomagnesaemia, and plasma levels of these ions should be checked. Severe hypomagnesaemia can cause hypocalcaemia due to decreased PTH release and activity. There is an association with diabetes mellitus, which should be considered. Measurement of 24-h urinary magnesium excretion can be useful in assessing the response to treatment.

Mild to moderate hypomagnesaemia

Treat the underlying cause.

Give oral replacement therapy with a magnesium salt.

Symptomatic severe hypomagnesaemia

Treat the underlying cause.

Give magnesium sulphate, 2–4 g of 50% solution (8.3–16.6 mmol) IV, diluted in saline or glucose intravenously (IV) over 30–60 min (for adults: 0.5 mmol/kg IV), but use caution if there is renal impairment.

Table 88.2 Causes of hypomagnesaemia.

Poor intake of magnesium
Alcoholism
Malnutrition

Gastrointestinal loss of magnesium
Malabsorption states
Acute pancreatitis
Proton pump inhibitors
Intestinal hypomagnesaemia with secondary hypocalcaemia
Chronic diarrhoea

Renal loss of magnesium
Drugs;
• Diuretics (loop and thiazide)
• Antibiotics (aminoglycoside, amphotericin, pentamidine)
• Calcineurin inhibitors
• Cisplatin
• Antibodies targeting epidermal growth factor (EGF) receptor (cetuximab, panitumumab, matuzumab)
Volume expansion
Uncontrolled diabetes mellitus
Hypercalcaemia
Acquired tubular dysfunction:
• Recovery from acute tubular necrosis
• Post-obstructive diuresis
• Post-renal transplantation
Genetic disorders:
• Bartter and Gitelman syndromes
• Familial hypomagnesaemia with hypercalciuria and nephrocalcinosis
• Autosomal dominant isolated hypomagnesaemia (Na-K-ATPase gamma subunit, Kv1.1 and cyclin M2 mutations)
• Autosomal recessive isolated hypomagnesaemia (EGF mutation)
• Renal malformations and early-onset diabetes mellitus (HNF1-beta mutation

Further reading

Agus ZS (2016) Mechanisms and causes of hypomagnesemia. *Current Opinion in Nephrology & Hypertension* 25, 301–307.
Ayuk J, Gittoes NJ (2014) Treatment of hypomagnesemia. *Am J Kidney Dis* 63, 691–695.
Jahnen-Dechent W, Ketteler M (2012) Magnesium basics. *Clin J Kidney* 5 (Suppl 1), i3–i14.

CHAPTER 89

Disorders of plasma phosphate concentration

MARTIN CROOK

Phosphate is a predominately intracellular anion with numerous physiological functions. It acts as a buffer, plays a central role in metabolic processes such as oxidative phosphorylation and glycolysis, as well as nucleotide pathways and nervous system conduction. Classification of plasma phosphate concentration is given in Box 89.1.

Hyperphosphataemia

Causes of hyperphosphataemia are given in Table 89.1. Pseudohyperphosphataemia can be due to phosphate leakage out of cells if the sample is haemolysed or delivery to the laboratory is delayed.

Box 89.1 Classification of plasma phosphate concentration.

Plasma phosphate concentration (mmol/L)	Classification	Clinical features
>3.0	Severe hyperphosphataemia	Hypocalcaemia, tetany
2.0–3.0	Moderate hyperphosphataemia	May be asymptomatic
1.2–2.0	Mild hyperphosphataemia	Usually asymptomatic
0.7–1.2	**Normal range**	
0.5–0.7	Mild hypophosphataemia	Usually asymptomatic
0.3–0.5	Moderate hypophosphataemia	May be asymptomatic
<0.3	Severe hypophosphataemia	Rhabdomyolysis, myopathy, seizures, coma Haemolysis, thrombocytopenia, cardiac arrhythmias Hypomagnesaemia, hypokalaemia

Acute Medicine: A Practical Guide to the Management of Medical Emergencies, Fifth Edition. Edited by David Sprigings and John B. Chambers.
© 2018 John Wiley & Sons Ltd. Published 2018 by John Wiley & Sons Ltd.

Table 89.1 Causes of hyperphosphataemia.

Acute phosphate load

Endogenous
  Rhabdomyolysis
  Tumour lysis syndrome
  Crush injury
  Malignant hyperpyrexia

Exogenous
  Phosphate-containing medications (laxatives, fosphenytoin)
  Intestinal uptake (vitamin D toxicity)

Cellular shift
  Acidosis, for example lactic acidosis or diabetic ketoacidosis

Decreased renal clearance
  Reduced glomerular filtration rate
  Acute kidney injury
  Chronic kidney disease

Increased tubular reabsorption
  Hypoparathyroidism or pseudohypoparathyroidism
  Acromegaly
  Bisphosphonates
  Vitamin D toxicity (also increases intestinal absorption)
  Familial tumoral calcinosis

Pseudohyperphosphataemia
  In vitro haemolysis
  Delayed sample delivery

Symptomatic severe hyperphosphataemia

Treat the underlying cause.

The major clinical consequence of severe hyperphosphataemia is hypocalcaemia (Chapter 87). The reason for this is that calcium phosphate precipitation into the tissues occurs when the phosphate and calcium plasma concentrations exceed their solubility product ([calcium] × [phosphate]).

In the presence of renal dysfunction and/or symptoms, a nephrologist's opinion and possible dialysis may be necessary. Consider oral phosphate-binding agents.

Mild to moderate hyperphosphataemia

Treat with oral phosphate-binding agents, for example magnesium hydroxide or calcium carbonate.

Hypophosphataemia

Causes of hypophosphataemia are given in Table 89.2.

Severe hypophosphataemia can cause numerous clinical features. These may include rhabdomyolysis, impaired skeletal muscle function, weakness and myopathy, impaired diaphragmatic contractility and difficulty weaning patients off mechanical ventilators and cardiomyopathy. Severe hypophosphataemia can provoke seizures, paraesthesiae, and renal tubular impairment and osteomalacia.

Table 89.2 Causes of hypophosphataemia.

Cellular shift
  IV glucose
  Metabolic or respiratory alkalosis
  Administration of insulin
  Refeeding syndrome

Inadequate intake of phosphate
  Starvation
  Malnutrition

Gastrointestinal loss of phosphate
  Malabsorption states
  Inhibition of phosphate absorption (e.g. antacids containing aluminium or magnesium, niacin)

Renal loss of phosphate
  Hypophosphataemic osteomalacia
  X-linked hypophosphataemia
  Oncogenic hypophosphataemia
  Paracetamol poisoning
  Fanconi syndrome

Others
  Severe liver disease
  Sepsis
  Hyperparathyroidism or parathyroid hormone-related peptide release

Other effects of severe hypophosphataemia include thrombocytopenia and haemolysis, as well as erythrocyte 2,3-DPG depletion, resulting in a shift in the haemoglobin/oxygen dissociation curve to the left (increasing its oxygen affinity).

Hypophosphataemia can be associated with hypomagnesaemia and hypokalaemia. A urine phosphate determination may help see if there is a renal cause of phosphate loss, for example Fanconi syndrome.

Symptomatic severe hypophosphataemia

Treat the underlying cause.

Give IV phosphate replacement:

- 9 mmol of monobasic potassium phosphate in half-normal saline by continuous IV infusion over 12 h or
- Phosphate Polyfusor® up to 50 mmol by continuous IV infusion over 24 h. This should not be given to patients with hypercalcaemia, because of the risk of metastatic calcification, or to patients with hyperkalaemia or hypernatraemia. Each 500 mL Polyfusor® contains: phosphate 50 mmol, potassium 9.5 mmol and sodium 81 mmol. In severe hypophosphataemia 20 mmol phosphate up to 0.5 mmol/kg of body weight may be given in up to a maximum of 50 mmol over 6–12 hours.

In addition to phosphate, measure plasma electrolytes, calcium, magnesium and renal function including eGFR, which must be monitored during therapy.

Mild to moderate hypophosphataemia

Treat the underlying cause.

Give oral phosphate (although gastrointestinal side-effects such as diarrhoea can be a problem and phosphate correction may be delayed), for example Phosphate-Sandoz® one tablet (containing phosphate

16.1 mmol, sodium 20.4 mmol, potassium 3.1 mmol) 8-hourly PO, which can be increased to maximum of 6 tablets daily, in divided doses, if tolerated.

Further reading

Crook MA (2014) Refeeding syndrome: problems with definition and management. *Nutrition* 30, 1448–1455.
Manghat P, Sodi R, Swaminathan R (2014) Phosphate homeostasis and disorders. *Ann Clin Biochem* 51, 631–656.

CHAPTER 90

Acute adrenal insufficiency

JAMES CRANE AND PAUL CARROLL

Consider the diagnosis in any patient with unexplained hypotension and suggestive clinical features (Table 90.1). Acute adrenal insufficiency most commonly occurs as an acute exacerbation of an underlying chronic or subacute insufficiency, triggered by concomitant illness such as infection.

- A high index of suspicion should be maintained in any patient with circulatory collapse particularly if not responsive to initial fluid resuscitation. Prompt recognition and glucocorticoid replacement may be a life-saving treatment in a critically unwell patient, and should not be delayed while awaiting test results.
- Patients on long-term corticosteroid therapy (prednisolone >5 mg daily or equivalent for ≥4 weeks) are at risk of glucocorticoid insufficiency if steroids are abruptly withdrawn.
- In secondary adrenal insufficiency (Table 90.2), haemodynamic compromise may not be accompanied by typical electrolyte disturbance as aldosterone is unaffected.

Priorities

In the patient presenting with acute circulatory collapse and suspected adrenal insufficiency (Tables 90.1 and 90.2), the following goals should be achieved in the first hour of treatment:

- Rapid assessment of airway, breathing, circulation and conscious level in a level 2 or 3 environment, with continuous monitoring of heart rate, blood pressure and oxygen saturation.
- Airway management by competent staff if the airway is compromised or the Glasgow Coma Scale score is less than 8.
- Supplemental oxygen if needed to maintain oxygen saturation >94%.
- Intravenous access, with blood sent for urgent investigation (Table 90.3).
- Fluid resuscitation with normal saline to correct the volume deficit.
- Place a bladder catheter for monitoring of urine output.
- Look for a MedicAlert® or similar bracelet/necklace as this may reveal the diagnosis.
- Give hydrocortisone 200 mg IV. Fludrocortisone is not required in addition, as this dose of hydrocortisone has sufficient mineralocorticoid action.
- Give a broad-spectrum antibiotic after taking blood and urine for culture, in case the trigger is infection.
- If the patient is well enough, take a detailed history for the symptoms of adrenal insufficiency and commonly associated disorders (Tables 90.1 and 90.2). Look for clinical signs, especially hyperpigmentation suggestive of elevated ACTH, to differentiate primary from secondary adrenal insufficiency. Hyperpigmentation is best seen over the palmar creases, knuckles, old scars and the oral mucosa.

Once stabilized, transfer the patient to an appropriate care area.

Acute Medicine: A Practical Guide to the Management of Medical Emergencies, Fifth Edition. Edited by David Sprigings and John B. Chambers.
© 2018 John Wiley & Sons Ltd. Published 2018 by John Wiley & Sons Ltd.

Table 90.1 Clinical features of adrenal insufficiency.

Primary (Addison's disease) and secondary adrenal insufficiency
Tiredness, weakness, anorexia, weight loss
Hypotension/postural hypotension
Nausea, vomiting, diarrhoea
Hyponatraemia, hypoglycaemia, mild normocytic anaemia, lymphocytosis, eosinophilia

Primary adrenal insufficiency and associated disorders only
Hyperpigmentation
Hyperkalaemia
Vitiligo
Autoimmune thyroid disease

Secondary adrenal insufficiency and associated disorders only
Pale skin without marked anaemia
Amenorrhea, decreased libido and potency
Scanty axillary and pubic hair
Small testicles
Secondary hypothyroidism
Headache, visual symptoms
Diabetes insipidus

Table 90.2 Causes of adrenal insufficiency.

Primary adrenal insufficiency	
Cause	**Examples**
Infective	Tuberculosis
	Fungal
Infiltrative	Sarcoidosis
	Metastatic disease
	Lymphoma
	Amyloid
	Haemochromatosis
Vascular (bilateral adrenal haemorrhage)	Anticoagulation
	Antiphospholipid syndrome
	Sepsis (Waterhouse-Friderichsen syndrome):
	• Meningococcal
	• Staphylococcal
Congenital	Congenital adrenal hyperplasia
	Congenital adrenal hypoplasia
	Adrenoleukodystrophy
Autoimmune*	Isolated autoimmune adrenalitis
	Autoimmune polyglandular syndromes
Iatrogenic	Bilateral adrenalectomy (for Cushing's disease, oncological resection)
	Drug-induced:
	• Antifungals (ketoconazole)
	• Metyrapone
	• Mitotane
	• Etomidate

(continued)

Secondary adrenal insufficiency[†]	
Cause	**Examples**
Infective	Tuberculosis
Infiltrative	Neurosarcoidosis
	Haemochromatosis
	Langerhans cell histiocytosis
Inflammatory/autoimmune	hypophysitis (lymphocytic, IgG4, immune checkpoint inhibitors, other)
	Isolated corticotroph autoimmunity
	Autoimmune polyglandular syndromes
Vascular	Sheehan's syndrome
	Pituitary apoplexy
Congenital	Various rare genetic or developmental defects
Neoplastic	Pituitary adenoma
	Metastasis
	Craniopharyngioma
	Pituitary carcinoma
	Meningioma
	Invasion of other intracranial tumour
Iatrogenic	Exogenous glucocorticoids
	Hypophysectomy
	Pituitary radiotherapy
	Radiation of other head and neck tumour
Unknown	'Empty sella syndrome'

[*] 90% of primary adrenal insufficiency is due to autoimmune adrenalitis.

[†] Secondary adrenal insufficiency is roughly twice as prevalent as primary. Exogenous glucocorticoid commonly causes transient adrenal insufficiency. The commonest cause of permanent secondary adrenal insufficiency is a pituitary tumour and consequent treatment, with sufficient damage to pituitary function to result in hypopituitarism.

Table 90.3 Urgent investigation in suspected acute adrenal insufficiency.

Creatinine, sodium and potassium, glucose[*]
Venous blood gases and lactate
Plasma cortisol[†]
Plasma corticotrophin (ACTH) (taken in EDTA tube, for later analysis; transport immediately to the laboratory for freezing)
Thyroid function tests
Full blood count
Coagulation screen
C-reactive protein
Blood culture
Urine microscopy and culture
Chest X-ray
ECG

[*] Typical biochemical findings in acute adrenal insufficiency are raised creatinine, low sodium (120–130 mmol/L), raised potassium (5–7 mmol/L), low glucose.

[†] The cortisol level at presentation may be difficult to interpret. In a critically ill patient, a level of <500 nmol/L is suspicious for insufficiency.

Box 90.1 Acute adrenal insufficiency – alerts

- Adrenal insufficiency can be a difficult diagnosis to make in an acutely unwell patient as the diagnostic tests are not valid in this population and apparently normal plasma cortisol level may not be appropriately elevated for the degree of metabolic stress present.
- Delay in administration of high-dose glucocorticoid leads to excess morbidity and mortality in critically unwell patients with adrenal insufficiency.
- Newly-diagnosed patients with adrenal insufficiency require careful education regarding sick-day rules and may need an emergency injection pack and training before discharge.

Further management

Steroid replacement

- If in doubt, hydrocortisone replacement should continue until adrenal sufficiency can be conclusively confirmed or excluded. In the acutely unwell patient, give hydrocortisone 50–100 mg 6-hourly IV or IM.
- After treatment of any underlying concomitant illness and when the patient is feeling well, parenteral hydrocortisone can be stepped down to a double-physiological dose of oral hydrocortisone, or approximately 40 mg daily in divided doses. When completely recovered, physiological replacement can commence.
- Mineralocorticoid replacement for primary adrenal insufficiency is normally achieved with a dose of fludrocortisone 50–200 µgm PO once daily, and is started at 100 µgm. Adequacy of dose can be assessed by an absence of clinical signs of hypovolaemia (e.g. postural hypotension) and normal electrolytes.

Making the patient safe for discharge

- Educating the patient on what to do in the presence of acute illness is of paramount importance and may be a life-saving intervention. Patient information resources can be found and reproduced free of charge at the website of the Addison's Disease Self-help Group, www.addisons.org.uk, and are based on the advice of an expert panel.
- Patients should be advised to double their hydrocortisone dose in the presence of febrile illness (temperature >37.5 °C), if on antibiotics or if undertaking very strenuous exercise. Patients should take 20 mg after vomiting and seek medical attention if vomiting more than once as parenteral hydrocortisone is likely to be required.
- If a cause of permanent adrenal insufficiency is confirmed, the patient should be strongly advised to wear an identity bracelet to alert health-care professionals to their condition and potential need for immediate hydrocortisone in the event of an emergency.

Confirming the diagnosis

When well, definitive determination of adrenal status can be sought. If primary adrenal insufficiency is suspected (ACTH elevated at presentation), a short Synacthen test is done (Table 90.4). Alternative investigations (e.g. an insulin stress test) may be necessary for secondary adrenal insufficiency; seek advice from an endocrinologist.

Determining the cause

- If primary adrenal insufficiency is confirmed, further investigations are required to elucidate the aetiology. The presence of adrenal autoantibodies suggests an autoimmune process that may be part of a polyglandular syndrome, and clinical features of other associated conditions should be sought (Table 90.2). Seek advice from an endocrinologist.

  If secondary adrenal insufficiency is identified, a thorough search for a history of exogenous steroid is the first step. Inhaled and topical steroids can be absorbed systemically in sufficient quantities to result in adrenal

Table 90.4 Short tetracosactrin (Synacthen) test.

- The test should be done when the patient has recovered from acute illness, as hydrocortisone (but not fludrocortisone) must be stopped for 24 h before the test. The patient should be resting quietly but need not fast prior to the test. Tetracosactrin may exacerbate bronchospasm in those with asthma. Oestrogens, for example in oral contraceptives, should be stopped six weeks before the test.
- Give 250 μgm of tetracosactrin IV or IM before 10 am. Measure plasma cortisol immediately before, and 30 and 60 min after the injection. Baseline plasma ACTH should also be measured.
- With normal adrenal function, the baseline plasma cortisol is over 140 nmol/L, and the 30 or 60-min level is over 500 nmol/L and at least 200 nmol/L above the baseline level. (note: cut off values are dependent on the assay used - check local values with your laboratory)
- In patients with primary hypoadrenalism, tetracosactrin does not stimulate cortisol secretion, because the adrenal cortex is already maximally stimulated by endogenous corticotropin. In severe secondary hypoadrenalism, plasma cortisol does not increase because of adrenocortical atrophy. However, in secondary hypoadrenalism which is mild or of recent onset, the test may be normal.

insufficiency if stopped abruptly. Glucocorticoids are also found in commercially available skin-lightening creams and are a common cause of Cushing's syndrome (followed by adrenal insufficiency after cessation) in certain demographic groups.

- In the absence of exogenous steroid, first-line investigations are directed at the pituitary gland. Seek advice from an endocrinologist.

Further Reading

Charmandari E, Nicolaides NC, Chrousos GP (2014) Adrenal insufficiency. *Lancet* 383, 2152–2167.
Society for Endocrinology. Endocrine Emergency Guidance. Emergency management of acute adrenal insufficiency (adrenal crisis) in adult patients. http://www.endocrineconnections.com/content/5/5/G1.

CHAPTER 91

Thyrotoxic storm

JAMES CRANE AND PAUL CARROLL

Consider the diagnosis in any patient with fever, abnormal mental state, sinus tachycardia or atrial fibrillation, who also has signs of thyrotoxicosis. Thyrotoxic storm is an acute life-threatening metabolic emergency caused by extremely high levels of thyroid hormone activity. If the diagnosis is suspected, antithyroid treatment must be started before biochemical confirmation. Adequate beta blockade to neutralize the associated autonomic overdrive is also essential.

Thyrotoxicosis is the syndrome resulting from supranormal thyroid hormone activity, and is usually the result of hyperthyroidism, defined as increased thyroid hormone production by the native thyroid gland. Causes are summarized in Table 91.1.

Priorities

Is this thyrotoxic storm?

- The diagnosis of thyrotoxic storm is clinical, and rests on the identification of actual or impending decompensation of organ function due to thyrotoxicosis (Table 91.2).
- Since thyroid storm represents the end of a spectrum of severity, and due to inter-patient differences in the tipping point between compensated organ stress and decompensated organ failure, the diagnosis may be difficult.

What has triggered the thyrotoxic storm?

- Thyrotoxic storm may occur in the course of the natural history of an underlying thyrotoxic process, but is more often related to decompensation caused by an intercurrent precipitant. This is most frequently an infective illness, but may also be surgery (particularly thyroid surgery or occasionally non-thyroid surgery), other critical illness or childbirth.
- Other iatrogenic causes include radioactive iodine therapy in patients with insufficiently controlled hyper-thyroidism, abrupt cessation of antithyroid medications (or non-adherence to these), administration of iodine-containing pharmaceuticals (e.g. amiodarone or contrast agents), induction of anaesthesia or repeated vigorous palpation of a Graves' goitre.

Immediate management

Thyrotoxic storm is an acutely life-threatening condition and must be managed in a level 2 or 3 (resuscitation area/ HDU/ICU) setting. The immediate management priorities in the first hour are:

- Rapid assessment of airway, breathing, circulation and conscious level. Continuous monitoring of blood pressure, heart rate and ECG.

Acute Medicine: A Practical Guide to the Management of Medical Emergencies, Fifth Edition. Edited by David Sprigings and John B. Chambers.
© 2018 John Wiley & Sons Ltd. Published 2018 by John Wiley & Sons Ltd.

Table 91.1 Causes of hyperthyroidism*.

Autoimmune	Graves' disease[†]
	Hashitoxicosis
	Postpartum thyroiditis
Infective	Subacute thyroiditis
	Pyogenic thyroiditis
Neoplastic	Solitary adenoma
	Toxic multinodular goitre
	Differentiated thyroid carcinoma (rare, mostly follicular)
Secondary	TSHoma
	Thyroid hormone resistance
	Hyperemesis gravidarum
	Hydatidiform mole/choriocarcinoma
Destructive	Amiodarone-induced thyrotoxicosis type 2 (AIT-2)
	Trauma
	Irradiation
	Lithium
Iodine excess	Amiodarone-induced thyrotoxicosis type 1 (AIT-1)
(Jod-Basedow phenomenon)	Iodine contrast
	Dietary (moving from iodine deficient to iodine rich area)

* Thyrotoxicosis is the syndrome resulting from supranormal thyroid hormone activity. It is usually the result of hyperthyroidism, defined as increased thyroid hormone production by the native thyroid gland. Other causes are oversupply of exogenous thyroid hormone in patients taking levothyroxine or other thyroid supplements, and very rarely, ectopic thyroid hormone production by an ovarian teratoma (struma ovarii).

[†] Pathognomonic features of Graves' disease include the presence of thyroid eye disease, pretibial myxoedema, thyroid acropachy, or a bruit over the thyroid gland.

- Airway management by competent staff if the airway is compromised or the Glasgow Coma Scale score is less than 8.
- Supplemental oxygen if needed to maintain arterial oxygen saturation 94–96%.
- Haemodynamic stabilization. Hypotension may be due to high output cardiac failure or a compromising tachyarrhythmia (usually supraventricular). DC cardioversion may well be unsuccessful for AF in a severely hyperthyroid patient. Unless there is clinical suspicion of underlying cardiomyopathy, rate-related failure may be managed with a short-acting beta blocker (e.g. IV esmolol) with prompt withdrawal if clinical state worsens. Patients with thyrotoxic storm and heart failure must be managed in a level 3 environment, with continuous BP and CVP monitoring.
- Assessment for common precipitants of thyrotoxic storm: sepsis, diabetic ketoacidosis, or myocardial infarction (see above). If identified, appropriate management should be initiated. When no precipitating factor is apparent, broad-spectrum antibiotics are warranted until intercurrent infection has been excluded. Other precipitating causes can be managed in the usual manner.
- Cooling measures should be employed to correct fever, initially with paracetamol 1000 mg PO/IV.
- Administer a non-cardioselective beta blocker, for example propranolol 40–80 mg PO. If rapid onset of action needed or if oral route unavailable due to reduced conscious level, intravenous esmolol 50–100 μgm/kg/min may be used. Consider an arterial line for continuous blood pressure monitoring if IV beta blockers initiated.
- Administer a thionamide to prevent further thyroid hormone production, for example propylthiouracil 500–1000 mg loading dose PO (followed by 250 mg 4-hourly). Carbimazole may also be used (20–30 mg every 4–6 h PO). There are no intravenous preparations but they may be given via nasogastric tube or rectally if there are concerns about absorption.

Table 91.2 Diagnosis of thyrotoxic storm.

Criteria	Points
Thermoregulatory dysfunction	
Temperature	
Less than 37.2 °C (99.0 °F)	0
37.2–37.7 °C (99.0–99.9 °F)	5
37.8–38.2 °C (100.0–100.9 °F)	10
38.3–38.8 °C (101.0–101.9 °F)	15
38.9–39.3 °C (102.0–102.9 °F)	20
39.4–39.9 °C (103.0–103.9 °C)	25
40.0 °C or higher (104 °F or higher)	30
Cardiovascular	
Heart Rate	
Less than 100	0
100–109	5
110–119	10
120–129	15
130–139	20
140 or higher	25
Atrial fibrillation	
Absent	0
Present	10
Congestive heart failure	
Absent	0
Mild	5
Moderate	10
Severe	20
Gastrointestinal/hepatic dysfunction	
Manifestation	
Absent	0
Moderate (diarrhoea, abdominal pain, nausea/vomiting)	10
Severe (jaundice)	20
Central nervous system disturbance	
Manifestation	
Absent	0
Mild (agitation)	10
Moderate (delirium, psychosis, extreme lethargy)	20
Severe (seizure/coma)	30
Precipitant history	
Status	
Present	0
Absent	10
Interpretation	
Total score	**Interpretation**
<25	Thyrotoxic storm unlikely
25–45	Impending thyrotoxic storm
>45	Thyrotoxic storm confirmed

Source: Burch HB, Wartofsky L (1993) Life-threatening hyperthyroidism: thyroid storm. *Endocrinol Metab Clin North Am* 22, 263–277. Reproduced with permission of Elsevier.

- Administer 100mg IV hydrocortisone to support circulation and reduce thyroid hormone action.
- Transfer to HDU/ICU for further management

Further management

- The ongoing management of thyroid storm is directed towards blocking further production of thyroid hormone, blocking its release, blocking conversion of T4 to active T3 and limiting the adrenergic effects of high thyroid hormone activity. Thionamide treatment should be continued. Propylthiouracil at a dose of 250 mg every 4–6 h has been the preferred agent due to its additional benefit in reducing conversion of T4 to T3. Recent concerns regarding an association between propylthiouracil and hepatitis should be taken into account and in patients with known liver disease or if liver function tests become abnormal, carbimazole 60–80 mg daily is an alternative. 'Cold' iodine (i.e. non-radioactive iodine) can be administered in the form of 3–5 drops of Lugol's solution (5% elemental iodine, 10% potassium iodide in distilled water) or a saturated solution of potassium iodide (SSKI), diluted in water three times daily, making use of the Wolff-Chaikoff effect in which high doses of iodine result in a blockade of the incorporation of iodine into thyroglobulin. Effectiveness of iodine solutions is time-limited to around ten days, after which the thyroid escapes this effect by down-regulating iodine transporters.
- A beta blocker should be administered to negate the catecholaminergic effects of thyrotoxicosis. Oral propranolol is most frequently used due to its additional capacity to block peripheral T4 to T3 conversion. The dose is titrated according to cardiovascular parameters. In thyrotoxic storm, 60–120 mg 6-hourly PO may be required. Glucocorticoids also reduce peripheral conversion of T4 to T3: hydrocortisone 100 mg 6-hourly IV would be a typical dose.
- In extreme, treatment refractory thyrotoxicosis, plasmapheresis has been used to clear circulating thyroid hormones to allow a window for emergency thyroidectomy to be performed safely.

Further reading

De Leo S, Lee SY, Braverman LE (2016) Hyperthyroidism.pdf *Lancet* 388, 906–918.
Sharp CS, Wilson MP, Nordstrom K (2016) Psychiatric emergencies for clinicians: The Emergency Department management of thyroid storm. *J Emerg Med* 51, 155–158.

CHAPTER 92

Myxoedema coma

JAMES CRANE AND PAUL CARROLL

At the extreme end of the hypothyroid spectrum lies the rare endocrine emergency of myxoedema coma, which has a prevalence of less than 1 per million per year, and is largely a disease of the elderly. The physical signs of hypothermia from whatever cause closely resemble those of myxoedema coma; however, if there is other evidence of hypothyroidism (Table 92.1), thyroid hormone and hydrocortisone (in case there is coexisting autoimmune adrenal insufficiency) should be given. Even with treatment, mortality is high.

Priorities

Is this myxoedema coma?
- Hypothermia and reduced conscious level are the cardinal features (although most patients are not actually comatose, i.e. Glasgow Coma Scale score <8).
- Bradycardia, bradypnoea and hypoxaemia are common.
- Hyponatraemia, hypercapnia, hypercalcaemia, hypoglycaemia and elevated creatinine kinase are often present.

What has caused myxoedema coma?
- Myxoedema coma is usually precipitated by an event causing an increased metabolic demand which outstrips the adaptive mechanisms compensating for chronic hypothyroidism, such as infection or trauma.
- Other triggers include cold weather, sedative agents, general anaesthesia, acute coronary syndrome and stroke.

Immediate management
- ABCDE assessment
  - Airway – may be compromised by oedema of the upper respiratory tract structures. Airway adjuncts or intubation may be required.
  - Breathing – ventilatory failure is usual and should be confirmed with arterial blood gas analysis. Assisted ventilation is often necessary for the first 24–48 h.
  - Circulation – cautious fluid resuscitation, bearing in mind the likely impairment of cardiac contractility, can be employed. Glucocorticoids should be administered (50–100 mg 6-hourly IV) as severe hypothyroidism may impair ACTH response to stress. The possibility of undiagnosed autoimmune adrenal insufficiency as a comorbidity must be recognized.
- Correct hypoglycaemia using intravenous glucose
- Identify the precipitant and initiate treatment. Investigation needed urgently is given in Table 92.2.

Acute Medicine: A Practical Guide to the Management of Medical Emergencies, Fifth Edition. Edited by David Sprigings and John B. Chambers.
© 2018 John Wiley & Sons Ltd. Published 2018 by John Wiley & Sons Ltd.

Table 92.1 Features suggesting myxoedema coma in the patient with hypothermia.

Preceding symptoms of hypothyroidism (weight gain with reduced appetite, dry skin and hair loss) or confirmed hypothyroidism
Previous radioactive iodine treatment or thyroidectomy for hyperthyroidism
Thyroidectomy scar
Hyponatraemia (plasma sodium <130 mmol/L)
Macrocytosis
Failure of core temperature to rise 0.5 °C per hour with external rewarming

- Infection may be occult and sepsis is unlikely to be accompanied by an elevated temperature. If in doubt, administer broad spectrum antibiotics.
- The ECG will be abnormal and usually shows bradycardia, small voltage QRS complexes and flattened or inverted T-waves. Varying degrees of heart block may be present. Measure the QTc interval, which may be prolonged, bringing a risk of polymorphic ventricular tachycardia (torsades de pointes; see Chapter 41). Assess for evidence of myocardial ischaemia or infarction.
- Cerebellar signs may be the result of severe hypothyroidism, but assess for evidence of an acute stroke.
- Assess for evidence of an upper gastrointestinal bleed.
- Obtain a collateral history – there will usually be a history of hypothyroidism or thyroid ablation.
- Review the drug history for new medications, which may have precipitated the acute presentation.
  Alert the critical care team and transfer to an appropriate ICU or HDU bed when stable.

Further management

Thyroid hormone replacement
- Restoration of thyroid hormone activity is essential. There is no high-grade evidence to suggest how this is best achieved. Replacement may be enteral or parenteral; with T4, T3 or both.
- Restoring normal target tissue thyroid hormone activity as soon as possible to reverse life-threatening disturbance of body systems must be weighed against the possibility of inducing fatal tachyarrhythmias

Table 92.2 Urgent investigation in suspected myxoedema coma.

Blood glucose
Creatinine and electrolytes
Plasma calcium and phosphate
Liver function tests
Creatine kinase
Full blood count
C-reactive protein
Arterial pH, gases and lactate
Blood and urine culture
Thyroid function tests (TSH, free T4, free T3)
Plasma cortisol
Plasma corticotrophin (ACTH) (taken in EDTA tube, for later analysis; transport immediately to the laboratory for freezing)
ECG
Chest X-ray
CT head

with rapid correction. The enteral route should lead to a less abrupt increase in circulating thyroid hormone levels and allows for the use of T4, which, by virtue of requiring peripheral conversion to T3 for maximal activity, gives a smoother tissue response. However, absorption may be impaired by oedema, slow transit or ileus. The intravenous route limits one to using T3 since intravenous preparations of T4 are not commonly available. The associated rapid increase in thyroid hormone receptor signalling may induce adverse cardiac events.

- The choice of treatment should be made on a patient-specific basis. The options are:
  - NG T4 alone
  - NG T4 plus T3
  - IV T3: typically 20 µgm/24 h

  T3 and T4 replacement should be carefully titrated against free thyroid hormone levels, which may be measured daily. Over-replacement risks tachyarrhythmia in what is likely to be a myopathic heart.

Supportive care

- Hypothermia should not be treated with external rewarming since this will induce peripheral vasodilatation, negating the compensatory diversion of blood flow to the vital organs.
- Glucocorticoids should be continued until coexisting adrenal insufficiency (Chapter 90) has been excluded by a short Synacthen test.
- Ongoing supportive management of organ failure (e.g. mechanical ventilation or vasopressors) while awaiting response to thyroid hormone replacement is a key determinant of outcome. The time to recovery may be variable depending on the duration of severe hypothyroidism.

Further reading

Chiong YV, Bammerlin E, Mariash CN (2015) Development of an objective tool for the diagnosis of myxedema coma. *Translational Research* 166, 233–243. http://doi.org/10.1016/j.trsl.2015.01.003.

CHAPTER 93

Pituitary apoplexy

JAMES CRANE AND PAUL CARROLL

Pituitary apoplexy is a rare clinical syndrome comprising sudden-onset severe headache accompanied by visual deficit, or extraocular muscle nerve palsy, or reduced conscious level. It may be misdiagnosed as meningitis or subarachnoid haemorrhage.

Pituitary apoplexy results from haemorrhage into or infarction of a pre-existing pituitary tumour, and is almost invariably associated with hypopituitarism. A prior diagnosis of pituitary tumour is usually absent, with the apoplexy representing the first presentation of a previously unrecognized tumour in 80% of cases.

Patients with pituitary apoplexy should, once stabilized, be transferred to a neurosurgical centre for the multidisciplinary management of an experienced pituitary surgeon, neuro-ophthalmologist and endocrinologist.

Priorities

Consider the diagnosis

- Headache is usually frontal, although may take any form. It is primarily caused by pressure effects in the pituitary fossa and often induces nausea and vomiting.
- If blood escapes into the subarachnoid space, this may be accompanied by meningism. Cranial nerve III, IV and VI palsies result from compression of the adjacent cavernous sinuses, and visual field/acuity deficits from compression of the optic chasm lying superior to the fossa. Haemorrhage and the resultant pressure effects may not be maximal at presentation and repeated examination is essential to detect progressive neurological deficit, the presence of which may trigger escalation to emergency neurosurgical intervention.
- Some degree of pituitary hormone insufficiency is a feature of most cases of apoplexy, with ACTH and consequently cortisol insufficiency being both common, and the most important of these. If severe enough this may manifest as haemodynamic instability, since the lack of glucocorticoid obtunds the pressor effect of catecholamine signals. Delay in glucocorticoid replacement in these patients may be fatal.
- Apoplexy may be precipitated by many factors; hypertension is the commonest. Conditions causing wide variations of blood pressure, including major surgery, are frequently implicated. Other known risk factors include head trauma, anticoagulant therapy or clotting disorders and pregnancy (especially in the peripartum phase, when pituitary apoplexy is known as Sheehan syndrome).

Resuscitate the patient

In the first hour of treatment the following goals should be achieved:

- Rapid assessment of airway, breathing, circulation and conscious level.
- Airway management by competent staff if the airway is compromised or the Glasgow Coma Scale score is less than 8.
- Supplemental oxygen, if needed to achieve arterial saturation 94–96%.

Acute Medicine: A Practical Guide to the Management of Medical Emergencies, Fifth Edition. Edited by David Sprigings and John B. Chambers.
© 2018 John Wiley & Sons Ltd. Published 2018 by John Wiley & Sons Ltd.

Table 93.1 Urgent investigation in suspected pituitary apoplexy.

Creatinine and electrolytes
Blood glucose
Venous blood gases and lactate
Baseline pituitary profile: cortisol, ACTH, TSH and free T4, prolactin, growth hormone, insulin-like growth factor-1, luteinizing hormone, follicular-stimulating hormone and testosterone (male) or oestradiol (female)
Full blood count
Coagulation screen
C-reactive protein
Blood culture
Urine microscopy and culture
Chest X-ray
ECG
MRI brain

- Fluid resuscitation in the shocked or otherwise haemodynamically compromised patient, with the addition of immediate administration of a sufficient dose of glucocorticoid on the presumption of ACTH insufficiency, for example 100–200 mg intravenous hydrocortisone to be followed by 50–100 mg every 6 h (preferably by intramuscular injection as this provides a predictable pharmacokinetic profile and therefore more consistent glucocorticoid activity when compared to intravenous boluses).
- Visual field examination by confrontation (with a red pin if available), Snellen chart visual acuity and cranial nerve III, IV, Va and VI examination. Document these clearly in the notes for later comparison.
- Request urgent dedicated pituitary imaging, preferably MRI as this is the most sensitive modality. General cerebral imaging not dedicated to the pituitary fossa cannot be relied upon to reveal the diagnosis, with CT demonstrating a pituitary mass in less than 80% of cases and pituitary haemorrhage in only 20%.
- Other investigation needed urgently is given in Table 93.1.

Further management

- Once stabilized, take a history, seeking symptoms of pituitary hormone insufficiency, including menstrual changes, sexual dysfunction, any constitutional changes in weight, skin, hair, bowel habit, energy levels and symptoms of specific hormone excess, including those of acromegaly, Cushing's syndrome, hyperprolactinaemia (galactorrhoea, oligomenorrhoea, hypogonadism) and thyrotoxicosis.
- You should liaise with the local centre of expertise to arrange a safe and early transfer. Images should be linked or downloaded to a suitable digital medium to travel with the patient.
- Specific, evidence-based indications for surgical intervention remain unclear, with a lack of randomized controlled trial data due to the rarity of the condition. Guidelines exist (see further reading), and in general those with a significant neuro-ophthalmic deficit and those with reduced conscious level require surgical decompression and those without can be managed conservatively. However, the decision to proceed either on a conservative or a surgical path must be taken by an experienced and multidisciplinary team of endocrinologists, neurosurgeons and ophthalmologists.
- Urine output should be carefully monitored and if averaging more than 200 mL/h for two consecutive hours may indicate posterior pituitary impairment and the onset of diabetes insipidus. Paired serum and urine osmolalities should be sent (and processed) urgently. If plasma osmolality is >285 mOsmol/L and urine osmolality is not more than this, desmopressin can be given, for example as a 1 μgm subcutaneous injection. A urinary catheter must be inserted for fluid balance monitoring.

Box 93.1 Pituitary apoplexy – alerts

- Consider pituitary apoplexy in any patient with sudden onset severe headache.
- Once stabilized, the patient with pituitary apoplexy should be managed by a specialist multi-disciplinary team of neurosurgeons, ophthalmologists and endocrinologists.
- Glucocorticoid replacement is a life-saving intervention and should be administered without delay in patients with cardiovascular compromise.

- In all but those with no adverse signs, hourly neurological assessment should be carried out (to include GCS and cranial nerve examination with visual fields) until stability has been established. Progression of neurological deficit is not uncommon and in these patients urgent neurosurgical intervention is likely to be required.
- Formal neuro-ophthalmological assessment in the form of visual fields (Humphrey or Goldmann perimetry) and gaze palsy assessment (e.g. Hess chart) should be completed as soon as is practicable and daily thereafter.
- If serial neurological examination reveals rapidly deteriorating signs or reducing conscious level, repeat contact with the neurosurgical team is required to arrange transfer for emergency surgery.

Further reading

Society for Endocrinology. Endocrine Emergency Guidance. Emergency management of pituitary apoplexy in adult patients. http://www.endocrineconnections.com/content/5/5/G12.

CHAPTER 94

Paraganglioma (phaeochromocytoma) crisis

JAMES CRANE AND PAUL CARROLL

Paragangliomas (phaeochromocytomas; see Box 94.1) can present with life-threatening catecholamine-induced crises:
- Hypertensive crisis (which may be complicated by encephalopathy, heart failure, myocardial infarction, or aortic dissection)
- Atrial and ventricular arrhythmias
- Hypotensive crisis (through poorly understood mechanisms)
- Multi-organ crisis, characterized by hyperpyrexia, encephalopathy, acute kidney injury and pulmonary oedema
    Crises may be triggered by administration of drugs, such as dopamine antagonists, tricyclic antidepressants, radiocontrast media or anaesthetic agents.
    Manipulation of the tumour is likely to trigger a crisis in a patient without sufficient alpha-adrenergic blockade and exclusion of catecholamine excess is necessary prior to surgery on any tumour located at a site typical for paragangliomas.

Priorities

In the patient presenting with a suspected catecholamine-induced crisis (Table 94.1), the following goals should be achieved in the first hour of treatment:
- Rapid assessment of airway, breathing, circulation and conscious level in a level 2 or 3 environment, with continuous monitoring of heart rate, blood pressure and arterial oxygen saturation. Consider an arterial line for invasive monitoring.

Box 94.1 Paragangliomas (phaeochromocytomas).

- These are tumours of chromaffin cells, derived from neural crest tissue.
- Most commonly occur in the adrenal medulla, in which instance they are called a phaeochromocytomas. Often secrete catecholamines (adrenaline, noradrenaline, dopamine) but may secrete other hormones as well.
- Usually sporadic, but are also associated with several genetic syndromes including multiple endocrine neoplasia (type 2A or 2B), von Hippel-Lindau disease, succinate dehydrogenase (SDH) mutations and neurofibromatosis type 1.
- Usually present between the ages of 20 and 50 years, with earlier presentation increasing the likelihood that they are due to one or other of the genetic syndromes.

Acute Medicine: A Practical Guide to the Management of Medical Emergencies, Fifth Edition. Edited by David Sprigings and John B. Chambers.
© 2018 John Wiley & Sons Ltd. Published 2018 by John Wiley & Sons Ltd.

Table 94.1 When to consider a catecholamine-induced crisis.

Severe hypertension
Headache, palpitation and sweating
Acute pulmonary oedema
Acute regional ischaemia (limb/mesenteric)
Encephalopathy with hypertension
Acute chest pain with hypertension
Heart failure with hypertension
Acute kidney injury with hypertension
Any acute presentation in a patient with known genetic associate: neurofibromatosis, von Hippel-Lindau, MEN 2,
previous paraganglioma (SDH mutation)

- Airway management by competent staff if the airway is compromised or the Glasgow Coma Scale score is less
  than 8.
- Supplemental oxygen if needed to maintain $SaO_2 > 94\%$.
- Intravenous access with blood sent for urgent investigation (Table 94.2).
- Assess for organ failure:
  - Cardiovascular – arrhythmias, heart failure, ischaemic stroke, intracranial bleed, vasospastic peripheral
    ischaemia, myocardial infarction, aortic dissection or aneurysmal rupture
  - Respiratory – pulmonary oedema
  - Neurological – encephalopathy
  - Renal – acute kidney injury
  - Haematolgical – disseminated intravascular coagulation
- In the absence of organ failure, see Further management for advice on commencing alpha blockade with oral
  phenoxybenzamine. If organ failure is present, intravenous alpha blockade may be necessary. Phentolamine is
  the preferred agent, delivered as a slow IV push of 1 mg over 1 min, with blood pressure monitoring via an
  arterial line. Caution is required; the circulating volume may be substantially reduced as a physiological
  response to increased vascular resistance. When reversed rapidly, a dramatic fall in blood pressure may ensue.

Table 94.2 Investigation of suspected catecholamine-induced crisis.

Urgent
ECG
Echocardiography
Chest X-ray
Arterial blood gases, pH and lactate (high lactate not necessarily indicative of ischaemic tissue, may be raised by direct
effect of catecholamines on cellular metabolism)
Blood metadrenaline, normetadrenaline and dopamine concentration
Full blood count
Coagulation screen
Biochemical profile
Triple phase adrenal CT scan (or in and out of phase adrenal MRI)

Later
Base of skull to pelvis imaging if adrenal imaging negative
Nuclear medicine imaging (^{123}I-mIBG)
Further investigation to be directed by neuroendocrine tumour multidisciplinary team

Intravenous alpha blockade must be accompanied by aggressive intravenous filling to replace this missing volume as the arterial resistance falls.

- Identify the precipitant and commence appropriate management.
- Involve a specialist endocrinology team at the earliest opportunity.

Further management

Biochemical confirmation

If organ failure is not present, confirmation of pathological elevation of catecholamines should be sought by measuring catecholamines or their metabolites (metanephrines) in the urine or blood. Plasma metanephrine levels are the most specific of these tests and less susceptible to the effects of intercurrent illness than levels of adrenaline or noradrenaline themselves. The vast majority of paragangliomas will secrete one or both of these hormones, pure dopamine-secreting paragangliomas are very rare.

Imaging

Dedicated cross-sectional imaging (CT or MRI) of the adrenal glands should be undertaken to localize the tumour. If negative, imaging from neck to pelvis is required.

Functional imaging is also useful as it may identify metastases and/or confirm uptake of a tracer by malignant paragangliomas, which may then be utilized in targeted radiotherapy should this be necessary post-surgery (peptide-receptor radionuclide therapy). ^{131}I-meta-IodoBenzylGuanidine (mIBG) is most commonly used.

Adrenergic blockade

Alpha blockade using phenoxybenzamine at an initial dose of 10 mg 12-hourly PO should be initiated once the diagnosis is confirmed. This carries a risk of inducing profound hypotension (see above) and is best undertaken as an inpatient. This allows for more rapid up-titration of the dose and more accurate fluid replacement as the degree of alpha blockade increases. The dose is sequentially increased until normotension is achieved or adverse effects (chiefly nasal congestion and postural hypotension) become intolerable.

Beta blockade to control tachycardia or tachyarrhythmia may safely be commenced once adequate alpha blockade is in place.

Multidisciplinary management

Early involvement of the surgical team to plan surgery is important, and management of paragangliomas is best under a multidisciplinary team of endocrinologists, endocrine surgeons, radiologists and nuclear medicine physicians.

Consider a genetic syndrome

In those with family history or who are aged <40, the possibility of a genetic syndrome should be considered. Evidence of neurofibromatosis type 1 (café-au-lait spots, cutaneous neurofibromata), multiple endocrine neoplasia type 2A (medullary thyroid cancer, hyperparathyroidism) or type 2B (as for type 2A plus Marfanoid habitus, and mucosal ganglioneuromas) and von Hippel Lindau (haemangioblastoma, renal cell cancer, pancreatic islet cell tumours) should be sought. If genetic testing confirms a diagnosis of these conditions or of SDH mutation, appropriate cascade screening of family members is necessary and referral to a clinical geneticist is required.

Further reading

Lenders JWM, Duh Q-Y, Graeme Eisenhofer G, et al. (2014) Phaeochromocytoma and paraganglioma: an Endocrine Society clinical practice guideline. *J Clin Endocrinol Metab* 99, 1915–1942.

Skin and Musculoskeletal

CHAPTER 95

Cellulitis and necrotizing fasciitis

David Sprigings and John L. Klein

Assessment of suspected cellulitis is given in Figure 95.1.

Box 95.1

Cellulitis is an acute spreading bacterial infection of the deeper dermis and subcutaneous tissue, typically of the lower leg, which may complicate a wound, ulcer, interdigital fungal infection or primary skin disorder. Predisposing factors include previous episodes of cellulitis, limb oedema and lymphoedema. *Streptococcus pyogenes* and *Staphylococcus aureus* are the commonest causative organisms.

Erysipelas is an acute bacterial infection of the upper dermis and epidermis, which may be clinically distinguished from cellulitis by a more clearly demarcated border between infected and healthy skin. Assessment and management is the same as for cellulitis.

Necrotizing fasciitis is a rapidly progressive infection of the deep fascia and muscle, and should be suspected in an ill patient with severe pain and marked local tenderness. In the later stages the skin may show blue-black discolouration and blistering. The majority of cases are polymicrobial and caused by anaerobes, Gram- negative bacilli and streptococci (not *S. pyogenes*). Most other cases are caused by *S. pyogenes* or *Clostridium perfringens* (gas gangrene). Management requires resuscitation, antibiotic therapy and urgent referral to an orthopaedic or plastic surgeon for consideration of debridement.

Priorities

Make a focused assessment and consider the differential diagnosis (Figure 95.1, Table 95.1). Bilateral cellulitis is very rare. Mark the margin of affected skin. Investigation required urgently is given in Table 95.2.

If cellulitis is the likely diagnosis, assess the severity of the illness, on the basis of the clinical features and comorbidities, and manage the patient accordingly (Tables 95.3 and 95.4).

If necrotizing fasciitis is suspected, give IV fluid, start antibiotic therapy (Table 95.4) and seek urgent advice from an orthopaedic or plastic surgeon, and a microbiologist.

Acute Medicine: A Practical Guide to the Management of Medical Emergencies, Fifth Edition. Edited by David Sprigings and John B. Chambers.
© 2018 John Wiley & Sons Ltd. Published 2018 by John Wiley & Sons Ltd.

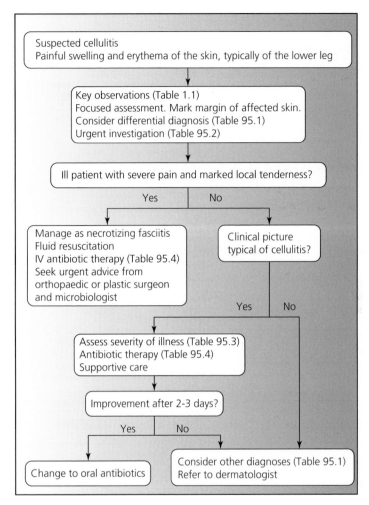

Figure 95.1 Assessment of suspected cellulitis.

Further management

Any underlying skin disorder should be treated. Seek advice from a dermatologist.

Supportive care of the patient with cellulitis of the lower leg includes:

- Elevation of the limb
- Use of a bed cradle
- Analgesia
- DVT prophylaxis
- Adequate hydration
- Treatment of comorbidities, for example diabetes

Clinical improvement is usually seen after 2–3 days, and with this, patients treated initially with IV antibiotic therapy can be switched to oral therapy, to complete a 7–14 day course. If there is no improvement at this time, other diagnoses should be considered and a dermatological opinion obtained.

Patients who have recurrent episodes of cellulitis should be considered for prophylactic antibiotic therapy: seek advice from a dermatologist.

Table 95.1 Disorders which may be mistaken for cellulitis.

Disorder	Distinguishing features
Necrotizing fasciitis	Ill patient
	Severe pain, disproportionate to physical signs
	Skin may be very tender, with blue-black discolouration and blistering
	Rapid clinical progression
Leg eczema (venous eczema or contact dermatitis) (NB cellulitis may complicate eczema)	Longer history
	May be bilateral (bilateral cellulitis is rare)
	No fever or systemic symptoms
	Itching rather than tenderness of the skin
	History of varicose veins or DVT
	Crusting or scaling (in cellulitis the skin is typically smooth and shiny)
Deep vein thrombosis (DVT) (NB cellulitis may complicate DVT)	Proximal margin of erythema usually not well demarcated
	If clinical setting suggests DVT (Chapter 56), duplex scan of leg veins needed to exclude this
Allergic reaction to insect sting or bite	No ascending lymphangitis
	Itching
Chronic oedema/ lymphoedema (NB cellulitis may complicate chronic oedema or lymphoedema)	Usually bilateral
	Erythema may be feature
	No fever
Gouty arthritis	Arthritis prominent
	Typically involves first metatarsophalangeal joint (Chapter 97)
Pyoderma gangrenosum	Rapidly enlarging painful ulcer
	Associated systemic disease (most often inflammatory bowel disease) in 50%

Table 95.2 Urgent investigation in suspected cellulitis or necrotizing fasciitis.

Full blood count
C-reactive protein
Electrolytes and creatinine
Blood culture (in class 3 or 4 illness (Table 95.3)
Microscopy and culture of blister fluid if present
Urgent Gram stain of debrided tissue (in necrotizing fasciitis)
Duplex scan if deep venous thrombosis is possible (Chapter 56)

Table 95.3 Cellulitis: assessment of severity of illness and management.

Class	Features	Management
1	No significant systemic illness No uncontrolled comorbidities	Oral antibiotic therapy (Table 95.4) Outpatient management
2	Significant systemic illness or comorbidity (e.g. peripheral arterial disease, morbid obesity)	IV antibiotic therapy (Table 95.4) Outpatient/inpatient management*
3	Haemodynamic instability or delirium Limb-threatening infection due to vascular compromise Comorbidities that may interfere with response to therapy	IV antibiotic therapy (Table 95.4) Inpatient management: level 1/HDU
4	Sepsis syndrome Suspected necrotizing fasciitis	IV antibiotic therapy (Table 95.4) Inpatient management: HDU/ICU

Source: Eron LJ (2000) Infections of skin and soft tissue: outcomes of a classification scheme. *Clinical Infectious Diseases* 31, 287 (A432). Reproduced with permission of Oxford University Press.
* Contraindications to outpatient management of patients with class 2 cellulitis:
- Penicillin/cephalosporin allergy
- Chronic liver or renal (CKD 4 or 5) disease
- Immunosuppression
- Facial or orbital cellulitis
- Non-compliance with outpatient management likely
- Unable to cope at home

Table 95.4 Initial antibiotic therapy in cellulitis and necrotizing fasciitis.

Setting	Organisms to be covered in addition to *Streptococcus pyogenes* and *Staphylococcus aureus*	Antibiotic therapy IV	
		Not allergic to penicillin	Penicillin allergy
Otherwise well	*Strep. pyogenes* is commonest causative organism, but *Staph. aureus* should also be covered if cellulitis is severe	Flucloxacillin	Clarithromycin or clindamycin
Diabetes with foot ulcer	Gram-negative and anaerobic bacteria	Co-amoxiclav	Clindamycin
Possible necrotizing fasciitis	Streptococci spp. Gram-negative and anaerobic bacteria	Piperacillin/tazobactam	Vancomycin or teicoplanin + gentamicin + metronidazole
Hospital- or nursing-home acquired	Meticillin-resistant *Staph. aureus* (MRSA)	Vancomycin or teicoplanin	Vancomycin or teicoplanin
Human bite	Mixed oral flora including anaerobes	Co-amoxiclav	Tetracycline + metronidazole

Further reading

Sartelli M, Malangoni MA, May AK, *et al.* (2014) World Society of Emergency Surgery guidelines for management of skin and soft tissue infections. *World Journal of Emergency Surgery* 9, 57. http://www.wjes .org/content/9/1/57 (open access).

Stevens DL, Bisno AL, Chambers HF, *et al.* Practice guidelines for the diagnosis and management of skin and soft tissue infections: 2014 Update by the Infectious Diseases Society of America. http://cid.oxfordjournals. org/content/59/2/e10.

CHAPTER 96

Erythroderma and toxic epidermal necrolysis

NEMESHA DESAI AND SESHI MANAM

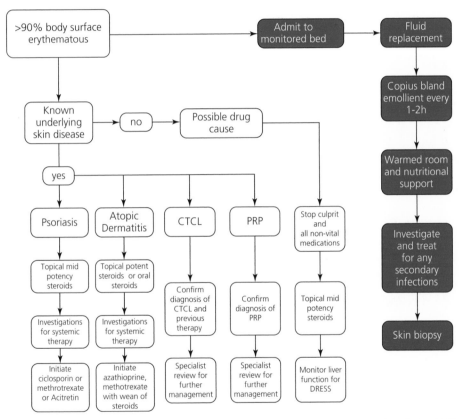

Figure 96.1 Management of erythroderma. CTCL, cutaneous T cell lymphoma; PRP, pityriasis rubra pilaris; DRESS, drug reaction with eosinophilia and systemic symptoms

Acute Medicine: A Practical Guide to the Management of Medical Emergencies, Fifth Edition. Edited by David Sprigings and John B. Chambers.
© 2018 John Wiley & Sons Ltd. Published 2018 by John Wiley & Sons Ltd.

Erythroderma

Erythroderma is redness of the skin involving more than 90% of the body surface area, and can be due to an underlying skin disease, or secondary to a systemic disorder.

- The aetiology is broad, including infection, new medication and even withdrawal of oral steroid in patients with psoriasis (Table 96.1).
- Erythroderma can extend rapidly and hence requires urgent assessment and intervention as seemingly well patients may decompensate abruptly due to the extent of skin barrier impairment.
- Patients are at risk of electrolyte derangement, hypovolaemia, high output cardiac failure, hypothermia and sepsis, thus fluid balance and close monitoring is required.
- Associated exfoliation of the skin contributes to hypoalbuminaema, hence nutritional support is important.

Table 96.1 Common causes of erythroderma.

Cause	Key points on history	Clinical features seen in particular disease	Important specific tests
Psoriasis	Personal or family history of psoriasis Recent oral steroids	Scalp scale, nail changes (pitting, onycholysis) Joint involvement Pustules	
Eczema		Lichenification of skin Periorbital disease	Serum IgE raised Eosinophilia
Drug-related	New medications in past eight weeks	Morbiliform rash Flexural erythema Pustules	Monitor eosinophils and liver function for DRESS*
Cutaneous T cell lymphoma (CTCL)		Generalized erythema	Circulating atypical T cells
Pityriasis rubra pilaris (PRP)		'Islands' of clear skin	

*DRESS, drug reaction with eosinophilia and systemic symptoms: a severe idiosyncratic drug reaction with a broad range of clinical features (which may include raised ALT) appearing 2 to 8 weeks after starting the causative drug.

Priorities

- Clinical assessment is given in Table 96.2 and investigation needed urgently in Table 96.3.
- Management is summarized in Figure 96.1. The erythrodermic patient should be managed in a monitored bed with close nursing input. Meticulous fluid balance must be maintained, taking into consideration insensible losses from the skin. The room should be warm and a Bair-Hugger blanket or equivalent applied, to prevent heat loss and maintain core temperature.
- Patients should be monitored closely for cutaneous and systemic sepsis and nutritional support initiated early.
- Copious bland emollient should be applied to whole body, 50:50 white soft paraffin/liquid paraffin is recommended.
- Discontinue unnecessary medications; any drug is a potential candidate. A mild potency topical steroid can be used on the body; potent topical steroids are not advised due to increased systemic absorption through the impaired skin barrier.
- If the underlying disease is identified on history or examination, specific treatment should be initiated. Management is otherwise guided by skin biopsy.

Table 96.2 Focused assessment of the patient with erythroderma.

History

Take a full medical and drug history, focusing on a personal and family history of underlying skin disease, atopy and new medications in the preceding eight weeks, to include topical agents, herbal and over-the-counter therapies.

Establish the timing of onset of the rash; drug reactions tend to evolve rapidly, whereas inflammatory skin disease may be more insidious.

Assess for cutaneous symptoms; skin pain may be experienced with drug rashes and unstable psoriasis, itch with atopic dermatitis.

Systemic symptoms should be sought including fever and prodromal flu-like illness.

Examination

Physiological observations and general examination

Examine the palms and nails

Inspect scalp, oral mucosa, natal cleft and genitalia in addition to the body skin. Observe carefully for pustules or vesicles. Multiple sterile micropustules are seen in erythrodermic psoriasis patients and drug reactions.

Examine for Nikolsky sign (see TEN skin failure).

Palpate for lymph nodes; widespread lymphadenopathy can occur in erythrodermic patients both as a non-specific reaction to the inflammatory process ('dermatopathic' lymphadenopathy) or secondary to the underlying aetiology (e.g. cutaneous T cell lymphoma).

In chronic erythroderma, ectropion, hair loss and thickening of the skin on the palms and soles is seen.

Table 96.3 Urgent investigation in erythroderma.

Full blood count

C-reactive protein

Sodium, potassium, urea and creatinine: to monitor for derangement secondary to fluid loss

Liver function tests: drug reactions are often associated with hepatic derangement

Blood culture

Skin swab to screen for secondary infections: bacterial and viral

ECG

Chest X-ray to assess for high-output cardiac failure

Skin biopsy should be performed if there is a negative history of established skin disease

- For a large proportion of erythrodermic patients, an aetiology is not found; for such patients continual emollients and topical steroids should be considered, alongside supportive therapy to prevent and monitor for complications.
  - For unstable psoriasis, systemic management can be considered in the acute setting, which includes ciclosporin (important contraindications include hypertension or renal impairment), methotrexate (liver screen and procollagen III must be checked prior to initiation) and acitretin (check liver function and lipids prior to treatment).

    For erythrodermic atopic dermatitis, potent topical steroids and oral steroids may be indicated.
  - Recurrent or chronic erythroderma may require second-line immunosuppressive agents in the subacute period to overlap with oral steroids.
  - Cutaneous T cell lymphoma (CTCL) requires specialist review for specific treatment. Pityriasis Rubra Pilaris (PRP) requires intensive topical steroids; second-line therapies include oral retinoids.

Table 96.4 Features of toxic epidermal necrolysis (TEN), Stevens-Johnson syndrome (SJS) and erythema multiforme major

	TEN	SJS	Erythema multiforme major
Percentage of body skin affected	>30%	10%	n/a
Initial skin lesions	Painful dusky erythematous cutaneous and mucosal skin	Erythema in mucous membranes	Dusky erythema
Skin signs	Mucosal involvement Full thickness epidermal necrosis resulting in friable bullae Nikolsky positive	Mucosal involvement Erosions and bullae	Targetoid skin lesions Mucosal involvement
Mortality	30%	<10%	Rare

Toxic epidermal necrolysis

Skin failure is defined as loss of normal barrier function, including loss of temperature control, percutaneous fluid, protein, electrolyte loss and mechanical barrier function.

Severe skin failure occurs in the setting of extensive cutaneous pathology of any aetiology, including erythroderma (see above), generalized blistering disorder and toxic epidermal necrolysis (TEN).

TEN is the most severe form of skin failure. It is rare, affecting 1–2 persons per million population per year and associated with significant morbidity and mortality. It is a severe muco-cutaneous reaction, usually drug-induced, characterized by fever, full thickness skin necrosis affecting more than 30% of the body surface area, erosion or ulceration of at least two mucous membrane sites (ocular, oral, anogenital) and variable systemic organ involvement.

TEN lies on a spectrum with Stevens-Johnson syndrome (SJS) and erythema multiforme major (see table 96.4). The aetiology is often drug-related (Table 96.5), rarely infections such as *Mycoplasma* and herpes simplex virus are implicated.

At risk individuals include the elderly (relating to polypharmacy), patients with systemic lupus erythematosus (SLE), HIV/AIDS and recipients of bone marrow transplants.

Table 96.5 Focused assessment in toxic-epidermal necrolysis.

History

A careful history of comorbidities and detailed drug history of the last eight weeks is imperative, including prescribed, over-the-counter and herbal therapies. Specific symptoms to support a diagnosis of incipient TEN include skin pain, involvement of the mucous membranes presenting as ocular pain, grittiness, photophobia, sore throat, odynophagia, dysuria and systemic malaise, specifically flu-like symptoms and fever. Muco-cutaneous symptoms in established disease include a spectrum of extensive blistering, erosions and haemorrhagic mucositis.

Examination

Careful skin and mucous membrane examination is required to assess the extent of involved sites. The skin may be friable and denude easily on examination; hence assistance will be required to minimize direct handling of the skin during examination. Assessment of the percentage body surface area involved should be made, to include erythema (which may take the appearance of subtle slate grey pigmentation in darker skin types or where full thickness skin necrosis is already established), erosions and bullae. Nikolsky sign is positive in TEN: gentle lateral pressure applied to the skin results in separation of the epidermis from the dermis. The ocular, oral, genital and urethral mucous membranes should be examined for involvement. Systemic examination should focus on respiratory and gastrointestinal systems, which may exhibit early involvement, although any organ can be involved.

The leading cause of death is secondary sepsis. Morbidity relating to chronic pain, stricturing of mucosal sites (e.g. urethral stenosis and vaginal synechiae causing chronic dyspareunia; ocular symblepharon, corneal scarring and sicca symptoms), oesophageal strictures and bronchiolitis obliterans can persists long after the acute cutaneous reaction has resolved.

Priorities

- Clinical assessment is given in Table 96.6 and investigation needed urgently in Table 96.7. The SCORTEN criteria predict mortality (Table 96.8).
- The mainstay of management is supportive with high level nursing care. The aims are: prevention of further skin injury, prevention of infection and maintenance of thermoregulation.

Table 96.6 Medications which are likely causative agents in toxic epidermal necrolysis/Stevens-Johnson syndrome.

Allopurinol
Aromatic anticonvulsants, for example phenytoin, carbamazepine, sodium valproate, phenobarbitone, lamotrigine
Antibiotics, for example amoxicillin, cotrimoxazole, ciprofloxacin, tetracyclines
HAART drugs, for example nevirapine
Analgesics, for example paracetamol, NSAIDs
Others: sulphasalazine, omeprazole, diuretics

Table 96.7 Urgent investigation in toxic epidermal necrolysis.

Full blood count
C-reactive protein
Creatinine and electrolytes
Full biochemical profile
Immunoglobulins
Mycoplasma serology
Blood culture
Skin swab to screen for secondary infections: viral and bacterial
Skin biopsy
ECG
Chest X-ray to assess for high-output cardiac failure

Table 96.8 SCORTEN scoring system for toxic epidermal necrolysis.

SCORTEN criteria	Points	Total SCORTEN score	Predicted mortality
Age >40 years	1	0–1	1–3%
Heart rate >120/min	1	2	12%
Comorbid malignancy	1	3	35%
Epidermal detachment >10% body surface area on day 1	1	4	58%
Serum urea >10 mol/L	1	5+	>90%
Bicarbonate level <20 mmol/L	1		
Serum glucose >14 mmol/L	1		

- Stop the suspected drug immediately. All drugs started within 7–21 days of the first manifestation of the skin eruption should be discontinued. Consider any drug started within the previous eight weeks as a candidate.
- Early referral to a multidisciplinary, high dependency/intensive care unit for 1:1 specialist nursing with aseptic technique and close monitoring of vital parameters and respiratory function.
- Nurse in a warmed room of 30–32 °C to reduce percutaneous heat loss, on a non-adherent bed lining such as Exu-dry* or Lyofoam* lined with copious bland emollient such as 50:50 white soft paraffin.
- Cover skin with copious bland emollient such as 50:50 white soft paraffin and liquid paraffin.
- Open denuded skin should be swabbed and covered with moist silicone dressings such as mepitel.
- Immediate referral to ophthalmology; ocular involvement requires lubricating eye drops and preservative free topical antibiotics/steroids.
- Careful fluid balance. Fluid requirements for TEN patients are usually two-thirds to three-quarters of those with burns covering the same area. Urinary catheters are effective in keeping urethra patent but meticulous aseptic technique must be observed on insertion.
- Regular oral toilette with sterile water and soft applicator sponge to remove crusts and exudates.
- Supplement nutrition with careful siting of a nasogastric tube.

Further management

There are few large clinical trials on TEN/SJS management, thus treatment remains supportive. Interest in intravenous immunoglobulin (IVIG) as a treatment for TEN has grown in the last decade. However, there are no firm conclusions on benefit.

Corticosteroids have shown benefit in limited studies; however, there is increased risk of infection and poor wound healing. Anti-TNF alpha agents, N-acetylcysteine and ciclosporin have been trialled in management of TEN. In the absence of high quality evidence supporting any single agent, therapy remains supportive, with vigilant prevention of secondary infection.

Further reading

Bastuji-Garin S, Fouchard N, et al. (2000) SCORTEN: A Severity-of-Illness Score for Toxic Epidermal Necrolysis. *Journal of Investigative Dermatology* 115, 149–153. DOI: 10.1046/j.1523-1747.

Creamer D, Walsh SA, Dziewulski P, et al. (2016) UK guidelines for the management of Stevens-Johnson syndrome/toxic epidermal necrolysis in adults 2016. *British Journal of Dermatology* 174, 1194–1227. http://www.bad.org.uk/shared/get-file.ashx?id=3968&itemtype=document.

Scwartz R. (2013) Toxic epidermal necrolysis Part II. Prognosis, sequelae, diagnosis, differential diagnosis, prevention, and treatment. *J Am Acad Dermatol* 69 (2), 182.

CHAPTER 97

Acute gout and pseudogout

Kᴇʜɪɴᴅᴇ Sᴜɴᴍʙᴏʏᴇ

Gout and pseudogout are the two most common crystal arthropathies. Gout is caused by deposition of monosodium urate monohydrate crystals, and pseudogout by calcium pyrophosphate crystals. Their epidemiology is summarized in Table 97.1.

Table 97.1 Epidemiology of gout and pseudogout.

	Gout	Pseudogout (calcium pyrophosphate dihydrate deposition (CPPD) disease)
Age	Predominantly 30–60 years, risk increases with advancing age	>60 years, risk increases in the elderly
Sex	Male predominance, post-menopausal women, very rare in premenopausal women	Male: female ratio 50:50
Risk factors	Conditions which promote hyperuricaemia, due to overproduction or under-excretion of urate Overproduction of urate Genetic diseases: • Hypoxanthine-guanine phosphoribosyltransferase deficiency (Lesch-Nyhan syndrome) • Superactivity of phosphoribosyl pyrophosphate synthetase (PRPP) High cell turnover: • Cell lysis from chemotherapy for malignancies • Lympho- and myelo-proliferative diseases Under-excretion of urate: • Chronic alcohol abuse (beer and hard liquor) • Renal insufficiency (also below) • Dehydration	Conditions that promote altered concentrations of calcium, inorganic pyrophosphate (PPi) and the solubility products of these ions Genetic diseases: • Mutations in the ANKH gene, leading to altered PPi metabolism (familial CPPD deposition disease) Metabolic conditions causing CPPD deposition: • Hyperparathyroidism • Haemochromatosis • Hypomagnesaemia • Hypophosphataemia • Familial hypocalciuric hypercalcaemia (The 5 Hs of CPPD disease)
Related comorbid conditions	Hypertension Diabetes mellitus Renal insufficiency Hypertriglyceridaemia Hypercholesterolaemia Obesity Anaemia	Hyperparathyroidism Haemochromatosis Hypomagnesaemia (Chapter 88) Hypophosphataemia (Chapter 89) Familial hypocalciuric hypercalcaemia
Dietary factors	Foods rich in purines such as red meat and sea food	No clear dietary causes

Acute Medicine: A Practical Guide to the Management of Medical Emergencies, Fifth Edition. Edited by David Sprigings and John B. Chambers.
© 2018 John Wiley & Sons Ltd. Published 2018 by John Wiley & Sons Ltd.

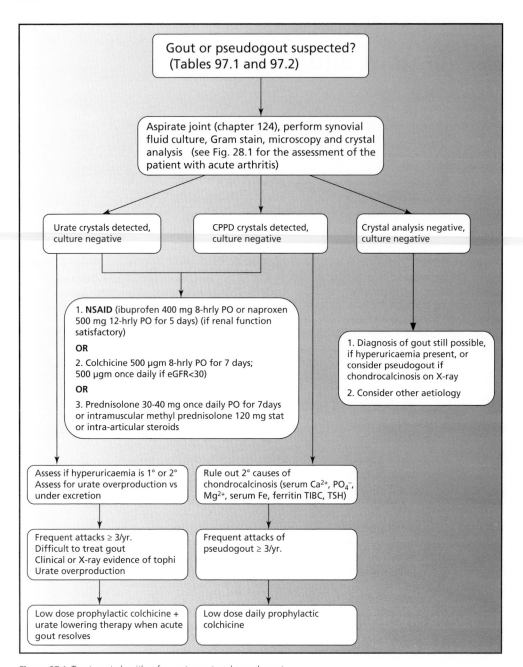

Figure 97.1 Treatment algorithm for acute gout and pseudogout.

Priorities

- Septic arthritis (Chapter 98) must be excluded in any patient presenting with an acute monoarthritis.
- The clinical assessment of a patient with suspected gout or pseudogout is given in Table 97.2 and investigation needed urgently in Table 97.3. Management is summarized in Figure 97.1.

Table 97.2 Focused assessment in suspected acute gout or pseudogout.

Element	Comment
Time course and duration of joint and other symptoms	In gout, attacks begin abruptly, usually overnight, and typically reach maximum intensity within 12 hours. In pseudogout, attacks may resemble those of acute gout or follow a sub-acute course over several days.
Pattern of joint involvement	In gout, the first MTP joint (podagra) is the initial joint involved in 50% cases and is eventually involved in >90% of cases. Monoarticular involvement occurs commonly, although polyarticular acute flares do occur. In pseudogout, large joint involvement such as the knee, wrist, elbow or ankle.
Context and comorbidities	See Table 97.1.
History of trauma	Trauma may cause agitation, with subsequent deposition of urate and CPPD crystals in patients with tophi and chondrocalcinosis, respectively.
Examination of involved joint(s)	Swelling, warmth, redness (sometimes resembling cellulitis) and tenderness.
Other signs	In gout, tophi may be present in the helix of the ear, fingers, toes, prepatellar bursa, olecranon bursa.
Fever	May be present in polyarticular presentations of gout or pseudogout (septic arthritis must be excluded).

Table 97.3 Urgent investigation for suspected acute gout or pseudogout.

X-ray of involved joints
Aspiration of involved joint (samples for crystal analysis, microscopy and culture)
Blood culture (×2) if febrile
Creatinine and electrolytes
Urate level (may be normal in acute gout; gout and pseudogout may coexist)
Full blood count

If pseudogout confirmed:
Bone profile: calcium and phosphate, alkaline phosphatase
Magnesium
Ferritin, serum iron and total iron binding capacity (to assess for haemochromatosis)
Thyroid stimulating hormone (hypothyroidism and pseudogout often coexist)
Parathyroid hormone levels (if hypercalcaemia)

Further reading

Dalbeth N, Merriman TR, Stamp LK. (2016) Gout. *Lancet* 388, 2039–2052.
Rosenthal AK, Ryan LM. (2016) Calcium pyrophosphate deposition disease. *N Engl J Med* 374, 2575–2584.

CHAPTER 98

Septic arthritis

KEHINDE SUNMBOYE AND JOHN L. KLEIN

Consider the diagnosis in any patient who has fever with joint pain and swelling, particularly if only one large joint is involved.

- Septic arthritis is typically mono-articular but can be poly-articular (15% of cases).
- The knee is the joint most commonly involved, followed by the elbow, shoulder and hip.
- *Staphylococcus aureus* is the causative organism in 50% of cases of native joint infection; other causative organisms include streptococci, gonococci and Gram-negative bacilli.
- Prosthetic joint infection is caused by a wider range of pathogens.

Priorities

Your clinical assessment should address the following points:

- Does the patient have arthritis or periarticular inflammation (bursitis, tendinitis or cellulitis)? Painful limitation of movement of the joint suggests arthritis. Causes of acute mono- or oligo-arthritis are given in Table 28.1 (p. 183).
- Is the patient at risk of septic arthritis? Septic arthritis usually follows an overt or occult bacteraemia (e.g. from infective endocarditis, pneumonia or IV drug use) in a patient at risk because of rheumatoid arthritis, the presence of a prosthetic joint, or immunosuppression (including anti-TNF therapy).
- Could this be a crystal arthritis (gout or pseudogout; Chapter 97): is there a history of previous similar attacks of arthritis?
- Could this be a reactive arthritis: is there an associated rash, diarrhoea, urethritis or uveitis?
- Could this be gonococcal arthritis (Table 98.1)?

Aspirate the joint (Chapter 124) and send synovial fluid for cell count (in an EDTA tube; normal cell count is <180/mm^3, most mononuclear); Gram stain; culture; and microscopy under polarized light for crystals. Other investigations needed urgently are given in Table 98.2.

- If you are not familiar with joint aspiration, ask the help of a rheumatologist or orthopaedic surgeon.
- Both crystal and septic arthritis give rise to a purulent effusion, although the white cell count is usually higher in septic arthritis (50,000–200,000/mm^3), with a polymorphonuclear cell count of >90%.
- Bloodstaining of the effusion is common in pseudogout but rare in sepsis.

Acute Medicine: A Practical Guide to the Management of Medical Emergencies, Fifth Edition. Edited by David Sprigings and John B. Chambers.
© 2018 John Wiley & Sons Ltd. Published 2018 by John Wiley & Sons Ltd.

Table 98.1 Comparison of gonococcal and non-gonococcal septic arthritis.

	Gonococcal septic arthritis	Non-gonococcal septic arthritis
Organisms	*Neisseria gonorrhoeae*	*Staphylococcus aureus* Beta-haemolytic streptococci *Streptococcus pneumoniae* Gram-negative rods
Patient profile	Young, healthy, sexually active	Elderly, rheumatoid arthritis, prosthetic joint, IV drug use, bacteraemia, immunosuppression
Initial presentation	Migratory polyarthralgia, tenosynovitis, dermatitis	Typically with a single hot, swollen, painful joint, but can be poly-articular (15% of cases)
Joints involved	Often poly-articular, especially knee and wrist	Knee joint most commonly involved, followed by the elbow, shoulder and hip
Other signs	Tenosynovitis, rash	Source of bacteraemia
Gram stain of synovial fluid	<25% positive	50–75% positive
Culture of synovial fluid	25% positive	85–95% positive
Blood culture	<10% positive	50% positive
Genitourinary culture (swab of urethra, cervix and anorectum)	80% positive	Not indicated

Table 98.2 Investigation in suspected septic arthritis.

Joint aspiration (Chapter 124)
X-ray joint for baseline
Blood glucose
Creatinine and electrolytes
Liver function tests
Full blood count
Erythrocyte sedimentation rate and C-reactive protein
Blood culture (×2)
Urine stick test, microscopy and culture
Swab of urethra, cervix and anorectum for culture and nucleic acid amplification test (NAAT) if gonococcal infection is possible

Further management

Organisms on Gram stain of synovial fluid, or high probability of septic arthritis

Start antibiotic therapy IV (Table 98.3).

- Intra-articular administration is not needed.
- The antibiotic regimen may need modification in the light of blood and synovial fluid culture results: discuss this with a microbiologist.
- Antibiotic therapy for non-gonococcal septic arthritis usually needs to be given for 2–4 weeks, initially IV, but may be switched to an appropriate oral agent in uncomplicated cases.
- Gonococcal arthritis may be cured with just 1–2 weeks of therapy.

Table 98.3 Initial antibiotic therapy for suspected native joint septic arthritis.

	Antibiotic therapy (IV, high dose)	
Organisms on Gram stain	**Not allergic to penicillin**	**Allergic to penicillin**
Gram-positive cocci	Flucloxacillin Vancomycin if MRSA suspected	Clindamycin
Gram-negative cocci	Ceftriaxone	Ceftriaxone (mild allergy) Seek expert advice if severe allergy
Gram-negative rods	Piperacillin-tazobactam	Ciprofloxacin
None seen	Flucloxacillin Vancomycin if MRSA suspected	Clindamycin

If septic arthritis is confirmed, seek advice on further management from a rheumatologist or orthopaedic surgeon.

- Daily aspiration of the joint until an effusion no longer re-accumulates is an acceptable approach where access to the joint is easy (e.g. the knee).
- Other larger joints (e.g. hip or shoulder) may be more effectively drained by arthroscopic washout.
- While the infection is resolving, the joint should be immobilized using a splint or cast.
- Physiotherapy should be started early.
- Give an NSAID for pain relief (e.g. indomethacin or diclofenac).
- In patients with gonococcal arthritis, a sexual health screen of the patient and his/her sexual partners should be offered.

No organisms on Gram stain of synovial fluid and low probability of septic arthritis

Consider the other causes of acute arthritis (Table 28.1).

- Pseudogout is the commonest cause of acute mono-or oligo-arthritis in the elderly.
  Hold off antibiotic therapy (pending the results of blood and synovial fluid culture for definite exclusion of infection).
- Treat with an NSAID, covered with a proton-pump inhibitor in the elderly or patients with previous peptic ulceration).
- If gout is confirmed (also check plasma urate) and fails to respond to an NSAID, use colchicine. Allopurinol should not be started until the acute attack has completely resolved.

Further reading

Sharff KA, Richards EP, Townes JM (2013) Clinical management of septic arthritis. *Curr Rheumatol Rep* 15, 332. DOI: 10.1007/s11926-013-0332-4.

CHAPTER 99

Acute vasculitis

RAASHID LUQMANI

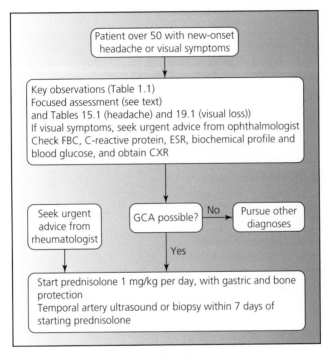

Figure 99.1 Management of suspected giant cell arteritis (GCA).

Consider vasculitis in the patient with systemic symptoms (e.g. fever, weight loss, malaise) and headache or evidence of organ dysfunction.

- The diagnosis of a specific vasculitis (Appendix 99.1) is based on the pattern of organ injury, characteristic features on imaging, the size of involved blood vessels and histological findings on biopsy.
- The commonest vasculitis in adults is giant-cell arteritis (GCA), usually presenting with new-onset headache in older people, associated with constitutional upset; it carries a significant risk (20–30%) of visual loss from ischaemic optic neuropathy, and so needs urgent assessment and treatment (Chapter 19).

Acute Medicine: A Practical Guide to the Management of Medical Emergencies, Fifth Edition. Edited by David Sprigings and John B. Chambers.
© 2018 John Wiley & Sons Ltd. Published 2018 by John Wiley & Sons Ltd.

Table 99.1 Typical presentations of acute vasculitis*.

Clinical problem	Typical features	Differential diagnosis (see also Table 99.3)
Headache (see also Chapter 15)	Unaccustomed, severe with tenderness over arteries and scalp. May be accompanied by visual disturbance, jaw or tongue claudication or aches and pains in muscles (polymyalgia).	Widespread causes: for example non-specific headache; cervical spondylosis; shingles; orbital cellulitis.
Neurological presentation with stroke (see also Chapters 14 and 65)	Headache Unilateral weakness Speech disturbance	Atherosclerotic stroke Haemorrhagic stroke Sub-arachnoid haemorrhage Meningitis Malignancy
Visual loss (see also Chapter 19)	Sudden loss of vision in one or both eyes	Non-arteritic ischaemic optic neuropathy Diabetic retinopathy Multiple sclerosis Severe hypertensive retinopathy Infection, for example CMV retinitis
Hearing loss	Sudden loss of hearing in one or both ears	Wax Trauma Drug toxicity Infection Cholesteatoma Ménière's disease
Haemoptysis (see also Table 99.2)	Cough Breathlessness Blood streaked sputum or more florid haemoptysis	Cancer Infection Exacerbation of bronchiectasis Anti-coagulant therapy
Upper respiratory chronic illness (see also Table 99.2)	Nasal crusting, hearing loss, sinusitis	Chronic sinusitis; infection; sarcoidosis; midline granuloma
Systemic illness with chest symptoms (see also Table 99.2)	Cough, breathless, haemoptysis with rash or fever or weight loss plus any other feature of active inflammation in different organ systems, for example microscopic haematuria, upper respiratory tract illness	Infection Sarcoidosis Malignancy Drug toxicity Multiple comorbidities
Acute abdominal pain (see also Chapter 21)	Claudicant ischaemic pain (after food) Blood stained stool/diarrhoea	Constipation Drug toxicity Diverticulitis Peptic ulcer Pancreatitis Malignancy Infection Inflammatory bowel disease
Unexplained renal impairment (see also Chapter 25 and Table 99.2)	Tiredness; anaemia; asymptomatic finding of hypertension and or haematuria and proteinuria	Diabetic nephropathy Obstructive uropathy Hypertensive renal failure Acute sepsis with low volume Drug toxicity
Proteinuria	Asymptomatic	Diabetes Reflux nephropathy Hypertension Infection Minimal change nephropathy

* This list is not exhaustive as vasculitis can affect any vascular bed.

- The main focus in the immediate management of suspected new-onset vasculitis is to contact a specialist in vasculitis for advice, while at the same time exploring the broad differential diagnosis (Tables 99.1–99.3). Clinical assessment of the patient and investigation are summarized in Tables 99.4 and 99.5.
- With the exception of suspected giant-cell arteritis, early intervention with high-dose corticosteroid therapy is rarely needed, and should not be given unless advised by a specialist in vasculitis.

Suspected giant-cell arteritis (GCA) (Figure 99.1; see also Chapter 19)

- Consider in any patient over 50 with new-onset headache (which will usually be of days or a few weeks in duration) or visual symptoms (amaurosis fugax, diplopia and partial or complete loss of vision (Chapter 19)).
- Associated symptoms include malaise, weight loss, jaw or tongue claudication and scalp tenderness. The temporal artery may be thickened, tender or non-pulsatile, and bruits may be heard over arteries of the head and neck.
- Check full blood count, C-reactive protein, ESR, biochemical profile and blood glucose. Obtain a chest X-ray (and ultrasonography of the temporal artery, if available).
- If the clinical picture is suggestive of GCA, and the C-reactive protein is raised, start prednisolone 1 mg/kg per day (max 60 mg per day) with gastric and bone protection.
- Arrange for a temporal artery biopsy or ultrasound to be done within seven days of starting prednisolone.
- Seek advice from a rheumatologist or vasculitis specialist on management and follow-up.

New presentation of suspected systemic vasculitis (Figure 99.2)

Principles of management
- Assess for other causes of the clinical presentation (e.g. infection; see Table 99.3).
- Look for evidence of organ-threatening or life-threatening disease, which may require admission to ICU or HDU for supportive care. Close observation and repeated re-examination of the patient with suspected systemic vasculitis is very important, as the clinical features may rapidly evolve.
- Contact a specialist in vasculitis for advice on management.
- Do not start corticosteroid or other anti-inflammatory treatment without advice from a specialist in vasculitis, as this may reduce the diagnostic yield of biopsy, and prevent the patient's inclusion in clinical trials of therapy.
- Biopsy of the affected organ is the most important test to organize; imaging may be an adequate substitute for some diseases (e.g. large-vessel vasculitis).

Table 99.2 Pulmonary-renal syndromes.

Feature	Goodpasture syndrome	Granulomatosis with polyangiitis	Microscopic polyangiitis	Systemic lupus erythematosus
Pulmonary haemorrhage	Usually present	Common	Common	Uncommon
Glomerulonephritis	Usually present	Usually present	Usually present	Usually present
Upper airway involvement	Not seen	Usually present	Uncommon	Uncommon
Rash	Very rare	Common	Common	Usually present
Arthralgia	Not seen	Common	Common	Usually present
High C-reactive protein/ ESR	Very rare	Usually present	Usually present	Usually present
Serology	Antiglomerular basement membrane antibody	c-ANCA Rarely, p-ANCA	p-ANCA, c-ANCA	Antinuclear antibody Anti-double-stranded DNA antibody Rarely, p-ANCA Low complement

ANCA, antineutrophil cytoplasmic antibodies; c-ANCA, antibodies with a cytoplasmic pattern of staining; p-ANCA, antibodies with a perinuclear pattern of staining; ESR, erythrocyte sedimentation rate.
From O'Sullivan, B.P. et al. (2002) Case records of the Massachusetts General Hospital (Case 30–2002): N Engl J Med 347, 1009–17.

Table 99.3 Differential diagnosis of systemic vasculitis.

Infectious diseases
- Sepsis with multiorgan failure
- Infective endocarditis
- Tuberculosis
- Falciparum malaria
- Mycoplasma and Legionella infection
- Syphilis, Lyme disease, leptospirosis
- Fungal infection (coccidiodomycosis, histoplasmosis)

Neoplastic diseases
- Metastatic cancer
- Cancer with paraneoplastic syndrome
- Acute leukaemia
- Lymphoma

Vascular diseases
- Multifocal embolism from the heart, for example infective endocarditis, atrial myxoma, intracardiac thrombus
- Aortic dissection with involvement of multiple branch arteries

Other disorders
- Disseminated intravascular coagulation (Appendix 102.1)
- Thrombotic thrombocytopenic purpura (Appendix 102.2)
- Drug toxicity (prescribed and recreational)
- Pre-eclampsia (Table 32.6)
- Systemic lupus erythematosus
- Antiphospholipid syndrome (recurrent venous or arterial thromboses, fetal loss, mild thrombocytopenia, anticardiolipin antibodies, lupus anticoagulant antibodies)

Table 99.4 Focused assessment of the patient with possible systemic vasculitis.

History

Take a full history, including any previous episodes (and especially note any current or recent therapy given for the previous episodes; this would ensure that consideration is given as to whether or not the current presentation is a flare, or intercurrent infection or other comorbidity).

Ask about illicit drug use.

Consider whether or not the patient's current symptoms fit with a pattern of previous features that might be in different systems (e.g. the patient may present with weight loss, fever and rash; however, they may have a history of chronic nasal discharge, hearing loss or neuropathy).

Pattern recognition is very important. Upper airway and lower airway features in combination typify granulomatosis with polyangiitis (GPA), a small-vessel vasculitis, which often involves the kidney, with asymptomatic haematuria and proteinuria. By contrast, upper airway involvement is not common in microscopic polyangiitis (MPA), where there is mainly lung and (usually asymptomatic) renal involvement.

Examination

Do a full physical examination, including weight (important in helping to make the diagnosis but also useful in calculating the dose of some treatments).

Assess eyes for redness and or tenderness, afferent pupillary defect or evidence of haemorrhage (request a slit lamp examination if uveitis is suspected).

Check for sensorineural hearing loss.

Inspect mouth for ulcers (and genital areas if symptoms of genital ulceration).

Look for evidence of infarcts, purpura, ulceration, gangrene or other skin lesions compatible with vasculitis.

Palpate for lymph node enlargement.

Check pulses in all four limbs and blood pressure in both arms (and legs if there appears to be a discrepancy in strength of pulses) especially if suspecting large vessel vasculitis. Feel for artery tenderness in suspected large vessel vasculitis.

Listen to large arteries for bruits.

Listen to the chest (e.g. pleural inflammation or effusion, consolidation) and heart (reduced sounds due to pericardial inflammation, murmurs, failure).

Feel the abdomen for organomegaly. Palpate and listen to the aorta.

Check for evidence of neuropathy or central nervous system involvement (cranial nerves, reflexes, power, sensation, orientation, speech).

Table 99.5 Investigation of the patient with suspected systemic vasculitis.

Needed urgently in all patients

Sodium, potassium, urea and creatinine

Blood glucose

Arterial blood gases and pH

Full blood count and film

Coagulation screen if the patient has purpura or jaundice, or the blood film shows haemolysis or a low platelet count

C-reactive protein

Blood culture (×2)

Urine stick test for glucose, blood and protein

Urine microscopy and culture

ECG

Chest X-ray

For later analysis

Full biochemical profile

Serum and urine protein electrophoresis

Serum complement and other immunological tests (antinuclear antibodies, antineutrophil cytoplasmic antibodies, antiglomerular basement membrane antibodies)

Echocardiography if clinical cardiac abnormality, major ECG abnormality or suspected endocarditis (Chapter 52)

Serology for HIV, hepatitis B and C

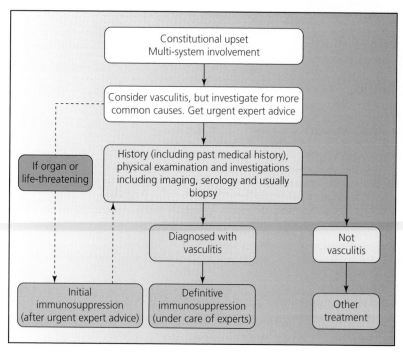

Figure 99.2 Initial management of suspected systemic vasculitis.

Appendix 99.1 The spectrum of systemic vasculitides

The vasculitides are a range of uncommon disorders characterized by inflammation of blood vessels, leading to organ damage. They can be defined as primary (occurring in isolation) or secondary to another condition (such as systemic lupus erythematosus or rheumatoid arthritis). Pathologically, vascular inflammation leads to narrowing or occlusion, resulting in tissue damage.

Many of the primary vasculitides are defined by the predominant vessel size involved: large-vessel vasculitis (typically giant cell arteritis (GCA) and Takayasu arteritis), medium-vessel vasculitis (polyarteritis nodosa (PAN) and Kawasaki disease (KD)) and small-vessel vasculitis, further grouped into the anti-neutrophil-cytoplasm-antibody (ANCA) associated diseases (granulomatosis with polyangiitis (GPA), microscopic polyangiitis (MPA) and eosinophilic granulomatosis with polyangiitis (EGPA), the immune-complex-associated diseases (cryoglobuli-naemic vasculitis, IgA vasculitis, hypocomplementaemic urticarial vasculitis) and anti-glomerular basement membrane antibody vasculitis.

Other forms of vasculitis do not fit into these patterns; they may be multi-system (e.g. Behcet syndrome), related to infection or affect single organs (e.g. central nervous system vasculitis).

The systemic vasculitides can present with a wide range of manifestations in specific organs. In many forms of vasculitis, constitutional features such as weight loss, fever and malaise are very common. The pattern for each form of vasculitis varies, but there is considerable overlap in some of these conditions. For example, ischaemic abdominal pain, colitis and pancreatitis occur in polyarteritis nodosa (PAN), but also in some of the small-vessel vasculitides. Eye involvement, typically episcleritis, scleritis or uveitis or occasionally retinal haemorrhage, occurs in different forms of small- vessel vasculitis.

Partly due to this overlap of features, but also the fact that we recognize potential cases of vasculitis at a much earlier stage than previously (and sometimes initiate treatment before confirming a diagnosis), for about 20% of cases it may not be possible to give a precise diagnostic label, other than calling it 'some sort of vasculitis'.

Although it is very tempting to start treatment for patients in whom you suspect a new diagnosis of systemic vasculitis, protocols for definitive therapy are complex. It is more likely that you will do harm than good by administering large doses of glucocorticoid therapy, so don't start these unless advised to do so by a vasculitis specialist.

Further reading

Buttgereit F, Dejaco C, Matteson EL, Dasgupta B (2016) Polymyalgia rheumatica and giant cell arteritis: a systematic review. *JAMA* 315, 2442–2458. DOI: 10.1001/jama.2016.5444.

Luqmani RA (2014) Vasculitis: an update. *British Journal of Hospital Medicine* 75, 432–439.

Vasculitis UK website: www.vasculitis.org.uk.

Vasculitis UK. Route map for vasculitis 2014. http://www.vasculitis.org.uk/content/downloads/r-m-july-2014.pdf.

Haematology and Miscellaneous

CHAPTER 100

Interpretation of full blood count and film

CLAIRE HARRISON

A full blood count (and film, if this shows abnormalities) is an inexpensive and highly informative investigation, with wide applicability. Normal values for the full blood count are given in Table 100.1. Clues from the blood film are summarized in Table 100.2.

Box 100.1 Findings on the full blood count.

Findings on the full blood count	Comment/table reference
Anaemia	Is this an isolated anaemia or are other cell lines affected? If an isolated anaemia, check the MCHC and MCV, and establish if the anaemia is: • Microcytic (Table 100.3) • Macrocytic (Table 100.4) • Normocytic (Table 100.5)
Polycythaemia (erythrocytosis)	This can be relative, as a result of haemoconcentration from dehydration or diuretic therapy, or absolute, due to an increase in red cell number (Table 100.6).
Abnormal white cell count	See Table 100.7.
Thrombocytopenia	See Tables 100.8 and 100.9. Bleeding disorders are discussed in Chapter 102. With platelet count: • $<50 \times 10^9$/L: there is excessive bleeding after surgery or trauma • $<20 \times 10^9$/L: spontaneous bleeding is common • $<10 \times 10^9$/L: spontaneous bleeding is usual
Thrombocytosis	This can be reactive (e.g. iron deficiency, bleeding, inflammation), or due to a primary haematological disorder, either isolated thrombocytosis (e.g. essential thrombocythaemia), or part of a myeloproliferative syndrome (e.g. chronic myeloid leukaemia).
Pancytopenia	Pancytopenia is a reduction in the numbers of circulating red blood cells, neutrophils and platelets. Production and destruction of blood cells is balanced in a steady state; either increased destruction, sequestration, or a generalized failure of production may result in pancytopenia. • Patients may present with mucosal bleeding, bruising or petechial haemorrhage due to thrombocytopenia (with spontaneous bleeding most likely once the platelet count drops below 20×10^9/L). • The risk of bacterial infection and neutropenic sepsis increases once the total neutrophil is below 1×10^9/L, and increases progressively in moderate and severe neutropenia ($<0.5 \times 10^9$/L). • Patients may also have symptomatic anaemia. See Table 100.10 and Chapter 101.

Acute Medicine: A Practical Guide to the Management of Medical Emergencies, Fifth Edition. Edited by David Sprigings and John B. Chambers.
© 2018 John Wiley & Sons Ltd. Published 2018 by John Wiley & Sons Ltd.

Table 100.1 Normal values for full blood count.

Variable	Unit	Normal range for males	Normal range for females
Haemoglobin	g/L	137–170	120–150
Red blood cell count	×10^{12}/L	4.4–5.8	3.95–5.15
Packed cell volume		0.40–0.55	0.36–0.47
Mean corpuscular volume	fl	80–100	80–100
Mean corpuscular haemoglobin	pg	27.0–32.0	27.0–32.0
Red-cell distribution width		11.0–16.0	11.0–16.0
White blood cell count	×10^9/L	4.0–11.0	4.0–11.0
Neutrophils	×10^9/L	1.5–7	1.5–7
Lymphocytes	×10^9/L	1.2–3.5	1.2–3.5
Monocytes	×10^9/L	0.2–1.0	0.2–1.0
Eosinophils	×10^9/L	0–0.4	0–0.4
Basophils	×10^9/L	0–0.2	0–0.2
Platelet count	×10^9/L	150–400	150–400

Source: Normal values of the Haematology Department, Guy's and St Thomas' Hospitals NHS Foundation Trust, UK.

Table 100.2 Clues from the blood film.

Finding	Interpretation/causes
Red cells	
Red cell aggregration	Rouleaux, seen in: • High polyclonal immunoglobulin (e.g. acute phase response) • Monoclonal immunoglobulin (paraprotein, e.g. myeloma) • High fibrinogen Agglutination, reflecting the presence of cold agglutinin, seen in: • Mycoplasma infection • Infectious mononucleosis • Lymphoproliferative disorder • Idiopathic
Fragmented red cells (schistocytes)	Microangiopathic haemolytic anaemia, seen in: • Disseminated intravascular coagulation • Thrombotic thrombocytopenic purpura/haemolytic uraemic syndrome • Systemic infection • Metastatic cancer • Severe preeclampsia/eclampsia • Severe hypertension with fibrinoid necrosis • Autoimmune/vasculitic disorders (e.g. systemic lupus erythematosus, systemic sclerosis, antiphospholipid syndrome) Haematopoietic stem-cell or organ transplantation Prosthetic heart valve Severe burns
'Bite cells' (keratocytes)	Acute haemolysis induced by oxidant damage (e.g. in glucose-6-phosphate dehydrogenase deficiency)
Target cells	Iron deficiency Thalassaemia Liver disease Post-splenectomy

Table 100.2 (*Continued*)

Finding	Interpretation/causes
Nucleated red cells	Marrow replacement, due to:
	• Carcinoma (most commonly of breast or prostate origin)
	• Myelofibrosis
	• Myeloma
	• Tuberculosis
Red cell inclusions – Howell-Jolly bodies	Post-splenectomy
White cells	
Blast cells	Leukaemias
	Lymphomas
	Marrow replacement (see above)
Platelets	
Platelet clumps	EDTA-induced platelet clumping may cause spurious thrombocytopenia
Other findings	
Abnormal cells	Lymphoma cells
	Plasma cells (myeloma)
Parasites	Malaria

Adapted from: Bain BJ (2005) Diagnosis from the blood smear. *N Engl J Med* 353, 498–507; Tefferi A, Hanson CA, Inwards DJ, *et al.* (2005) How to interpret and pursue an abnormal complete blood cell count in adults. *Mayo Clinic Proc* 80, 923–936.

Table 100.3 Microcytic anaemia (MCV <80 fl).

Cause	Clues from full blood count and film	Other blood results	Causes/comment
Iron deficiency	Increased red-cell distribution width Anisocytosis Increased platelet count Pencil cells	Low iron Increased total iron binding capacity Low transferrin saturation Low ferritin	Commonest cause of microcytic anaemia, caused by blood loss, inadequate dietary intake of iron, or malabsorption of iron (e.g. coeliac disease)
Anaemia of chronic disease (ACD)	Film usually unremarkable	Low iron Low/normal transferrin Normal/increased ferritin	~20% ACDs are microcytic
Thalassaemia	Polychromasia Target cells	Normal ferritin Haemoglobin electrophoresis normal in alpha-thalassaemia trait and abnormal in beta-thalassaemia trait and other thalassaemia syndromes. Haemoglobin gene sequencing frequently used to establish diagnosis.	RBC frequently elevated and MCH less than 27. Haematocrit usually >30% and MCV <75 fl in beta thalassaemia trait.
Sideroblastic anaemia	Siderocytes may be seen: hypochromic red cells with basophilic stippling that stains positive for iron (Pappenheimer bodies)	Increased ferritin	Rare; comprises both hereditary and acquired forms.

Table 100.4 Macrocytosis (MCV >100 fl).

Cause	Clues from full blood count and film	Other blood results	Causes/comment
Drug-induced	Usually unremarkable	No specific abnormality	Many drugs, for example azathioprine, zidovudine
B12/folate deficiency	Oval macrocytic red cells, hypersegmented neutrophils, pancytopenia	Low serum B12/red cell folate Positive intrinsic factor antibodies in pernicious anaemia	B12 deficiency: pernicious anaemia/malabsorption Folate deficiency: inadequate dietary intake/malabsorption
Haemolysis	See Table 100.5		
	Haemolytic anaemia usually normocytic but can be macrocytic if there is marked reticulocytosis		
Primary bone marrow disorder	Other cytopenias Leukocytosis Monocytosis Thrombocytosis Blast cells	No specific abnormality	Myelodysplasia, leukaemia
Alcohol	Alcohol excess may also cause lymphopenia and thrombocytopenia	Abnormal liver function tests, with raised AST (> ALT) and gamma GT	See Chapter 106, Alcohol-related problems in acute medicine
Hypothyroidism	Usually unremarkable	Raised TSH, low free T4/free T3	Hypothyroidism may also cause normocytic anaemia
Chronic liver disease	Associated thrombocytopenia may be seen in cirrhosis with portal hypertension and splenomegaly	Abnormal liver function tests/ prothrombin time	See Chapter 77.

Table 100.5 Normocytic anaemia (MCV 80 – 100 fl).

Cause	Clues from full blood count and film	Other blood results	Causes/comment
Bleeding	Polychromasia Anisocytosis	Falling haemoglobin without evidence of haemolysis	Occult bleeding may occur from gut or into retroperitoneal space
Haemolysis	Polychromasia (reflecting increased reticulocyte count) Spherocytes Keratocytes ('bite' cells, due to acute haemolysis induced by oxidant damage, as may occur in G6PD deficiency) Fragmented red cells seen in microangiopathic haemolytic anaemia (Table 100.2)	Increased unconjugated bilirubin, increased lactate dehydrogenase (LDH) and reduced serum haptoglobin seen in haemolysis of all causes Positive Coombs' test or DAGT in autoimmune haemolysis	Haemolysis is due either to abnormalities of red cells (e.g. G6PD deficiency, sickle cell anaemia) or to extrinsic factors (immune and non-immune causes)
Anaemia of chronic disease	Film usually unremarkable	Normal/increased ferritin Abnormalities related to underlying cause	Seen in acute and chronic infection, cancer, renal failure, inflammatory disorders (e.g. rheumatoid arthritis, SLE), endocrine disorders, and chronic rejection after solid-organ transplantation
Bone marrow disorder	Other cytopenias Leukocytosis Monocytosis Thrombocytosis Blast cells	Paraproteinaemia in myeloma	Myelodysplasia, myeloma, leukaemia

Table 100.6 Polycythaemia (erythrocytosis).

Mechanism of polycythaemia	Diseases
Erythropoietin secretion due to chronic tissue hypoxia	Chronic obstructive pulmonary disease with respiratory failure
	Obesity-hypoventilation syndrome
	Right-to-left intracardiac shunts
	Pulmonary arteriovenous malformations
	High altitude
	Red cell defects
	High oxygen-affinity haemoglobins
	Chronic carbon monoxide poisoning
	Congenital methaemoglobinaemia
Erythropoietin secretion not due to hypoxia	Renal cell carcinoma
	Cerebellar haemangioblastoma
	Hepatocellular carcinoma
	Uterine fibroids
	Phaeochromocytoma
	Polycystic kidney disease
	Chuvash polycythaemia (VHL gene mutation)
Germline and somatic mutational causes of polycythaemia	Polycythaemia vera (JAK2 mutation)
	Idiopathic familial polycythaemia
	Bisphosphoglycerate mutase (BPGM) deficiency
	Activating mutations of the erythropoietin receptor (EPOR gene)
Hormonal stimulus	Androgens
	Anabolic steroid
	Cushing's syndrome
Haemoconcentration	Dehydration
	Diuretic therapy

Table 100.7 White blood cell abnormalities.

Finding	Possible causes
Neutrophilia	Sepsis
	Metastatic cancer
	Acidosis
	Corticosteroid therapy
	Smoking
	Trauma, surgery, burn
	Myeloproliferative disorders
Neutropenia (see Chapter 102)	Myelosuppressive chemotherapeutic agents
	Idiosyncratic reaction to drug (e.g. carbimazole)
	Infections (e.g. viral, severe bacterial, HIV)
	B12 and folate deficiency
	Systemic lupus erythematosus
	Felty syndrome
	Haematological disorders (e.g. leukaemia)
	Ethnic neutropenia (Afro-Caribbean origin is often associated with neutrophilis as low as 0.8×10^9/L
Lymphocytosis	Infections (e.g. infectious mononucleosis)
	Lymphoproliferative disorders (e.g. chronic lymphocytic leukaemia, lymphoma)

(continued)

Table 100.7 (*Continued*)

Finding	Possible causes
Lymphopenia	Infections (e.g. viral, HIV, severe bacterial)
	Immunosuppressive therapy
	Systemic lupus erythematosus
	Alcohol excess
	Chronic renal failure
	Lymphoma
Monocytosis	Infections
	Myeloproliferative disorders (e.g. chronic myelomonocytic leukaemia)
	Metastatic cancer
Eosinophilia	Drug allergy
	Parasitic infestation
	Haematological disorders (e.g. lymphoma, leukaemia, hypereosinophilic syndrome)
	Churg-Strauss vasculitis
	Disorders with eosinophilic involvement of specific organs
	Adrenal insufficiency (see Chapter 90)
	Atheroembolism

Table 100.8 Causes of thrombocytopenia.

Setting	Common causes
Acute admission	Sepsis
	Acute alcohol toxicity
	Drug-induced thrombocytopenia
	Immune thrombocytopenic purpura*
	Thrombotic thrombocytopenic purpura (Table 100.9)
Inpatient	Sepsis
	Disseminated intravascular coagulation (Appendix 102.1)
	Drug-induced thrombocytopenia
	Post-transfusion purpura
Inpatients with cardiac disease	Use of platelet glycoprotein IIb/IIIa-receptor antagonists
	Use of adenosine diphosphate-receptor antagonists (e.g. clopidogrel)
	Heparin-induced thrombocytopenia (Appendix 102.3)
	Post-cardiopulmonary bypass
	Use of intra-aortic balloon pump
Pregnancy and post-partum	Gestational thrombocytopenia
(Table 100.9)	Immune thrombocytopenic purpura (ITP)
	HELLP syndrome (Haemolysis, Elevated Liver enzymes, Low Platelet count)
	Disseminated intravascular coagulation (Appendix 102.1)
	Thrombotic thrombocytopenic purpura (Appendix 102.2)
Outpatient	Myelodysplasia
	Leukaemia
	Hypersplenism
	Immune thrombocytopenic purpura*
	Antiphospholipid-antibody syndrome
	Vitamin B12 deficiency

*Immune thrombocytopenic purpura (idiopathic thrombocytopenic purpura, ITP) is diagnosed when there is isolated thrombocytopenia, with no other cause of thrombocytopenia evident (after bone marrow aspiration to rule out marrow disorders, and testing for HIV).

Table 100.9 Causes of thrombocytopenia in pregnancy and post-partum.

Cause	Comment
Gestational thrombocytopenia	Incidence is ~5% of pregnancies May be mild form of ITP Diagnosed when there is: • Mild thrombocytopenia (platelet count typically >70 × 10⁹/L) • No past history of thrombocytopenia (except during a previous pregnancy) • No other cause for thrombocytopenia is evident • Spontaneous resolution after delivery
Immune thrombocytopenic purpura (ITP)	ITP is more likely than gestational thrombocytopenia if thrombocytopenia occurs during early pregnancy or if the platelet count is <50 × 10⁹/L Exclude other causes of thrombocytopenia Discuss management with a haematologist
HELLP syndrome (Haemolysis, Elevated Liver enzymes, Low Platelet count)	Usually complicates severe pre-eclampsia, although 15–20% of patients do not have elevated liver enzymes Features are: • Microangiopathic haemolytic anaemia • Serum lactate dehydrogenase (LDH) >600 units/L • Serum aspartate transaminase (AST) >70 units/L Platelet count <100 × 10⁹/L Management is as for pre-eclampsia
Disseminated intravascular coagulation	See Appendix 102.1 May be caused by amniotic fluid embolism, placental abruption or sepsis Treat underlying disorder Consider blood product replacement and coagulation inhibitor therapy Seek advice from a haematologist See Appendix 102.2
Thrombotic thrombocytopenic purpura	Features supporting diagnosis of TTP rather than HELPP syndrome: • Absence of preceding hypertension/proteinuria • Severe thrombocytopenia • Fragmented red cells (schistocytes) (microangiopathic haemolytic anaemia) • Absence of liver function abnormalities • Normal prothrombin and activated partial thromboplastin times Treatment is with plasma exchange TTP is not improved by delivery of foetus

Table 100.10 Causes of pancytopenia.

Mechanism of pancytopenia	Causative diseases*
Reduced synthesis (bone marrow failure)	Chemo/radiotherapy Marrow infiltration due to non-haematological malignancy Haematological malignancy Megaloblastic anaemia Panhypopituitarism Idiopathic aplastic anaemia

(continued)

Table 100.10 (Continued)

Mechanism of pancytopenia	Causative diseases[*]
Increased destruction	Splenic sequestration (e.g. due to splenomegaly of any aetiology)
	Drug-induced immune destruction
	Haemophagocytic syndrome/macrophage activating syndrome
	HIV infection
Complex pathology	Hepatitis B/C
	Paroxysmal nocturnal haemoglobinuria
	Systemic immune disorders (e.g. SLE)
	Storage disorders

[*] See Table 101.5 for clues from the blood film.

Further reading

Butt NM, Lambert J, Ali S, *et al.* (2016) Guideline for the investigation and management of eosinophilia: A British Society for Haematology Guideline. http://www.bcshguidelines.com/documents/BCSH_Eosinophilia_Guideline_FINALresubmissioncopy_12th_Oct_2016.pdf.

George JN, Nester CM (2014) Syndromes of thrombotic microangiopathy. *N Engl J Med* 371, 654–666.

Hesdorffer CS, Longo DL (2015) Drug-induced megaloblastic anemia. *N Engl J Med* 373, 1649–1658.

Hill QA, Stamps R, Massey E, Grainger JD, Provan D, Hill A, on behalf of the British Society for Haematology (2016) The diagnosis and management of primary autoimmune haemolytic anaemia. http://www.bcshguidelines.com/documents/AIHA_Primary_Guideline_BSH_website.pdf.

Lopez A, Cacoub P, Macdougall IC, Peyrin-Biroulet L (2016) Iron-deficiency anaemia. *Lancet* 387, 907–916.

Steensma DP (2015) Myelodysplastic syndromes: diagnosis and treatment. *Mayo Clin Proc* 90, 969–983.

CHAPTER 101

Pancytopenia and febrile neutropenia

DEBORAH HAY

Pancytopenia may be due to inadequate or defective production of blood cells (bone marrow failure), increased destruction or complex mechanisms (see Table 100.10).

- Where marrow synthesis is adequate but peripheral counts are low, increased cellular consumption is likely to be responsible, and the focus of further investigation shifts to include any cause of splenomegaly, autoimmune disorders both primary and secondary, and the macrophage-activating syndrome seen in cases of extreme sepsis and in severe exacerbations of rheumatological disease.
- The commonest cause of pancytopenia presenting to the emergency department or general medical take is the expected and transient consequence of recently delivered chemotherapy (Table 101.1). While this is unlikely to be a diagnostic challenge, there is significant potential risk to the patient from neutropenic sepsis, which requires prompt empirical treatment.

Priorities

Immediate clinical assessment

- Assess for fever >37.5 °C.
- Assess for circulatory compromise (sepsis/symptomatic anaemia/occult haemorrhage – NB avoid rectal examination in neutropenic patients).
- Assess for evidence of bleeding, for example petechiae, bruising, mucosal blood blisters.
- Assess for lymphadenopathy, splenomegaly and hepatomegaly.
- Assess for sources of infection, for example indwelling venous catheters.

Immediate management and urgent investigation

- Alert the haematologist on-call (Figure 101.1).
- Secure venous access and obtain blood samples for first-line investigation (see Table 101.2).
- Fluid resuscitation if haemodynamically compromised.
- Septic screen for patients with febrile neutropenia, including aseptic sampling of any indwelling lines for culture (Table 101.3).
- Broad-spectrum empiric antibiotic treatment if neutropenic and febrile (>37.5 °C). Agents are likely to include piperacillin/tazobactam as recommended by NICE guidelines, but will be determined by local hospital microbiology policy.

Acute Medicine: A Practical Guide to the Management of Medical Emergencies, Fifth Edition. Edited by David Sprigings and John B. Chambers.
© 2018 John Wiley & Sons Ltd. Published 2018 by John Wiley & Sons Ltd.

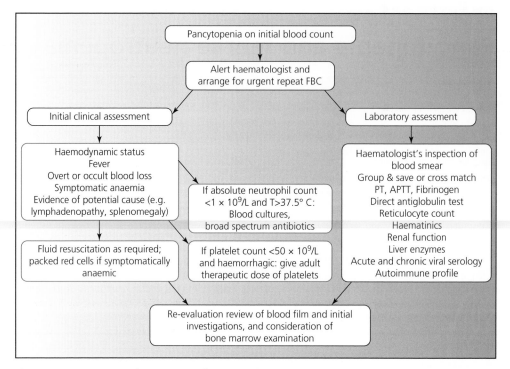

Figure 101.1 Assessment and management of pancytopenia.

- If haemorrhagic:
  - Adult therapeutic dose of platelets if count $<50 \times 10^9$/L
  - Cryoprecipitate if fibrinogen <1 g/L
  - Fresh frozen plasma (FFP) if PT and APTT >1.5× upper limit of normal
- Packed red cells if symptomatically anaemic.

  NB: Some haematological malignancies and exposure to some chemotherapy agents necessitate the use of irradiated packed red cells and platelet concentrates (Table 101.4).

Table 101.1 Drugs associated with cytopenias.

Myelosuppressive chemotherapy	Drugs causing idiopathic marrow aplasia or cytopenias
Chemotherapeutic agents including: • Alkylating agents • Topoisomerase inhibitors • Nucleoside analogues • Some newer 'targeted' agents	Many drugs implicated, including: • Chloramphenicol • Gold • Carbamazepine • Non-steroidal anti-inflammatory drugs (NSAIDs) • Carbimazole • Sulphonamides

Table 101.2 Urgent investigation in patients with pancytopenia of unknown aetiology.

Test	Rationale
Repeat full blood count	To exclude artefactual result (e.g. blood from drip stream, clotted sample)
Reticulocyte count	A low reticulocyte count in the context of pancytopenia suggests a defect in the marrow rather than a peripheral consumptive problem
Blood film for attention of haematologist	Critical to assess for morphological diagnostic clues (e.g. leukaemic blast cells)
Group and save, direct antiglobulin test	In case transfusion is required; the DAT will be positive in autoimmune haemolytic anaemia (e.g. Evans syndrome)
Serum B12 and folate	To exclude remediable deficiencies resulting in megaloblastic anaemia
Serum ferritin	Likely to be elevated in acute infection/inflammation; grossly elevated in haemophagocytic syndrome
ALT, ALP, bilirubin, albumin	May be abnormal in acute hepatitis, EBV and CMV infection; unconjugated hyperbilirubinaemia also seen in haemolysis
LDH	Typically elevated in haemolysis, B12 and folate deficiency, high grade lymphoma, hepatitis
PT, APTT, fibrinogen	To assess for disseminated intravascular coagulation
Acute viral serology (EBV, CMV IgM and IgG)	Potential causes of unexplained acute onset pancytopenia
Chronic viral serology (HIV, Hepatitis B/C)	Each can cause pancytopenia; recognized association between hepatitis and marrow aplasia
Autoimmune profile	Rare presentation of SLE, and other connective tissue disorders
Lipid profile	Elevated triglycerides in haemophagocytic syndrome

DAT, direct antiglobulin test; ALT, alanine transaminase; ALP, alkaline phosphatase; LDH, lactate dehydrogenase; PT, prothrombin time; APTT, activated partial thromboplastin time; EBV, Epstein-Barr virus; CMV, cytomegalovirus; HIV, human immunodeficiency virus; SLE, systemic lupus erythematosus.

Table 101.3 Further investigation in febrile neutropenia.

Peripheral blood culture (×2)
Blood culture from indwelling venous catheters
Urine microscopy and culture
Stool culture if clinically appropriate
Chest X-ray

Table 101.4 Transfusion for patients with bone marrow failure: when to use irradiated blood products.

Disorders*	Chemotherapy/immunosuppression agents*
Hodgkin lymphoma	Fludarabine
Patients <6 months post allogeneic bone marrow transplant	Cladribine
Patients with chronic graft-versus-host disease post allogeneic transplant	Deoxycoformicin
	Clofarabine
Patients <3 months post autologous transplant (high dose therapy and stem cell rescue)	Bendamustine
	Alemtuzumab (Campath)
T lymphocyte immunodeficiency syndromes	Anti-thymocyte globulin

*Blood bank and the duty clinical haematologist on call should be contacted for advice.

Patients needing admission

- Pancytopenia itself is not an absolute indication for admission: many patients who are receiving outpatient chemotherapy regimens will have intermittent and expected periods of pancytopenia that are safely managed in the community with regular attendance at day treatment units for blood product support. In this setting, platelets are typically given when the count falls to 10×10^9/L, and packed red cells when the haemoglobin falls below 80 g/L.
- Patients receiving myelosuppressive chemotherapy should be counselled by their coordinating physician to seek urgent medical attention if they develop a fever or any symptoms suggestive of infection. Regular and frequent follow-up is critical in this setting.
- Admission is indicated for patients with febrile neutropenia (absolute neutrophil count $<1 \times 10^9$/L, temperature $>37.5\,°C$), and these patients should be carefully monitored for signs of deterioration, especially while antibiotic treatment is empirical. Those with febrile neutropenia as a result of chemotherapy should be managed by their coordinating specialty team, but any delay in the administration of antibiotics should be avoided.
- For patients with unexplained pancytopenia, admission is likely to be required to permit a comprehensive evaluation (see below, including Table 100.2).
  - Where the initial investigations suggest a primary haematological cause (e.g. acute leukaemia evident on the peripheral blood film) admission should be under the care of the haematologist.
  - Where no cause is identified from the first-line investigations, admission under the general medical service is appropriate, with haematological guidance for empirical management and further investigation.
- Patients with mild pancytopenia in whom an indolent course can be clearly established from historic blood results may be suitable for discharge and further evaluation by the haematology service as an outpatient; seek advice from a haematologist.

Monitoring and escalation of care

- Intensive support should be requested for patients with febrile neutropenia who remain hypotensive or haemodynamically unstable despite aggressive fluid resuscitation and broad-spectrum antibiotic treatment.
- Where patients have an indwelling tunnelled venous catheter (for the delivery of chemotherapy), consideration should be given to whether this constitutes the source of infection. Erythema along the line of the tunnel, discharge from the tunnel exit point and rigors on flushing of the line may all suggest local infection, and removal of the line is likely to be needed.
- In patients where the cause of bone marrow failure is secondary to chemotherapy, close liaison with the coordinating specialty team is essential to establish long-term prognosis and appropriate ceilings of care.

Further management

Clinical assessment

Once the patient is stabilized, an initial assessment of the possible causes of pancytopenia can be undertaken. For those with a known likely explanation (e.g. recent chemotherapy) this should include:

- Details of the diagnosis
- The status of the disease (e.g. newly diagnosed, induction chemotherapy, in remission)
- Duration of treatment
- Nature of the chemotherapy given
- Date of most recent treatment
- Antimicrobial prophylaxis received

These factors will affect management by determining the choice of blood product and may also influence the antimicrobial agents used for the treatment of neutropenic fever.

Patients who have been exposed to prolonged and/or repeated periods of neutropenia may have fungal as well as bacterial infection.

In heavily immunosuppressed patients, the possibility of pneumocystis infection or CMV reactivation should also be considered.

For seriously ill or unstable patients, early liaison with the physicians coordinating the patient's care is vital to establish any previous history or infection, and any previously isolated organisms.

For patients with new or unexplained pancytopenia, the history should elicit the following:
- Features to suggest occult malignancy: weight loss, fevers, night sweats, focal symptoms
- Current and recently prescribed medications and over-the-counter treatments (Table 101.1)
- Risk factors for blood-borne viruses (HIV, hepatitis B and C)
- Travel history (e.g. leishmaniasis, malaria; see Chapter 33)
- History of thrombosis (malignancy, paroxysmal nocturnal haemoglobinuria)
- Features of haemoglobinuria (paroxysmal nocturnal haemoglobinuria)
- Recent jaundice (hepatitis-associated aplasia)
- Occupational history and exposure to toxins (e.g. solvents, pesticides)
- Especially for children: family history of marrow failure, anaemia or malignancies

The features on physical examination of a patient with unexplained pancytopenia will include pallor, petechiae and bruising. However, features to suggest an underlying aetiology may be much more subtle. In cases where the pancytopenia arises due to accelerated consumption, there is likely to be splenomegaly; features suggesting an underlying cause for splenomegaly (e.g. liver disease, lymphoma, connective tissue diseases) must also be sought.

Where there is inadequate marrow production due to marrow infiltration, there may be physical evidence to suggest a primary malignancy (with prostate, breast, lung and renal tumour being typical primary sites for marrow metastases). Clonal haematological disorders suppressing normal haemopoiesis may also give signs on examination, including lymphadenopathy and splenomegaly. Rarely, hypopituitarism can give rise to marrow aplasia, and it is worth considering features due to both hormone deficiency and local effects in the region of the pituitary fossa.

Patients presenting (typically in childhood) with the rare congenital and inherited bone marrow failure syndromes may also have characteristic features on clinical examination, including skeletal abnormalities, short stature and changes in skin pigmentation.

In many cases, however, the clinical examination will yield no clues to the cause of pancytopenia, and the ultimate diagnosis will require specific haematological investigation.

Investigation

After the first-line investigations described above, specialized haematological input is needed. Clues on the peripheral blood film may guide a working differential (Table 101.5), but patients with persistent pancytopenia of unknown aetiology are very likely to require examination of the bone marrow in order to obtain a diagnosis. An opinion on the morphological appearance of the marrow aspirate may be available as soon as one hour following the bone marrow biopsy. A more detailed evaluation of any abnormal cell population seen in either the peripheral blood or marrow aspirate can be obtained using immunophenotyping by flow cytometry.

A bone marrow trephine offers complementary information, and allows assessment of a more representative section of marrow including the distribution of cells and the presence or absence of fibrosis. Detailed immunostaining protocols allow the identification of haemopoietic and infiltrating cell types, even when their appearance is atypical. However, since these samples require extensive laboratory manipulation and specialist interpretation, information from a trephine will not be available to inform immediate management.

Table 101.5 Pancytopenia: clues from the peripheral blood film.

Diagnosis	Typical blood film findings
Acute leukaemia	Pancytopenia, with or without a population of blast cells
	Specific morphological features may help differentiate between myeloid and lymphoblastic leukaemia, and may raise the suspicion of acute promyeloblastic leukaemia
Lymphoma	Variable; possible circulating lymphoma cells (e.g. CLL, mantle cell lymphoma, hairy cell leukaemia); possible leucoerythroblastic change (nucleated red blood cells, myelocytes)
Myelofibrosis	Cytopenias with prominent red cell changes, including teardrop poikilocytes, nucleated red cells
Myelodysplasia	Variable red cell size and shape; hypogranular and abnormally segmented neutrophils
Metastatic malignancy	Leucoerythroblastic film (nucleated red blood cells, myelocytes)
B12 or folate deficiency	Oval macrocytes, hypersegmented neutrophils
Liver disease	Macrocytosis, target-form red cells
Acute viral infection (EBV, CMV)	Atypical lymphocytes; polychromasia/spherocytes if haemolysis

Lymphadenopathy is best assessed by cross-sectional imaging such as CT, or PET-CT, which may provide additional information about the site and nature of malignant disease.

Problems

Artefacts

Occasionally, samples are reported as pancytopenic simply because a clot is present in the tube. Drawing blood from a site proximal to an intravenous infusion is another potential error that might lead to the false impression of pancytopenia (though here, biochemical results would also be markedly abnormal). An urgent repeat plus blood film is always warranted – although where the clinical picture fits there should be no delay in emergency management.

Acute infection

Infections that have been termed the 'mononucleosis syndromes' – including acute EBV and CMV infection – can sometimes produce a clinical picture of alarming severity, especially in adults. Complications may include haemolysis, immune thrombocytopenia and immune neutropenia, and the combination of pancytopenia with atypical lymphocytes in the peripheral blood film can raise concerns of high-grade haematological malignancy. Many cases also feature lymphadenopathy and splenomegaly, and it is easy to expose the patient to a bone marrow examination that is both unnecessary and potentially very easy to misinterpret. The monospot test is useful, especially in adults, but not uncommonly gives false negative results in children with acute EBV infection; consequently, specific viral serology and PCR testing are indicated where these infections form part of the differential diagnosis.

Acute promyelocytic leukaemia (APML)

Although rare, this subtype of acute myeloid leukaemia is worth particular mention due to its association with disseminated intravascular coagulation. Patients may present with signs of haemorrhage, including widespread purpura, gum bleeding, epistaxis and intracranial bleeding. It is for the emergency diagnosis of this condition above all others that a haematologist will review the blood film of a pancytopenic patient urgently, at any time of day or night.

APML is the consequence of a chromosomal translocation that involves the retinoic acid receptor gene (*RARα*). For this reason, treatment with all-*trans* retinoic acid (ATRA) can promote differentiation of the leukaemic cells, reducing the risk of haemorrhage. For any patient in whom APML is considered after inspection of the peripheral blood film, immediate treatment with ATRA is indicated.

Macrophage-activating syndrome

This umbrella term refers to a constellation of clinical features, including persistent fever, cytopenias, consumptive coagulopathy, deranged liver function, gross hyperferritinaemia and hypertriglyceridaemia. The underlying pathophysiology is most clearly defined in the rare familial haemophagocytic syndrome where perforin or Munc gene mutations result in dysregulation of cytotoxic immune functions. However, acquired haemophagocytic syndrome is also described, and can be triggered by infections such as HIV, EBV and CMV, and by malignancies, notably aggressive lymphomas. It is also seen in association with connective tissue disorders. The uncontrolled T cell proliferation and macrophage activation that characterize this syndrome are associated with a high mortality. Although rare, this syndrome and its associated disorders should be considered in patients with persistent pancytopenia and unremitting fevers, despite appropriate antimicrobials.

Further reading

Klastersky J, de Naurois J, Rolston B, *et al*. (2016) Management of febrile neutropaenia. ESMO Clinical Practice Guidelines. *Ann Oncol* 27 (suppl 5), v111–v118. https://annonc.oxfordjournals.org/content/27/suppl_5/v111.full.pdf+html.

Weinzierl EP, Arber DA (2013) The differential diagnosis and bone marrow evaluation of new-onset pancytopenia. *Am J Clin Pathol* 139, 9–29. http://ajcp.oxfordjournals.org/content/ajcpath/139/1/9.full.pdf.

CHAPTER 102

Bleeding disorders

CLAIRE HARRISON

Consider a bleeding disorder (Table 102.1) in the patient with spontaneous, prolonged or disproportionate bleeding.

Drugs are the commonest cause of an acquired bleeding disorder.

Priorities

1 Make a clinical assessment and take a detailed drug history. Is there a known inherited disorder, past or family history of abnormal bleeding?
2 If the patient has had previous significant injury, surgery, tooth extraction or childbirth without abnormal bleeding, an inherited disorder of haemostasis is unlikely.
3 Check a full blood count, blood film and coagulation screen (including fibrinogen level): see Chapter 100 for interpretation of full blood count and film; interpretation of the coagulation screen is summarized in Table 102.2. Check renal and liver function. Other investigations will be determined by the clinical context.

Further management

1 Further management is directed at the underlying disorder. Seek expert advice from a haematologist on management and haemostatic support, particularly in the event of unexplained bleeding, positive family history, prior bleeding and for help with blood product support.
2 Clinical features and management of disseminated intravascular coagulation, thrombotic thrombocytopenic purpura and heparin-induced thrombocytopenia are summarized in Appendices 102.1–102.3.

Acute Medicine: A Practical Guide to the Management of Medical Emergencies, Fifth Edition. Edited by David Sprigings and John B. Chambers.
© 2018 John Wiley & Sons Ltd. Published 2018 by John Wiley & Sons Ltd.

Table 102.1 Causes of abnormal bleeding.

Cause	Comment
Inherited disorders of haemostasis	These are rare in acute medicine If the patient has had previous significant injury, surgery, tooth extraction or childbirth without abnormal bleeding, an inherited disorder of haemostasis is unlikely
Acquired disorders of haemostasis	
Direct effect of drugs	
Warfarin	Inhibits vitamin K-dependent gamma-carboxylation of coagulation factors II, VII, IX and X
Direct-acting oral anticoagulants (e.g. dabigatran, rivaroxaban, apixaban)	These drugs are direct inhibitors of factor Xa
Unfractionated heparin	Inhibits thrombin
Low-molecular-weight heparins	Inhibit factor Xa and thrombin
Thrombolytic agents (e.g. alteplase)	Activate plasminogen and thus the fibrinolytic system
Antiplatelet agents (e.g. aspirin, clopidogrel, ticagrelor)	Inhibit platelet aggregation
Platelet glycoprotein IIb/IIIa-receptor antagonists	Inhibit platelet aggregation
Other causes	
Thrombocytopenia	See Tables 100.7 and 100.8. Platelet count: • $<50 \times 10^9$/L: excessive bleeding seen after surgery or trauma • $<20 \times 10^9$/L: spontaneous bleeding is common • $<10 \times 10^9$/L: spontaneous bleeding is usual
Platelet dysfunction	Most often due to drugs, notably antiplatelet agents, but also NSAIDs and beta-lactam antibiotics Also seen in advanced renal failure and myelodysplasia
Coagulation factor deficiency or inhibitor	See Table 102.2. Acquired inhibitors are antibodies to coagulation factors, which may be idiopathic or associated with malignancy, autoimmune disorders, pregnancy and clonal lymphoma proliferative disorders (e.g. Waldenstrom macroglobulinaemia) Typically presents with bleeding into muscles or large ecchymoses
Vessel disorder	Corticosteroid therapy, scurvy

Table 102.2 Acquired causes of prolonged prothrombin time (PT) and activated partial thromboplastin time (APTT).

PT	APTT	Cause
Prolonged	**Normal**	Warfarin or other vitamin K antagonist therapy
		Vitamin K deficiency
		Liver disease
		Acquired factor VII deficiency
		Inhibitor of factor VII
Normal	**Prolonged**	Heparin therapy
		Inhibitors of factors VIII, IX, XI or XII
		Acquired von Willebrand disease (usually associated with autoimmune or clonal proliferative disorders)
		Lupus anticoagulant (associated with thrombosis)
Prolonged	**Prolonged**	Liver disease
		Disseminated intravascular coagulation
		Excess heparin
		Excess warfarin or other vitamin K antagonist therapy (ingestion of rat poison)
		Heparin + warfarin therapy
		Primary amyloidosis-associated factor X deficiency
		Inhibitors of prothrombin, fibrinogen or factors V or X
Variable	**Variable**	The direct-acting oral anticoagulants (dabigatran, rivaroxaban and apixaban) have variable effects on the PT and APTT, depending on the drug, its concentration (the dose-response is not always linear) and the particular laboratory assay. If you have a patient taking one of these drugs who is bleeding, always consult a haematologist. A reversal agent for dabigatran is now available (idarucizumab). See Chapter 103.

Table 102.3 Diagnosis of heparin-induced thrombocytopenia (HIT): the 4T score.

Category	2 points	1 point	0 points
Thrombocytopenia	Platelet count fall >50% and platelet nadir $\geq 20 \times 10^9$/L	Platelet count fall 30–50% or platelet nadir 10–19×10^9/L	Platelet count fall <30% or platelet nadir $<10 \times 10^9$/L
Timing of platelet count fall	Clear onset between days 5 and 10 or platelet fall ≤ 1 day (prior heparin exposure within 30 days)	Consistent with days 5–10 fall, but not clear (e.g. missing platelet counts) or onset after day 10 or fall ≤ 1 day (prior heparin exposure 30–100 days ago)	Platelet count fall <4 days without recent heparin exposure
Thrombosis or other sequelae	New thrombosis (confirmed) or skin necrosis at heparin injection sites or acute systemic reaction after intravenous heparin bolus	Progressive or recurrent thrombosis or non-necrotizing (erythematous) skin lesions or suspected thrombosis (not proven)	None
Other causes for thrombocytopenia	None apparent	Possible	Definite

Total points:
$\leq 3 =$ **low probability of HIT**
4–5 = intermediate probability of HIT
$\geq 6 =$ **high probability of HIT**
Source: Lo GK, Juhl D, Warkentin TE, Sigouin CS, Eichler P, Greinacher A (2006) Evaluation of pretest clinical score (4 Ts) for the diagnosis of heparin-induced thrombocytopenia in two clinical settings. *J Thromb Haemost* 4, 759–65. Reproduced with permission of John Wiley & Sons.

Appendix 102.1 Disseminated intravascular coagulation (DIC)

Element	Comment
Causes	Sepsis
	Trauma (major injury, head injury, fat embolism)
	Malignancy (e.g. acute myeloid leukaemia)
	Obstetric complication (amniotic fluid embolism, placental abruption)
	Immune-mediated disorder (e.g. anaphylaxis, haemolytic transfusion reaction, transplant rejection)
	Other causes include giant haemangioma, abdominal aortic aneurysm, snake venom, amphetamine poisoning, cardiac arrest, drowning and heat stroke
Clinical features	Bleeding from skin and mucosae (nose and gums)
	Bleeding from surgical incisions, wounds, venepuncture sites
	Acute kidney injury
	Jaundice Acute respiratory distress syndrome (ARDS) due to diffuse alveolar haemorrhage
	Delirium, seizures
	Adrenal insufficiency (adrenal haemorrhage)
	Purpura fulminans
Full blood count and film	Thrombocytopenia
	Fragmented red cells (schistocytes) in ~50%
Blood results	Prolonged prothrombin and activated partial thromboplastin times
	Low fibrinogen concentration
	Raised concentration of fibrin degradation products/D-dimer
Differential diagnosis	Thrombotic thrombocytopenic purpura (Appendix 102.2)
	Chronic DIC (Trousseau syndrome)
	Acute liver failure
	Decompensated chronic liver disease
	HELLP syndrome of pregnancy (haemolysis, elevated liver enzymes, low platelet count) (see Table 100.8)
	Amyloidosis
Management	Seek urgent advice from a haematologist
	Treatment is of the underlying disorder
	Consider blood product replacement therapy if the patient is actively bleeding or requires an intervention

Appendix 102.2 Thrombotic thrombocytopenic purpura

Element	Comment
Patient characteristics	Rare disorder (incidence ~1 per 100,000 per year)
	Idiopathic TTP most often seen in black women with obesity
	TTP may be associated with autoimmune disorders (SLE, antiphospholipid antibody syndrome, scleroderma), pregnancy, and with drugs (e.g. quinine, clopidogrel, cancer chemotherapy)
Clinical features	Weakness
	Nausea, vomiting, abdominal pain
	Fever
	Neurological abnormalities (fits, fluctuating focal deficits) (present in ~50%)
	Acute kidney injury (in ~30%)

(continued)

Appendix 102.2 (*Continued*)

Element	Comment
Full blood count and film	Anaemia
	Thrombocytopenia
	No leucopenia
	Fragmented red cells (schistocytes) characteristic
	Increased reticulocyte count
Blood results	Normal prothrombin and activated partial thromboplastin times
	Increased LDH and unconjugated bilirubin (reflecting haemolysis)
	Raised creatinine in ~30%
Differential diagnosis	Disseminated intravascular coagulation (Appendix 102.1)
	In pregnant women, pre-eclampsia/eclampsia and HELLP syndrome (Table 100.8)
	Evans syndrome
	Autoimmune haemolysis
	Immune thrombocytopenic purpura
Management	Seek urgent advice from a haematologist
	Do not transfuse platelets
	Plasma exchange until platelet count normal
	Add corticosteroid if no underlying cause found

Appendix 102.3 Heparin-induced thrombocytopenia

Element	Comment
Clinical features	Recognized by a falling platelet count (platelet count falls by >50% to <150 × 10^9/L) in a patient receiving unfractionated or (much more rarely) low-molecular-weight heparin, with or without previous exposure to heparin.
	Thrombotic complications (venous and arterial) occur in 20–50%. Bleeding is rare.
	Probability of diagnosis can be assessed by 4T score (Table 102.4).
	Diagnosis proved by the presence of heparin-dependent antibodies.
Differential diagnosis	Sepsis
	Post-transfusion purpura
	Thrombocytopenia caused by other drugs
Management	Seek urgent advice from a haematologist
	Stop heparin
	Use alternative anticoagulant therapy with direct-acting thombin inhibitor (e.g. bivalirudin) or heparinoid (danaparoid) if needed
	The platelet count typically recovers within 4–14 days after stopping heparin
	The risk of thrombosis persists for up to several weeks

Further reading

British Committee for Standards in Haematology: Haemostasis and thrombosis guidelines. http://www
.bcshguidelines.com/4_haematology_guidelines.html?dtype=Haemostasis%20and%20Thrombosis
&dpage=0&sspage=0&ipage=0#gl.

CHAPTER 103

Management of anticoagulation

CATHERINE HILDYARD

Box 103.1

Heparin	An endogenously produced polysaccharide with anticoagulant effects. The form of heparin used clinically is derived from pig or cow intestines. Unfractionated heparin is comprised of different length polysaccharides. Low-molecular-weight heparin (LMWH) is purified to contain the shorter polysaccharides only. Heparins act indirectly by binding to the endogenous anticoagulant anti-thrombin III (AT), enhancing its inhibition of clotting factors. LMWH's predominant anticoagulant effect is mainly through inhibition of factor X, in comparison with unfractionated heparin, which also causes inhibition of thrombin (factor IIa) (Table 103.3). Fondaparinux which consists only of the AT binding domain, has pure anti-factor Xa activity.
Warfarin and other vitamin K antagonists (VKAs)	Deplete the level of the reduced form of vitamin K in the liver, which is required for activation of vitamin K-dependent coagulation factors (factors II (prothrombin), VII, IX and X).

Indications for anticoagulation

In most indications for anticoagulation (Table 103.1), there is broadly equal efficacy and safety of different anticoagulants, and choice may be based on patient and clinician preference. For some indications, and in some clinical contexts, one form of anticoagulation is preferred.

Heparins (Table 103.2 and 103.3)

Table 103.4 provides a regimen for administering unfractionated heparin by infusion, and Table 103.5 shows enoxaparin (a LMWH) dosing by body weight for the treatment of deep vein thrombosis/pulmonary embolism and acute coronary syndrome.

Warfarin and other vitamin K antagonists

As vitamin-K dependent activation occurs at the time of protein synthesis, VKAs do not affect the function of clotting factors that have already been synthesized. While factor VII has a short half-life (around 4–6 h), other factors, for example prothrombin, have a longer half-life (around three days). This means that although the INR may reach therapeutic levels, warfarin does not have a fully effective anticoagulant effect until at least five days after the drug has been started and must be given with LMWH/UFH cover.

The CHA_2DS_2VASc score (Table 103.6) estimates annual risk of stroke or systemic thromboembolism in nonvalvar AF (Table 103.7). All patients with AF, whether paroxysmal, persistent or permanent are at increased

Acute Medicine: A Practical Guide to the Management of Medical Emergencies, Fifth Edition. Edited by David Sprigings and John B. Chambers.
© 2018 John Wiley & Sons Ltd. Published 2018 by John Wiley & Sons Ltd.

Table 103.1 Indications for anticoagulation and recommended anticoagulant.

Indication	Heparins Low-molecular-weight heparin (LMWH) Unfractionated heparin (UFH)	Vitamin K antagonists (VKAs)	Direct-acting oral anticoagulants (DOACs)
Prevention of VTE post-operatively, in hospital inpatients or in patients with high risk of recurrent VTE	Yes	No	Yes
Treatment of VTE	Yes	Yes	Yes
Treatment of VTE in disseminated malignancy	Yes	No	No
Treatment of unstable angina/NSTEMI	Yes	No	No
Atrial fibrillation (AF)	Yes	Yes	Yes
Prevention of mechanical-heart-valve-associated thromboembolic events and thrombosis	No	Yes	No
Bioprosthetic valve replacements in the first three months after surgery	No	Yes	No
Acute peripheral arterial occlusion	Yes (UFH)	No	No
As adjunct to thrombolytic therapy with alteplase	Yes (UFH)	No	No

VTE, venous thromboembolism.

Disseminated malignancy, low-molecular-weight heparin (LMWH) preferred over vitamin K antagonists (VKAs). Direct-acting oral anticoagulants (DOACs) not currently licensed.

Chronic kidney disease stages 4 and 5; estimated glomerular filtration rate (eGFR) <30 mL/min), warfarin or unfractionated heparin (UFH) is preferred over LMWH and DOACs because of predominantly hepatic metabolism. The DOACs are licensed in patients with eGFR 15–30 mL/min at reduced doses.

Table 103.2 Comparison of unfractionated heparin and low-molecular-weight heparin (LMWH).

	Unfractionated heparin	LMWH
Route of administration	Intravenous	Sub-cutaneous
Time to peak action	Immediate onset Time to peak action 2–4 h	3–5 h
Half-life	45 min–1 h	2 h
Metabolism/excretion	Metabolized in reticulo-endothelial system and liver	Metabolized in the liver and excreted by the kidney (approx. 40% renal clearance)
Advantages	More rapid offset may be safer peri-operatively and in bleeding	Wider therapeutic window; therefore does not require monitoring Easier to administer on outpatient basis Lower risk of HIT* and osteoporosis
Disadvantages	Narrow therapeutic window necessitating monitoring Higher risk of HIT*	Longer half-life
Dose adjustments in renal impairment	Nil required	If CrCl <30 mL/min, monitor anti-Xa levels and adjust dose accordingly
Monitoring	1.5–2.5x mid point of normal APTT range or anti-Xa levels if abnormal baseline APTT	Anti-Xa levels: only in severe renal impairment, extremes of body weight, if clot extension occurs while on treatment

* HIT, heparin induced thrombocytopenia.

Table 103.3 Commonly used LMWH products and their anti-Xa activity per mg.

Preparation	Anti-Xa activity/mg
Enoxaparin	100 units/mg
Dalteparin	156 units/mg
Tinzaparin*	70–120 units/mg

*Each formulation contains different anti-factor Xa activity and therefore doses are not interchangeable.

Table 103.4 Unfractionated heparin by infusion.

Loading dose
5000 units IV over 5 min

Infusion
20,000 units made up in saline to 40 mL (500 units/mL). Start the infusion using a syringe pump:

Patient weight (kg)	Heparin dose (480 units/kg/day)	Heparin infusion rate (mL/h)
>70	33,600	2.8
60	28,800	2.4
50	24,000	2.0

Check the activated partial thromboplastin time (APTT) at 4–6 h. Ensure that the request form clearly states the patient is receiving heparin.

Adjust the dose as follows:

Activated partial thromboplastin (APTT) time (target 1.5–2.5 × control)	Action
>5	Stop for 1 h then reduced infusion rate by 1.0 mL/h.
4.1–5	Reduce infusion rate by 0.6 mL/h
3.1–4	Reduce infusion rate by 0.2 mL/h.
2.6–3	Reduce infusion rate by 0.1 mL/h.
1.5–2.5	No change. Recheck APTT in 10 h
1.2–1.4	Increase infusion rate by 0.4 mL/h.
<1.2	Increase infusion rate by 0.8 mL/h.

After each change in infusion rate, recheck APTT in 4–6 h, and every 24 h if stable.
Check the platelet count daily. Heparin-induced thrombocytopenia (HIT), which may be complicated by thrombosis, is most likely to occur 5–10 days after starting heparin. Stop heparin immediately and take advice from a haematologist if there is a significant fall in platelet count. See p. 580 Table 102.3 and p. 582 appendix 102.3 for further information on the diagnosis of HIT.

risk of thromboembolism. Anticoagulation should be considered with a score of ≥2 depending on concurrent risks including the HASBLED score (Table 103.8) which estimates the annual risk of major bleeding for patients on warfarin for atrial fibrillation (Table 103.9). 'Major bleeding' in the original study was defined as bleeding requiring hospitalization and/or blood transfusion and/or a drop in haemoglobin >20 g/L. Unfortunately, patients at the highest risk of stroke in AF are often also at the highest risk of bleeding. A risk score of 3 or more is considered high risk for bleeding and use of anticoagulation is cautioned.

Table 103.5 Example of LWMH dosing: enoxaparin for the treatment of deep vein thrombosis/pulmonary embolism (DVT/PE) and acute coronary syndrome (ACS).

Weight (kg)	Dose for DVT/PE treatment	Dose for ACS treatment
	Subcutaneous administration	Subcutaneous administration
40	60 mg once daily	40 mg twice daily
45	70 mg once daily	45 mg twice daily
50	75 mg once daily	50 mg twice daily
55	85 mg once daily	55 mg twice daily
60	90 mg once daily	60 mg twice daily
65	100 mg once daily	65 mg twice daily
70	105 mg once daily	70 mg twice daily
75	114 mg once daily	75 mg twice daily
80	120 mg once daily	80 mg twice daily
85	126 mg once daily	85 mg twice daily
90	135 mg once daily	90 mg twice daily
95	144 mg once daily	95 mg twice daily
100	100 mg once daily	100 mg twice daily
105	160 mg once daily	105 mg twice daily
110	165 mg once daily	111 mg twice daily
115	175 mg once daily	115 mg twice daily
120	180 mg once daily	120 mg twice daily
125	185 mg once daily	126 mg twice daily

Table 103.6 CHA$_2$DS$_2$VASc score (estimates the annual risk of stroke or systemic thromboembolism in non-valvular AF).

	Variable	Score
C	**Congestive heart failure** or left ventricular systolic dysfunction	1 for yes
H	**Hypertension**	1 for yes
	Blood pressure consistently above 140/90 mmHg (or treated hypertension on medication)	
A$_2$	**Age >75 years**	2 for yes
D	**Diabetes mellitus**	1 for yes
S$_2$	Prior **stroke or TIA or systemic thromboembolism**	2 for yes
V	**Vascular disease** (peripheral arterial disease, coronary artery disease, aortic atheroma)	1 for yes
A	**Age 65–74 years**	1 for yes
Sc	**Sex category**	1 for female
	Total score	0–9
	(as age <65 scores 0, age 65–74 scores 1 and age ≥75 scores 2)	

Table 103.10 lists some of the more common clinical conditions affecting the anticoagulant response to warfarin and Table 103.11 shows a practical method of starting warfarin.

Duration of anticoagulation following VTE and predicting risk of recurrence

At least three months of anticoagulation is advised following of deep venous thrombosis (DVT) and pulmonary embolism (PE). In general, VTE **provoked** by a reversible risk factor (see Chapter 56) has a low probability of

Table 103.7 Cumulative CHA$_2$DS$_2$VASc score and risk of stroke or systemic thromboembolism.

Cumulative CHA$_2$DS$_2$ VASc score	Annual risk of stroke or systemic thromboembolism (%)
0	0.3
1	1.3
2	2.2
3	3.2
4	4
5	6.7
6–8	9.8
9	15.2

Table 103.8 **The HAS-BLED score** (estimates the annual risk of major bleeding for patients on warfarin for atrial fibrillation).

	Variable	Score
H	**Hypertension**	1 for yes, 0 for no
	Systolic BP >160 mmHg	
A	**Abnormal renal or liver function**	1 for yes, 0 for no
	Renal disease:	1 for yes, 0 for no
	Dialysis, transplant or serum creatinine >200 micromol/L	
	Liver disease:	
	Cirrhosis, serum bilirubin >2× normal or AST/ALT/alkaline phosphatase >3× normal	
S	**Stroke history**	1 for yes, 0 for no
B	**Bleeding risk**	1 for yes, 0 for no
	Prior major bleeding or predisposition to bleeding	
L	**Labile INR**	1 for yes, 0 for no
	Time in therapeutic range <60%	
E	**Elderly**	1 for yes, 0 for no
	Age >65	
D	**Drug/alcohol history**	1 for yes, 0 for no
	Medication usage predisposing to bleeding (antiplatelet agents, NSAIDs)	1 for yes, 0 for no
	Alcohol consumption ≥8 units/week	
	Total score	0–9

Table 103.9 Cumulative HAS-BLED score and risk of major bleeding.

HAS-BLED score (1–9)	Annual risk of major bleeding (%)
0	0.9
1	3.4
2	4.1
3	5.8
4	8.9
5–9	9.1

Table 103.10 Clinical conditions affecting the response to warfarin*.

Increased anticoagulation
Impaired liver function
Heart failure
Acute kidney injury or chronic kidney disease
Malabsorptive states
Hyperthyroidism

Decreased anticoagulation
Hypothyroidism
Transfusion of whole blood or fresh frozen plasma
Diet high in vitamin K (green vegetables)
Hereditary resistance to warfarin

* Drug interactions with warfarin are common and can be serious. When starting or stopping a treatment in a patient taking warfarin, check the list in the *British National Formulary* for an interaction.

Table 103.11 Starting warfarin.

Day	International Normalized Ratio (INR), best checked 09.00–10.00 h	Dose of wafarin (mg) to be given that evening (17.00–18.00 h)
1	1.4 or above	Establish cause of coagulation disorder
		Do not start warfarin before discussion with a haematologist
	<1.4	10
2	<1.8	10
	1.8	10
	<1.8	5
3	<2.0	10
	2.0–2.1	5
	2.2–2.3	4.5
	2.4–2.5	4
	2.6–2.7	3.5
	2.8–2.9	3
	3.0–3.1	2.5
	3.2–3.3	2
	3.4	1.5
	3.5	1
	3.6–4.0	0.5
	>4.0	Give none
4	<1.4	Ask advice from a haematologist
	1.4	8
	1.5	7.5
	1.6–1.7	7
	1.8	6.5
	1.9	6
	2.0–2.1	5.5
	2.2–2.3	5
	2.4–2.6	4.5
	2.7–3.0	4
	3.1–3.5	3.5
	3.6–4.0	3
	4.1–4.5	Miss 1 day, then give 2 mg
	>4.5	Miss 2 days, then give 1 mg

Source: Fennerty A, Campbell IA, Routledge PA, *et al.* (1988) Anticoagulants in venous thromboembolism. *British Medical Journal* 297, 1285–8. Reproduced with permission of BMJ Publishing Group Ltd.

recurrence and anticoagulation can be safely stopped after this point. Conversely, if there is an irreversible risk factor, for example incurable disseminated malignancy, indefinite anticoagulation should be considered.

Discuss with a haematologist whether to continue anticoagulation beyond 3 months in **unprovoked** VTE is a difficult one and the advice of a haematologist should be sought. Various factors are normally taken into account, including whether this was a recurrent event; the age and sex of the patient (increased chance of recurrence in patients under the age of 50 years and in males); and post-treatment D-dimer (increased risk of recurrence if elevated). Thrombophilia testing may be considered, **once the patient has completed three months of anticoagulation**, in individuals with a strong family history of VTE or in young patients with recurrent events, but is not recommended in unselected individuals as it is a poor determinant of risk of recurrence. Thrombophilia testing in the acute setting is **not recommended** as results may be affected by acute VTE and by anticoagulation.

National guidelines currently recommend a CT chest/abdomen/pelvis to investigate potential underlying malignancy in all patients over the age of 50 who present with apparently unprovoked VTE, and those under the age of 50 with any index of suspicion raised by clinical history and examination, chest X-ray and urine dipstick testing. Indiscriminate CT scanning of older patients has recently been challenged on the basis of more up-to-date evidence. Hospitals will often have their own local policy.

Direct-acting oral anticoagulants (DOACs)

DOACs are becoming increasingly popular and widely available. They are known as **direct-acting** oral anti-coagulants as they act through direct inhibition of procoagulant factors in the clotting cascade.

They combine the advantages of a convenient oral preparation without need for monitoring, because of a wide therapeutic range and similar pharmacokinetic and pharmacodynamic effects in different individuals. Disadvantages include difficulties in monitoring anticoagulant effect and the fact that they remain harder to reverse than VKAs and heparins, although this is changing as reversal agents are being rapidly developed. They are not recommended for all anticoagulation indications (see Table 103.1). The properties of dabigatran, rivaroxaban and apixaban are compared in Table 103.12.

There are circumstances in which monitoring of DOAC levels may be required (see Table 103.13) and all hospital laboratories should have this capacity. It should be noted that the prothrombin time (PT) and activated partial thromboplastin time (APTT) cannot be used to reliably assess the intensity of anticoagulation.

Table 103.12 Comparison of direct-acting oral anticoagulants.

	Dabigatran	Rivaroxaban	Apixaban
Mechanism	Inhibition of IIa	Inhibition of Xa	Inhibition of Xa
Onset of action	2–3 h post dose	2–3 h post dose	2–3 h post dose
Half-life	12–17 h	7–9 h	9–14 h
Metabolism	20% hepatic; 80% renal	75% hepatic; 25% renal	75% hepatic; 25% renal
Effect on PT (at peak concentration)	Normally <1.5	1.3–1.6	Often normal
Effect on APTT (at peak concentration)	Normally increased	APTT ratio 1.4–1.6	Normally some prolongation
Effect on thrombin time (TT)	Very prolonged	Unaffected	Unaffected
Measurement of anticoagulant effect	Modified thrombin time	Anti-Xa assays	Anti-Xa assays

Table 103.13 Circumstances when measurements of DOACs may be necessary (BSH).

Spontaneous/traumatic haemorrhage
Following suspected overdose
When patients are taking another interacting drug
When patients develop a new thrombosis while on the anticoagulant
When emergency surgery is required
At extremes of body weight
When intestinal adsorption may be a problem

Table 103.14 Dosing of direct oral anticoagulants by indication.

	Dabigatran	Rivaroxaban	Apixaban
Acute VTE	150 mg BD following 5 days of LMWH/UFH	Day 1–21: 15 mg BD Day 22: 20 mg OD	Days 1–7: 10 mg BD Day 7: 5 mg BD
Prevention of recurrent VTE	150 mg BD 110 mg BD*	20 mg OD	2.5 mg BD (after 6 months of 5 mg BD completed)
Thromboprophylaxis	220 mg OD 150 mg OD*	10 mg OD	2.5 mg BD
Atrial fibrillation	150 mg BD 110 mg BD*	20 mg OD	5 mg BD 2.5 mg BD†

*A dose of 150 mg OD for thromboprophylaxis or 110 mg BD for AF/recurrent VTE should be considered in patients >75 years or patients with eGFR <50 mL/min.
†The reduced doses of apixaban and dabigatran in atrial fibrillation are recommded for patients with two of the following: age >60 years, weight <60 kg, serum creatinine >133 micromol/L.

DOACs can be switched to and from heparin on the next scheduled dose. When converting from a DOAC to warfarin, a two-day overlap period should be ensured. When converting from warfarin to a DOAC, the INR should be less than 2.

DOACs have fewer clinically significant drug interactions than warfarin. However, concomitant use of certain drugs should be avoided. Dabigatran, rivaroxaban and apixaban are substrates for the P-gp efflux transporter and the CYP3A4 enzyme complex. Strong inhibitors of these metabolic pathways, such as azole antifungals, HIV protease inhibitors and the immunosuppressants, cyclosporine and tacrolimus are contraindications to use of the DOACs. Use in patients taking weaker inhibitors, for example amiodarone, pozaconazole, quinidine, verapamil and ticagrelor is cautioned. Strong inducers, such as St John's Wort, carbamazepine and phenytoin are also contraindicated. The advice of a pharmacist should be sought.

The dosing of DOACs by indication is shown in Table 103.14.

Management of bleeding in a patient taking an anticoagulant or antiplatelet drug

General measures are summarized in Table 103.15, and specific measures in Tables 103.16–103.18.

Table 103.15 Management of bleeding in a patient taking an anticoagulant or antiplatelet drug.

General measures

Stop the anticoagulant drug

Document the timing and amount of the last drug dose and presence of pre-existing renal or hepatic impairment

Estimate the half-life and length of functional defect induced by the drug

Assess the source of bleeding

Request full blood count, prothrombin time, activated partial thromboplastin time, thrombin time, fibrinogen concentration, creatinine concentration

If available, request a specific laboratory test to measure the antithrombotic effect of the drug

Correct haemodynamic compromise with intravenous fluids and red cell transfusion

Apply mechanical pressure, if possible

Use endoscopic, radiological or surgical measures to achieve haemostasis

Source: British Society for Haematology. Reproduced with permission of John Wiley & Sons.

Table 103.16 Specific measures according to the anticoagulant/antiplatelet agent.

Anticoagulant/antiplatelet	Specific measures
Heparins	
Unfractionated heparin by continuous IV infusion (half-life 1–2 h)	Stop the infusion.
	For rapid reversal in major bleeding, give IV protamine sulphate.
	1 mg protamine neutralizes 80–100 units of heparin.
	If the infusion has been stopped for 30 min or longer, give protamine 25 mg IV by slow injection over 10 min.
	If the infusion has only just been stopped, give protamine 50 mg IV by slow injection over 10 min.
Low-molecular-weight (LMW) heparin	Stop the LMW heparin.
	Check FBC, coagulation screen and fibrinogen.
	Check anti-Xa level.
	If last dose of LMW heparin was <8 h, give protamine.
	1 mg per 100 anti-Xa units of LMW heparin IV, by slow injection over 10 min.
	Consider rFVIIa if there is continued life-threatening bleeding despite protamine sulphate and the time-frame suggests there is residual effect from the LMW heparin contributing to bleeding.
Warfarin and other vitamin K antagonists	For rapid reversal in major bleeding or in head injury*, give prothrombin complex (contains factor IX, together with variable amounts of factors II, VII, and X), available from CSL Behring (Beriplex® P/N) and octapharma (Octaplex®)): give Beriplex or Octaplex 50 units/kg (to a maximum single dose of Beriplex 5000 units or Octaplex 3000 units). Fresh frozen plasma produces suboptimal anticoagulation reversal and should only be used if prothrombin complex is not available.
	Give vitamin K 5–10 mg IV by slow injection.
	For non-major bleeding give 1–3 mg intravenous vitamin K (correction of the INR is seen within 6–8 h; this has a faster time to effect than oral administration).

(continued)

Table 103.16 (*Continued*)

Anticoagulant/antiplatelet	Specific measures
Direct-acting oral anticoagulants	
Dabigatran	Stop dabigatran and ascertain time of last dose.
	Seek advice from a haematologist.
	Consider use of PRAXBIND (idaracizumab): 5 mg bolus by IV injection.
	Consider use of PCC, APCC and rFVIIa.
Rivaroxaban/apixban	Stop drug and ascertain time of last dose.
	Seek advice from a haematologist.
	Consider use of PCC, APCC, rFVIIa.
Antiplatelet agents, for example aspirin, clopidogrel, ticagrelor	Transfuse 2–3 units of platelets.

NB Protamine is contraindicated if the patient has fish allergy. Protamine can cause hypotension, bradycardia and anaphylaxis. At high concentration (if >50 mg administered), it has an anticoagulant effect.

* In head injury sufficient to cause facial or scalp laceration, bruising or haematoma, arrange for urgent CT head. If there is a suspicion of intracerebral bleed, reverse warfarin before the results of the CT head and INR are known. Even in patients with a normal CT head, a supra-therapeutic INR should be corrected with oral or IV vitamin K because of the risk of delayed bleeding. Adapted from: British Society for Haematology.

Table 103.17 Management of over-anticoagulation in a patient taking warfarin or another vitamin K antagonist who is *not* bleeding.

INR	Action
<5	Reduce maintenance dose
5–8	Omit 1–2 doses and reduce maintenance dose
>8	Give 1–5 mg oral vitamin K

Adapted from: British Society for Haematology.

Table 103.18 Safe timing of invasive procedures in patients on anticoagulation.

Anticoagulant	Safe interval between last dose and procedure	Safe interval between procedure and recommencing anticoagulation
Prophylactic LMWH	12 h	4 h
Treatment dose LWMH	24 h	6–8 h
Unfractionated heparin	2–4 h	2–4 h
Rivaroxaban/apixaban	24 h	6–8 h
Dabigatran	24 h	6–8 h

Warfarin and other vitamin K antagonists

Bleeding complications increase significantly when the international normalized ratio (INR) is >5, and rise exponentially above this. Management depends on the INR and according to the presence and severity of bleeding.

The risk of bleeding for patients on warfarin is increased by trauma, age, instability in INR, alcohol-use disorder and organ failure.

Full reversal of anticoagulation in a patient with a mechanical prosthetic heart valve carries a risk of valve thrombosis: discuss management with a haematologist and cardiologist.

If there is unexpected bleeding at therapeutic INR, a structural lesion (e.g. carcinoma of bladder or large bowel) should be investigated for.

Direct-acting oral anticoagulants (DOACs)

Because of the short half-life of these agents, minor bleeding occurring on DOACs can normally be managed by withholding further doses and following general supportive measures. However, more serious or life-threatening bleeding is harder to manage and the advice of a haematologist should be sought.

If bleeding occurs within two hours of the last dose, activated charcoal may be used to prevent intestinal adsorption. Haemodialysis may be partially effective in removing dabigatran but not the other DOACs, because of dabigatran's relatively low binding to plasma proteins.

Prothrombin complex concentrate (PCC), activated prothrombin complex concentrate (APCC) and recombinant FVIIa have all been used in *in vitro* and in animal studies, with partial reversal of anticoagulant effect of the DOACs, but their efficacy in human subjects is not confirmed.

Idaracizumab (Praxbind) is a newly developed and approved monoclonal antibody fragment that binds to and rapidly reverses the anticoagulant effects of dabigatran. Specific antidotes to anti-Xa inhibitors are in development.

Antiplatelet agents

Antiplatelet agents, for example the COX inhibitor, aspirin, and P2Y12 antagonists such as clopidogrel, prasugrel and ticagrelor, cause irreversible platelet inhibition, and therefore, despite their short half-lives, have a prolonged inhibitory effect (up to seven days).

Glycoprotoein IIb/IIIa inhibitors, that block fibrinogen mediated platelet aggregation, for example abcixamab and tirofiban, have a much shorter duration of action (<1 day). Abcixamab can cause profound thrombocytopenia.

Some types of elective surgery, especially cardiac surgery, are performed with the patient still on aspirin, because of the risk of adverse events when the drug is stopped.

Platelet transfusion of 2–3 units should be considered to treat major bleeding that occurs while on antiplatelet agents, or to prevent this during surgery.

Safe timing of invasive procedures in patients on anticoagulation

Apart from in an emergency, for example insertion of a central line in a critically unwell patient, it is safer to allow anticoagulants to be metabolized/excreted rather than attempting to reverse them before a planned invasive procedure (e.g. lumbar puncture, chest drain, ascitic drain), as reversal agents are potentially pro-thrombotic and may expose the patient unnecessarily to plasma products. Safe timing of a procedure requires a knowledge of when the last dose of anticoagulant was taken, the half-life of the drug, the excretion pathway, and any factors in the patient that may alter this, for example deranged renal function.

Further reading

Kearon C, Akl EA, Ornelas J, *et al.* (2016) Antithrombotic therapy for VTE disease: CHEST guideline and expert panel report. *Chest* 149, 315–352.

Keeling D, Tait RC, Watson H. (2016) Peri-operative management of anticoagulation and antiplatelet therapy: A British Society for Haematology Guideline (2016). http://www.bcshguidelines.com/documents/Peri-Op_Wiley_final__01091.pdf.

Mega JL, Simon T (2015) Pharmacology of antithrombotic drugs: an assessment of oral antiplatelet and anticoagulant treatments. *Lancet* 386, 281–291.

CHAPTER 104

Acute painful sickle cell crisis

Jo Howard

Consider painful sickle cell crisis if there is acute pain in the spine, abdomen, chest or joints in a patient of Afro-Caribbean, Arabic or Indian origin. Management is summarized in Figure 104.1.

Priorities

1 Make the diagnosis

- Most patients with sickle cell disease who are having an acute painful crisis will recognize their pain as typical in character and location. If the patient says the pain is unlike their usual sickle pain, consider alternative diagnoses. See the relevant chapters for other causes of acute pain in the chest (Chapter 7), abdomen (Chapter 21), joints (Chapter 28), spine (Chapter 29) and limbs (Chapter 30).
- If the patient does not have a prior diagnosis of sickle cell disease, confirm the diagnosis with a full blood count, blood film and high-pressure liquid chromatography (HPLC) or haemoglobin electrophoresis. Patients with HbSS will usually have Hb 60–90 g/L, but in other genotypes it may be 90–130 g/L. The blood film will show sickle cells, target cells and irregularly contracted or boat cells. Sickle solubility test is positive in sickle trait as well as in sickle cell disease, so if negative will exclude the diagnosis, but if positive does not confirm it.

2 Relieve pain

- Establish the patient's previous requirement for analgesia and how much has been taken in the past 24 h. Most patients will know their usual analgesic regimen or have an individual pain protocol.
- Offer pain relief within 30 min of arrival at hospital (as per NICE guidance). Monitor the level of pain with an age-appropriate pain assessment tool.
- For severe pain or for moderate pain which has not responded to initial analgesia, offer a bolus of strong opioid, for example morphine 5–10 mg SC, IV or PO; oxycodone 2.5–5 mg can be used if morphine-intolerant, with monitoring of oxygen saturation and sedation score.
- For moderate pain where the patient has not yet received any analgesia offer a weak opioid (e.g. codeine).
- All patients should be offered regular paracetamol, NSAID and weak opioid unless contraindicated.
- Do not use pethidine for treatment of acute painful sickle cell crisis because of the risk of fits.

3 Look for precipitating factors and treat these

- Focus the history and examination on detecting evidence of infection, as this is the most common precipitating factor. Patients with sickle cell disease are effectively splenectomized and thus at particular risk of infection with encapsulated bacteria: pneumococcus, meningococcus and H. influenzae type B.
- Low-grade fever may occur without infection (reflecting tissue necrosis).
- Take appropriate microbiological samples (blood, urine and sputum samples and viral swabs), other blood tests and arrange a chest X-ray (Table 104.1).

Acute Medicine: A Practical Guide to the Management of Medical Emergencies, Fifth Edition. Edited by David Sprigings and John B. Chambers.
© 2018 John Wiley & Sons Ltd. Published 2018 by John Wiley & Sons Ltd.

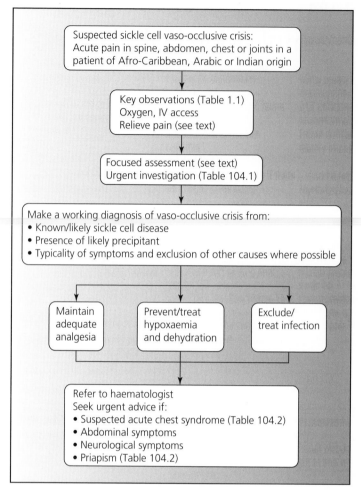

Figure 104.1 Assessment and management of acute painful sickle cell crisis.

Table 104.1 Urgent investigation of suspected painful sickle cell crisis.

Full blood count, blood film, reticulocyte count*

Confirmatory diagnosis (high pressure liquid chromatography) if patient not known to have sickle cell disease or new to hospital[†]

Transfusion compatibility testing (group and screen) if the patient new to hospital or if severely unwell and transfusion may be indicated

Blood culture, urine microscopy and culture and viral screening if patient febrile

Chest X-ray if patient febrile or hypoxic

Arterial blood gases (if oxygen saturation <95%, chest X-ray shadowing or respiratory symptoms)

Electrolytes and creatinine

Liver function tests

C-reactive protein

---

*Blood film in sickle cell disease (homozygous SS): normochromic normocytic anaemia; raised reticulocyte count; Howell-Jolly bodies (reflecting hyposplenism) in adults, usually sickle cells. Numerous target cells may indicate HbSC.

[†] Solubility test indicates the presence of HbS, and is therefore positive in both homozygotes (SS) and heterozygotes (AS, sickle cell trait) and also in compound heterozygotes (S Beta thalassaemia, HbSC).

Table 104.2 Other acute complications of sickle cell disease.

Complication	Clinical features and management
Acute chest syndrome	Chest symptoms or signs with a new infiltrate on chest X-ray.
	It is impossible to distinguish vaso-occlusive infarction from pneumonia with certainty and you should assume that both are present.
	Arterial blood gases are a useful tool for assessing severity and should be done if SaO_2 is <94% on air or >3% below baseline.
	Treat with antibiotics and oxygen to maintain SaO_2 >94%.
	If PaO_2 <9 kPa on air, intervention with transfusion and/or invasive respiratory support should be considered. In this situation haematology and high dependency teams should be consulted.
Stroke	Acute neurological symptoms may indicate infarctive or haemorrhagic stroke, both of which are common in patients with sickle cell disease.
	Arrange urgent CT.
	Exchange transfusion may be required: seek advice from a haematologist.
Priapism	Painful and persistent penile erection.
	If not adequately treated, it may result in permanent erectile failure.
	Initial treatment includes exercise, encourage urination, fluid replacement and pain relief. Oral etilefrine may be of help.
	If >1 h duration and no response to initial management, contact urologist for consideration of penile aspiration.
Splenic sequestration	Common in children. Rapid enlargement of spleen and fall in haemoglobin. Treated supportively with blood transfusion.
Aplastic crisis	Acute anaemia due to parvovirus B19 infection. Characterized by low reticulocyte count. Treated supportively with blood transfusion.

- Antibiotic therapy should be started after cultures have been taken. Use a broad-spectrum penicillin and macrolide if there are chest symptoms; antibiotic choice should depend on local microbiology advice.
- Other precipitating factors include stress, cold weather and dehydration.

4 **Refer to a haematologist for urgent advice if the patient has:**
- Chest, abdominal or neurological symptoms (Table 104.2)
- Priapism
- Pain which is atypical or does not respond to usual analgesia

Further management

Titration of analgesia
- Assess adequacy of pain relief using a pain assessment tool every 30 minutes until pain is relieved and at least four-hourly thereafter. If the patient has ongoing severe pain, offer repeated bolus doses of analgesic.
- Consider Patient Controlled Analgesia (PCA) if repeated bolus doses of analgesic are needed.
- Consider a long-acting opioid (e.g. morphine sulphate modified release).
- Monitor the patient for adverse effects of opioid with repeat observations (including sedation score) hourly for first six hours and at least four-hourly thereafter.
- Refer for haematology review.

Supportive care
- Monitor the patient for other sickle complications, including acute chest syndrome, throughout hospital admission.

- Give an oral laxative, antiemetic and antipruritic while receiving opioid analgesia.
- Consider venous thromboembolism risk and prescribe appropriate prophylaxis.
- Fluids can be taken orally in most patients. Aim for an intake of 3 L/day (in adults). IV fluids should be given if the patient has clinical signs of dehydration, vomiting, diarrhoea, abdominal pain or is unable to take adequate oral fluids.

Blood transfusion

- Blood transfusion is not usually indicated for treatment of a simple painful crisis.
- A decreased haemoglobin (below the patient's baseline) may be caused by increased haemolysis, splenic sequestration (raised reticulocyte count) or aplastic crisis (parvovirus infection, decreased reticulocyte count).
- Do not transfuse without discussion with a haematologist.
- If blood is required please let the transfusion laboratory know that this is for a sickle cell patient and ensure that the blood is matched for full Rh and Kell type.

Reducing analgesia

- Reduce doses of analgesia once pain is under control.
- Introduce oral analgesics as soon as possible, at least 24 h before discharge.

Further reading

Howard J, Hart N, Roberts-Harewood M, *et al.* on behalf of the BCSH Committee (2015) Guideline on the management of acute chest syndrome in sickle cell disease. *British Journal of Haematology*, 169, 492–505. http://onlinelibrary.wiley.com/doi/10.1111/bjh.13348/epdf.

National Institute for Care and Health Excellence (2012) Sickle cell disease: managing acute painful episodes in hospital. Clinical guideline (CG143). https://www.nice.org.uk/guidance/cg143.

CHAPTER 105

Complications of cancer

John B. Chambers and Janine Mansi

Patients with cancer often present acutely, with:

- Complications or progression of cancer (Table 105.1)
- Complications of chemotherapy (Table 105.2) or radiotherapy (Table 105.3)
- New symptoms, with a range of diagnostic possibilities (Tables 105.4–105.10)
    Seek urgent help from the oncology team if the patient is critically ill or you suspect:
- Neutropenic sepsis (Chapter 101)
- Spinal cord compression (Chapter 70)
- Superior vena caval obstruction (Table 105.5)
    Otherwise refer for advice the next day.
    Where possible, before contacting your oncology team, establish:
- The primary origin and staging of the tumour including known spread
- The type and timing of chemotherapy and radiotherapy
- The presence of comorbidities

Table 105.1 Complications or progression of cancer.

Complication	Reference
Superior vena caval (SVC) obstruction	Table 105.5
Upper airway obstruction	Chapter 59
Acute kidney injury	Chapter 25
Bowel obstruction	Chapter 21
Delirium	Chapter 4
Paraneoplastic neurological syndromes	
Pleural effusion	Chapter 12
Cardiac tamponade	Chapter 54
Ascites	Chapter 24
Hyponatraemia	Chapter 85
Hypercalcaemia	Chapter 87
Raised intracranial pressure	Chapter 72
Spinal cord compression	Chapter 70
Deep vein thrombosis	Chapter 56
Pulmonary embolism	Chapter 57

Acute Medicine: A Practical Guide to the Management of Medical Emergencies, Fifth Edition. Edited by David Springings and John B. Chambers.
© 2018 John Wiley & Sons Ltd. Published 2018 by John Wiley & Sons Ltd.

Table 105.2 Complications of chemotherapy.

Complication	Comment
Neutropenic sepsis	Consider neutropenic sepsis in any patient who has received chemotherapy in the previous six weeks and is feeling unwell. Manage as neutropenic sepsis if the temperature is >38 or <36 °C and neutrophil count is <0.5 × 10^9/L. Antibiotic therapy should be given within 1 h of presentation. See Chapter 101.
Tumour lysis syndrome	Results from metabolic derangements as a consequence of tumour breakdown: hyperuricaemia, hyperkalaemia, hyperphosphataemia, hypocalcaemia, uraemia. Usually occurs 12–72 h after start of treatment and presents with lethargy, nausea, vomiting, fluid overload, muscle cramps, cardiac arrythmias, tetany, seizures, syncope or even sudden death. Management: • Hyperuricaemia is best prevented through appropriate use of prophylactic agents, such as xanthine oxidase inhibitors or the newer agent rasburicase. • Appropriate rehydration to reduce acute kidney injury, which may be multifactorial (dehydration, obstructive nephropathy, intrarenal calcification, nephrotoxic drugs). • Management of hypophosphataemia if phosphate level exceeds 2.1 mmol/L. Oral phosphate binding resins may be required. See Chapter 89. • Hypocalcaemia is usually managed with calcium gluconate 50–100 mg/kg cautiously if symptomatic. Need to avoid precipitation of calcium phosphate. See Chapter 87. • Severe hyperkalaemia may require insulin/glucose infusion. See Chapter 86. • Renal replacement therapy may be necessary if uncontrolled hyperkalaemia, hyperphosphataemia or severe acute kidney injury occurs.
Cardiac toxicity	Heart failure: anthracyclines, for example doxorubicin; HER2 receptor inhibitors, for example trastuzumab Acute coronary syndrome: fluorouracil, vincristine Arrhythmia: cisplatinum; alkylating agents, for example cyclophosphamide
Systemic hypertension	Monoclonal antibodies, for example bevacizumab Tyrosine kinase inhibitors, for example sunitinib
Adverse effects of antiangiogenic therapy	Clinical features which may precipitate emergency admission: • Haematological: haemorrhage, neutropenia, thrombocycopenia, thromboembolic events • Gastrointestinal: diarrhoea, dyspepsia, perforation, stomatitis, nausea and vomiting • Cardiovascular: hypertension, cardiac failure • Renal: proteinuria • Cerebrovascular: posterior reversible encephalopathy syndrome Management: Seek urgent advice from a consultant with experience in the management of anti-angiogenic therapy
Abnormal liver function	See Chapter 77
Acute kidney injury	Idiosyncratic: methotrexate, temsirolimus, targeted molecules Dose-dependent: bleomycin, carmustine, busulfan, chlorambucil, taxanes
Thyroid dysfunction	See Chapters 91 and 92
Diabetes	Secondary to corticosteroid therapy See Chapter 82.
Skin abnormalities, for example hand-foot syndrome	Clinical features: Progressive erythema of hands and feet (plantar-palmer erythema) which may progress to pain, cracking or blistering of skin and eventually desquamation with concomitant progressive functional impairment. Management: Stop cytotoxic therapy. Emollients should be applied liberally and frequently. Give antibiotics if secondary infection occurs. Pyridoxine 50–100 mg 8-hourly PO may be helpful. Other skin abnormalities (allergic/hypersensitivity reactions, maculopapular/acneiform rashes may also occur) with certain drugs. See Chapter 26 for assessment of rash.

Table 105.2 (*Continued*)

Complication	Comment
Diarrhoea	See Table 105.7 and Chapter 22.
Posterior reversible encephalopathy syndrome	Also known as posterior leucoencephalopathy syndrome, can present with visual symptoms, increasing confusion, generalized headaches, seizures and hypertension
	May be caused by gemcitabine, cytarabine, cisplatin, bevacizumab, ciclosporin, sunitinib. The diagnosis is confirmed by brain MRI (excluding other possible causes such as brain metastases, intracerebral haemorrhage or infarction) with hyperintense lesions involving the parieto-occipital regions.
	Management:
	Stop the causative agent.
	Closely monitor and treat hypertension, seizures and ensure close monitoring of fluid balance. Symptomatic improvement usually occurs over several days.
	Radiological resolution takes longer.
Lung toxicity	Antibiotics: bleomycin, mitomycin C
	Alkylating agents: carmustine, busulfan
	Antimetabolites: methotrexate, fludarabine
	Taxanes: paclitaxel, docetaxel
	Targeted agents: gefitinib, everolimus, temsirolimus

Table 105.3 Complications of radiotherapy.

Complication	Comment
Pneumonitis	Early: radiation pneumonitis
	Late: radiation-related pulmonary fibrosis
	Clinical features: breathlessness with or without a dry cough.
	Often there may be no clinical signs, but there may be fine crackles.
	Chest X-ray may be normal or show some interstitial shadowing.
	CT chest: ground glass shadowing within the area of the radiotherapy.
	Differential diagnosis includes infection, pulmonary embolism, progression of disease.
	Management: corticosteroids and oxygen.
	Symptoms should improve, but if fibrosis occurs then long-term oxygen may be required.
Head and neck mucositis	Clinical features: oral ulcers, difficulty swallowing, pain
	Management: if patients are unable to manage oral intake, then a percutaneous endoscopic gastrostomy or nasogastric tube may be required.
	Pain relief with opioids.
	Oral hygiene.
Skin toxicity	Clinical features: usually occurs 10–14 days after the start of radiotherapy.
	Symptoms can range from discomfort, erythema to ulceration and functional impairment.
	Secondary infection can occur, causing cellulitis.
	Management: moisturisers, analgesia and treatment of secondary infection (bacterial or fungal).
Pelvic toxicity	Clinical features: acute effects: bowel (diarrhoea and gastrointestinal mucositis), bladder (dysuria, frequency) and skin toxicity
	Late effects: sexual dysfunction, impaired fertility, dysfunction of bowel (urgency and frequency of defaecation) and bladder (rarely incontinence).
	Psychological distress.
	Management: supportive treatment for acute bowel toxicity including hydration and antidiarrhoeal agents (ensure no superadded infection e.g. *C difficile*; see Chapter 22).
	Bladder: oral fluids are important although patients may try to avoid this to reduce the urinary frequency.
Central nervous system toxicity	Clinical features: neurological symptoms can be related to toxicity of treatment or due to disease progression.
	Symptoms of radiation toxicity include nausea, vomiting, somnolence and rarely an encephalopathy.
	Management: symptomatic, corticosteroids (e.g. dexamethasone 8–16 mg daily PO with gastroprotection) may be helpful with encephalopathy.

Table 105.4 Causes of breathlessness in the patient with cancer.

Cause	Onset and progression	Associated clinical features	Investigation	Management options
Upper airway obstruction (Chapter 59)	Relentless progression. May rapidly progress to complete occlusion of airway.	Stridor, wheeze	Flow-volume loop Flexible laryngoscopy CT	Corticosteroids Debulking of intraluminal lesions using endobronchial therapies Stenting of extrinsic compression Radiotherapy
Acute superior vena caval obstruction	Rapid onset and progression of dyspnoea.	Facial swelling Distension of the neck veins Prominent chest wall veins	Ultrasound CT	See Table 105.5
Bronchial obstruction causing lung collapse/consolidation	Gradual onset. Progression over days.	Reduced chest movements, dullness to percussion, breath sounds reduced on affected side.	Chest X-ray Bronchoscopy	Laser therapy Stenting
Pleural effusion (Chapter 12)	Insidious onset. Slow progression over days to weeks.	Reduced chest movements, marked dullness to percussion, breath sounds reduced on affected side.	Chest X-ray Ultrasound Cytology	Aspiration Pleurodesis
Cardiac tamponade (Chapter 54)	Insidious onset. Progression over days to weeks.	Raised jugular venous pressure Pulsus paradoxus	Echocardiography	Pericardiocentesis Pericardial window
Lymphangitis carcinomatosa	Insidious onset. Relentless progression.	Basal crackles	Chest X-ray CT (high-resolution)	Corticosteroids Chemotherapy
Progression of disease			Chest X-ray, CT	
Heart failure		See Chapter 48	BNP/NTproBNP Echocardiogram See Table 105.3	
Radiation pneumonitis **Chemotherapy-induced pneumonitis**	Acute onset Cough		Chest X-ray, CT See Chapters 62 and 63	Dexamethasone
Pneumonia **Pulmonary embolism (Chapter 55)**				Anticoagulation (Chapter 103)

CT, computed tomography; BNP, brain natriuretic peptide; NTproBNP, N-terminal pro-BNP.

Table 105.5 Acute superior vena caval (SVC) obstruction.

Element	Comment
Causes	Two-thirds of cases due to cancer: lung cancer (72%); lymphoma (12%); other cancers (16%) One-third of cases due to non-malignant causes, most often thrombosis associated with intravenous catheter or leads of pacemaker/ICD
Clinical features	Swelling of the face or neck (80%), often with cyanosis or plethora Swelling of the arm (70%) Breathlessness (65%) Cough (50%) Distended neck veins and prominent chest wall collateral veins
Diagnosis	Chest X-ray usually abnormal in cancer-related SVC obstruction, with mediastinal widening (in two-thirds) and pleural effusion (in one-quarter). CT with contrast for definitive diagnosis, or MRI if contrast administration contraindicated
Management of SVC obstruction due to cancer	Seek expert advice Obtain tissue for histological/cytological diagnosis Corticosteroids if suspected lymphoma or thymoma (as steroid-responsive) Radiotherapy/chemotherapy as appropriate to cancer type Stent placement if severe symptoms requiring urgent relief of obstruction

CT, computed tomography; ICD, implantable cardioverter-defibrillator; MRI, magnetic resonance imaging; SVC, superior vena cava.

Table 105.6 Causes of vomiting in the patient with cancer.

Syndrome	Causes	Management	
		First line	Second line
Meningeal irritation or stretch	Intracranial tumour causing raised intracranial pressure Meningeal infiltration by tumour Skull metastases	Dexamethasone Radiotherapy	Add cyclizine or levomepromazine
Abdominal and pelvic tumour	Mesenteric metastases Liver metastases Retroperitoneal cancer Ureteric obstruction	Cyclizine Stent to relieve obstruction	Levomepromazine Treat underlying cause
Malignant bowel obstruction	*Mechanical obstruction* – intrinsic or extrinsic by tumour *Functional obstruction* – intestinal motility disorder caused by malignant involvement of blood supply, bowel muscle or nerves, or paraneoplastic neuropathy	Haloperidol or cyclizine Dexamethasone	Reduce gastric secretions: ranitidine or octreotide Treat underlying cause
Gastric stasis	Opioids and anticholinergic drugs Mechanical resistance to emptying: ascites, hepatomegaly, peptic ulcer, gastritis, tumour Paraneoplastic autonomic failure causing gastroparesis	If starting opioids – metoclopramide or haloperidol	Levomepromazine
Chemically/ metabolically induced	Drugs – opioids, anti-epileptics, cytotoxics, antibiotics, digoxin. Metabolic, for example hypercalcaemia Toxins, for example bacterial exotoxins, tumour necrosis	Treat underlying cause Haloperidol	Cyclizine
Movement-related nausea and vomiting	Abdominal tumours	Levomepromazine	Hyoscine hydrobromide (transdermal patch is an alternative route of administration)
Tumour lysis syndrome		See Table 105.2	

Table 105.7 Causes of diarrhoea in the patient with cancer*.

Cause	Comment	Management
Infection	*C difficile* infection (see Chapter 22)	Oral metronidazole or vancomycin Stop potential causative antibiotics Stop chemotherapy
Mucositis due to chemotherapy	Direct toxicity to mucosa often two weeks after treatment Common after 5-fluorouracil, irinotecan, capecitabine	Mouthwashes with anaesthetic Antifungals Adequate hydration – may require intravenous fluids if unable to swallow
Previous pelvic radiotherapy	See Table 105.3	
GI surgery	As a result of obstruction, altered gastric emptying, altered bile salt flow, bacterial overgrowth, hepatic insufficiency	Seek advice from a gastroenterologist

* Admit if there are adverse features: fever, neutropenia, blood or mucus in stool, dehydration, vomiting, poorly controlled diabetes.
- Start IV fluids
- Start octreotide 100–150 µgm SC daily
- Send stool samples including for *C. difficile* toxin

If there is bloody diarrhoea, neutropenia and right lower quadrant pain and tenderness, manage as neutropenic sepsis.

Table 105.8 Causes of delirium in the patient with cancer.

As well as other causes of delirium (Chapter 4), consider in particular:

Opioid-induced neurotoxicity (may present with agitated confusion: reduce dose of opioid, ensure adequate hydration, use haloperidol if needed to treat agitation)

Brain or meningeal metastases

Hyponatraemia

Hypercalcaemia

Hypomagnaesaemia

Paraneoplastic syndrome

Table 105.9 Causes of pain in the patient with cancer: due to the cancer.

Tissue affected	Mechanism of pain	Characteristics of pain/comments
Bone	Tumour in bone stretching periosteum Pathological fracture caused by lysis of bone by tumour	Continuous, dull, poorly localized pain, worsened by weight bearing or by straining the bone. Severe pain worsened by the slightest passive movement.
Pleura and peritoneum	Infiltration of pleura or peritoneum by tumour	Well-localized sharp pain provoked by inspiration. Non-malignant causes are common (e.g. pulmonary embolism and pneumonia).
Visceral pain	Pain from deep structures of chest, abdomen, or pelvis	Pain poorly localized to the affected viscera and may refer to other sites. May be tender to palpation over affected organ. Non-malignant causes are common.

Table 105.9 (*Continued*)

Tissue affected	Mechanism of pain	Characteristics of pain/comments
Nerve compression pain	Compression of nerve by tumour or bone	Pain may be continuous (e.g. tumour compression) or intermittent (e.g. skeletal instability), but only investigation will differentiate the cause. Reduced sensation or paraesthesiae are common.
Neuropathic pain	Altered spinal and central neurotransmitter levels caused by nerve damage	Unpleasant sensory change (e.g. burning, cold, numb, stabbing) in the distribution of a peripheral nerve or nerve root. Often accompanied by hypersensitivity or allodynia (pain on light touch). May involve the sympathetic system and have a vascular distribution accompanied by sympathetic changes (pallor or flushing, sweating or absence of sweating).
Central nervous system	Spinal cord compression (Chapter 70)	Spinal pain is usually first feature. Motor and sensory signs occur later. Sphincter disturbance is a late sign.
	Cerebral metastases	Headache on lying flat, vomiting, drowsiness, focal neurological deficit.

Table 105.10 Causes of pain in the patient with cancer: other causes.

Mechanism	Comment
Chemotherapy	Severe mucositis can occur as a toxicity of chemotherapy. Peripheral neuropathy, may take longer to develop and very slow to improve. Extravasation of chemotherapy, a rare event.
Radiotherapy	Can cause inflammation and ulceration of exposed mucous membranes (e.g. gut, vagina and bladder). Myelopathy may occur following radiation of the cervical and thoracic spinal cord (tends to develop weeks after treatment and may take up to six months to resolve).
Hormonal therapy	Tumour flare may occur transiently with initiation of luteinizing hormone releasing hormone (LHRH) therapy in patients with prostate cancer. Tumour flare may also occur with hormonal treatment of breast cancer, predominantly tamoxifen.
Indirectly related to cancer	For example pulmonary embolism, peptic ulceration, constipation, infection, pressure ulceration.
Other causes	For example pre-existing arthritis.

Further reading

Marshall E, Young A, Clark PI, Selby S (eds) (2014) *Problem Solving in Acute Oncology*. Published in association with the Association of Cancer Physicians. Clinical Publishing. Oxford.

CHAPTER 106

Alcohol-related problems in acute medicine

DAVID SPRIGINGS

Table 106.1 Taking an alcohol history.

Information needed	Questions to ask
Average weekly alcohol consumption and pattern of drinking • One unit of alcohol equals 10 mL by volume (8 g by weight) of pure alcohol. • The percentage alcohol by volume (abv) of any drink equals the number of units in 1 L of that drink (e.g. a bottle (750 mL) of wine (12% abv) contains 9 units). • Higher-risk drinking is defined as regularly consuming >50 units/week for men and >35 units/week for women.	Do you ever drink alcohol? What do you usually drink? How many times each week do you drink? How much do you have on these occasions? Are there times when you drink more heavily than this?
Is there alcohol dependence?	Do you drink every day? What time of day is your first drink? If you do not drink for a day or miss your first drink of the day, how do you feel? How would you rate alcohol as one of your priorities? Is it sometimes hard to think of anything else? Have you ever needed medication to stop drinking?
Has alcohol caused medical, psychiatric or social problems?	Has alcohol ever caused you any problems in the past? What were these? Has anyone close to you expressed worries about your drinking? Did this cause difficulties between you? Are you concerned about your alcohol use? Has alcohol ever affected your work or ability to sort things out at home? Has alcohol ever got you into trouble with the police (e.g. drink-driving offence)? Is your alcohol use leaving you short of money?

Source: McIntosh C, Chick J (2004) Alcohol and the nervous system. *J Neurol Neurosurg Psych* 75 (III), 16–21. Reproduced with permission of BMJ Publishing Group Ltd.

Acute Medicine: A Practical Guide to the Management of Medical Emergencies, Fifth Edition. Edited by David Sprigings and John B. Chambers.
© 2018 John Wiley & Sons Ltd. Published 2018 by John Wiley & Sons Ltd.

Table 106.2 Common acute medical problems in the patient who drinks heavily.

System	Problems
Neuropsychiatric	Alcohol withdrawal syndrome
	Major seizures related to alcohol withdrawal Wernicke encephalopathy (thiamine deficiency)
	Polyneuropathy
	Depression/anxiety Self-poisoning
Respiratory	Pneumonia (including aspiration pneumonia)
	Smoking-related disorders (~80% of patients with alcohol dependence smoke)
Cardiovascular	Acute atrial fibrillation
	Alcoholic cardiomyopathy
Liver and pancreas	Alcoholic hepatitis
	Acute pancreatitis
	Cirrhosis
	Decompensated chronic liver disease
Alimentary tract	Variceal bleeding
	Alcoholic gastritis
	Poor diet with consequent vitamin deficiencies
Musculoskeletal	Myopathy
	Fractures
Haematological	Macrocytosis
	Anaemia
	Thrombocytopenia
	Leucopenia

Table 106.3 Management of alcohol withdrawal syndrome and Wernicke encephalopathy.

Problem	Features	Management
Alcohol withdrawal syndrome	Signs of autonomic hyperactivity (appear within hours of the last drink, usually peaking within 24–48 h): tremor, sweating, nausea, vomiting, anxiety, agitation Alcohol withdrawal delirium (delirium tremens): acute confusional state, auditory and visual hallucinations, marked autonomic hyperactivity Delirium tremens may be complicated by hyperthermia, hypovolaemia, electrolyte derangement and respiratory infection	Manage severe alcohol withdrawal syndrome on the high-dependency unit General supportive measures: fluid replacement if needed; exclusion of hypoglycaemia; treatment of intercurrent illness (e.g. pneumonia, alcoholic hepatitis); vitamin supplements (vitamin B compound, strong, two tablets daily, thiamine 100 mg 12-hourly PO, and vitamin C 50 mg 12-hourly PO) Mild or moderate withdrawal symptoms: treat with reducing doses of oral chlordiazepoxide Severe withdrawal symptoms: treat initially with IV lorazepam (monitor respiratory rate and oxygen saturation)
Seizures related to alcohol withdrawal	One to six tonic-clonic seizures without focal features which begin within 48 h of stopping drinking May occur up to seven days after stopping drinking if the patient has been taking benzodiazepines	Usually brief and self-limiting and do not require specific treatment. Consider lorazepam to reduce the risk of further seizures. If frequent or prolonged, manage as status epilepticus (Chapter 16). Avoid phenytoin. Exclude/treat hypoglycaemia
Wernicke encephalopathy	Confusional state Nystagmus VI nerve palsy (unable to abduct the eye) Ataxia with wide-based gait; may be unable to stand or walk	Treat with IV thiamine (Pabrinex IV high-potency injection, containing thiamine 250 mg per 10 mL (two ampoules): two pairs of ampoules 8-hourly for two days, then one pair daily for five days, followed by oral thiamine. IV Pabrinex should be given by infusion over 30 min; may cause anaphylaxis.

Further reading

Connon JP, Haber PS, Hall WD (2016) Alcohol use disorders. *Lancet* 387, 988–998.

Simpson SA, Wilson MP, Nordstrom K (2016) Psychiatric emergencies for clinicians: Emergency Department management of alcohol withdrawal. *J Emerg Med* 51, 269–273.

CHAPTER 107

Hypothermia

DAVID SPRIGINGS

Hypothermia is most often seen in the elderly (usually as a consequence of acute illness) and in those living rough (due to the combination of alcohol and cold exposure). Management is summarized in Figure 107.1.

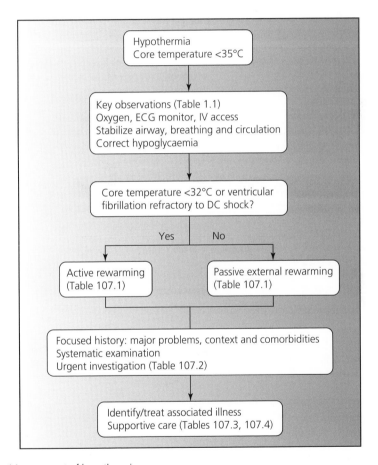

Figure 107.1 Management of hypothermia.

Acute Medicine: A Practical Guide to the Management of Medical Emergencies, Fifth Edition. Edited by David Sprigings and John B. Chambers.
© 2018 John Wiley & Sons Ltd. Published 2018 by John Wiley & Sons Ltd.

Table 107.1 Rewarming methods.

Method	Comment
Passive external rewarming	Indicated for mild hypothermia (core temperature 32–35 °C)
	Nurse in a side room heated to 20–30 °C on a ripple mattress with the blankets supported by a bed cage
	Give warmed, humidified oxygen by facemask IV fluids can be warmed (38–42 °C)
	Aim for a slow rise in core temperature around 0.5 °C per hour
Active rewarming methods	Indicated for moderate (<32–28 °C) and severe (<28 °C) hypothermia
Forced air warming blanket (Bair-Hugger)	Rewarms by blowing air of up to 43 °C into a blanket that lies on or surrounds the patient; may be available in theatre suite
	Rate of rewarming faster than with passive external rewarming; may result in hypotension
Inhalation of warmed oxygen via endotracheal tube	Oxygen is warmed in a waterbath humidifier
	Monitor the gas temperature at the mouth and maintain it around 44 °C: this will require modification of most ventilators
Other methods of active rewarming	Peritoneal dialysis/haemodialysis
	Cardiopulmonary bypass
	Extracorporeal membrane oxygenation

Table 107.2 Urgent investigation in hypothermia.

Blood glucose (raised blood glucose (10–20 mmol/L) is common (due to insulin resistance) and should not be treated with insulin because of the risk of hypoglycaemia on rewarming)

Creatinine and electrolytes (renal failure may be due to hypovolaemia/hypotension and rhabdomyolysis)

Liver function tests

Creatine kinase

Full blood count

C-reactive protein

Arterial pH, gases and lactate (severe hypothermia results in metabolic acidosis)

Blood and urine culture

Thyroid function (if age >50 or suspected thyroid disease) (for later analysis)

Blood and urine for toxicology screen if no other cause for hypothermia is evident

ECG (Figure 107.2)

Chest X-ray

X-ray pelvis and hips if history of a fall or clinical signs of fractured neck of femur

Table 107.3 Management of hypothermia.

Problem	Comment/management
Deranged blood glucose	Treat hypoglycaemia Raised blood glucose (10–20 mmol/L) is common (due to insulin resistance) and should not be treated with insulin because of the risk of hypoglycaemia on rewarming.
Arrhythmias	Ventricular fibrillation may occur at core temperatures below 28–30 °C. Precipitants include central vein cannulation, chest compression, endotracheal intubation and IV injection of epinephrine. DC countershock may not be effective until core temperature is >30 °C. Continue cardiopulmonary resuscitation for longer than usual (as hypothermia protects the brain from ischaemic injury) Sinus bradycardia does not need treatment: temporary pacing is only indicated for complete heart block Atrial fibrillation and other supraventricular arrhythmias are common and usually resolve as core temperature returns to normal
Hypovolaemia/hypotension	Most hypothermic patients are volume depleted (due in part to cold-induced diuresis) If chest X-ray does not show pulmonary oedema, start an IV infusion of normal saline 1 L over 4 h via a warming coil; further fluid therapy should be guided by the blood pressure, central venous pressure and urine output.
Acute kidney Injury	Bladder catheter to monitor urine output. See Chapter 25.
Sepsis	Pneumonia is a common cause and complication of hypothermia: give co-amoxiclav 1.2 g IV or cefotaxime 1 g IV once blood cultures have been taken. Further doses need not be given until the core temperature is >32 °C.
Cause of hypothermia	Hypothermia in the elderly is often the consequence of acute illness (e.g. pneumonia, stroke, myocardial infarction, fractured neck of femur). Consider poisoning with alcohol or psychotropic drugs if no other cause of hypothermia is evident.

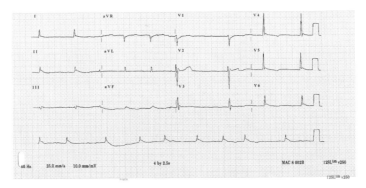

Figure 107.2 ECG in hypothermia (core temperature 30 °C) showing bradycardia, prolongation of ECG intervals, and elevation of the J point in the chest leads giving a J or Osborne wave.

Table 107.4 Monitoring in hypothermia.

Continuous display
ECG
Arterial oxygen saturation by pulse oximeter

Check hourly
Conscious level until fully conscious
Rectal temperature
Respiratory rate
Blood pressure: if systolic BP falls below 100 mmHg reduce the rate of rewarming and give further IV fluid
Central venous pressure (NB do not put in a central line until core temperature is >30 °C as it may precipitate ventricular fibrillation)
Urine output

Check four-hourly
Blood glucose

Further reading

European Resuscitation Council Guidelines (2015) https://cprguidelines.eu/.
Paal P, Gordon L, Strapazzone G, *et al*. (2016) Accidental hypothermia – an update. *Scandinavian Journal of Trauma, Resuscitation and Emergency Medicine* 24, 111. DOI: 10.1186/s13049-016-0303-7 (open access).

CHAPTER 108

Drowning

Francesca Garnham

Drowning is defined as a process resulting in primary respiratory impairment from submersion or immersion in a liquid medium, and is the third commonest cause of accidental death worldwide. The pathophysiology of drowning is summarized in Figure 108.1.

Box 108.1 Drowning – alerts.

> Pitfalls in the management of the patient after drowning include:
>   Missing airway obstruction
>   Missing cervical spine injury or head injury
>   Missing occult haemorrhage
>   Missing the cause of drowning: you should consider alcohol or substance use, epilepsy,
>   acute coronary syndrome, primary arrhythmia (e.g. congenital long QT syndrome), diabetes
>   with hypoglycaemia, or attempted suicide

Priorities

- If there is cardiorespiratory arrest, resuscitate along standard lines. Clear the airway, removing mud and other foreign bodies. Immobilize the cervical spine if trauma is possible or there is no adequate history of the event.

Table 108.1 Clinical assessment of the patient after drowning.

Circumstances of drowning
Quality of water: salt or fresh; clean or contaminated
Immersion/submersion time
CPR required?
- Time to return of spontaneous circulation
- Time to first spontaneous gasp
Alcohol or substance use
Evidence of suicidal intent?
Age
Comorbidities
Current symptoms
Physiological observations and systematic examination (ABCDE method)

Acute Medicine: A Practical Guide to the Management of Medical Emergencies, Fifth Edition. Edited by David Sprigings and John B. Chambers.
© 2018 John Wiley & Sons Ltd. Published 2018 by John Wiley & Sons Ltd.

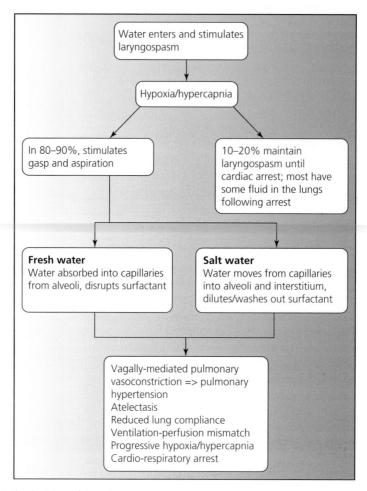

Figure 108.1 Pathophysiology of drowning.

- Maintain a clear airway (Chapter 111), with endotracheal intubation if the patient is comatose (Glasgow Coma Scale score <9). Treat bronchospasm using an inhaled beta agonist. If still hypoxic, consider continuous positive airway pressure (CPAP) or bilevel positive airways pressure (BiPAP) if awake and compliant (see Chapter 112).
- If systolic BP is <80 mmHg in sinus rhythm and the chest is clear, give 500 mL IV crystalloid over 30 min, with further fluid as needed up to 2 L.
- Treat seizures with IV lorazepam (see Chapter 16)
- Check blood glucose and correct hypo- or hyperglycaemia (Chapters 81 and 82).

Key points in the clinical assessment are given in Table 108.1, and investigations needed urgently in Table 108.2.

Table 108.2 Urgent investigation after drowning.

Full blood count (haemorrhage, haemolysis)
Coagulation screen
Electrolytes and creatinine
Glucose (hypo- or hyperglycaemia may be present)
Creatine kinase
Urine stick test for myoglobinuria
Blood alcohol level and urine toxicology screen
ECG (may have changes due to cold (Figure 107.1), myocardial ischaemia, channelopathy (e.g. long QT syndrome), arrhythmia)
Chest X-ray (aspiration, oedema or signs of a foreign body (e.g. segmental atelectasis))
Arterial blood gases and pH
CT head if there are signs of head injury, reduced conscious level or cause of drowning is unclear
Trauma imaging as indicated

Further management

Admit or discharge?

- Discharge following observation for 6–8 h (as acute respiratory distress syndrome may develop over this period) if there is no or only minor immersion/submersion injury at presentation, as evidenced by:
  - Clear history of only brief immersion/submersion
  - Normal conscious level
  - No significant injuries
  - No bronchospasm, tachypnoea or dyspnoea
  - Normal arterial oxygen saturation breathing air and normal arterial blood gases
  - No comorbidities
    Those discharged should be advised to return if they develop cough, dyspnoea or fever.
- Patients with moderate immersion/submersion injury (hypoxaemia corrected by oxygen 35–60%, normal conscious level) should be admitted to a high-dependency unit. Those with severe immersion injury (hypoxaemia despite breathing oxygen 60% or more, or reduced conscious level) should be admitted to an intensive care unit. Monitoring is summarized in Table 108.3.

Table 108.3 Monitoring after drowning with moderate or severe immersion injury.

Respiratory rate
Arterial oxygen saturation
End-tidal CO_2
Heart rate
Blood pressure
ECG
Urine output
Temperature
Conscious level (Glasgow Coma Scale score)
Blood glucose

Table 108.4 Clinical features at presentation after drowning indicating a poor prognosis.

Duration of submersion >5 min
Respiratory or cardiac arrest
Time to effective basic life support >10 min
Resuscitation duration >25 min
Glasgow Coma Scale score <5
Comorbidities and advanced age

Hypoxia

- This may be due to airway obstruction, brain injury, acute respiratory distress syndrome or pneumonia.
- Consider early intubation and mechanical ventilation. High levels of PEEP may be needed due to reduced lung compliance. After endotracheal intubation, insert a nasogastric or orogastric tube to decompress the stomach.
- Bronchoscopy or bronchial lavage may be required to remove foreign bodies and clear debris from the airways.
- Consider extracorporeal membrane oxygenation if adequate oxygenation cannot be achieved by ventilation.

Hypotension

Rewarming causes vasodilation and the patient is likely to require additional fluid resuscitation. If systolic BP remains <90 mmHg despite adequate filling, use ino-pressor therapy (Chapter 2).

Hypothermia

- Hypothermia should be corrected by rewarming: see Chapter 107.
- After cardiopulmonary arrest, hypothermic patients should not be rewarmed to more than 36 °C, and fever should be prevented, for neuroprotection. Body temperature should be maintained at 36 °C for 24 h in patients with moderate coma (some motor response), and no evidence of cerebral oedema on CT scan; a target temperature of 33 °C should be considered for patients with deep coma (loss of motor response or brainstem reflexes), or evidence of cerebral oedema on CT.

Acute kidney injury

- Acute kidney injury may be due to hypoxaemia, hypotension or rhabdomyolysis.
- Management of acute kidney injury is detailed in Chapter 25.

Prophylactic antibiotic or steroid therapy?

There is no benefit from prophylactic corticosteroid or antibiotic therapy unless near drowning occurred in highly contaminated water. In these cases start antibiotic and consider antifungal therapy to cover likely organisms.

Other injuries

Advice should be sought from the appropriate specialist.

Estimating prognosis

Clinical features indicating a poor prognosis are listed in Table 108.4; survival is possible despite these features, especially if hypothermic on arrival.

Further reading

Bierens JJLM, Lunetta P, Tipton M, Warner DS (2016) Physiology of drowning: a review. *Physiology* 31, 147–166. DOI: 10.1152/physiol.00002.2015.
European Resuscitation Council Guidelines (2015) https://cprguidelines.eu/.
WHO website http://www.who.int/mediacentre/factsheets/fs347/en/.

CHAPTER 109

Electrical injury

FRANCESCA GARNHAM AND DAVID SPRIGINGS

Electrical injury is caused by generated electrical current passing through the body, and may include burns, coagulation necrosis of limb arteries, rhabdomyolysis and cardiac arrhythmias (see Table 109.1).

Electrical burns can be direct-contact (potentially causing damage from entry to exit point, with a need to consider the tissues and organs between these two points), electrical arcs (which may cause thermal, flame and direct-current burns), flame (with ignition of clothing) or flash (current does not usually enter the body, but can cause large-surface-area burn, usually only partial thickness) (see Table 109.2).

Management of severe electrical injury consists of resuscitation, with vigorous fluid administration, supportive care on an ICU and involvement of surgical colleagues (plastic, vascular and orthopaedic) to address specific complications (see Table 109.3).

Table 109.1 Effects of electrical injury.

Feature	Lightning	High voltage	Low voltage
Voltage, V	$>30 \times 10^6$	>1000	<600
Current, A	>200,000	<1000	<240
Duration	Instantaneous	Brief	Prolonged
Type of current	DC	DC or AC	Mostly AC
Cardiac arrest	Asystole	Ventricular fibrillation	Ventricular fibrillation
Respiratory arrest	Direct CNS injury	Indirect trauma or titanic contraction respiratory muscles	Tetanic contraction of respiratory muscles
Muscle contraction	Single	Single (DC), tetanic (AC)	Tetanic
Burns	Rare, superficial	Common, deep	Usually superficial
Rhabdomyolysis	Uncommon	Very common	Common
Blunt injury (cause)	Blast effect (shock wave)	Fall (muscle contraction)	Fall (uncommon)
Acute mortality	Very high	Moderate	Low

AC, alternating current; CNS, central nervous system; DC, direct current.

Source: Koumbourlis AC (2002) Electrical injuries. *Crit Care Med* 30, S424–30. Reproduced with permission of Wolters Kluwer Health, Inc.

Acute Medicine: A Practical Guide to the Management of Medical Emergencies, Fifth Edition. Edited by David Sprigings and John B. Chambers.
© 2018 John Wiley & Sons Ltd. Published 2018 by John Wiley & Sons Ltd.

Table 109.2 Investigation after electrical injury.

Blood glucose
Electrolytes and creatinine
Creatine kinase
Troponin
Urine stick test for myoglobinuria
Full blood count
Arterial blood gases and pH
ECG
Chest X-ray
CT/MRI if neurological or ocular injury
Echocardiography if arrhythmia, abnormal ECG or elevated troponin

Table 109.3 Management after electrical injury.

Complication of electrical injury	Comment/management
Burns	Seek advice on management from burns unit
	Patients with burns above the neck may have associated airway/lung injury with respiratory failure
Musculoskeletal injuries	Refer to plastic/orthopedic surgeon
	Fractures, spinal injury, periosteal burns, destruction of bone matrix and osteonecrosis may occur
	Deep electrothermal tissue injury may result in oedema and compartment syndrome
Neurological and ocular injury	Manifestations of electrical injury include paralysis, autonomic dysfunction, secondary complications such as head or spinal injury, ruptured eardrum, hyphema and vitreous haemorrhage
	Arrange CT/MRI if there is evidence of neurological/ocular injury
Cardiac injury	Cardiac contusion may occur
	Incidence of arrhythmia following electrical injury is ~15%, most benign and transient (atrial arrhythmias, first and second-degree atrioventricular block and bundle branch block)
	Monitor ECG; request echocardiography if plasma troponin is raised or if there is significant arrhythmia
Acute kidney injury	May occur due to hypovolaemia (from extravasation of fluid) and rhabdomyolysis (from muscle injury) (Appendix 25.1)
	Fluid resuscitation
	See Chapter 25 for management of acute kidney injury
Injury to abdominal viscera	Damage is uncommon
	Refer to general surgeon if suspected

Further reading

European Resuscitation Council Guidelines (2015) https://cprguidelines.eu/.

CHAPTER 110

Palliative and end-of-life care

LOUISE FREE

Palliative care

Pain management

- Diagnose the cause and consider specific treatment (e.g. antibiotics for cellulitis, fixation of pathological fracture), combined with adjuvant therapy if indicated.
- Pain may be 'total pain' – a combination of psychological, social, spiritual as well as physical pain – therefore, addressing these factors is also important.
- Consider non-pharmacological management of pain alongside analgesics (e.g. heat/cool pads, TENS, complementary therapy).
- Prescribe 'by mouth (oral), by the clock (regularly) and by the ladder' (WHO ladder) (Figure 110.1). Adjuvants (Table 110.1) may be added at any step of the ladder.
- If prescribing opioids, co-prescribe antiemetic and laxative.

Persisting or increasing pain

- Give regular four-hourly doses of immediate-release morphine 5–10 mg PO (lower if the patient is elderly, frail, has liver disease or renal impairment) with equal doses of one-sixth of the total daily dose for breakthrough pain.
- Once a stable daily dose is established, maintenance should be with a modified release preparation.
- Review daily requirements after 24–48 h and adjust the regular and breakthrough doses as needed.
- If the oral route is not possible, drugs may need to be given subcutaneously (SC) via syringe driver using the same principles.

Breathlessness*

- Diagnose the cause and consider specific treatment, if appropriate (Table 110.2).
- Consider non-pharmacological measures before pharmacological therapy (Table 110.3).

Nausea and vomiting*

- Diagnose the cause and consider specific treatment.
- Consider non-pharmacological measures (e.g. reassurance, positioning, placement of a nasogastric tube).
- Ensure appropriate route of administration (parenteral if drug not being absorbed enterally).
- Use stepwise approach to management: start with most appropriate narrow-spectrum antiemetic and either switch to an alternative or add in a second if symptomatic control not achieved (Table 110.4).

---

* Adapted from Beynon T (2014): Guy's, King's and St Thomas's School of Medicine Clinical Teaching Resource: Palliative Care and Symptom Assessment.

Acute Medicine: A Practical Guide to the Management of Medical Emergencies, Fifth Edition. Edited by David Sprigings and John B. Chambers.
© 2018 John Wiley & Sons Ltd. Published 2018 by John Wiley & Sons Ltd.

Box 110.1 Palliative care

'Palliative care is an approach that improves the quality of life of patients and their families facing the problems associated with life-threatening illness, through the prevention and relief of suffering by means of early identification and impeccable assessment and treatment of pain and other problems, physical, psychosocial and spiritual.'

World Health Organization (2013)

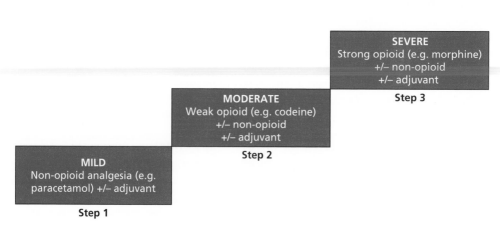

Figure 110.1 WHO Analgesic Ladder.

Table 110.1 Adjuvant analgesics.

Class of drugs	Indication	Example	Adverse effects/comments
Non-steroidal anti-inflammatory drugs (NSAIDs)	Inflammation Bone metastases Soft tissue infiltration	Individual drug choice based on patient's risk factors and adverse effect profile of drug Use PPI cover	Peptic ulceration, bleeding and perforation Arterial thrombosis Renal impairment Fluid retention Avoid in elderly
Steroids	Inflammation Soft tissue infiltration Bone metastases Nerve compression Liver capsule pain Raised intracranial pressure	Dexamethasone (4–8 mg daily, morning dose to reduce insomnia) Titrate down to lowest dose that controls pain Short course with PPI cover	GI irritation and bleeding Fluid retention Cushingoid appearance Diabetes Candidiasis Osteoporosis
Anti-muscarinics	Smooth muscle colic	Hyoscine butylbromide	Dry mouth, constipation, urinary retention, blurred vision, flushing, tachycardia

Table 110.1 (*Continued*)

Class of drugs	Indication	Example	Adverse effects/comments
Bisphosphonates	Painful bone metastases	Various regimens (usually IV infusion)	Hypocalcaemia Flu-like symptoms Osteonecrosis of the jaw (need dental review before commencing)
Neuropathic agents			
Gabapentin	Neuropathic pain (Anticonvulsant)	300 mg PO with starting dose at night and titrate by 300 mg/24 h every 2–3 days (Slower titration in elderly/frail: 100 mg at night and titrate by 100 mg/24 h every 2–3 days)	Mild sedation Tremor Confusion Reduce dose in renal impairment
Pregabalin	Neuropathic pain (Anticonvulsant)	75 mg 12-hourly PO starting dose and titrate at intervals of 3–7 days, in debilitated patients start with 25–50mg BD.	Dizziness, drowsiness (usually improve) Confusion, tremor, dry mouth Reduce dose in renal impairment
Amitriptyline	Neuropathic pain (antidepressant)	10 mg PO with starting dose at night and titrate up after 3–7 days if tolerated	Sedation, dizziness, confusion, dry mouth, constipation, urinary retention Caution in heart failure

Table 110.2 Specific causes of breathlessness and their management.

Cause	Management
Hypoxia	Oxygen (see Chapter 118)
Infection	Antibiotics (see Chapters 62 and 63)
Pulmonary embolism	Anticoagulation (see Chapter 103)
Bronchospasm	Beta-2 agonist by nebuliser (see Chapters 60 and 61)
Pleural effusion	Drainage of effusion (see Chapters 12 and 122)
Heart failure	Diuretic, ACE-inhibitor (see Chapters 47 and 48)
Anaemia	Blood transfusion
Pericardial effusion	Pericardiocentesis (chapter 120)

Table 110.3 Management of breathlessness.

Non-pharmacological measures

Sit the patient up (increases vital capacity and reduces abdominal splinting)
Arrange cool airflow over the patient's face with a fan or by opening a window
Maintain a calm empathic approach and presence
Reassurance
Physiotherapy
Breathing/relaxation exercises
Activity pacing
Complementary therapies

(*continued*)

Table 110.3 (*Continued*)

Pharmacological therapy

Oxygen	May be helpful if patient is hypoxic (i.e. arterial SaO_2 <92%)
Beta-2 agonists	Give salbutamol by inhaler or nebuliser if there is bronchospasm.
Opioids	Start with oral morphine 1 mg as required, if tolerated and beneficial then consider using this regularly every 4 hrs and as required.
	After 2 days: calculate the total dose given over 24 hrs, and use this to recalculate the 4-hourly dose (the new 4-hourly and 'as required' dose is one-sixth of the new total daily dose).
	Once a stable dose has been reached, this can be converted to once- or twice-daily modified-release morphine.
	If the patient is already on regular (analgesic) morphine: increase the dose of regular morphine by 30–50% every 2–3 days until symptoms are controlled, or adverse effects prevent further dose increases.
Anxiolytics	If anxiety-related breathlessness, consider use of long-term anxiolytic (e.g. citalopram).
	For panic-related breathlessness in patient approaching end of life then consider use of low dose lorazepam (0.5 mg to 1 mg up to 12-hourly).

Table 110.4 Antiemetic therapy.

Drug	Receptors	Indications	
Cyclizine	H_1/Muscarinic-ACh	Raised intracranial pressure Motion sickness Inoperable bowel obstruction	
Metoclopramide – central and peripheral action **Domperidone** – peripheral action only	D_2/$5HT_4$	Gastric stasis Gastric irritation Inoperable bowel obstruction if no colic	
Haloperidol	D_2	Opioid induced Metabolic causes Inoperable bowel obstruction	
Ondansetron	$5HT_3$	Chemo/RT Gastric irritation	
Hyoscine butylbromide	Muscarinic-ACh	Inoperable bowel obstruction with colic	
Levomepromazine	D_2/H_1/ Muscarinic-ACh	Broad-spectrum antiemetic, often third-line use	

RT, radiotherapy.

Table 110.5 Common causes of agitation in palliative care and their management.

Identify and treat underlying cause

Pain	Adverse effect of drugs (e.g. opioid toxicity)
Infection	Brain or meningeal metastases
Urinary retention	Electrolyte disorder
Constipation	(e.g. hyponatraemia, hypercalcaemia)
Hypoglycaemia	Paraneoplastic effect

Non-pharmacological measures
Reassure patient and their family
Move to quiet side-room
Nurse in a moderately-lit room

Pharmacological therapy
Only if absolutely necessary; choose doses according to age and physical condition
Haloperidol 1.5–3 mg (0.5–1 mg elderly) once daily at night or 12-hourly (oral or SC)
Benzodiazepine, for example lorazepam 0.5–1 mg sublingual as needed sublingual up to 12-hourly or midazolam 2.5–5 mg SC 12-hourly.

Agitation and delirium

- Common causes and their management are summarised in Table 110.5. Refer also to Chapter 4.
- Terminal agitation describes the condition when a patient is dying and no clear cause can be found for agitation, or agitation is likely to be due to a number of factors which it may not be appropriate to investigate.
- Contact specialist palliative care team for advice if the patient is not settling.

End-of-life care

Recognise the patient is dying
Signs that are commonly seen in the last few days of life include:
- Rapid deterioration in condition (often day by day) despite active treatment
- Increasing weakness – bed-bound, requiring help with personal care
- Barely able to take liquids and unable to take medicines by mouth
- Impaired concentration, muddled thinking and difficulty sustaining conversation
- Increasing drowsiness

Consider potentially reversible disorders contributing to the patient's deterioration
These include infection, acute kidney injury, hypercalcaemia, opioid toxicity, and oversedation. You must decide if treatment is appropriate and whether specialist opinion should be sought.

Communicate with the patient and their family
You should speak to the patient and those close to the patient, involving a translator if needed. Assess the patient's insight into their condition. If the patient does not have capacity, you should consult with those close to the patient and the multidisciplinary team, and make decisions in the best interests of the patient.

Make a plan of care

Elements that should be included in an individualised plan of care are summarised in Table 110.6.

- If the patient is on regular medications for symptom control but is becoming unable to swallow, or is at risk of not absorbing drugs, convert these to subcutaneous administration, for example continuous subcutaneous infusion via syringe driver.
- Ensure the patient has anticipatory subcutaneous symptom control medications written up as required. The as required opioid prescription should be one-sixth of total daily dose of regular opioid.

Table 110.6 Elements that should be included in an individualised plan of care for a patient nearing the end of life.

Review the patient's preferred place of death: is it appropriate or possible to transfer the patient to this place?
Review resuscitation status and ceiling of treatment and ensure up-to-date documents are in the medical record.
Consider deactivation of ICD if present: contact the cardiology service.

Review current medications and discontinue non-essential drugs.
Consider plan for management of diabetes: seek advice from diabetes service (see Further reading).
If the patient is unable to take medication by mouth, give essential medications subcutaneously.
Prescribe as required medications for anticipatory symptom control according to local guidelines (Table 110.7).

Decide if artificial nutrition and hydration should be continued.
Encourage oral intake if not harmful to patient.

Discontinue inappropriate interventions (e.g. observations, turning regimens).
Ensure regular care of the mouth and pressure areas.

Assess and meet the spiritual and psychological needs of the patient and those close to the patient.
Find out how those close to the patient wish to be informed of the patient's death.

Table 110.7 Common symptoms in dying patients for which anticipatory as-required prescribing is appropriate.

Symptom	Drug	Dose for subcutaneous administration*	Comment
Pain	Morphine[†]	2–5 mg up to 2-hourly	
Restlessness or agitation	Midazolam	2–5 mg up to 2-hourly	
Breathlessness	Morphine[†]	1–2 mg up to 2-hourly	
Nausea and vomiting	Haloperidol	0.5–1.5 mg up to 8-hourly	
Retained bronchopulmonary secretions	Glycopyrronium	200–400 µgm up to 4-hourly	

* Usual starting dose in opioid-naive patient with normal renal function; lower doses may be required for elderly or frail patients. For patients with liver or renal impairment (eGFR <50), consult local guidelines or contact palliative care team for advice.
† Opioid drug conversions are given in Table 110.8.

Table 110.8 Opioid drug conversions.

SC morphine is twice as strong as PO morphine
PO oxycodone is twice as strong as PO morphine
SC oxycodone is twice as strong as PO oxycodone
SC diamorphine is three times as strong as PO morphine

PO morphine to SC morphine	÷ 2	for example 10 mg PO morphine = 5 mg SC morphine
PO morphine to PO oxycodone	÷ 2	for example 10 mg PO morphine = 5 mg PO oxycodone
PO oxycodone to SC oxycodone	÷ 2	for example 10 mg PO oxycodone = 5 mg SC oxycodone
PO morphine to SC diamorphine	÷ 3	for example 15 mg PO morphine = 5 mg SC diamorphine

- Review PRN requirement after 24 hrs: if three or more doses were required, consider the need for a continuous subcutaneous infusion, if not already in place.
- If the patient has reliable IV access and difficult to control symptoms (e.g. pulmonary oedema), then the continued use of IV administration (e.g. for diuretics) may be appropriate.

Keep good notes
Details of the plan of care, and summaries of conversations with the patient and family members should be documented in the medical record.

Review the patient
The patient should be seen at least daily; plans should be reviewed. Consider if specialist palliative care advice is needed.

After death
The body of the deceased person should be cared for in accordance with their spiritual and cultural beliefs. Bereavement support should be offered to close family members.

Further reading

Blinderman CD, Billings JA (2015) Comfort care for patients dying in the hospital. *N Engl J Med* 373, 2549–2561.

Diabetes UK (2013). End-of-life diabetes care. Available online at: http://www.diabetes.org.uk/upload/Position%20statements/End-of-life-care-Clinical-recs111113.pdf.

General Medical Council (2010). Treatment and care towards the end of life: good practice in decision making.

National Institute for Health and Care Excellence. Care of dying adults in the last days of life (2015) NICE guideline (NG31). https://www.nice.org.uk/guidance/ng31?unlid=976936892016102725548.

CHAPTER 111

Medicolegal issues in acute medicine

TOM LLOYD AND ANGELIQUE MASTIHI

Autonomy and the right to self-determination are fundamental to the doctor-patient relationship. Consent is therefore required before any examination, investigation or treatment. Failure to obtain consent could open the doctor to a criminal charge of assault or battery, or a finding of misconduct by the regulator.

Age and capacity

The legal age of capacity in England, Wales and Northern Ireland is 18 years, when an individual is assumed to be a competent adult capable of consenting to or refusing treatment, unless other factors prevent them from making informed decisions. The Family Law Reform Act 1969 made provisions for those aged 16 and 17 years; asserting the presumption that the majority of young people had capacity to provide affirmative consent (assent) to investigation or treatment deemed in their best interests, but that could be overruled in exceptional circumstances. In Scotland the age of consent is 16.

Assessment of mental capacity

This can be carried out by any clinician not just psychiatrists or consultants, and must follow the principles set down within the Mental Capacity Act (MCA) 2005. There is a presumption that adults have capacity to make decisions, and therefore unless there is evidence to the contrary, this would be the starting point. Capacity is time and decision-specific, so someone may lack capacity to make one decision but be able to make another. The assessment is in two parts:
- Does the person have 'impairment of, or a disturbance in the functioning of, the mind or brain'? It does not matter whether this is temporary or permanent.
- Does the impairment mean that the person cannot make the decision in question at the time it needs to be made?
  The capacity to make an informed decision depends on the patient:
- Understanding and believing the information relevant to the decision
- Retaining the information

Box 111.1 Valid consent.

For consent to be valid, three criteria must be met:
- The patient must have the mental capacity to make the decision.
- The patient must be fully informed.
- The patient's decision should be voluntary and made without coercion.

Acute Medicine: A Practical Guide to the Management of Medical Emergencies, Fifth Edition. Edited by David Sprigings and John B. Chambers.
© 2018 John Wiley & Sons Ltd. Published 2018 by John Wiley & Sons Ltd.

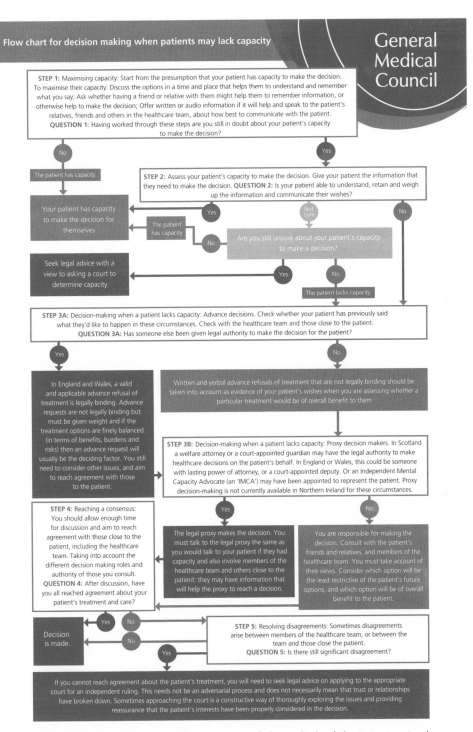

Figure 111.1 Flow chart for decision-making when patients may lack capacity, in relation to treatment and care towards the end of life.
Source: General Medical Council UK. Treatment and care towards the end of life: decision making. http://www .gmc-uk.org/guidance/ethical_guidance/end_of_life_care.asp. Reproduced with permission of GMC.

Table 111.1 The legal framework in which patients are treated. (England & Wales)

Common Law	A number of cases have set out the principles of consent and confidentiality enshrined in professional standards and Government guidelines.
Mental Capacity Act (2005) (MCA) (England & Wales)	The Act, which was enacted in October 2007, was largely based on previous common law and sets down the framework for decision making. It is supported by a Code of Practice and imposes a duty on health-care professionals to follow that code.
	The Code helpfully defines capacity, how it is assessed and how decisions should be made on behalf of those who lack capacity, whether temporarily or permanently, to ensure any steps taken are in the best interests of the individual.
Mental Health Act (2007) (MHA) (England & Wales)	The Act sets down the circumstances in which an individual maybe detained and treated for a mental health condition. It may only be used where it is required to protect the individual or others from serious harm.
	Detention under the Act does not create an assumption of lack of capacity. Therefore, any treatment decisions that do not relate to the patient's mental health disorder requires their consent unless it can be demonstrated they lack the capacity to make that specific decision.

- Using the information to weigh up the pros and cons
- Communicating the decision (although this does not have to be verbally)

A patient is not treated as lacking capacity simply because the doctor or family thinks the decision is unwise.

The unconscious patient or those that lack capacity

In these circumstances, the doctor needs to act in the patient's 'best interests'. The MCA and accompanying code of practice put an onus on the doctor to consult widely to discover whether the patient has any previously expressed wishes. The doctor should avoid making assumptions about the person's past quality of life. If a decision can wait, and it is anticipated that the individual will gain capacity, then the decision should be deferred to allow the patient to decide for themselves. If the decision cannot wait, you should consult the following if they exist:

- Anyone previously named by the patient to consult if they lose capacity
- A close relative or carer
- An attorney appointed under the Lasting Power of Attorney
- Any deputy appointed under the Court of Protection

All reasoning at arriving at a decision should be recorded. This should include who was spoken to and what information was considered. Whilst any medical decisions rest with the doctor, if there is disagreement between you and an attorney under the Lasting Power of Attorney or a family member, and the decision can be safely deferred without harm to the patient then the doctor can:

- Involve an independent medical capacity advocate (IMCA; see below) to act on behalf of the person who lacks capacity to make the decision
- Get a second opinion
- Hold a formal or informal 'best interests' case conference
- Attempt some form of mediation
- Ultimately, if all other attempts to resolve the dispute have failed, the Court of Protection may need to be involved. You would need to approach your hospital solicitors.

The General Medical Council (UK) has issued guidance on decision making when a patient may lack capacity, in relation to treatment and care towards the end of life, summarized in Figure 111.1.

Self-harm

A particular challenge is those patients who present having attempted suicide. You cannot assume that this action renders an individual incapable of making decisions for themselves, and therefore a rapid assessment of capacity in relation to the specific treatment is required. As discussed, a competent adult may refuse life-saving treatment. If they lack capacity, then treatment can be given in their best interests. It is important that assessments and decision making is clearly documented.

There is often confusion between the Mental Health Act and Mental Capacity Act (Table 111.1) The Mental Health Act can be used to detain a patient, should they have a mental health disorder that puts themselves or others at risk of serious harm, but it only allows for the assessment and treatment of the mental illness, and does not allow all medical investigations and treatment. If a patient presents with a possible psychiatric condition, they may require treatment for the condition and therefore close liaison with the psychiatric team would be advisable.

Independent Mental Capacity Advocates (IMCA)

In the acute setting, if time allows, an IMCA may need to be involved with a patient who lacks capacity for decision making, when there is no one else appropriate to consult except paid staff. The MCA code of practice describes three decisions:
- Providing, withholding or stopping serious medical treatment
- Placing people into accommodation (for example a care home or a long-stay hospital)
- Moving people to different long-stay accommodation
    If in doubt, you should discuss your thoughts with an IMCA.

Advance directives

There is no set format for an advance directive. It is valid and should be respected if:
- It is written or verbal (unless concerning life-sustaining treatment, in which case it must be written)
- It is applicable to the specific situation in hand
- The person lacks the capacity to make a decision at the time of consideration
    An advance directive cannot refuse basic care to keep the patient comfortable, but can refuse artificial nutrition and hydration, and other life-sustaining treatment. It must be:
- Written and signed by the patient
- Signed by a witness
- Include a clear statement that the person understands the risk of refusing the treatment
- Be applicable to the specific clinical setting in hand

Lasting Power of Attorney

An individual may appoint a Lasting Power of Attorney (LPA) to make decisions on their behalf when they no longer have capacity. There are two types of LPA: (1) Financial and Property; (2) Personal Welfare. An attorney holding a Personal Welfare LPA can make medical decisions on behalf of a patient if:
- The patient does not have capacity to make the specific decision
- There is no advanced directive, made by the patient, about this particular decision
- It does not relate to life-sustaining treatment
- The patient is not detained under the Mental Health Act

They cannot however:
- Demand treatment that the medical staff feel is inappropriate
- Prohibit life-sustaining treatment, unless, when making the LPA, there was a specific direction applicable to this situation

If there is any disagreement between an attorney or the medical staff as to what the patient's best interests might be, then the case can be brought before the Court of Protection. You will need to discuss this with your hospital's solicitor.

In the absence of a Personal Welfare LPA, an attorney holding the Financial and Property LPA may be considered close to the patient, so that their view on a patient's past wishes should be considered in any discussions of best interests.

Deprivation of Liberty

The Mental Capacity Act Deprivation of Liberty Safeguards (MCA DOLS) provides a legal framework to safeguard the interests of vulnerable individuals, ensuring that any restriction to their movement is kept to the minimum, and their independence maximized as much as is possible. The Supreme Court recently clarified that there is a deprivation of liberty in circumstances where a person is under continuous supervision and control and is not free to leave, and the person lacks capacity to consent to these arrangements. When a hospital identifies that a person who lacks capacity is being deprived of their liberty, they must apply to the local authority for an authorization of deprivation of liberty. Your hospital will have a local procedure to follow in these circumstances.

The patient should be fully informed

The General Medical Council and the courts expect a patient to be given sufficient information to make a decision. Always remember that consent is a process, not a piece of paper, and should include:
- Ensuring that information is easy to understand
- Involving other members of the healthcare team if appropriate
- Ensuring you present the information in a balanced way
- Providing written material or other aids as necessary to assist with the discussion
- Taking into account the nature of the patient's condition, and presenting the relevant risks and benefits
- Checking understanding of risk, because it is possible the patient may interpret the information differently to you
- Discussion of possible serious adverse events of the proposed intervention, however unlikely

The consent process can be delegated to someone who may not be able to perform the intervention or procedure, or will not be doing so. However, this person must be suitably trained and have adequate knowledge about the risks and benefits, and understand their responsibilities to the patient.

Confidentiality

Doctors have a duty to keep information about their patients confidential. Care should be taken whenever communicating verbally or in writing that information is not inadvertently provided to others who are not entitled to know it. Information should not be shared without the consent of the patient. If consent is refused, or the patient lacks capacity, a number of points need to be considered to decide if disclosure is justified. This is normally whether it is in the patient's best interests or in the public interest. Public interest disclosure could be justified if relevant information could prevent harm to a third party or aid the detection, investigation or prosecution of a serious crime. Care should be employed when providing information to relatives to ensure that it is what the patient may have wished.

Confidentiality may be inadvertently breached when:

- Doctors talk about patients in areas where others can overhear, for example the hospital cafeteria
- Medical handover sheets are left in public places
- The data security policy of the Trust is not followed
- Doctors take patient-identifiable information out of the the the work place, such as on memory sticks, to prepare a presentation at home

Further reading

Confidentiality. General Medical Council 2009. http://www.gmc-uk.org/guidance/ethical_guidance/confidentiality.asp.

Department of Health. Reference guide to consent for examination and treatment. 2nd edn 2009. Department of Health. https://www.gov.uk/government/uploads/system/uploads/attachment_data/file/138296/dh_103653__1_.pdf.

GMC guidance: 'Consent: patients and doctors making decisions together'. http://www.gmc-uk.org/guidance/ethical_guidance/consent_guidance_index.asp.

Mental Capacity Act 2005. Assessments under the Deprivation of liberty Safeguards (MCA DOLS) http://www.medicalprotection.org/uk/resources/factsheets/england/england-factsheets/uk-mental-capacity-act-2005-assessments-under-the-deprivation-of-liberty-safeguards-(mca-dols).

Mental Capacity Act 2005. Code of Practice. Department of Constitutional affairs 2007. https://www.gov.uk/government/uploads/system/uploads/attachment_data/file/497253/Mental-capacity-act-code-of-practice.pdf.

Techniques and Procedures in Acute Medicine

CHAPTER 112

Airway management

Matthew Frise

Management of the upper airway, which runs from the mouth and nose to the carina, has two fundamental aims:
- Maintenance of a patent passage for free movement of gas between the atmosphere and the aveoli.
- Prevention of soiling of the lungs by vomitus or other material.

Non-invasive techniques

Manual manipulation of the airway

Head tilt and chin lift – can be enough to relieve airway obstruction in a patient with reduced consciousness (Figure 112.1).

Jaw thrust – preferred if there is concern over an unstable cervical spine (Figure 112.2).

Suction
- If vomit, secretions, or other debris is present in the oropharynx, these can be removed with a wide-bore rigid Yankauer sucker, to relieve obstruction and prevent aspiration.
- A flexible suction catheter can also be passed through an oro- or nasopharyngeal airway.
- Care must be taken not to cause mucosal injury and bleeding; provoking vomiting or laryngospasm are also risks in semi-conscious patients.

Oropharyngeal airway
- In an unconscious patient, obstruction may occur in an anatomically normal airway owing to loss of muscle tone with collapse at the level of the soft palate, epiglottis or tongue base. An oropharyngeal (Guedel) airway may restore airway patency sufficiently for spontaneous or bag-mask ventilation.
- The length should approximate to that from the angle of the mandible to the incisors; insert with the concavity facing the palate and rotate 180° into final position (Figure 112.3).
- Obstruction may be worsened if the epiglottis is pushed against the laryngeal inlet or the tongue displaced posteriorly; laryngospasm may also result – try a smaller size or nasopharyngeal airway if so.

Nasopharyngeal airway
- As an alternative to the oropharyngeal airway, a soft lubricated tube may be inserted into the nostril. Remember that that the floor of the nose is horizontal.
- Often better tolerated in patients with a reduced conscious level than the oropharyngeal airway.
- Epistaxis may result, and if too long, laryngospasm and vomiting are risks, as with an oropharyngeal airway.
- Contraindicated in patients with known or suspected base of skull fracture.

Acute Medicine: A Practical Guide to the Management of Medical Emergencies, Fifth Edition. Edited by David Sprigings and John B. Chambers.
© 2018 John Wiley & Sons Ltd. Published 2018 by John Wiley & Sons Ltd.

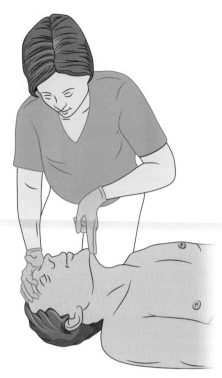

Figure 112.1 Head tilt and chin lift. (Redrawn from European Resuscitation Council Guidelines for Resuscitation 2005)

Bag-mask ventilation

- Rather than an airway management technique per se, this is a treatment for inadequate ventilation, usually in an unconscious patient with upper airway obstruction.
- Inadequate ventilation due to a poor seal can be improved by repositioning or a two-handed technique (Figure 112.4); bearded and edentulous patients can be a particular management problem. Keep well-fitting dentures in place.

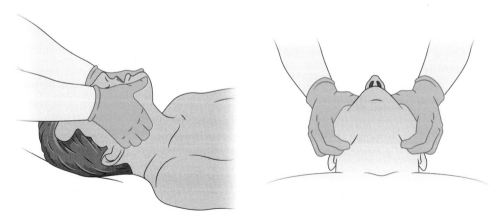

Figure 112.2 Jaw thrust. (Redrawn from European Resuscitation Council Guidelines for Resuscitation 2005)

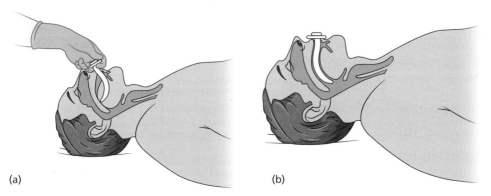

(a)   (b)

Figure 112.3 Insertion of an oropharyngeal (Guedel) airway. The device may be inserted upside-down (a) before rotation into final position (b). (Redrawn from European Resuscitation Council Guidelines for Resuscitation 2005)

- Some devices feature a positive end-expiratory pressure (PEEP) valve, which is very useful for managing airway obstruction due to laryngospasm.
- Over-ventilation may cause barotrauma, pneumothorax or cardiovascular compromise and should be avoided; gastric insufflation increases the risk of vomiting and aspiration. Aim for a tidal volume of 6–10 mL/kg.

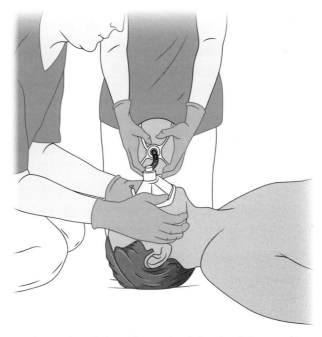

Figure 112.4 Two-person bag-mask ventilation with a two-handed mask technique to achieve a good seal. Note the positioning of the patient's head and the use of jaw thrust. (Redrawn from European Resuscitation Council Guidelines for Resuscitation 2005)

Supraglottic airway: laryngeal mask airway (LMA™) and i-gel®

- The LMA is inserted blindly into the oropharynx to sit over the laryngeal inlet, with an inflatable low-pressure seal. It is not a definitive airway and does not allow ventilation with high airway pressures nor provide the same level of protection against soiling as a cuffed endotracheal tube (ETT).
- Even in inexperienced hands the rate of successful insertion is high, making LMAs very useful in the emergency setting. ALS guidance now recommends that an LMA is preferred initially over attempted endotracheal intubation in the management of cardiorespiratory arrest.
- The i-gel® – like an LMA but with a soft, non-inflatable cuff – is increasingly used in preference to the classical LMA. Familiarize yourself with the particular supraglottic airways available on your cardiac arrest trolleys in advance of needing one.
- Supraglottic airways are not helpful if there is obstruction at or below the larynx.

Endotracheal intubation

A GCS of ≤8 is often taken as an indication to intubate a patient for airway protection, but this practice originates from work in trauma patients. Any degree of impairment of consciousness is associated with increased risk of aspiration pneumonia, though many medical patients in this category may reasonably be managed in a closely monitored environment with equipment and personnel on hand to intervene if necessary. Testing the gag reflex is not useful for predicting aspiration risk.

Endotracheal intubation provides a definitive airway, permitting mechanical ventilation (with high airway pressures if needed) and protection from aspiration, and is therefore considered a gold standard. However, there are several caveats:

- Cardiac arrest – guidance now emphasizes the harm that may result from interruption of cardiac massage by repeated intubation attempts; the LMA is preferred unless a critical care physician or anaesthetist is immediately on hand.
- Mechanical UAO – airway anatomy may be seriously distorted, leading to difficult intubation. The decision to sedate, paralyse and attempt endotracheal intubation with direct laryngoscopy should only be taken by a clinician with appropriate expertise.
- The comatose patient – if airway protection is the primary aim, intubation may be straightforward, but measures to reduce the risk of aspiration during the procedure should be employed. These include cricoid pressure during a rapid-sequence induction (RSI) and placement of a nasogastric tube to empty the stomach beforehand; though this has the potential itself to provoke vomiting and aspiration.

If intubation is performed, it is essential to confirm correct tube placement by a combination of methods rather than any one in isolation:

- Direct visualization – the tube is seen to pass between the vocal cords.
- Measurement of expired carbon dioxide by capnography – many resuscitation trolleys include indicator devices that can be attached to the endotracheal tube to detect carbon dioxide. Beware false-positive results from initial breaths after oesophageal intubation with an insufflated stomach, and false-negative results in cardiac arrest.
- Auscultation over the epigastrium and the thorax bilaterally.
- Portable CXR – to confirm where the tip of the tube lies and exclude complications such as pneumothorax.
  Complications of endotracheal intubation:
- Failure
- Inadvertent oesophageal intubation – devastating if unrecognized
- Laryngeal trauma
- Aspiration
- Cardiovascular instability from laryngeal stimulation and anaesthetic drugs

- Post-extubation airway obstruction
- Laryngeal and tracheal stenosis (late)

The Combitube (oesophageal-tracheal double-lumen airway) has been developed to have the benefits of a cuffed ETT but with easy insertion. It is blindly inserted into the oropharynx and ventilation can be delivered via either of two ports, depending on where the device has settled. If unfamiliar with this device it is better to use an LMA.

Surgical airway

Surgical techniques to establish an airway are appropriate in the acute setting if other approaches have failed or are contraindicated, or in the presence of upper airway obstruction that is unlikely to resolve quickly. A formal surgical tracheostomy may also be fashioned if there is an anticipated need for prolonged mechanical ventilation or tracheal toilet, and avoids the need for sedative and analgesic medication to promote ETT tolerance. For management of the patient with complications relating to an existing tracheostomy, and details of emergent surgical airway techniques, see Chapter 59 which discusses the approach to the patient with upper airway obstruction.

Further reading

Bernhard M, Benger JR (2015) Airway management during cardiopulmonary resuscitation. *Curr Opin Crit Care* 21, 183–187. DOI: 10.1097/MCC.0000000000000201.

Davies JD, Costa BK, Asciutto AJ (2014) Approaches to manual ventilation. *Respir Care* 59, 810–822. DOI: 10.4187/respcare.03060.

Lighthall G, Harrison TK, Chu LF (2013) Videos in clinical medicine: Laryngeal mask airway in medical emergencies. *N Engl J Med* 369, e26. http://www.nejm.org/doi/full/10.1056/NEJMvcm0909669.

Ortega R, Mehio AK, Woo A, Hafez DH (2007) Videos in clinical medicine. Positive-pressure ventilation with a face mask and a bag-valve device. *N Engl J Med* 357, e4. http://www.nejm.org/doi/full/10.1056/NEJMvcm071298.

CHAPTER 113

Non-invasive ventilation

Christopher Turnbull

Non-invasive ventilation (NIV) refers to systems which support gas exchange between the atmosphere and the lungs without the need for endotracheal intubation or tracheostomy.

The two main uses of NIV in acute medicine are:

- Management of acute type 2 respiratory failure (T2RF) complicating an exacerbation of chronic obstructive pulmonary disease (COPD) (Chapter 61; Figure 61.1), when it can reduce the need for invasive ventilation and improve survival.
- Management of patients with chronic T2RF maintained on home NIV presenting with worsening respiratory failure.

Less commonly, acute decompensated T2RF is the first presentation of chronic diseases causing T2RF (kyphoscoliosis, spinal injuries, neuromuscular diseases, e.g. motor neuron disease, or morbid obesity) and may require similar management with NIV.

Contraindications to the use of NIV are summarized in Table 113.1. When a relative contraindication is present, NIV may be considered on the ward, if invasive ventilation and ICU care is inappropriate.

NIV is often ineffective in treating severe hypoxaemia, as oxygen delivery is not controlled and depends on the pressure settings of the machine.

Non-invasive ventilation in exacerbation of COPD

NIV should be considered for respiratory acidosis which persists despite maximal medical therapy given within 60 min of admission (pH 7.25–7.35, PaCO$_2$ >6 kPa (>45 mmHg)). The patient should be conscious and cooperative, and the treatment should be in keeping with the patient's wishes.

Immediate maximal medical therapy consists of:

- Salbutamol 2.5–5 mg by nebulizer
- Ipratropium 500 µgm by nebulizer
- Prednisolone 30 mg PO (hydrocortisone 100 mg IV if oral route not possible)
- Antibiotic therapy where indicated
- Controlled oxygen using a Venturi system (see Chapter 118)

Before starting NIV, a plan of management should be decided and documented, with consultant involvement. Options include:

- Requires immediate intubation and ventilation
- Suitable for NIV and suitable for escalation to intensive care treatment/intubation and ventilation if required
- Suitable for NIV but not suitable for escalation to intensive care treatment/intubation and ventilation
- Not suitable for NIV but for full active medical management
- Palliative care agreed as most appropriate management

Acute Medicine: A Practical Guide to the Management of Medical Emergencies, Fifth Edition. Edited by David Sprigings and John B. Chambers.
© 2018 John Wiley & Sons Ltd. Published 2018 by John Wiley & Sons Ltd.

Table 113.1 Contraindications to NIV.

Absolute contraindications to NIV	Relative contraindications to NIV
Impending respiratory arrest*	Confusion or agitation
Upper airway obstruction*	Diagnosis of pneumonia
Glasgow Coma Scale score <8*	Severe hypoxaemia
Respiratory rate <8 breaths/min*	Haemodynamic instability
Asthma*	Copious respiratory secretions
Undrained pneumothorax	Vomiting
	Bowel obstruction
	Facial burns or trauma
	Upper airway or upper GI surgery
	Arterial pH < 7.25

* In all these settings invasive ventilation should be considered.

Set-up of non-invasive ventilation

NIV should be prescribed by a doctor trained in the use of NIV, and delivered in a setting where it can be managed by experienced staff (e.g. nurses and NIV physiotherapists working in ICUs, HDUs, acute medical units or respiratory wards).

NIV typically refers to bi-level ventilation delivering two set pressures:
- IPAP: the inspiratory positive airways pressure that delivers the pressure support required to ventilate the patient
- EPAP: the expiratory positive airways pressure that recruits under-ventilated areas of the lungs and holds the airways open

The set-up of bilevel NIV is summarized in Table 113.2.

CPAP is another form of NIV that provides one fixed pressure and is used mainly to improve oxygenation in type 1 respiratory failure due to cardiogenic pulmonary oedema (Chapter 47).

Up to 30% of patients are unable to tolerate NIV; the set-up is crucial to its success. Time spent with the patient in the first 30 min helps to reassure the patient and prevents future problems.

Management of the patient receiving non-invasive ventilation

- Patients receiving NIV outside HDU/ICU should have continuous ECG and pulse oximetry monitoring for the first 12 h, and physiological observations recorded every 15 min for the first 2 h.

Table 113.2 Checklist for set-up of NIV (bi-level NIV).

Explain the treatment to the patient.
Use a well-fitting full-face mask (sized to the patient, small, medium or large).
Start at low pressures tolerated by most patients:
- IPAP of 10 cm H_2O
- EPAP of 4 cm H_2O

Other settings at default levels.
Allow the patient to hold the mask over their face without the straps tightened.
Tighten the straps to form a seal around the face, but not so tight as to squash the membranes of the mask.
Increase the IPAP in increments of 2–5 cm H_2O approximately 5 cm H_2O every 10 min to a target IPAP of 20 cm H_2O or to the maximum tolerated by the patient. In general, an EPAP of 4–8 cm H_2O should be adequate for patients with exacerbation of COPD; EPAP >10 cm H_2O is poorly tolerated.

- An arterial blood gas should be repeated 1 and 4 h after initiating NIV to assess response: if the patient is clinically better and blood gases are improved then continue with current pressures; if the patient is deteriorating or failing to improve adequately it may be necessary to escalate to invasive ventilation at this stage.
- Problem solving is summarized in Table 113.3.

Weaning of non-invasive ventilation

- In general, patients require NIV for 48–72 h after presentation:
  - Day 1 continual NIV with breaks for meals, drinks, administration of medications by mouth or nebulizer
  - Day 2 NIV for 16 h
  - Day 3 NIV for 12 h including 6–8 h overnight
  - Discontinue NIV day 4 unless continuing therapy indicated
- Some patients will self-wean earlier and others may need longer. Weaning should be guided by clinical impression and blood gases.
- Failure to wean or recurrent admissions with decompensated T2RF are indications for consideration of long-term home NIV.

Problems

Higher pressures needed

Some patients (e.g. obstructive sleep apnoea, obesity hypoventilation syndrome) may require a higher EPAP to maintain adequate ventilation. Consider higher EPAP of 8–12 cm H_2O and also increase the IPAP aiming for a difference between EPAP and IPAP of ≥ 10 cm H_2O where tolerated.

Table 113.3 Problem-solving in NIV.

If the patient receiving NIV is not improving, consider:

Chest physiotherapy, if the patient has copious secretions.

Is medical therapy maximal? Nebulizers can be entrained into the NIV circuit but in general, where possible, should be given off NIV as the delivery rate is not controlled on NIV.

Has a complication such as pneumothorax or aspiration pneumonia developed?

Consider whether the oxygen delivery is excessive; oxygen can be added at a flow rate of 1–4 L/min, target arterial oxygen saturation of 88–92%.

Check NIV is working:

- Switched on
- Connected
- Not alarming
- Delivering a pressure at the mask end

Check for a mask leak, and if present adjust the mask. Loosen straps and reseat the mask. Do not simply tighten the straps, as this can squash the membranes and increase the risk of nasal bridge ulceration. Nasogastric tubes, if needed, should be fine-bore to reduce mask leak.

Persistent hypercapnia, when none of the above applies, is likely to be due to inadequate ventilation. If continuing with ward based NIV in general the next step would be to increase the IPAP by an increment of 2–5 cm H_2O (most machines deliver a maximal IPAP of ~30 cm H_2O).

In the case of persistent hypoxia consider increasing the FiO_2 or increasing the EPAP.

Arterial blood gases should be rechecked one hour after changing NIV settings.

Breathing asynchrony

Breathing asynchrony, one of the commonest reasons for patients failing on NIV, is when the patient's breathing is not coordinated with the NIV. From the end of the bed, look for chest wall movements and timing of breathing with NIV. If asynchrony is detected, seek expert help. Changes can be made to trigger sensitivity, inspiratory and expiratory times and back-up breathing rate as appropriate.

Nasal bridge ulceration

Ulceration of the skin of the nasal bridge from a tightly or poorly-fitting mask is a common problem. Regular checks of skin integrity should be performed, as well as checking for mask leak, as air leaks can cause corneal injury. If there is incipient ulceration, consider changing to a different mask interface such as nasal cushions or pillows and seeking advice from a tissue viability team.

Admissions in patients on long-term home NIV

Increasing numbers of patients are being cared for in the community with home NIV. It is important to review the ventilatory status as part of any admission in this group:
- Assess for symptoms of excessive daytime sleepiness (indicative of sleep fragmentation)
- Ask about early morning headaches (indicative of persisting hypercapnia)
- Enquire about snoring whilst on NIV (may suggest inadequate pressures to keep the upper airways patent)
- Check daytime arterial oxygen saturation: are the oxygen saturations < 92% on air?
    These features may indicate inadequate treatment. Check arterial or capillary blood gases and seek specialist advice.
    When admitted with unrelated problems, patients have occasionally had their NIV omitted in error. Ongoing NIV is crucial to prevent decompensation, and should be continued unless a contraindication has developed.
    Use the patient's own NIV where possible. Inform the respiratory team/team responsible for their NIV therapy. In those who have presented with worsening/decompensated T2RF, both the respiratory and intensivecare teams should be involved as appropriate. The reasons for deterioration include:
- Presenting condition worsens respiratory function, for example pneumonia
- Decreased use of NIV prior to admission, for example because of vomiting
- NIV not tolerated
- NIV interface no longer adequate
- High mask leak
- Settings no longer adequate, for example following weight gain
- Worsening of underlying condition
    Identify and treat the underlying cause and consider either increasing the hours of NIV usage or increasing the NIV pressure settings.
    Many patients on NIV have a poor prognosis because of the underlying diagnosis:
- Check if they have advanced care plans
- Check current or previously expressed wishes about future treatments, such as 24 h-a-day NIV use, invasive ventilation and resuscitation
- Consider palliative care involvement
- NIV can be weaned in end-of-life care if wished by the patient and a protocol for weaning NIV in this setting should be followed

Further reading

Davidson AC, Banham S, Elliott M, *et al*. (2016) British Thoracic Society/Intensive Care Society Acute
  Hypercapnic Respiratory Failure Guideline Development Group. 2016 BTS/ICS Guidelines for the ventilatory
  management of acute hypercapnic respiratory failure in adults. *Thorax* 71, ii1–ii35. https://www.brit-
  thoracic.org.uk/document-library/clinical-information/acute-hypercapnic-respiratory-failure/bts-guidelines-
  for-ventilatory-management-of-ahrf/.
Kelly CR, Higgins AR, Chandra SN (2015) Videos in clinical medicine. Non-invasive positive-pressure ventilation.
  N Engl J Med 372, e30. http://www.nejm.org/doi/full/10.1056/NEJMvcm1313336.

CHAPTER 114

Ultrasonography in acute medicine

JOHN B. CHAMBERS, NADIA SHORT, AND LUNA GARGANI

Emergency ultrasonography is useful for the presentations in Table 114.1.

- It is more accurate than a chest X-ray for the detection of pleural fluid. It can be used to guide chest drain insertion for those who have approved British Thoracic Society training (Chapter 122).
- A bladder scan as part of the abdominal examination can assess the amount of urine in the bladder pre- and post-voiding.
- Ultrasonography can also be used to identify peripheral veins for venepuncture or cannulation, or central veins for the insertion of central lines (Chapter 116).
- Practical aspects are summarized in Table 114.2.

Surgical applications (e.g. diagnosis of ruptured abdominal aortic aneurysms or traumatic intraperitoneal bleeds) are not described in this chapter.

Cardiac scan

- The ALS mnemonic '4Hs and 4Ts' (Table 114.3) summarizes the potentially reversible causes of hypotension, shock and cardiac arrest (Chapters 2 and 6). The findings in these conditions are shown in Table 114.4.
- In a cardiac arrest the cardiac scan can be performed in the 5s pulse check of the Advanced Life Support Resuscitation Council algorithm of 'non-shockable' rhythms.
- A motionless, asystolic heart at CPR is associated with a positive predictive value of 97% death.
- Cardiac ultrasonography at the time of chest pain may help to exclude myocardial ischaemia and to differentiate between an acute coronary syndrome and pericarditis (Chapter 7). Note that:
  - Left ventricular wall-motion analysis can be difficult and should be performed by an accredited echocardiographer.
  - The cardiac scan should be interpreted within the clinical context, including troponin levels.

Box 114.1 Ultrasonography in acute medicine

- Portable and hand-held devices allow echocardiography to be used as an extension of the clinical examination, providing bedside information about the heart, lungs and abdomen.
- These scans guide immediate management and the need for further tests.
- They do not replace definitive ultrasound scans and are potentially dangerous if the operator is not adequately trained and supervised.

Acute Medicine: A Practical Guide to the Management of Medical Emergencies, Fifth Edition. Edited by David Sprigings and John B. Chambers.
© 2018 John Wiley & Sons Ltd. Published 2018 by John Wiley & Sons Ltd.

Table 114.1 Indications for emergency ultrasonography.

Clinical scenario	Cardiac scan	Thoracic scan	Abdominal scan
Cardiac arrest/peri-arrest/hypotension/shock	+	(+)*	(+)†
Pulmonary oedema	+	+	
Breathlessness/hypoxaemia	+	+	
Lower respiratory tract infection	+	+	
Chest pain	+	(+)	
Abdominal pain			+†

*To exclude tension pneumothorax.
†In suspected rupture of abdominal aortic aneurysm.

Table 114.2 Practical guide to emergency ultrasonography.

Always optimize gain, depth and window sector size.

Cardiac scan

Probe:
• Cardiac

Positioning:
• Left lateral
• Supine (subcostal view)

Views:
• Parasternal long-axis
• Parasternal short-axis
• Apical four-chamber
• Subcostal

Uses:
Loading conditions
Critical pathology in four areas of the heart:
• The left ventricle
• The right ventricle
• Valve stenosis and regurgitation
• Pericardial effusion

Abdominal scan
Probe:
• Curved

Positioning:
• Supine

Views:
• Central abdominal
• Left lower lateral

Uses:
• Ascites and paracentesis

Thoracic scan

Probe:
• Cardiac: for B-lines and pleural effusion
• Curved: for all purposes
• Linear: for pleura and detect pneumothorax

Positioning:
• Seated forward with arms folded on pillow for pleural effusion
• Any position for pulmonary oedema
• Supine/near-to-supine for pneumothorax

Views:
• Posterior approach for pleural effusion
• Anti-dependent zones for pneumothorax (anterior sagittal, second intercostal space, mid-clavicular line)
• Dependent zones for cardiogenic pulmonary oedema

Uses:
• Pleural effusions
• Pulmonary oedema (cardiogenic, non-cardiogenic)
• Consolidation
• Pneumothorax

Bladder scan
Probe:
• Curved

Positioning:
• Supine with full bladder

Views:
• Pelvis – sagittal
  – transverse

Uses:
• Incomplete voiding
• Reduced urine output vs catheter blockage

Table 114.3 Reversible causes of hypotension/shock/cardiac arrest.

---

4 Ts
- *Tamponade – cardiac
- *Thrombosis – coronary or pulmonary
- Toxins
- *Tension pneumothorax

4 Hs
- *Hypovolaemia
- *Hypoxia
- Hyper/hypokalaemia/metabolic
- Hypothermia

---

* Recognized appearances on ultrasonography can guide immediate treatment.

- In suspected pulmonary embolism (Chapter 57):
  - The signs in Table 114.4 can be used to prove the working diagnosis sufficient to give immediate thrombolysis in a critically ill patient.
  - Sometimes the presence of RV dilatation can suggest the need for inpatient care in patients apparently suitable for outpatient care using clinical scoring systems.
- In hypotension (Chapter 2), a cardiac scan is useful to detect hypovolaemia (flat IVC) and cardiac dysfunction.
- In patients with suspected exacerbation of COPD (Chapter 61), LV systolic dysfunction is either the correct diagnosis or an associated diagnosis in up to 20% of cases.

Thoracic scan

- A thoracic emergency scan does not substitute for a standard thoracic ultrasound scan for pleural diseases as defined by British Thoracic Society (BTS) guidelines.
- A BTS approved ultrasound course is mandated before performing interventions such as chest drain insertion under real-time ultrasound.
- A thoracic scan can aid management by the detection of:
  - Pleural effusion (Chapter 12). Ultrasound is more accurate than a chest X-ray on which lobar collapse and elevated hemidiaphragm may mimic a pleural effusion.
  - Consolidation (Chapters 61 and 62).
  - Pneumothorax (Chapter 64).
  - Pulmonary oedema (Chapters 47–49).
- Normal aerated lung reflects ultrasound poorly and is characterized by A lines (Table 114.5) (Figure 114.1 (a)). The scatter of ultrasound causes a 'snow-storm' appearance.
- A wet lung reflects ultrasound and is characterized by 'B-lines' (Table 114.5, Figure 114.1 (b)):
  - Identifying whether A or B lines are present helps differentiating between COPD and heart failure with pulmonary oedema.
  - The absence of multiple bilateral B lines excludes cardiogenic pulmonary oedema with negative predictive value of 100%.
  - Acute respiratory distress syndrome/acute lung injury (Table 47.1) are characterized by non-homogeneously distributed B-lines and lung consolidations.

Abdominal scan

- In a tense distended abdomen ultrasound can confirm the presence of ascites immediately.
- Points on the examination are given in Table 114.6.

Table 114.4 The cardiac scan in cardiac arrest/shock: appearances in the 2Ts and 2Hs pathologies.

Tamponade – cardiac	• Echo free space around the heart (ends anterior to the descending thoracic aorta) • RV collapse during diastole • Heart 'swinging' during cardiac cycle • Dilated IVC with <50% collapse
Thrombosis – coronary	Direct results of myocardial infarction: • Regional LV wall-motion abnormality • Global LV dysfunction Acute complications of myocardial infarction: • Flail mitral valve • Ventricular septal rupture
Thrombosis – pulmonary	Right ventricular dysfunction: • Right ventricular dilatation • Free wall hypokinesis • Paradoxical septal motion • D-shaped LV in parasternal short-axis view Severe tricuspid regurgitation (with PASP <60 mmHg) IVC dilated and unreactive Thrombus may rarely be visible in the right heart or pulmonary artery
Hypotension	Signs of underfilling/hypovolaemic shock: • Markedly reduced end-diastolic chamber size reflecting reduced filling • Hyperdynamic wall motions of both ventricles with ventricular walls 'kissing' during systole • Flat inferior vena cava Sepsis – as above +/–: • LV dilated and hypokinetic • RV dilated and hypokinetic Cardiogenic causes: • LV global or regional dysfunction • Severe valve lesions such as severe aortic stenosis • Obstructed or regurgitant prosthetic valve • hypertrophic cardiomyopathy Aortic dissection involving aortic root: • Severe aortic regurgitation • Dilated aortic root • Intimal tear sometimes visible • There may be associated cardiac tamponade
Hypoxaemia	Pulmonary oedema (Pleural fluid and B-lines may be visible also by cardiac probe): • LV global or regional dysfunction discussed above • Severe valve lesions discussed above • Sepsis discussed above Pulmonary embolism – see above

• Unless there is marked splenomegaly, the left lateral flank is the preferred site for a diagnostic ascitic tap or paracentesis, aiming for an area between the anterior abdominal wall and the dark hypoechogenic fluid, and having confirmed that there is no bowel or other organ in the proposed track.

Bladder scan

• The bladder produces a posterior acoustic shadow. Scan suprapubically in midline both longitudinally and transversely.

Table 114.5 Appearances of A- and B-lines on thoracic scan.

	A-lines (Figure 114.1 (left))	B-lines (Figure 114.1 (right))
Appearance	Normal horizontal reverberation artefact, parallel to the pleural line	Pathological vertical reverberation artefact, arising from the pleural line
Interpretation	Normal lung Asthma COPD	Fluid-thickened interstitium: pulmonary oedema; or Collagen-thickened interstitium: pulmonary fibrosis

Table 114.6 The abdominal scan in suspected ascites (Chapter 24).

Suggests ascites
- Dark and hypo-echoic appearances in the flanks
- Loops of gas-filled bowel afloat around the centre/periumbilical region

Points of concern before ascitic tap
- Hepatomegaly or enlarged gallbladder
- Splenomegaly
- Full bladder. A common mistake is to insert a needle into the fluid of the bladder, so ensure several planes of view are evaluated before proceeding in real-time. It is also sensible to ask the patient to void beforehand.
- Measure the fluid in two planes to get a better idea of depth.

- A bladder scan is useful for:
  - Obese elderly males where clinical assessment for urinary retention due to prostatic hypertrophy can be difficult.
  - Post-voiding volumes when uncertainty about incomplete bladder emptying exists.
  - Confused patients who cannot tell you when they were last able to pass urine.
  - In acute kidney injury (Chapter 25).

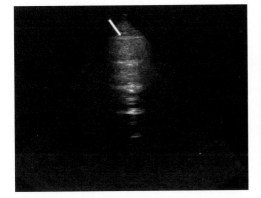 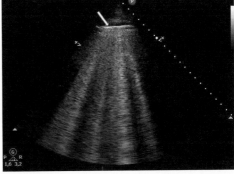

Figure 114.1 Appearances of A-lines (left) and B-lines (right) on thoracic scan. The bright white line (arrowed) is the visceral pleura. A-lines are normal horizontal reverberation artefacts, and B-lines are pathological vertical reverberation artefacts. See also Table 114.5.

Further reading

Gargani L, Volpicelli G (2014) How I do it: Lung ultrasound. *Cardiovascular Ultrasound* 12, 25. http://www.
cardiovascularultrasound.com/content/12/1/25.

Hothi SS, Sprigings D, Chambers J (2014) Point-of-care ultrasound in acute medicine – the quick scan. *Clinical
Medicine* 14, 608–611.

Lancellotti P, Price S, Edvardsen T, *et al.* (2015) The use of echocardiography in acute cardiovascular care:
Recommendations of the European Association of Cardiovascular Imaging and the Acute Cardiovascular
Care Association. *European Heart Journal – Cardiovascular Imaging* 16, 119–146. http://ehjcimaging.
oxfordjournals.org/content/ejechocard/16/2/119.full.pdf.

CHAPTER 115

Reading a chest X-ray

Reading a chest X-ray (also called a chest radiograph) is a fundamental skill for all doctors. During busy shifts it can be tempting to leap to the obvious abnormality. However, applying a systematic approach (Table 115.1) will ensure you never miss the more subtle abnormalities, and do not draw false conclusions from a technically poor film. This approach is by no means prescriptive, but should be a good initial guide to developing your own individual method.

Table 115.2 summarizes common normal variants. Commonly encountered pathological findings are addressed in Tables 115.3–115.12.

Table 115.1 Systematic approach to the chest X-ray.

Question	Comments
1. **Do I have the correct patient?**	Important to check and at this point also check clinical information provided.
2. **Is there satisfactory inspiration?**	The anterior end of the left sixth rib reaches the level of the dome of the diaphragm.
	Key point: Poor inspiration can cause the heart to appear enlarged and cause vessel crowding at the bases, mimicking consolidation.
	Exception: When seeking a small pneumothorax this is best seen on full expiration.
3. **Is the patient rotated?**	This can be assessed by comparing the medial ends of the clavicles to the margins of the vertebral body at the same level.
	Key point: The mediastinum and hila can be distorted with rotation, sometimes giving the false appearance of possible enlargement or a mass.
The inside out approach	
4. **Is the trachea central?**	Important to note as deviation can occur in many pathologies.
5. **Is the heart enlarged?**	In an adult, the cardiothoracic ratio should be less than 50% on a PA radiograph.
6. **Are the heart borders clearly visible and well defined?**	If not, there is a high probability that there is pathology in the immediately adjacent lung.
7. **What is the position, size and density of the hila?**	The left hilum should be at the same level or higher than the right, but NEVER lower than the right.
	The hilar density on each side should be similar.
The lungs	
8. **Size?**	Look for signs of hyper-expansion (>7th anterior rib intersects the diaphragm at the mid-clavicular line). May also see flattening of the diaphragms.
9. **Lung markings clearly visible?**	If lung markings are not clearly visible, consider pneumothorax or lung collapse.
10. **Any features of collapse/consolidation?**	See below.

(continued)

Acute Medicine: A Practical Guide to the Management of Medical Emergencies, Fifth Edition. Edited by David Sprigings and John B. Chambers.
© 2018 John Wiley & Sons Ltd. Published 2018 by John Wiley & Sons Ltd.

Table 115.1 (*Continued*)

Question	Comments
11. Are all borders clearly visible (e.g. costophrenic, cardiophrenic)	If borders are obscured, consider if there is a fluid level, for example in pleural effusion or evidence of lobar collapse.
	The silhouette sign:
	This is when an intrathoracic lesion touching a border of the heart, aorta or diaphragm will obliterate that border on the chest radiograph.
12. Have I checked the hidden areas?	These are the lung apices; behind the heart; the hila and below the domes of the diaphragm.
	These are the sites where lesions are most commonly overlooked.
13. Is there an old image I can compare this to?	
14. Finally ask yourself, have I addressed the patient's clinical problem?	

Table 115.2 Common normal variants.

Variant	Comments
Azygos lobe	This is created when a laterally displaced azygos vein makes a deep fissure in the upper part of the lung. On the chest radiograph this is seen as a fine line that crosses the apex of the right lung.
Pectus excavatum	The right heart border can be ill defined. The silhouette sign is apparent, appearing as consolidation or atelectasis of the middle lobe.
Cervical rib	A supernumerary rib that arises from a cervical vertebra (usually the seventh).
Pericardial fat	Loss of clarity of the heart borders without any alveolar opacity in the context of an asymptomatic patient.
Dextrocardia	Always check that the image is the correct way around before making this assumption.

Common Pathology

Table 115.3 Hilar enlargement.
The position of the hilum often changes in lobar collapse (see Table 115.8 and Figure 115.1).

Differential diagnosis of hilar enlargement	
Unilateral	**Bilateral**
Infection, TB	Sarcoidosis
Vascular: pulmonary artery stenosis	Vascular: pulmonary artery hypertension
Pulmonary artery aneurysm	
Tumour: Lymph nodes (due to bronchial carcinoma, lymphoma or extrathoracic metastases)	

Table 115.4 Mediastinal mass.

Compartment	Chest X-ray appearance	Common causes	Comments
Anterior	These masses lie adjacent to the heart. They may efface a heart border or the margin of the ascending aorta.	• Thyroid mass • Thymoma • Teratoma • Lymphoma	In general, lymphadenopathy from any cause can occur in the anterior mediastinum.
Middle	These masses may splay the carina or efface a normal hilar shadow.	• Lymphadenopathy • Central lung tumours • Oesophageal lesions	
Posterior	These masses will displace either or both of the paravertebral stripes laterally. They may also widen the space between adjacent ribs and erode into ribs and or vertebrae.	• Spinal/paraspinal abscess • Neurogenic tumours	Look for abnormalities in the intervertebral discs and vertebral bodies. Look for rib splaying +/– vertebral body erosion.

Table 115.5 Pneumomediastinum.

- Mediastinal gas can cause the central part of the diaphragm to be visualized (this is not normally the case).
- A rim of air around the heart appears as a lucent black halo surrounding the heart.
- Streaks of gas in the neck or soft tissues of the chest wall.
- Air around the pulmonary artery (and/or its main branches) or around the arteries arising from the aortic arch appear as black rings.

Table 115.6 Cardiac silhouette.
The density of the cardiac shadow should be equal on both sides of the spine. If there is any difference in density consider pneumonia, lower lobe collapse or a lower lobe mass on the denser side.

Abnormality	Comment
Pericardial effusion	Appearance difficult to distinguish from chamber enlargement. Changes in cardiac size or shape occur once 250–500 mL of fluid has accumulated. **The most important sign is that there is rapid alteration in heart size or shape without any changes in the lungs.**
Left ventricular failure	**Early features:** • Cardiomegaly • Upper lobe vessels are wider than lower lobe vessels • Oedema: poorly defined hilar vessel margins • Oedema: septal lines • Small bilateral pleural effusions **Later features:** • Interstitial shadowing • Alveolar shadowing • Pleural effusions of increasing size

Table 115.7 Alveolar and interstitial lung disease.

	Alveolar disease	Interstitial lung disease
Definition	Alveolar spaces are filled with material, for example blood, pus, water or protein.	The supporting tissue surrounding the alveoli and the alveolar walls are affected due to oedema, inflammation or fibrotic thickening.
Chest X-ray appearance	• Fluffy/blobby • Poorly defined margins • Segmental/lobar/diffuse	• Small nodules • Linear/reticular shadows +/− septal lines • Reticulo-nodular • Honey-combing • Usually diffuse
Differential diagnosis	**Dominant alveolar pattern** • Pulmonary oedema • Lobar pneumonia • Haemorrhage • Adenocarcinoma in situ • Early adult respiratory distress syndrome • Aspiration pneumonia	**Dominant interstitial pattern** • Pulmonary oedema • Viral pneumonia • Pulmonary fibrosis • Sarcoidosis • Lymphangitis carcinomatosis

General features of lobar collapse:

- Features of volume loss such as displaced fissure, hilum, trachea or mediastinum and occasional elevation of hemidiaphragm.
- Over-inflation of adjacent unaffected lobe.

Specific features of collapse according to the involved lobe (see Figure 115.1).

Collapsed lobe	Chest X-ray features
Right lower lobe	• Oblique fissure moves posteriorly and medially • Right hilum depressed • Medial aspect of right hemidiaphragm obscured • Lateral margin of adjacent vertebrae effaced
Left lower lobe	• Oblique fissure moves posteriorly and medially • Left hilum lies at a lower level than usual • Medial aspect of the left hemidiaphgram obscured • Lateral margin of adjacent vertebrae effaced
Middle lobe	• Horizontal fissure moves inferiorly (NB this fissure is not always visible) • Blurring of right heart border • Sometimes there is increased density in the collapsed lobe
Right upper lobe	• Horizontal fissure moves superiorly • Right hilum elevated • Increased density of collapsed lung • **Golden S sign:** Can occur when a tumour at the right hilum is the cause of lobar collapse
Left upper lobe	• Veil-like density covering most of left hemithorax • Left heart border obscured • Left hilum elevated • **Luftsichel sign:** crescenteric lucency around left side of aortic knuckle.

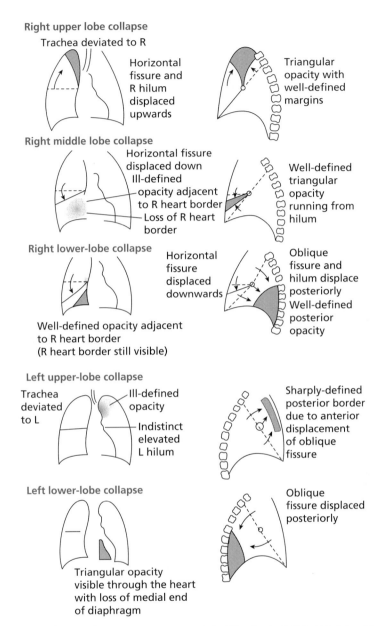

Right upper lobe collapse
Trachea deviated to R

Horizontal fissure and R hilum displaced upwards

Triangular opacity with well-defined margins

Right middle lobe collapse

Horizontal fissure displaced down
Ill-defined opacity adjacent to R heart border
Loss of R heart border

Well-defined triangular opacity running from hilum

Right lower-lobe collapse

Horizontal fissure displaced downwards

Well-defined opacity adjacent to R heart border (R heart border still visible)

Oblique fissure and hilum displace posteriorly
Well-defined posterior opacity

Left upper-lobe collapse

Trachea deviated to L
Ill-defined opacity
Indistinct elevated L hilum

Sharply-defined posterior border due to anterior displacement of oblique fissure

Left lower-lobe collapse

Oblique fissure displaced posteriorly

Triangular opacity visible through the heart with loss of medial end of diaphragm

Figure 115.1 Patterns of lobar collapse. Source: Longmore, Oxford Handbook of Clinical Medicine, 5th edition, 2001. Reproduced with permission of Oxford University Press.

Approach to the chest x ray of a patient in Intensive Care

- Check the position of all lines and tubes
- Check the lungs, pleura and mediastinum
- Always compare the present chest radiograph with the immediately preceding one and then with an earlier one
- Chest radiographs in intensive care tend to be bedside AP projections that magnify the heart and the mediastinum.

Table 115.8 Lobar collapse.

Lobar collapse can often be easily missed. Collapse essentially refers to volume loss and is also termed 'atelectasis'.

There are three main disease processes that can result in lobar collapse; these are summarized below. In this chapter we will mainly focus on the most common: obstructive.

Mechanism of lobar collapse	Definition
Obstructive	Intrinsic occlusion by tumour, mucous plug or foreign body
Compressive	Compression by pleural fluid, pneumothorax or adjacent intrapulmonary space occupying lesion
Cicatrization	Fibrotic contraction due to pulmonary fibrosis, tuberculosis or radiotherapy

Table 115.9 Lung nodules and masses.

Nodule (<3 cm 2D diameter)	Mass (>3 cm 2D diameter)	Multiple masses
Benign Subpleural lymph node Perifissural nodule Granuloma – fungal/TB Hamartoma	**Benign** Hamartoma Granuloma	**Benign** Infection, TB, fungal, Histioplasmosis, septic emboli
Malignant Lung carcinoma Lung metastasis	**Malignant** Lung carcinoma Lung metastasis	Sarcoidosis Wegener's granulomatosis Rheumatoid nodules
		Malignant Lung metastases

Table 115.10 Pleural diseases.

Abnormality	Comments	
Pleural effusion	200–300 mL of fluid required before it becomes visible on a chest radiograph	
Pleural opacities	**Solitary**	**Multiple**
	Fluid collection: • Loculated pleural effusion • Organized empyema • Haematoma	Pleural plaques: secondary to asbestos exposure Mostly seen posteriorly and laterally, mainly affecting the lower third of the thorax
	Tumour: mesothelioma Metastases Lipoma Solitary fibrous tumour of pleura	Fluid collection: loculated pleural effusion Tumour: mesothelioma Metastases
Pleural calcification	**Unilateral**	**Bilateral**
	Infection (TB) Empyema Haemorrhagic effusion	Asbestos related pleural plaques where the calcification is:

Table 115.10   (*Continued*)

Abnormality	Comments		
	Talc inhalation	• Bilateral and extensive • Usually covers the dome of the diaphragm • Unilateral in 25% of cases	

Pneumothorax	**Spontaneous – primary**
	Subpleural blebs common in:
	• Adults 20–40 y
	• Male: female 6:1
	• No known lung disease. A subpleural bleb is an outpouching of the alveolar wall that thins the visceral pleural membrane. In general, blebs are present at the lung apices only.
		Spontaneous – secondary
		Lung disease:
		• COPD/asthma
		• Cavitating pneumonia
		• Pleural metastases
		• Cystic disease, for example lymphangio-leiomyomatosis (LAM), Langerhans cell histocytosis X (LCH)
			Traumatic/iatrogenic
			• Blunt/penetrating trauma
			  • CVP line placement
			  • Lung biopsy
			  • Aspiration of pleural fluid
			• Thoracic surgery
			• Mechanical ventilation
			• Smoking cocaine/marijuana

Table 115.11 Chest wall and abdomen.
To assess the ribs more easily, rotate the image through 90° and then 180°. This will remove other distracting anatomy and allow the rib outline to stand out.

Abnormality	Comments
Rib fractures	Callus formation may create a mass-like appearance sometimes warranting a CT to confirm the diagnosis
Free air under the diaphragm	Sign of perforation of intra-abdominal viscus

Table 115.12 Diffuse lung shadowing.

Diagnosis	Chest X-ray features
Pneumonia **Acute Respiratory** **Distress Syndrome** **(ARDS)**	• Patchy areas of consolidation with sparing of some areas • Predominantly interstitial shadowing with rapid development into alveolar pattern • Widespread opacities throughout all lung fields, central and peripheral • Proximal pulmonary vessels remain well defined • Chest radiograph appearance may be delayed by 12 h or more from the onset of symptoms • Appearances may persist for days after clinical improvement • Pleural effusions are rare
Cardiogenic pulmonary oedema	• Cardiomegaly • Changes predominantly at the lung bases • Blurred margins and hilar vessels • Appearances clear rapidly in response to treatment • Pleural effusions are common

Further reading

De Lacey G, Morley S, Berman L (2008) *The Chest X-ray: A Survival Guide*. Elsevier Health Sciences.

Radiology Masterclass website. Tutorial on chest X-ray anatomy. http://radiologymasterclass.co.uk/tutorials/chest/chest_home_anatomy/chest_anatomy_start.html.

Radiopaedia.org is a free educational radiology resource with one of the web's largest collections of radiology cases and reference articles. http://radiopaedia.org/.

Webb WR, Higgins CB (2016) *Thoracic Imaging: Pulmonary and Cardiovascular Radiology*, 3rd edition. Lippincott Williams and Wilkins.

CHAPTER 116

Central vein cannulation

SANDEEP HOTHI AND DAVID SPRIGINGS

Indications, contraindications and potential complications are given in Table 116.1.

The use of ultrasound to guide central vein cannulation increases the success rate of the procedure from 60% to >90%, and reduces the complication rate from 30% to <10%. Ultrasound should be used when available and for elective procedures. For central vein cannulation in an emergency, the most rapid and safest method should be selected, depending on the operator's experience, patient factors and ultrasound availability.

Equipment needed is given in Table 116.2. You will need at least one assistant to monitor the patient during the procedure and assist with the equipment.

Choosing the approach

The internal jugular, femoral and subclavian veins are the veins most commonly used for central access.

- Cannulation of the internal jugular vein is generally associated with fewer complications than with the subclavian vein, and is the recommended approach in patients with a bleeding tendency (because of the risk of uncontrollable bleeding from inadvertent puncture of the subclavian artery) or respiratory failure (because of the greater risk of pneumothorax with subclavian access). The right internal jugular vein is preferable to the left as it is contralateral to the thoracic duct, and the circulation of the dominant cerebral hemisphere in the right-handed.
- Cannulation of the femoral vein may be the preferred approach if rapidity of access is paramount (e.g. for placement of a temporary pacing lead in a haemodynamically unstable patient), or if central venous access is required during cardiopulmonary resuscitation. Its drawbacks are a higher rate of infection, venous thrombosis and restricted mobility of the leg.
- An antecubital fossa vein can be used to place a central line for infusions, but manipulation of a pacing lead via this route can be very difficult. Use of antecubital and forearm veins should be avoided in patients with advanced renal disease as they may be needed for arterio-venous fistula formation.

Ultrasound-guided cannulation of the internal jugular vein

Preparation

1 Confirm the indications for the procedure. Explain the procedure to the patient and obtain consent.
2 Prepare the surroundings: clear the bedside and remove the bed head; adjust the bed height so that the operator is comfortable; ensure adequate lighting; position your trolley, clinical waste bowl and ultrasound device.
3 Prepare the patient: connect ECG and oxygen saturation monitors; give oxygen via a mask (which will lift the drape off the face). Remove the pillow and place an absorbent pad placed under the neck and shoulder. Lie the patient supine with head-down tilt (Trendelenburg position) unless not tolerated, for example due to pulmonary oedema or other respiratory compromise. The head-down tilt is important to reduce the risk of air embolism, particularly for jugular venous access (as opposed to femoral access).

Acute Medicine: A Practical Guide to the Management of Medical Emergencies, Fifth Edition. Edited by David Sprigings and John B. Chambers.
© 2018 John Wiley & Sons Ltd. Published 2018 by John Wiley & Sons Ltd.

Table 116.1 Central vein cannulation: indications, contraindications and potential complications.

Indications

Measurement of central venous pressure (CVP):
- Transfusion of large volumes of fluid required (the fluid itself can be given faster via a large-bore peripheral IV cannula)
- Fluid challenge in patients with oliguria or hypotension
- To exclude hypovolaemia when clinical evidence is equivocal

Monitoring venous oxyhaemoglobin saturation

Cardiac output monitoring with a pulmonary artery catheter

Insertion of a temporary pacing lead (see Chapter 119) or pulmonary artery catheter

IVC filter placement

Administration of some drugs (e.g. epinephrine, norepinephrine and dopamine) and IV feeding solutions, which have to be given via a central vein

Renal replacement therapy and plasmapheresis

No suitable peripheral veins for IV infusion

Pacemaker/cardiac device placement

Contraindications

Bleeding disorder (including platelet count $<50 \times 10^9$/L, INR >1.5, receiving oral anticoagulant or anticoagulant-dose heparin, during or after thrombolytic therapy): discuss management with a haematologist. If central venous access is needed urgently, before the bleeding disorder can be corrected, use the femoral vein in preference to the internal jugular vein.

Prohibitive anatomic distortion

Local infection

Potential complications

During placement

Arterial puncture or laceration, which in the case of the carotid artery may lead to haematoma formation in the neck, with compromise of the airway. Seek vascular surgical advice.

Pneumothorax (via internal jugular or subclavian vein) or tension pneumothorax

Haemothorax

Cardiac tamponade (can be caused by central venous catheter introduced by any route, if its tip lies below the pericardial reflection and it perforates the vessel wall; least likely via internal jugular vein).

Injury to adjacent nerves

Air embolism

After placement

Infection

Venous thrombosis

---

4 Visualize the internal jugular vein with ultrasound. The vein can be distinguished from the artery by compressibility and phasic change with respiration of the former (Figures 116.1 and 116.2). If the internal jugular vein is relatively flat (i.e. central venous pressure is low), head-down tilt or peripheral IV administration (if not contraindicated) may increase its calibre.

Table 116.2 Central vein cannulation: equipment.

Ultrasound machine

Sterile sheath for ultrasound probe and sterile ultrasound gel

Central venous catheter set containing the appropriate catheter length, number of lumens and lumen diameters

---

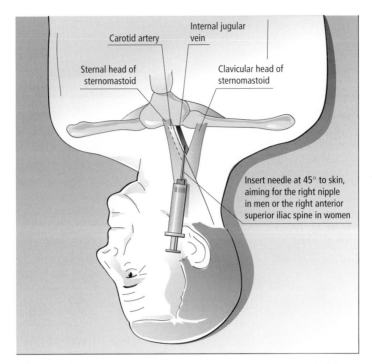

Carotid artery

Internal jugular vein

Sternal head of sternomastoid

Clavicular head of sternomastoid

Insert needle at 45° to skin, aiming for the right nipple in men or the right anterior superior iliac spine in women

Figure 116.1 Relations of the right internal jugular vein. Ultrasound-guided puncture of the internal jugular vein is the recommended method. Landmark-guided puncture, as depicted, may be chosen in an emergency by an experienced operator.

5 Open the procedure pack onto the trolley by the bedside. Scrub up in an aseptic manner and don hat, mask, gown and gloves. Prepare the skin with chlorhexidine or povidone-iodine and apply drapes. Put the windowed drape over the target area, and additional drapes to cover the end of the bed and to bridge from the bed to the procedure trolley.

6 Open the sterile sheath for the ultrasound probe. Identify the open (distal) end and place sterile ultrasound gel inside it. Your assistant should hold the probe vertically by its cable and lower it into the open end of the sheath. Then unfurl the sheath along the probe and secure the open end over the probe with a sterile elastic band/tape, ensuring that the sheath is flush with the probe face.

7 Reconfirm the location of the internal jugular vein with the sheathed probe. Assess the distance from the skin to the vein. Plan your vein puncture site and 'upstream' skin puncture site guided by the depth of the skin to the vein.

8 Anaesthetize the skin with 2 mL of lidocaine 1% using a 25 G (orange) needle. Ensure that the skin bleb will cover the area needed for sutures. Then infiltrate a further 2–3 mL of lidocaine along the planned needle path.

9 While the local anaesthetic is taking effect, prepare the venous catheter. Flush all lumens with normal saline. Leave the central lumen open for passage of the guidewire but cap the other ports. Flush the dilator with normal saline. Ensure the guidewire flows freely from its coil. Prepare a sterile site adjacent to the patient where you can conveniently put the guidewire with the straightener for the J tip in place. Have the skin blade and dilator close to hand.

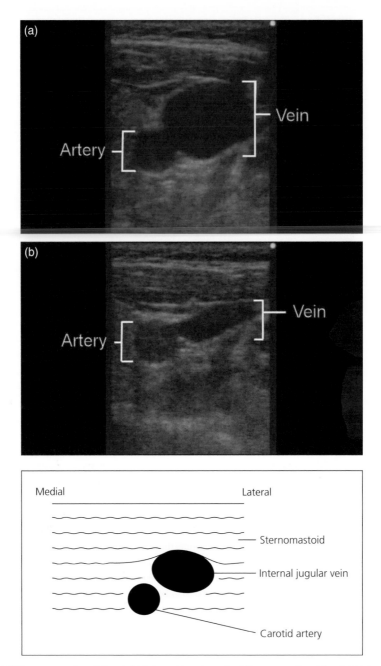

Figure 116.2 Ultrasonography of the right internal jugular vein. Ultrasonography of the right internal jugular vein, before (a) and after (b) compression by the ultrasound probe. The vein can be distinguished from the artery by its compressibility. The depth from the skin to the anterior wall of the vein averages 11 mm (range 6–18 mm). The vein is usually 10 mm in diameter, but its calibre is reduced in volume-depletion. Head-down tilt or volume loading increases the diameter of the vein and facilitates venepuncture.

Venepuncture

10 Mount the needle for the central vein puncture on a 10 mL syringe containing 5 mL of normal saline and flush it. Ensure that the needle is not put on too tightly. Taking the probe in your left hand, visualize the vein at the target puncture site.

11 With the syringe and needle in your right hand, puncture the skin upstream of the probe and then stop. Angle the probe towards the needle and identify the needle artefact. Adjust the needle angle to ensure the artefact is in line with the centre of the vein. Slowly advance the needle with continuous gentle aspiration. Monitor and adjust the probe angle to track the needle tip if feasible. Venepuncture is indicated by aspiration of venous blood or visualized puncture of the vein. Stop advancing the needle and re-aspirate to confirm you are in the vein.

12 Hold the needle steady in position and carefully place the ultrasound probe on a sterile surface. Then use your left hand to stabilize the needle at the skin. Check again by aspiration that the needle is still in the vein. Remove the syringe while supporting the needle. Blood should drip from the needle. If it does not, then cover the hub of the needle with your thumb and use a clean syringe to aspirate venous blood. If blood cannot be aspirated, leave the needle in place and rescan the vein. Do not alter the angle of the needle while within the skin/soft tissue – doing so can result in laceration injuries.

If you are not sure if the needle is in the vein or the artery, either aspirate blood and check oxygen saturation, or connect to a pressure transducer.

Placing the catheter

13 Having confirmed you are in the vein, pick up the guidewire and gently advance it (J end leading) into the needle and vein. Take care not to displace the needle while you are doing this. If resistance is felt, withdraw the guidewire slightly, depress the needle hub to reduce the angle into the vein and try again to pass the wire. If it still will not pass, remove the guidewire and re-aspirate to check the needle is indeed in the vein. Pass the guidewire to just beyond the 20 cm marking. Withdraw the needle over the guidewire and cover the puncture site with a piece of gauze, held in place with your left hand.

14 Use the blade to make a short incision along the guidewire at the site of skin puncture to allow passage of the dilator and catheter.

15 Mount the dilator on the guidewire and advance it with gentle rotation and forward pressure to insert it to a depth of 3–4 cm. There is no need to insert the whole length of the dilator: doing so risks perforation of the vein.

16 Remove the dilator keeping the guidewire in place and again cover the puncture site with gauze. Mount the catheter onto the guidewire and advance it with gentle rotation and forward pressure to insert it to a depth of around 12 cm. Remove the guidewire. If blood cultures are required, take them at this point. Aspirate the central lumen to confirm venous blood and then flush with normal saline. Close the port with a sterile bung. Confirm satisfactory placement of the catheter with ultrasound.

17 Apply suture wings to the catheter as it exits the skin and suture through each wing hole, taking care that the sutures are placed deeply and not tied too tightly.

18 Remove the sterile drape from around the catheter and clean the skin with wet gauze to remove any blood. Blot with dry sterile gauze. Use an alcohol swab to clean the skin and the line, and when the alcohol has dried, cover the skin puncture site with a bio-occlusive dressing. A second dressing should be used to support the upper part of the catheter.

Final points

19 Remove all drapes and sit the patient up. Check that the dressings are satisfactory. Clear up and dispose of sharps safely. Arrange a chest X-ray to confirm the position of the catheter. The tip of the catheter should be at or above the carina to ensure that it lies above the pericardial reflection.

20 Write a note of the procedure in the patient's record, documenting technique (i.e. ultrasound-guided or not), vein used, any complications and post-procedure chest X-ray findings. If the catheter needs to be used

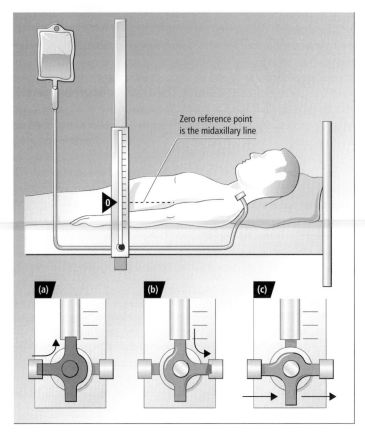

Figure 116.3 Method of measuring central venous pressure (CVP). CVP line with the position of the three-way tap for: (a) priming the manometer; (b) reading the CVP; and (c) fluid infusion. Adapted from: Davidson TI (1987) *Fluid Balance*. Oxford: Blackwell Scientific Publications.

immediately, use pressure monitoring to confirm the location is venous and not arterial before any infusion is started (Figure 116.3).

Troubleshooting
Frequent ventricular extrasystoles or ventricular tachycardia during procedure may indicate that the tip of the guidewire has passed across the tricuspid valve into the right ventricle: draw it back.

Landmark-guided technique for cannulation of the femoral vein

1 Lie the patient flat. The leg should be slightly abducted and externally rotated. Identify the femoral artery below the inguinal ligament: the femoral vein usually lies medially (Figure 116.4). Shave the groin. Prepare with skin with chlorhexidine or povidone-iodine and apply drapes.
2 Infiltrate the skin and subcutaneous tissues with 5–10 mL of lidocaine 1%. Nick the skin with a small scalpel blade. Place two fingers of your left hand on the femoral artery to define its position. Holding the syringe in

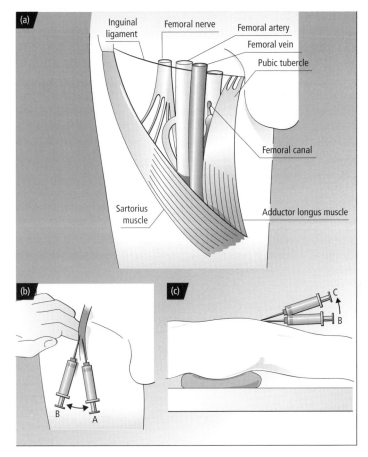

Figure 116.4 Right femoral vein puncture. Panel (a) depicts the anatomy of the femoral vein; and panels (b) and (c), the technique of femoral vein puncture. See text for details. Source: Rosen M, *et al.* (1993) *Handbook of Percutaneous Central Venous Catheterization*, 2nd edn. London: WB Saunders. Reproduced with permission of Elsevier.

your right hand, place the tip of the needle at the entry site on the skin. Move the syringe slightly laterally, and advance the needle at an angle of around 30° to the skin whilst aspirating for blood. The vein is usually reached 2–4 cm from the skin surface.

3 If the vein is not found, withdraw slowly whilst aspirating. Flush the needle to make sure it is not blocked. Try again, aiming slightly to the left or right of your initial pass.

The above method can be easily supplemented for use with ultrasound guidance and this is recommended wherever possible.

Management of central venous catheters

- Minimize the duration for which the catheter is kept in situ.
- Daily inspection of the entry site.
- Regular dressing changes.
- Aseptic technique whenever using or handling the catheter.
- Use heparinized catheter lock solutions.

Catheter infection

Staphylococcus aureus and *Staph. epidermidis* are the commonest pathogens, but infection with Gram-negative rods and fungi may occur in immunocompromised patients.

If the catheter is obviously infected (tenderness, erythema and purulent discharge at the skin exit site), the catheter must be removed and the tip sent for culture. If the patient is febrile or has other signs of sepsis, take blood cultures (one via the catheter and one from the peripheral vein) and start antibiotic therapy.

Initial treatment should be with IV vancomycin or teicoplanin (to cover methicillin-resistant *Staph. aureus* (MRSA) plus gentamicin if Gram-negative infection is possible.

If cultures show *Staph. aureus* infection with bacteraemia, IV antistaphylococcal therapy should be given for two weeks. For *Staph. epidermidis* and Gram-negative infection, give IV therapy until the patient has been afebrile for 24–48 h. For *Pseudomonas* infection, give IV therapy for 7–10 days. Seek advice from a microbiologist.

If the catheter is possibly infected (fever or other systemic signs of sepsis, but the skin exit site is clean), take blood cultures (one via the catheter and one from the peripheral vein). The decision to remove the catheter before culture results are back depends on the likelihood of it being infected, how long the catheter has been in and if there is another source of infection. If both blood cultures grow the same organism, the catheter must be removed and antibiotic therapy given as above.

Further reading

Ortega R, Song M, Hansen CJ, Barash P (2010) Videos in clinical medicine. Ultrasound-guided internal jugular vein cannulation. *N Engl J Med* 362, e57. http://www.nejm.org/doi/full/10.1056/NEJMvcm0810156.

Smith RN, Nolan JP (2013) Central venous catheters. *BMJ* 347, f6570. DOI: 10.1136/bmj.f6570

CHAPTER 117

Arterial blood sampling and cannulation

DAVID GARRY

Arterial blood sampling

Equipment

Arterial sampling requires an arterial blood gas syringe, a needle (20, 23 or 25 G) and a dressing to apply to the site.

Preparation

1 Explain the procedure to the patient and obtain consent.
  - When the radial artery or the dorsalis pedis artery are used then the collateral circulation should be checked prior to puncture.
  - The Allen test is used prior to radial artery puncture. Both the radial and ulnar arteries are occluded, with the fist clenched and elevated. Once the blood has drained, the fist is opened and lowered and the ulnar artery is released. Patency of the ulnar artery is assumed if colour returns to the hand within six seconds.
  - In dorsalis pedis artery puncture, the dorsalis pedis artery can be occluded, and the capillary refill time of the big toe can be observed.
  - Ultrasonography can be used to locate the artery if it is difficult to palpate.
2 Local anaesthesia (a few mL of 1% or 2%) should be considered as it reduces pain without making the procedure more difficult, and may reduce vasospasm.
3 Wear adequate protection (gown and gloves, consider eye protection), observe strict hand hygiene and prepare the skin with chlorhexidine.

Technique

4 The artery should be located by gentle palpation with the second and third finger of the non-dominant hand. The syringe can be held like a dart, and the artery is usually punctured at an angle of approximately 45°, about 1 cm away from the operator's fingers. The blood will fill the syringe on its own (usually 2–3 mL), the needle should then be removed and firm pressure should be applied to the area for several minutes.
5 The needle should be disposed of immediately according to local policy in a sharps bin. Some syringes have a safety cover to enclose the needle; if present this should also be applied.

Specimen care and transport

Arterial blood samples are collected in pre-heparinized syringes to prevent clot formation. The majority of the heparin should be disposed of prior to arterial puncture (heparin can be acidic), and any excess air present in the

Acute Medicine: A Practical Guide to the Management of Medical Emergencies, Fifth Edition. Edited by David Sprigings and John B. Chambers.
© 2018 John Wiley & Sons Ltd. Published 2018 by John Wiley & Sons Ltd.

syringe after blood collection should be expelled (it can cause a falsely high PaO$_2$ and a falsely low PaCO$_2$). If a point-of-care machine is not available for immediate analysis, the sample should be placed on ice and analysed within 15 min (to minimize oxygen consumption within the sample).

Interpretation of results

See Chapters 37 and 117.

Arterial cannulation

Indications, contraindications and potential complications are summarized in Table 117.1. Explain the procedure to the patient and obtain written consent, if the circumstances permit. Arterial cannulation is a sterile procedure, and requires appropriate hand hygiene and the wearing of hat, gown and gloves.

Table 117.1 Arterial cannulation: indications, contraindications and potential complications.

Indications

Blood sampling

When frequent sampling is indicated it may be preferable to insert an arterial catheter rather than performing serial needle punctures.

Haemodynamic monitoring

- In certain patient groups (large arm circumference, arrhythmias, extremes of blood pressure) it can be difficult to obtain reliable non-invasive blood pressure readings.
- Provides beat-to-beat blood pressure measurement for patients with haemodynamic instability or during therapeutic manipulation of the cardiovascular system.
- Reduces the risk of neuropraxias and tissue damage when frequent blood pressure measurements are needed over a long period of time.
- The waveform can be analysed to provide additional haemodynamic information, such as cardiac output by pulse contour analysis or thermodilution techniques.

Contraindications

Absolute

- Risk of, or actual limb ischaemia
- Infection at site of puncture
- Known aneurysm or pseudoaneurysm of artery

Relative

- Coagulopathy/bleeding disorder
- Planned procedure at the same arterial site (e.g. angiogram, creation of an arterio-venous fistula)

Potential complications

- Arterial vasospasm
- Bruising/haematoma/persistent bleeding
- Infection
- Air embolism
- Accidental intra-arterial injection
- Formation of arterial aneurysm, pseudo-aneurysm or arterio-venous fistula
- Distal limb ischaemia
- Damage to local structures
- Blood loss from repeated sampling
- Uncontrolled bleeding from an arterial catheter circuit left open to air
- Loss of the guidewire into the artery if Seldinger technique is used for catheter insertion

Table 117.2 Selection of artery for cannulation.

Artery	Anatomy/considerations
Radial artery	Located at the distal end of the radius between the tendons of brachioradialis and flexor carpi radialis.
	Technically easy to cannulate, success rates up to 92%.
	Extensive collateral circulation should be provided via the ulnar artery and the palmar arch.
Brachial artery	Located at the medial side of the antecubital fossa overlying the lateral border of the brachial muscle.
	No collateral circulation.
Axillary artery	Located in the intramuscular groove between the coracobrachial and triceps muscles.
	Technically difficult to cannulate.
	Extensive collateral circulation.
	Axillary arterial pressure accurately reflects aortic pressure in patients with low-output states.
Femoral artery	Located in a neurovascular bundle between the femoral vein and the femoral nerve.
	Technically easy to cannulate, even in patients with shock.
	Risk of retroperitoneal haemorrhage if artery is perforated.
	Femoral arterial pressure accurately reflects aortic pressure in patients with low output states.
Dorsalis pedis	Located lateral to the extensor hallucis longus tendon.
	Collateral circulation.
	Systolic blood pressure at this site is higher than in the aorta because of distal pulse wave amplification, but mean arterial pressure is similar.

Choice of artery

See Table 117.2. There are no firm data that one site is superior to another. The radial artery is often used as a first choice due to the relative ease of insertion. As the blood pressure wave spreads distally from the heart, there is an increase in systolic and decrease in diastolic blood pressure from distal pulse wave amplification. This can result in an elevated reading in the systolic blood pressure from a dorsalis pedis catheter, but the mean arterial pressure should remain similar to that in the aorta.

Equipment

Assemble the following equipment:

- An arterial catheter. This is usually 20 or 22 G, as larger sizes have a higher risk of thrombosis and smaller sizes can lead to excessive damping of the blood pressure trace.
- A short and stiff piece of tubing to connect the catheter to the pressure transducer. It is important to use the correct tubing as it is specifically designed to reduce damping.
- A pressure transducer, which is in continuity with the blood inside the artery via a continuous column of saline. The transducer contains a strain gauge that converts the pressure wave into an electrical signal. A cable is then used to transfer this signal to a microprocessor and a display.
- A flushing system. This is a bag of normal saline that is connected to the fluid filled tubing via a flush system. The bag of saline is pressurized to 300 mmHg, allowing a continuous infusion of 2–4 mL/h to maintain patency of the arterial catheter. It also contains a flushing device to allow for a high pressure flush of fluid to the system.

Most systems incorporate several three-way taps. The bungs on the taps are often designed with holes in them; these must be replaced prior to use to preserve a closed system.

Technique

Catheter insertion is similar to arterial sampling, but the artery is approached at a shallower angle and in line with the course of the artery.

Once the tip of the needle is inside the artery, it should be advanced slightly to ensure that the plastic catheter is also located in the artery. At this point, the catheter should be gently passed over the needle, and into the artery. The needle should then be removed, and the catheter can be connected to the tubing.

An alternative design uses a guidewire; the artery is cannulated with a needle (once again at a shallow angle), and the guidewire is threaded down the needle into the artery. The needle is then removed, and the catheter is passed over the wire. The wire is removed and the catheter is attached to the tubing. If this technique is being used it is imperative not to insert the wire too far, and to always hold onto it to avoid the risk of losing the wire into the arterial system. Newer designs are available that use an incorporated guidewire.

Whichever system is used, it is imperative to secure the catheter with a suitable dressing and/or sutures.

Further reading

Ailon J, Mourad O, Chien V, Saun T, Dev SP (2014) Videos in clinical medicine. Ultrasound-guided insertion of a radial artery catheter. *N Engl J Med* 371, e21. http://www.nejm.org/doi/full/10.1056/NEJMvcm1213181.

CHAPTER 118

Arterial blood gases, oxygen saturation and oxygen therapy

David Sprigings

Table 118.1 Overview.

Feature	Comment
Normal values	In a person breathing air (FiO_2 21%), normal arterial oxygen tension (PaO_2) is >10.7 kPa and normal arterial oxygen saturation (SaO_2) is >93%.
	Arterial oxygen tension and oxygen saturation are related by the oxyhemoglobin dissocation curve.
	Normal arterial carbon dioxide tension (PaO_2) is 4.7–6.0 kPa.
Determinants of arterial oxygen tension	• Inspired oxygen concentration (FiO_2)
	• Alveolar ventilation (determined by tidal volume, dead space and respiratory rate)
	• Diffusion of oxygen from alveoli to pulmonary capillaries
	• Distribution and matching of lung ventilation and pulmonary blood flow (V/Q matching) (see Table 118.2)
Pulse oximetry	Arterial oxygen saturation can be measured non-invasively by pulse oximetry, although this method does not always give accurate readings (Table 118.3)
	Remember that pulse oximetry does not give information about arterial PCO_2 or pH
	Arterial blood gases and pH should be checked if arterial oxygen saturation by oximetry is <92%, or if there are clinical features of respiratory failure (Chapter 11)
Respiratory failure	Arterial hypoxaemia is defined as an arterial PaO_2 <10.7 kPa, and respiratory failure as an arterial PaO_2 <8 kPa, breathing air.
	Respiratory failure is subdivided according to the arterial carbon dioxide tension ($PaCO_2$). Type 1 respiratory failure is when arterial $PaCO_2$ is normal or low (<6 kPa), and type 2 respiratory failure is when arterial $PaCO_2$ is high (>6 kPa)
	See Chapter 11.
Oxygen therapy and delivery devices	Oxygen should be given to patients with hypoxaemia (oxygen saturation by oximetry <92%), hypotension, low cardiac output, respiratory distress or cardiorespiratory arrest. See Figure 118.1.
	Where possible, arterial blood gases should be measured before oxygen is started.
	Oxygen should be prescribed as carefully as any other drug, specifying the delivery device to be used and the oxygen flow rate.
	Commonly used oxygen delivery devices are described in Table 118.4.
	Initial FiO_2 should be 40–60%, except for patients with type 2 respiratory failure ($PaCO_2$ >6 kPa) who should start with 24% oxygen, and patients with cardiorespiratory arrest who should receive ~100% oxygen.
	Arterial blood gases should be checked within 1 h of starting oxygen, and FiO_2 adjusted accordingly. The target is a PaO_2 of >8 kPa or SaO_2 >92%.
Ventilatory support	See Chapters 11 and 116.

Acute Medicine: A Practical Guide to the Management of Medical Emergencies, Fifth Edition. Edited by David Sprigings and John B. Chambers.
© 2018 John Wiley & Sons Ltd. Published 2018 by John Wiley & Sons Ltd.

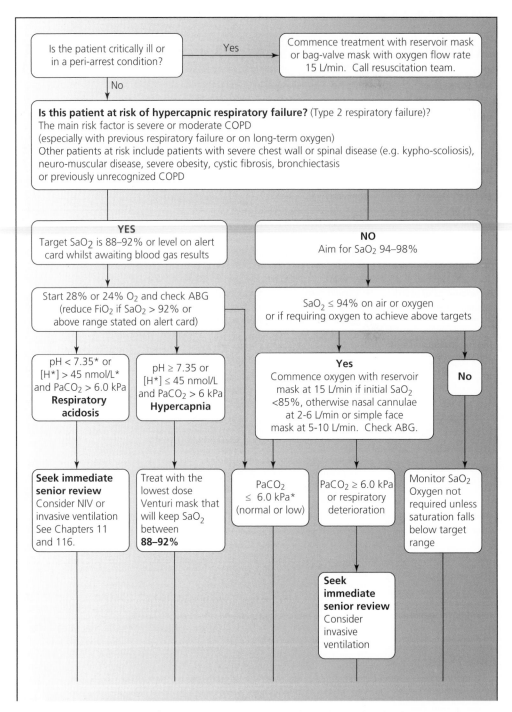

Figure 118.1 Oxygen prescription for acutely hypoxaemic patients in hospital. Reproduced with permission from: O'Driscoll R, Howard L, Earis J, Mak V, on behalf of the BTS Emergency Oxygen Guideline Group (2015) *BTS Guidelines for oxygen use in adults in healthcare and emergency settings.*

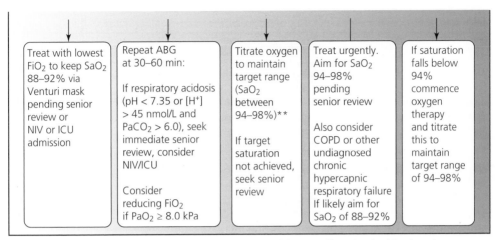

| Treat with lowest FiO$_2$ to keep SaO$_2$ 88–92% via Venturi mask pending senior review or NIV or ICU admission | Repeat ABG at 30–60 min: If respiratory acidosis (pH < 7.35 or [H$^+$] > 45 nmol/L and PaCO$_2$ > 6.0), seek immediate senior review, consider NIV/ICU Consider reducing FiO$_2$ if PaO$_2$ ≥ 8.0 kPa | Titrate oxygen to maintain target range (SaO$_2$ between 94–98%)** If target saturation not achieved, seek senior review | Treat urgently. Aim for SaO$_2$ 94–98% pending senior review Also consider COPD or other undiagnosed chronic hypercapnic respiratory failure If likely aim for SaO$_2$ of 88–92% | If saturation falls below 94% commence oxygen therapy and titrate this to maintain target range of 94–98% |

Any increase in FiO$_2$ must be followed by repeat ABG in 1 h (or sooner if conscious level deteriorates)
If pH is <7.35 ([H] > 45 nmol/L) with normal or low PaCo$_2$, investigate and treat for metabolic acidosis and keep SaO$_2$ 94–98%
**Repeat ABG in 30–60 min for all patients at risk of type 2 respiratory failure (even if initial PaCO$_2$ is normal)

Figure 118.1 *Continued.*

Table 118.2 Estimation of the alveolar–arterial oxygen difference.

1. Establish FiO_2, the fractional concentration of oxygen in inspired gas (0.21 in air)
2. Measure PaO_2 and $PaCO_2$, the partial pressures of oxygen and carbon dioxide (in kPa) in arterial blood
3. Estimate the partial pressure of oxygen in alveolar gas (PAO_2) from the simplified form of the alveolar gas equation:
$PAO_2 = [PiO_2 - (PaCO_2/R)] = [(94.8 \times FiO_2) - (PaCO_2/R)]$
where PiO_2 is the partial pressure of inspired oxygen and R is the respiratory quotient (can be taken to be 1). The table below shows the PiO_2 for a given FiO_2:

FiO_2	0.21	0.24	0.28	0.31	0.35	0.40	0.60	1.0
PiO_2	19.9	22.8	26.5	29.4	33.2	37.9	56.9	94.8

4. Subtract PaO_2 from PAO_2 to give the alveolar–arterial oxygen difference (A–a gradient). Normal values are given below:

Age (years)	Normal PaO_2 (kPa)	Normal A – a gradient (kPa)
20	13.2	1.8
40	12.5	2.5
60	11.9	3.1
80	11.3	3.7

5. An increased alveolar-arterial oxygen difference indicates V/Q mismatching: this may reflect a range of pulmonary and pulmonary vascular disorders, for example acute asthma, pneumonia, pulmonary oedema and pulmonary embolism

Table 118.3 Pulse oximetry: causes of inaccurate reading.

- Probe not properly on finger
- Motion artefact
- Poor perfusion of finger
- Venous congestion
- Hypothermia
- Intense ambient light
- Abnormal haemoglobin (carboxyhaemoglobin, methaemoglobin, sickle haemoglobin)
- Severe anaemia (Hb <50 g/L)

Table 118.4 Oxygen delivery devices.

Device	Indication	Concentration of O$_2$ delivered	Advantages	Disadvantages
Facemask with reservoir bag (O$_2$ flow rate 10–15 L/min)	Cardiorespiratory arrest or peri-arrest, when high concentration of O$_2$ essential	>80%	Highest O$_2$ concentration delivered	Some rebreathing of CO$_2$, with risk of CO$_2$ retention in type 2 respiratory failure
Low-flow mask (e.g. Hudson)	Type 1 respiratory failure	28–60%, depending on the O$_2$ flow rate, degree of leakage between the mask and face, and ventilatory minute volume	Simple and cheap No need to change mask if FiO$_2$ has to be changed	FiO$_2$ provided by a given O$_2$ flow rate is variable At flow rates <5 L/min, significant rebreathing may occur, with risk of CO$_2$ retention in type 2 respiratory failure
High-flow mask (Venturi principle)	Type 2 respiratory failure, and when accurate FiO$_2$ is needed	24%, 28%, 35%, 40% and 60%, determined by the Venturi valve (colour coded) used and the O$_2$ flow rate	Delivers an accurate FiO$_2$ Reduces the risk of CO$_2$ retention in type 2 rate respiratory failure; 60% mask is useful in type 1 respiratory failure when hypoxaemia persists despite 10 L/min O$_2$ flow rate via low-flow mask	Uncomfortable to wear for long periods New valve needed if FiO$_2$ has to be changed
Nasal cannulae	Patients with COPD or recovering from other causes of respiratory failure	Depends on the O$_2$ flow rate and ventilatory minute volume; 2 L/min gives an FiO$_2$ of roughly 25–30%	Prevents rebreathing and so reduces the risk of CO$_2$ retention in type 2 respiratory failure Comfortable to wear for long periods	Nasal irritation with flow rates >3 L/min

COPD, chronic obstructive pulmonary disease.

Further reading

British Thoracic Society Emergency Oxygen Guideline Group. BTS Guidelines for oxygen use in adults in healthcare and emergency settings 2015. https://www.brit-thoracic.org.uk/standards-of-care/guidelines/bts-guideline-for-emergency-oxygen-use-in-adult-patients/.

CHAPTER 119

Temporary cardiac pacing

SANDEEP HOTHI AND DAVID SPRIGINGS

Temporary cardiac pacing is the electrical stimulation of the heart to induce contraction. It can be achieved via several routes: transvenous, epicardial, transoesophageal and external (transcutaneous). This chapter describes temporary transvenous and external cardiac pacing.

Temporary transvenous cardiac pacing

Indications, contraindications and potential complications of temporary transvenous pacing are summarized in Table 119.1.

- Where permanent pacing is indicated, it should be performed instead, unless delay in achieving this is anticipated or contraindications to early permanent pacing are present (e.g. sepsis).
- Equipment needed is given in Table 119.2. You will need at least one medical or nursing assistant, to monitor the patient during the procedure and assist with the equipment, and a radiographer to set up and operate the X-ray screening.

Preparation

1 Confirm the indications for the procedure. Check there is no major contraindication to central vein cannulation. Decide on the route of venous access. Choose the femoral vein in preference to the internal jugular vein if the patient is haemodynamically unstable (especially if you have limited experience, as placement of the lead via the femoral vein is usually easier) or has received thrombolysis. Ensure that a defibrillator and other resuscitation equipment are to hand.

2 Explain the procedure to the patient, and obtain consent, unless the situation precludes this. Check that the bed is suitable for X-ray screening and that the screening equipment can obtain satisfactory access to the patient.

3 Connect an ECG monitor (making sure the leads are off the chest, so that they are not confused with the pacing lead when screening) and put in a peripheral venous cannula. Give supplemental oxygen via nasal cannulae or a mask, with continuous monitoring of oxygen saturation by oximetry. If sedation is needed, give midazolam 2 mg (1 mg in the elderly) IV over 30 s, followed after 2 min by increments of 0.5–1 mg if needed (usual range 2.5–5 mg).

4 Put on mask, gown and gloves. Prepare the skin with chlorhexidine or povidone-iodine and apply drapes to a wide area. Unpack the pacing lead and check that it will pass down the central venous catheter.

Cannulation of a central vein

5 See Chapter 116 for a detailed description of central vein cannulation.

Acute Medicine: A Practical Guide to the Management of Medical Emergencies, Fifth Edition. Edited by David Sprigings and John B. Chambers.
© 2018 John Wiley & Sons Ltd. Published 2018 by John Wiley & Sons Ltd.

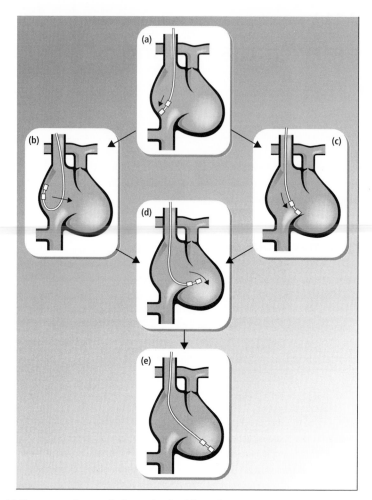

Figure 119.1 (a) Placement of a ventricular pacing lead from the superior vena cava (via the internal jugular or subclavian veins). (a) The lead is advanced to the low right atrium. (b) Further advancement produces a loop or bend in the distal lead, which is then rotated medially. (c) Alternatively, the lead in low right atrium deflects off the tricuspid annulus directly into the right ventricle. (d) Superior orientation of the lead tip in the ventricle requires clockwise torque during advancement to avoid the interventricular septum. (e) Final lead position in the right ventricular apex. The catheter position in (b) is suitable for atrial pacing.

Placement of the lead (Figures 119.1 and 119.2)

6 Advance the lead into the right atrium and direct it towards the apex of the right ventricle (just medial to the lateral border of the cardiac silhouette): it may cross the tricuspid valve easily.

7 If you have difficulty, form a loop of lead in the right atrium. With slight rotation and advancement of the lead, the loop should prolapse across the tricuspid valve.

8 Manipulate the lead so that the tip curves downwards at the apex of the right ventricle and lies in a gentle S-shape within the right atrium and ventricle. Displacement of the lead may occur if there is too much or not enough slack.

9 Ask your assistant to attach the terminal pins of the pacing lead to the connecting lead and pacing box.

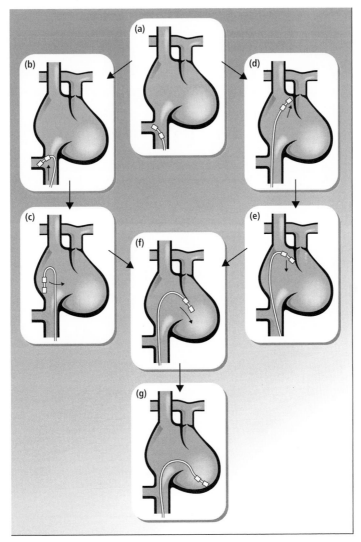

Figure 119.1 (b) Placement of a ventricular pacing lead from the inferior vena cava (via the femoral vein).
(a) The lead is advanced to the hepatic vein. (b) The lead tip engages in the proximal hepatic vein and is advanced further. (c) A loop or bend is formed in the distal lead, which is then rotated medially. (d) Alternatively, the lead is advanced to the high medial right atrium. (e) With advancement, a bend is formed in the lead, which is then quickly withdrawn or 'snapped' back to the level of the tricuspid orifice. (f) After crossing the tricuspid valve, the lead is advanced with counterclockwise torque to avoid the interventricular septum. (g) Final lead position in the right ventricular apex. The lead positions in (c) and (d) can be used for atrial pacing. Source: Ellenbogen KA (ed). Cardiac Pacing. Boston: Blackwell Scientific Publications, 1992; 178–9. Reproduced with permission of John Wiley & Sons.

Checking the threshold

10 Set the box to 'demand' mode, with a pacing rate faster than the intrinsic heart rate. Set the output at 3 V. This should result in a paced rhythm. If it does not, you need to find a better position. Before moving from a position that may have taken a long while to achieve, make sure the problem is not due to loose contacts: check these are all secure.

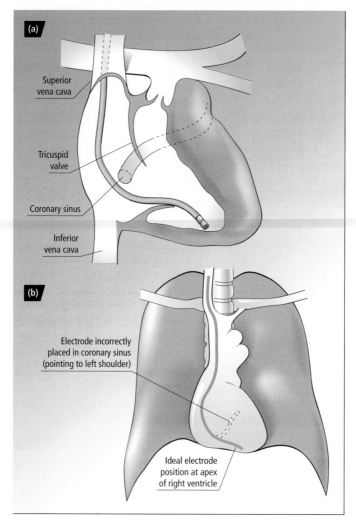

Figure 119.2 Lead position for temporary pacing: (a) anatomy; and (b) screening.

11 Progressively reduce the output until there is failure to capture: the heart rate drops abruptly and pacing spikes are seen but not followed by paced beats. A threshold of <1 V is ideal. A threshold a little above this is acceptable if the lead position is stable.

12 Check the stability of the lead position. Set the box at a rate faster than the intrinsic heart rate, with an output of 1 V (or just above threshold). Ask the patient to cough forcefully and breathe deeply. Watch the monitor for loss of capture.

Final points

13 Set the output at more than three times the threshold or 3 V, whichever is higher. Set the mode to 'demand'. If the patient is now in sinus rhythm at a rate of >50/min, set a back-up rate of 50/min. If there is atrioventricular block or bradycardia, set at 70–80/min (90–100/min if there is cardiogenic shock).

14 Remove the insertion sheath, with screening of the lead and counter-advancement if needed to prevent displacement. If the sheath has a haemostatic valve, it can be left in place.

Table 119.1 Temporary cardiac pacing: indications, contraindications and potential complications.

Indications

Bradycardia/asystole (sinus or junctional bradycardia or second/third-degree atrioventricular (AV) block) associated with haemodynamic compromise and unresponsive to atropine (Chapter 44).

After cardiac arrest due to bradycardia/asystole.

To prevent perioperative bradycardia. Temporary pacing is indicated in:

- Second-degree Mobitz type 2 AV block or complete heart block
- Sinus/junctional bradycardia or second-degree Mobitz type I (Wenckebach) AV block or bundle branch block (including bifascicular and trifascicular block) only if there is a history of syncope or presyncope

Atrial or ventricular overdrive pacing to prevent recurrent monomorphic ventricular tachycardia (Chapter 40) or polymorphic ventricular tachycardia with preceding QT prolongation (torsade de pointes) (Chapter 41).

Contraindications

Risks of temporary pacing outweigh benefits: for example rare symptomatic sinus pauses, or complete heart block with a stable escape rhythm and no haemodynamic compromise. Discuss management with a cardiologist. Consider using standby external pacing system instead of transvenous pacing.

Prosthetic tricuspid valve.

Complications

Complications of central vein cannulation (Chapter 116), especially bleeding in patients with acute coronary syndromes treated with thrombolytic therapy.

Cardiac perforation by pacing lead (may rarely result in cardiac tamponade).

Arrhythmias (atrial and ventricular, including tachycardia and ventricular fibrillation) during placement of pacing lead.

Infection of pacing lead.

---

15 Suture the lead (or sheath if left in place) to the skin close to the point of insertion and cover it with a dressing. The rest of the lead should be looped and also sutured to the skin. An air and water occlusive dressing is then applied over the entry site to the skin.

16 Clear up and dispose of sharps safely. Arrange a chest X-ray to confirm satisfactory lead position and exclude a pneumothorax.

17 Document the procedure including: indications/access/threshold/final pacemaker box settings/any complications/post-procedure chest X-ray findings/plan of management.

18 Establish continuous ECG monitoring. RV apical pacing should result in QRS complexes of left bundle branch block morphology with superior axis (positive in leads I and aVL).

Aftercare

19 Check the pacing threshold daily. The threshold usually rises to 2–3 times its initial value over the first few days after insertion because of endocardial oedema. The commonest reason for failure to capture and/or sense after the procedure is lead displacement.

20 If infection related to the lead is suspected, see p. 664.

Table 119.2 Temporary transvenous pacing: equipment.

Temporary pacing lead (a 6 French lead is easier to manipulate than a 5 French one, but its greater stiffness increases the risk of cardiac perforation)

Pacing box and connecting lead

Central vein cannulation pack, central venous sheath (one French size larger than the pacing lead to be used) and ultrasound device for central vein imaging

Suture

Local anaesthesia

X-ray screening equipment

Troubleshooting

The pacing lead cannot be advanced into the heart

This can happen if you have cannulated the carotid artery rather than the internal jugular vein: the pacing lead bounces off the aortic valve. Ask advice from a senior colleague or cardiologist. If inadvertent arterial cannulation is confirmed, withdraw the lead and sheath and apply pressure over the vessel to achieve haemostasis.

A pacing lead placed via the femoral vein will usually pass easily up the iliac veins and inferior vena cava, with a little manipulation, but may keep diving into other veins. Reducing the curve on the end of the lead may make this less likely to happen.

Tachyarrhythmias

Ventricular extrasystoles and non-sustained ventricular tachycardia are common as the lead crosses the tricuspid valve and do not require treatment. If there is sustained ventricular tachycardia, withdraw the pacing lead and it will usually terminate.

Ventricular fibrillation may occur with manipulation of the lead in the right ventricle, especially in patients with acute coronary syndromes, and requires defibrillation and other standard measures.

If ventricular tachycardia recurs after placement, check that the position of the lead is still satisfactory and that excess slack has not formed in the area of the tricuspid valve.

Failure to capture

Causes include:
- Contacts not secure: check these.
- Pacing lead not in right ventricle: it may be in the right atrium, in the coronary sinus (a lead in the coronary sinus points towards the left shoulder) or in the splenic vein (with femoral vein access). Ask advice from a senior colleague or cardiologist.
- Pacing lead has perforated the right ventricle. This may cause pericardial chest pain and diaphragmatic pacing at low output (3 V or less). Withdraw the lead and reposition it. Be aware that cardiac tamponade may occur following cardiac perforation but is rare.

External cardiac pacing

Indications are as for transvenous pacing. Consider sedation if the patient is awake as the procedure is uncomfortable: it is therefore more appropriate as a backup prior to transvenous or permanent pacing.
- Apply the large chest wall electrodes to the chest cavity in the anteroposterior positions.
- Connect to external pacing system. Commence at highest output. Then determine threshold by reducing in 5–10 mA steps until loss of capture. The lowest current output that causes capture is the threshold.
- Set the device to 5–10 mA above the threshold. Choose pacing mode: demand usually preferable to fixed.
- Change pads every 4–5 hours to minimize skins burns.

Further reading

The Task Force on cardiac pacing and resynchronization therapy of the European Society of Cardiology (ESC) (2013) 2013 ESC Guidelines on cardiac pacing and cardiac resynchronization therapy. *European Heart Journal* 34, 2281–2329.

CHAPTER 120

Pericardial aspiration (pericardiocentesis)

Sandeep Hothi and David Sprigings

Indications, contraindications and potential complications are summarized in Table 120.1.

Imaging with echocardiography is recommended to guide pericardiocentesis, and can be used in one of three ways: imaging before advancement of the needle, to establish the anatomy; imaging before and intermittently during advancement of the needle; continuous imaging throughout the procedure. Unless pericardiocentesis is required in the setting of actual or incipient cardiac arrest, the procedure should be done in a cardiac catheterization room with immediate access to X-ray screening (fluoroscopy) if needed.

Equipment needed is given in Table 120.2. You will need at least two assistants, to monitor the patient during the procedure and assist with the equipment.

Technique

Preparation

1 Confirm the indication for the procedure. Check for contraindications, though these are relative if there is cardiac tamponade. Obtain the informed consent of the patient. Blood should be sent for group and screen. Ensure that a defibrillator and other resuscitation equipment is to hand.

2 The patient should be sitting up at 30–45 degrees, so that the pericardial effusion pools anteriorly and inferiorly. The main approach is subcostal (Figure 120.1). Choose the approach with the largest thickness of effusion (this should be 2 cm or greater), and decide on the optimum needle trajectory, avoiding the liver or lung. Measure the depth from the skin surface to the pericardial effusion and mark the planned puncture site with an indelible marker.

3 Connect an ECG monitor and put in a peripheral venous cannula. Give supplemental oxygen via nasal cannulae or mask, with continuous monitoring of oxygen saturation by oximetry. If sedation is required, midazolam may be considered, balanced against the risks of respiratory depression. Give 2 mg (1 mg in elderly) IV over 30 s, followed after 2 min by 0.5–1 mg increments if sedation is not adequate (usual range 2.5–5 mg).

4 Put on hat, mask, sterile gown and gloves. Prepare the skin from mid-chest to mid-abdomen with chlorhexidine or povidone-iodine and apply drapes to a wide area.

Acute Medicine: A Practical Guide to the Management of Medical Emergencies, Fifth Edition. Edited by David Sprigings and John B. Chambers.
© 2018 John Wiley & Sons Ltd. Published 2018 by John Wiley & Sons Ltd.

Table 120.1 Pericardial aspiration: indications, contraindications and potential complications.

Indications

Cardiac tamponade (Chapter 54). Echocardiography must be done first to confirm the presence of a pericardial effusion unless there is cardiac arrest from presumed tamponade.

Pericardial effusion due to suspected bacterial pericarditis (p. 342).

To establish the cause of a moderate or large pericardial effusion, when other investigations have failed to do so.

Contraindications

Pericardial effusion of less than 2 cm thickness without haemodynamic compromise: discuss management with a cardiologist.

Bleeding disorder/coagulopathy (including platelet count $<50 \times 10^9$/L, INR >1.5, or receiving oral anticoagulant or anticoagulant-dose heparin): discuss management with a haematologist.

Associated aortic dissection or myocardial rupture: drainage may aggravate bleeding.

Potential complications (incidence in patients without contraindications <5%)

Penetration of a cardiac chamber (usually right ventricle) (may result in acute tamponade).

Laceration of an artery (coronary, left internal thoracic, intercostal, intraabdominal (may result in acute tamponade)).

Arrhythmia

Pneumothorax

Perforation of stomach or colon (with subcostal approach)

Vasovagal reaction

Failure of the procedure

Infection

INR, international normalized ratio.

Pericardiocentesis

5 Anaesthetize the skin at the planned puncture site with a 25 G (orange) needle, and then use a 21 G (green) needle to infiltrate local anaesthetic along the intended needle track towards the effusion. With the left parasternal approach, a green needle is usually long enough to enter the effusion. Allow the local anaesthetic time to work and then make a small skin incision with a scalpel at the puncture site.

6 Advance the needle into the pericardial space.

Table 120.2 Equipment needed for pericardiocentesis.

Syringes: 10 mL and 50 mL

Long needle (e.g. 7–10 cm, 18 G).

Scalpel

Guidewire (e.g. 80 cm, 0.035″ diameter, with J end)

Dilator (7 French)

Pigtail catheter (e.g. 40 cm long, 7 French diameter, multiple side holes)

Drainage bag and connector; three-way tap

Sterile drapes

Suture

Dressing

Sets containing the required kit are commercially available

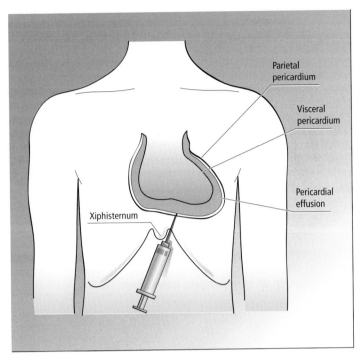

Figure 120.1 Anatomy of the pericardial space and pericardiocentesis. The pericardial sac contains the heart and the roots of the great vessels. It has two layers, a serous visceral layer (also known as epicardium when it comes into contact with the myocardium) and a fibrous parietal layer, and encloses the pericardial cavity. Pericardiocentesis can be done by subcostal, left parasternal and apical approaches (see text). For the subcostal approach (illustrated), the needle is introduced 1 cm below the left xiphocostal angle, and then advanced slowly at an angle of 30° to the skin, aiming for the left shoulder.

Subcostal approach: attach the long needle to a 10 mL syringe containing lidocaine 1% and introduce 1 cm below the left xiphocostal angle. Then advance slowly at an angle of 30° to the skin, along the anesthetized track, aiming for the left shoulder, with continuous aspiration and intermittent injection of lidocaine.

Other approaches are possible and are described below, but should only be used by cardiologists / cardiac surgeons with appropriate training.

Left parasternal approach: the needle is attached to a 10 mL syringe containing lidocaine and inserted at 90° to the skin over the superior margins of the fifth or sixth rib adjacent to and within 1 cm, or 3–5 cm lateral to, the left sternal margin (avoiding the LIMA).

Apical approach: insert the needle over the superior rib margins in the fifth to seventh left interspace over the cardiac apex.

7 When you aspirate pericardial fluid, advance the needle a couple of mm further, then remove the syringe and introduce about 20 cm of the guidewire (J end leading). See section on Troubleshooting below if you are not sure whether the fluid is haemorrhagic pericardial effusion or blood.

8 Pass the dilator over the guidewire to dilate the subcutaneous track and pericardium (taking care not to advance it further into the effusion) and then remove the dilator.

9 Put the pigtail catheter on the guidewire and advance it over the guidewire and into the pericardial space, so that around 20 cm of the catheter is within the pericardium. It helps to keep the guidewire fairly taut.

10 Remove the guidewire and aspirate 50 mL or more via the catheter. Take specimens for microscopy, culture and cytology. Attach the connector and drainage bag to the catheter via a three-way tap. If the indication for pericardiocentesis was cardiac tamponade, aspirate as much fluid as possible.

11 Insert a skin suture and loop it over the catheter several times, tying it each time, or use a device to anchor and support the catheter as it exits the skin.

Final points

12 Dispose of sharps safely. Arrange a chest X-ray to exclude pneumothorax. Check with echocardiography the size of the residual effusion.

13 Document the procedure in the patient's record, including: indications/approach/appearance of pericardial fluid/samples sent/any complications/post-procedure chest X-ray findings/post-procedure echocardiographic findings/management plan.

Aftercare

14 Leave the catheter on free drainage. Analgesia may be needed to relieve pericardial pain. Remove the catheter within 72 h to prevent infection.

15 Further management depends on the aetiology of the effusion.

Troubleshooting

You cannot enter the effusion

- Check that the diagnosis is correct and that the effusion does not look solid or loculated.
- Consider using an alternative approach, provided the effusion is >2 cm thickness.

The pigtail catheter will not pass over the guidewire into the pericardial space

- Check that the guidewire is correctly positioned within the cardiac shadow (use fluoroscopy to image the guidewire).
- Check that the guidewire is held taut and not looped.
- Repeat the dilatation of the subcutaneous track.

You aspirate heavily bloodstained fluid

- The possibilities are: haemorrhagic effusion (common in malignancy or Dressler syndrome); venous puncture; right heart puncture; or laceration of a coronary artery with haemopericardium.
- Keep hold of the needle, but remove the syringe and empty it into a clean pot. Blood will clot, but even heavily bloodstained effusion will not.
- Inject 10 mL of an agitated 9.5 mL 0.9% saline/0.5 mL solution (rapidly mixed using a three-way tap to create microbubbles) through the exploring needle to determine the space within which the needle tip resides under echocardiographic imaging.
- If you are still in doubt, compare the haematocrit of the fluid with that of a venous sample (both sent in ethylene diaminetetra-acetic acid (EDTA) tubes), or connect to a pressure monitor: right ventricular penetration is shown by a characteristic waveform.

Further reading

Fitch MT, Nicks BA, Pariyadath M, McGinnis HD, Manthey DE. (2012) Videos in clinical medicine. Emergency pericardiocentesis. *N Engl J Med* 366, e17. http://www.nejm.org/doi/full/10.1056/NEJMvcm0907841.

The Task Force for the diagnosis and management of pericardial diseases of the European Society of Cardiology (ESC). 2015 ESC Guidelines for the diagnosis and management of pericardial diseases. http://www.escardio.org/static_file/Escardio/Guidelines/Publications/PERICA/2015%20Percardial%20Web%20Addenda-ehv318.pdf.

CHAPTER 121

DC cardioversion

SANDEEP HOTHI AND DAVID SPRIGINGS

The management of arrhythmias is described in Chapters 39–44. Indications, contraindications and potential complications of DC cardioversion are summarized in Table 121.1. Equipment needed is given in Table 121.2. Haemodynamic compromise with tachyarrhythmias at rates less than 130/min should prompt consideration of other causes, such as hypovolaemia, sepsis, pulmonary embolism or heart failure.

Technique in haemodynamically stable patients

Preparation

1 Attach an ECG monitor and record a 12-lead ECG. Check the arrhythmia. General aspects of the preparation of the patient before cardioversion of atrial fibrillation or flutter are summarized in Table 121.3. Contact an anaesthetist to discuss the anaesthetic management and timing of the procedure. Discuss the procedure with the patient and obtain consent.

2 Put in a peripheral venous cannula, give supplemental oxygen via nasal cannulae or a facemask, and monitor arterial oxygen saturation by oximetry. Check the blood pressure. Check that the defibrillator, resuscitation equipment and drugs are to hand.

3 Lay the patient down and change the ECG leads from the bedside monitor to the defibrillator. Adjust the leads until the R waves are significantly higher than the T waves and check that the synchronizing marker falls consistently on the QRS complex and not the T wave. Place self-adhesive defibrillator pads on the sternum and over the cardiac apex (check this). Elevate the bed so that the airway is easily accessible.

4 The anaesthetist administers general anaesthesia or deep sedation.

Countershock

5 When the patient is anaesthetized, charge the defibrillator and deliver an appropriate charge to cardiovert the arrhythmia (Table 121.4). If the first shock fails to restore a sinus rhythm, deliver a second and if needed a third shock, at higher energy. The operator should call to all staff that the defibrillator is being charged and again before delivering the shock, and should look to make sure that no one is in contact directly or indirectly with the patient before the shock is delivered.

Aftercare

6 Record a 12-lead ECG. Consider prophylactic antiarrhythmic therapy to maintain the sinus rhythm. Write a note of the procedure in the patient's record, documenting: indications/anaesthetic technique/shocks delivered/any complications/post-procedure rhythm/plan of management.

7 Continue heparin/warfarin/DOAC anticoagulation for at least one month (or indefinitely if indicated) after successful cardioversion of atrial fibrillation or flutter of more than 48 h duration.

Acute Medicine: A Practical Guide to the Management of Medical Emergencies, Fifth Edition. Edited by David Sprigings and John B. Chambers.
© 2018 John Wiley & Sons Ltd. Published 2018 by John Wiley & Sons Ltd.

Table 121.1 DC cardioversion: indications, contraindications and potential complications.

Indications

Conversion of ventricular and supraventricular tachyarrhythmias

Contraindications

When another treatment is better (e.g. pharmacological cardioversion) or there is acceptance of supraventricular arrhythmia with rate control. Seek advice from a cardiologist about the management of haemodynamically stable tachyarrhythmias before cardioversion.
Digoxin toxicity
Hypokalaemia (plasma potassium <3.5 mmol/L)
Thyrotoxicosis if in atrial fibrillation (cardioversion unlikely to be successful without correction of thyrotoxicosis)

Potential complications

Tachyarrhythmias:
Ventricular: non-sustained VT (5%); sustained VT; VF (especially if the shock is delivered during the vulnerable phase of the cardiac cycle: its delivery should be synchronized with the QRS complex to avoid this)
Atrial: SVT (30%), sinus tachycardia, AVNRT, atrial flutter
Bradyarrhythmias (0.9%) – transient LBBB, high degree AV block, asystole. These may uncommonly require atropine or temporary pacing whether externally or transvenous. Risk factors: antiarrhythmic drugs.
ST elevation and T wave changes. These are non-specific and by themselves do not indicate an acute coronary syndrome.
Interference with settings of permanent pacemakers and implantable cardioverter-defibrillators (these should be checked post-cardioversion)
Thromboembolism – pulmonary or systemic. More likely in atrial fibrillation or flutter. Incidence 5.3% if not anticoagulated, <1% if adequately anticoagulated (see Table 121.3). The cause can be dislodgement of exiting thrombus or more usually de novo thrombus due to atrial stunning.
Complications of general anaesthesia/sedation
Skin burns from shocks – consider prophylactic topical hydrocortisone or topical NSAID
Myocardial necrosis – minimal necrosis, typically with higher energy levels. Usually asymptomatic with mild troponin or CK-MB rise.
Myocardial dysfunction – global LVSD (stunning), atrial stunning
Pulmonary oedema (rarely), transient hypotension (often fluid responsive)

Considerations for specific arrhythmias and circumstances

Synchronized DCCV may not be possible (very rapid VT) or dangerous (polymorphic VT) with risk of VF. In these situations, defibrillation should be performed as there is a risk of inducing VF with synchronized DCCV.

Patients with permanent pacemakers/ICDs/CRT devices – place pads in the antero-posterior position with both at least 12 cm from the generator. Use lowest indicated energy setting. Obtain a device check after DCCV.

ICD/CRT-D – cardioversion may be performed by the device using a device programmer. Avoids risk of injury to the system and of skin burns. However, consumes significant device energy.

Digoxin toxicity induced arrhythmias: digoxin toxicity is a relative contraindication to DCCV as it can exacerbate electrically induced arrhythmias. Correct hypokalaemia in all cases. Conservatively manage nodal

Table 121.2 Assistance/equipment.

An anaesthetist and anaesthetic equipment
Defibrillator and resuscitation equipment
Availability of advanced life support medications
One assistant to monitor the patient and help with equipment

Table 121.3 Checklist before DC cardioversion of haemodynamically stable atrial fibrillation or flutter.

Anticoagulation

Arrhythmia reliably known to be of less than 48 h duration:
Moderate to high-risk patients: these patients have a CHA_2DS_2-VASc score ≥1 and should have IV heparin, LMWH or a licensed DOAC commenced before DCCV and continued long term.
Lower risk patients: CHA_2DS_2-VASc score = 0; as well as patients with very high bleeding risk do not require anticoagulation prior to DCCV. It is unclear whether four weeks of anticoagulation should be given post successful DCCV in this group.

Arrhythmia of uncertain duration or more than 48 h duration:
Oral anticoagulation (warfarin with INR >2.0 for three weeks and on the day of DCCV, or licensed NOAC) should be given for at least three weeks before, and continued for at least one month after cardioversion.
Alternatively, a TOE-guided approach can be considered in those anticoagulated for less than three weeks pre-DCCV. A short period of anticoagulation is administered: LMWH or unfractionated heparin (bolus + infusion for APTT 1.5–2.0 times control) plus simultaneous PO warfarin initiation; or at least four doses dabigatran 150 mg bd or apixaban 5 mg bd without any heparin; or five days of warfarin pre-TOE with INR 2.0–3.0 on procedure day. TOE can then guide DCCV after excluding thrombus in left and right atrium, their appendages, and the LV. Post-procedural anticoagulation is continued for at least one month.
INR, international normalized ratio.

Plasma potassium
Check this is >3.5 mmol/L. Correct hypokalaemia before cardioversion (Chapter 86)

Digoxin
Check that there are no features to suggest toxicity (nausea, slow ventricular response, frequent ventricular extrasystoles) and that if the dose is high (>250 μgm/day), renal function is normal.

Thyroid function
Check that thyroid function is normal: cardioversion of atrial fibrillation due to thyrotoxicosis (which may be otherwise occult) is unlikely to be successful.

Tachybrady syndrome
Consider placing a temporary pacing lead or having an external pacing system on stand-by, as asystole or severe bradycardia may follow DC cardioversion.

Nil by mouth
Water up to 2 h before anaesthesia.
Food and other drinks up to 6 h before anaesthesia.

Table 121.4 Cardioversion of arrhythmias: charges.

Arrhythmia	First shock (J)		Second and third shocks (J)	
	Monophasic	Biphasic	Monophasic	Biphasic
Ventricular arrhythmias				
Ventricular fibrillation or pulseless ventricular tachycardia	360	200	360	200
Other ventricular tachycardias	200	100–200	360	200
Atrial arrhythmias				
Atrial fibrillation	200	120–150	360	200
Atrial flutter	100	50–100	200	150
Other supraventricular arrhythmias	100	70–120	200	150

or atrial tachycardia. SVTs: ideally defer DCCV until digoxin levels are normal and use the lowest indicated energy level. VT: consider IV lidocaine pre-shock and use the lowest indicated energy level.

Pregnancy – DCCV can be performed for the mother. Fetal heart rate monitoring is recommended.

Atrial fibrillation with potentially reversible causes, such as infection, pericarditis, post-operative, pulmonary embolism or hyperthyroidism may not benefit from acute DCCV whilst the exacerbating factor is still present, unless there is haemodynamic compromise, due to the increased chance of recurrence or failure.

Further reading

Page RL, Joglar JA, Caldwell MA, *et al.* (2016) 2015 ACC/AHA/HRS guideline for the management of adult patients with supraventricular tachycardia: a report of the American College of Cardiology/American Heart Association Task Force on Clinical Practice Guidelines and the Heart Rhythm Society. *J Am Coll Cardiol* 67, e27–115.

The Task Force for the management of patients with ventricular arrhythmias and the prevention of sudden cardiac death of the European Society of Cardiology (ESC) (2015) 2015 ESC Guidelines for the management of patients with ventricular arrhythmias and the prevention of sudden cardiac death. *Eur Heart J* 36, 2793–2867. DOI: 10.1093/eurheartj/ehv316

The Task Force for the management of atrial fibrillation of the European Society of Cardiology (ESC) (2016). 2016 ESC Guidelines for the management of atrial fibrillation developed in collaboration with EACTS. *European Heart Journal*. Published online 27 August 2016. Add citation at proof stage.

CHAPTER 122

Insertion of an intercostal chest drain

JOHN CORCORAN

Indications, contraindications and potential complications of intercostal chest drain (ICD) insertion are summarized in Table 122.1. One assistant is required to monitor the patient and assist with the equipment (Table 122.2).

- You should only insert an intercostal chest drain (ICD) if you have received appropriate training or are being supervised by someone who has been appropriately trained. ICD insertion is potentially associated with significant morbidity and even mortality.
- Whenever possible, the decision to place an ICD, and the type of drain to be used, should be discussed with a chest physician or thoracic surgeon.
- Many patients with symptomatic pleural disease should be managed without an ICD. Often, simple pleural aspiration (thoracocentesis) will suffice and allow the patient to be managed as an outpatient or day case.
- Pleural interventions, including intercostal chest drain (ICD) insertion, should not be performed out of hours unless it is a clinical emergency (i.e. a patient with significant physiological compromise and/or symptoms). If an out-of-hours intervention is necessary, it is worth considering whether thoracocentesis will provide adequate treatment and be safer than insertion of an ICD.
- Pleural interventions should be performed using full aseptic technique in a dedicated clean room (e.g. procedural suite, operating theatre) to reduce the risk of iatrogenic infection. A procedure should only be performed at the bedside in a clinical emergency when it is unsafe to move the patient elsewhere.
- Informed written consent should be taken from all patients undergoing any pleural intervention, including ICD insertion, unless it is a clinical emergency and the planned treatment may be lifesaving.
- The use of thoracic ultrasonography is strongly recommended. The marking of a site remotely for subsequent thoracocentesis or chest drain insertion in a separate clinical area (e.g. 'X marks the spot' in radiology, prior to chest drain insertion on a medical ward) is not recommended, as it can provide false reassurance and is no more accurate than a 'blind' intervention.
- There is no evidence to support the routine use of thoracic ultrasonography prior to pleural intervention for a pneumothorax. The operator should utilize an anatomical landmark technique (i.e. 'triangle of safety' for ICD insertion, Figure 122.1).

Technique

Preparation

1 Confirm the indications for the procedure. Review the relevant imaging (e.g. chest X-ray) and if appropriate perform thoracic ultrasonography to define the location and anatomy of the effusion.
   Explain the procedure to the patient and obtain written consent where possible (see above).
2 Assemble the equipment, including an appropriately sized chest tube, and ensure that any connections fit, for example for the underwater seal (Figure 122.2).

Acute Medicine: A Practical Guide to the Management of Medical Emergencies, Fifth Edition. Edited by David Sprigings and John B. Chambers.
© 2018 John Wiley & Sons Ltd. Published 2018 by John Wiley & Sons Ltd.

Table 122.1 Insertion of a chest drain: indications, contraindications and potential complications.

Indications

Pneumothorax (see Chapter 64). Chest drain insertion is indicated as the first-line intervention for:

- Pneumothorax in any ventilated patient
- Tension pneumothorax (following on from initial needle decompression)
- Large symptomatic spontaneous secondary pneumothorax
- Large symptomatic recurrent or persistent pneumothorax (following thoracocentesis)

Consider thoracocentesis as the first-line intervention in:

- Symptomatic spontaneous primary pneumothorax of any size
- Small symptomatic spontaneous secondary pneumothorax in patients under 50 years

Pleural effusion (see Chapter 12). Chest drain insertion is indicated as the first-line intervention for:

- Pleural infection, that is, complicated parapneumonic effusion or empyema (following diagnostic thoracocentesis)
- Symptomatic malignant pleural effusion where the intention is to perform a subsequent pleurodesis
- Traumatic haemothorax

Consider thoracocentesis as the first-line intervention in:

- Pleural effusion of unknown cause, for diagnostic purposes (small volume thoracocentesis, that is, usually between 20 and 50 mL pleural fluid)
- Large symptomatic pleural effusion for therapeutic purposes (large volume thoracocentesis, that is, usually up to 1.5L pleural fluid depending on patient's symptoms)

Contraindications

Uncertain diagnosis (e.g. emphysematous bulla misdiagnosed as pneumothorax; elevated hemidiaphragm, lung collapse or lung consolidation misdiagnosed as pleural effusion).

Evidence of lung adherent to the chest wall on imaging studies.

Coagulopathy including INR (international normalized ratio) >1.5, platelet count $<50 \times 10^9$/L, recent use of thrombolytic or anticoagulant therapy; any concerns should prompt discussion with a haematologist before going ahead with the procedure.

Potential complications

Failure of treatment

Pain

Malposition of the ICD

Damage to viscera

Bleeding, including from intercostal vessels, during or following ICD insertion

Infection (wound or intrapleural) following ICD insertion

Drain dislodgement or blockage following ICD insertion

Re-expansion pulmonary oedema following ICD insertion and re-expansion of the collapsed lung

3 Connect the patient to appropriate monitoring, including ECG, blood pressure and pulse oximetry. Give supplemental oxygen via nasal cannulae or a mask if indicated. Ensure the patient has venous access (e.g. peripheral cannula).

4 Consider pre-medication with either an opioid analgesic (e.g. morphine 2.5 mg IV) or an anxiolytic (e.g. midazolam 1–2 mg IV), taking care particularly in patients who are elderly and/or at particular risk of respiratory compromise (e.g. chronic obstructive pulmonary disease). Reversal agents (i.e. naloxone or flumazenil) should be immediately available if required.

5 Ensure the patient is comfortable and in a position (Figure 122.3) that allows access to the site where the chest drain is to be inserted. This will usually be within the 'triangle of safety' (Figure 122.1).

6 Put on a surgical hat, mask, gown and gloves. Prepare the skin with chlorhexidine or povidone-iodine and apply drapes.

Table 122.2 Insertion of a chest drain: equipment needed.

Surgical hat and mask
Sterile gloves and gown
Antiseptic solution for skin preparation (e.g. chlorhexidine in alcohol)
Sterile drapes
Sterile gauze swabs
Local anaesthetic (1% lidocaine)
Appropriate syringes and needles (18–25 G)
Sutures and dressings to secure the chest drain
Scalpel/surgical blade
Closed drainage system (e.g. connecting tubing, sterile water and kit for underwater seal)
Chest tube of appropriate size (see below) with equipment for insertion using either Seldinger technique or blunt dissection:
- Small-bore chest drains (8–14 French) are sufficient for most pleural conditions (including pleural infection, free-flowing pleural effusion and pneumothorax) and are associated with a lower risk of complications.
- Large-bore chest drains (>14 French) are specifically indicated in the context of, for example trauma and haemothorax, and may be useful in cases where the initial use of a small-bore drain has been unsuccessful.

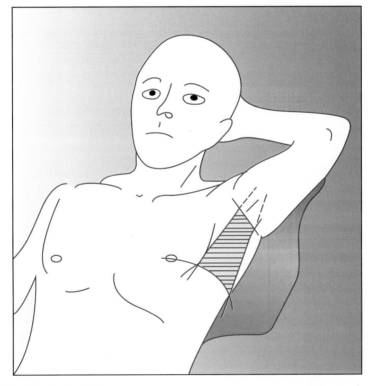

Figure 122.1 The 'triangle of safety'.
The triangle of safety is bordered anteriorly by the lateral edge of pectoralis major, laterally by the lateral edge of latissimus dorsi, inferiorly by the line of the fifth intercostal space and superiorly by the base of the axilla.
Source: BTS Pleural Disease Guidelines (2010) *Thorax* 65 (Suppl. II), ii61–76. Reproduced with permission of BMJ Publishing Ltd.

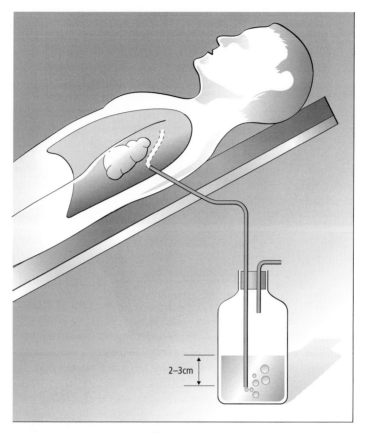

Figure 122.2 Intercostal chest drain attached to underwater seal.

The end of the tube is 2–3 cm below the level of the water in the bottle. If intrapleural pressure becomes negative, water rises up the tube, only to fall again when the intrapleural pressure falls towards atmospheric. The system operates as a simple one-way valve, allowing either air or fluid within the pleural space to drain out safely. Once a pneumothorax or effusion has resolved, the water level will generally be slightly negative throughout the respiratory cycle and reflect the normal fluctuation in intrapleural pressure. (Adapted from Brewis RAL (1985) *Lecture Notes on Respiratory Diseases*, 3rd edn. Oxford: Blackwell Scientific Publications, p. 290.)

7 Draw up 20 mL of 1% lidocaine. Generous use of local anaesthetic (up to 3 mg/kg lidocaine), focusing on highly innervated areas such as the skin, periosteum and parietal pleura will reduce the risk of patient discomfort during the procedure. Infiltrate the skin with 3–4 mL using a 25 G (orange) needle, then change to a 18 G (green) needle in order to infiltrate the subcutaneous tissues.

8 Advance the needle into the thorax (passing just superiorly to the lower rib of the intercostal space) until air or fluid is aspirated, then withdraw slightly in order to infiltrate 5 mL at the parietal pleural surface. Withdraw the needle completely, infiltrating a further 5–10 mL in and around the needle track as you withdraw. If you have been unable to freely aspirate air or fluid from the pleural space, do not proceed further at this site and seek advice from a senior colleague.

Seldinger technique

9 Advance the introducer needle mounted on a 10 mL syringe into the pleural space (again, passing just superiorly to the lower rib of the intercostal space) and confirm free aspiration of air or effusion. Pass the

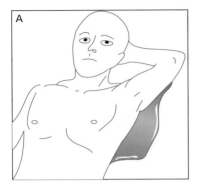
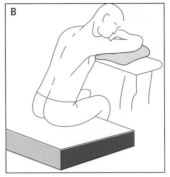
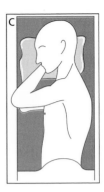

Figure 122.3 Common patient positions for chest drain insertion.
(A) Semi-reclined with hand behind head. (B) Sitting up leaning over a table with padding. (C) Lateral decubitus position.
Source: From BTS Pleural Disease Guidelines (2010) *Thorax* 65 (Suppl. II), ii61–76. Reproduced with permission of BMJ Publishing Ltd.

guidewire, J end first, through the needle into the pleural space; ideally, this should be directed apically for a pneumothorax or posterobasally for an effusion.

10 Remove the needle and then pass the dilator(s) over the guidewire to dilate a track for the chest tube. A small incision (5 mm) may be needed initially to help with passing the dilator through the skin and subcutaneous tissue. Always keep hold of the distal end of the guidewire, and do not insert the dilator any further into the chest than is necessary to breach the parietal pleural surface.

11 Pass the chest tube over the guidewire into the pleural space. In an adult of normal size, around 15 cm of drain will usually lie within the chest. The depth to which a chest tube is inserted is determined by the need to ensure the side holes on the tube are well within the chest, otherwise subcutaneous emphysema will result. Remove the guidewire and any stiffening device/dilator used to help introduce the chest tube, leaving the tube itself in place.

12 Attach the underwater seal bottle to the chest tube.

13 Secure the chest tube in position using a non-absorbable 1/0 suture passed through the adjacent skin and subcutaneous tissues and then wrapped and tied several times around the tube (Figure 122.4). Place a pad of gauze between the patient's skin and the tube, then further anchor the tube to the chest wall using tape or other adhesive dressing.

Blunt dissection technique

The use of small-bore drains (8–14 French) inserted with a Seldinger technique is now the most common mode of chest drain insertion, and is sufficient for most effusions and pneumothoraces. Large-bore drains (>14 French) inserted with a blunt dissection technique are used less frequently than before, but are still seen in emergency trauma or thoracic surgical cases.

9a Make a 1 cm incision with a scalpel in line with and just above the edge of the lower rib of the intercostal space. Place two interrupted 3/0 non-absorbable sutures across the incision. These should be left loose so the tube can pass, and will be tied when the tube is removed. Place a separate 1/0 non-absorbable suture through the skin and subcutaneous tissues above the incision, which will be used to anchor the chest tube later (Figure 122.4).

10a Using a Spencer Wells or similar straight forceps, enlarge the track down to and through the pleura so that the tube will pass with a snug fit. Note that the forceps should always be removed in an open position during the process of blunt dissection to prevent accidental avulsion of any structures, for example blood vessels.

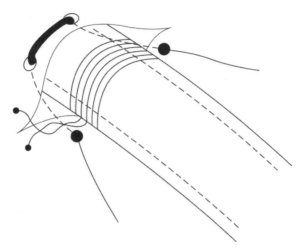

Figure 122.4 Stay and closing sutures for a chest drain. Source: BTS Pleural Disease Guidelines (2003) *Thorax* 58 (Suppl. II), ii53–9. Reproduced with permission of BMJ Publishing Ltd.

Once a track has been created, this should be explored with a finger to ensure there are no underlying organs that might be damaged during subsequent chest tube insertion.

11a Remove the chest tube from any trocar (a trocar should never be used to guide a chest tube due to the high risk of damaging underlying structures) and, holding the tip of the tube with the forceps, gently pass the tube into the pleural space. The tube should ideally be directed apically for a pneumothorax and posterobasally for an effusion. In an adult of normal size, around 15 cm of the chest tube will usually lie within the chest. The tube must be inserted far enough so that the side holes are well within the chest, otherwise subcutaneous emphysema will result. Excessive force should never be required during drain insertion – if the tube does not pass easily then withdraw and seek advice from a senior colleague.

12a Attach the underwater seal bottle to the chest tube.

13a Secure the chest tube in position with the 1/0 suture wrapped and tied several times around it. Place a pad of gauze between the patient's skin and the tube, then further anchor the tube to the chest wall using tape or other adhesive dressing.

Final points

14 Remove the drapes and ensure the patient is able to sit up comfortably. Check that the chest tube is well anchored, all connections are secure and the dressings are satisfactory. Clear up and dispose of all sharps safely. Arrange a chest X-ray to check the position of the chest tube. The procedure should be fully documented in the patient's record, including as a minimum: indications; approach; chest tube size; technique used; pre-medication and local anaesthetic used; any complications; post-procedure chest X-ray findings; further management plan.

15 Ensure that the patient has regular analgesia prescribed whilst the chest drain remains in situ; assuming no contraindications this should include regular paracetamol (1 g four times daily) and non-steroidal anti-inflammatory drugs as a minimum. Opioid analgesia may also be necessary on a regular or as required basis; this should be reviewed daily to ensure the patient is pain free.

Aftercare

16 Small-bore drains (8–14 French) require regular flushing (e.g. 20 mL normal saline three times daily) to prevent them becoming blocked.

17 If draining a pleural effusion, no more than 1.5 L should be drained in the first hour. After one hour, the rest of the fluid may be drained slowly (e.g. a further 1.0 L every 2–3 h) as clinically indicated. Controlling the rate and volume of fluid drainage in this way is necessary to reduce the risk of causing re-expansion pulmonary oedema. Drainage of fluid should also be stopped immediately if the patient develops worsening cough, chest pain or breathlessness. These symptoms may indicate the presence of unexpandable lung, or predict an increased risk of developing re-expansion pulmonary oedema. Further medical assessment should occur before drainage of fluid is started again.

18 If draining a pneumothorax, the chest tube should never be clamped as long as it continues to bubble, due to the risk of potentially causing a tension pneumothorax. A chest X-ray should be repeated 24 h after chest tube insertion to assess for re-expansion of the lung.
   - If the lung has re-expanded fully and the chest tube/underwater seal is no longer bubbling when the patient breathes and coughs forcefully, then this implies resolution of the pneumothorax with no ongoing air leak. It may therefore be appropriate to remove the chest tube in discussion with a chest physician or thoracic surgeon.
   - If the lung has not re-expanded fully and/or the chest tube/underwater seal continues to bubble when the patient breathes and/or coughs forcefully, then this implies a continued air leak. In these circumstances it may be appropriate to apply low-pressure, high-volume suction (e.g. using a Vernon-Thompson pump) via the underwater seal at a level of 10–20 cm H_2O. This decision should be made by an experienced specialist clinician, that is, a chest physician or thoracic surgeon.

19 When removing a chest drain, consider pre-medication with an opioid analgesic. Remove the dressings, then cut and remove the suture which has anchored the drain. The drain should be briskly withdrawn while the patient performs a Valsalva manoeuvre or during expiration. An assistant should apply a gauze swab to the drain site immediately after removal. Small-bore drains inserted using a Seldinger technique do not usually require a suture to close the incision at the insertion site and a simple sterile adhesive dressing will suffice. For large-bore drains inserted using blunt dissection, the two interrupted 3/0 sutures should be tied to close the incision before covering with a simple sterile adhesive dressing. These closing sutures should be removed after one week.

20 The patient should have specialist follow-up with either a chest physician or thoracic surgeon, ideally within two weeks of discharge from hospital and with a repeat chest X-ray taken prior to the appointment.

Troubleshooting

Pain
- Pain around the site of chest drain insertion is common post-procedure and should be managed with regular analgesia (see above).
- If the pain is distant to the insertion site (e.g. referring to the ipsilateral shoulder) this may relate to the drain tip position. A chest X-ray should be reviewed and if appropriate (e.g. chest tube tip seen to lie against the mediastinum) the tube should be withdrawn slightly.

Fluid level in underwater seal does not move with breathing (not 'swinging')
- Check for kinking of the tube, usually seen due to angulation of the ribs where the tube enters the chest, and if necessary release the dressings or withdraw the tube slightly.
- Small-bore chest tubes should be flushed regularly as part of routine aftercare (see above) to prevent blockage. Occasionally it may be appropriate to replace a small-bore chest tube that has become blocked with a larger tube, although this should be discussed with a specialist beforehand.
- The drain may be in the wrong position or dislodged – this can be confirmed on either chest X-ray or clinical assessment (e.g. drainage holes may be partially or wholly extrapleural), in which case the tube should be removed and replaced with another if clinically necessary.

Surgical emphysema
- It is normal to have a small amount of localized subcutaneous air at the drain insertion site.
- Increasing surgical emphysema may indicate malposition of the tube with a drainage hole in a subcutaneous position; if so, a new tube must be inserted.

Non-resolving pneumothorax
- This may present as failure of the lung to re-expand following chest tube insertion and/or continued bubbling from the chest tube/underwater seal. Assuming the chest tube is well positioned and patent, this indicates an ongoing air leak from the underlying lung parenchyma.
- Some cases may resolve with application of suction (see above), but all patients with a non-resolving pneumothorax should be discussed with an appropriate specialist (chest physician or thoracic surgeon).

Further reading

BTS Pleural Disease Guideline 2010 British Thoracic Society Pleural Disease Guideline Group: a sub-group of the British Thoracic Society Standards of Care Committee https://www.brit-thoracic.org.uk/document-library/clinical-information/pleural-disease/pleural-disease-guidelines-2010/pleural-disease-guideline/.

Corcoran JP, Hallifax RJ, Talwar A, *et al.* (2015) Intercostal chest drain insertion by general physicians: attitudes, experience and implications for training, service and patient safety. *Postgrad Med J* 91, 244–250.

CHAPTER 123

Lumbar puncture

KANNAN NITHI

Indications, contraindications and complications of lumbar puncture are summarized in Table 123.1. You will need one assistant to monitor the patient during the procedure and assist with the equipment (Table 123.2).

Technique (Figures 123.1 and 123.2)

Preparation

1 Confirm the indications for the procedure and check there are no contraindications. Explain the procedure to the patient and obtain written consent.

2 Move the patient to the edge of the bed on the left side if you are right handed (Figure 123.1) The thoracolumbar spine should be maximally flexed, that is, knees and hips flexed as much as possible. It does not matter if the neck is not flexed. Place a pillow between the knees to prevent torsion of the spine.

3 Define the plane of the iliac crests, which runs through L3/L4. The spinal cord in the adult ends at the level of L1/L2. Choose either the L3/L4 or L4/L5 spaces. Mark the space using your thumbnail or an indelible marker.

4 Put on gloves. Prepare the skin with chlorhexidine over the intended puncture site and surrounding area, and apply a drape. It helps to place an additional drape on top of the patient so that you can recheck the position of the iliac crest if necessary.

5 Draw up lidocaine 1%, assemble the manometer and undo the tops of the bottles. Check that the stylet of the needle moves freely. Place everything within easy reach.

6 Stretch the skin over the chosen space with the finger and thumb of your left hand, placed on the spinous processes of the adjacent vertebrae (Figure 123.2). Put 1–2 mL of lidocaine in the skin and subcutaneous tissues with a 21 G (orange) needle.

Lumbar puncture

7 Place the spinal needle on the mark, bevel uppermost, and advance it towards the umbilicus, taking care to keep it parallel to the ground.

8 The interspinous ligament gives some resistance, and you should notice increased resistance as you go through the tough ligamentum flavum. There is usually an obvious 'give' when the needle is through this. The dura is now only 1–2 mm away. Advance in small steps, withdrawing the stylet after each step.

9 Cerebrospinal fluid (CSF) should flow freely once you enter the dura. If the flow is poor, rotate the needle in case a nerve root is lying against it.

Measuring the opening pressure and collecting CSF

10 Connect the manometer and measure the height of the CSF column (the opening pressure). The patient should uncurl slightly and try to relax at this stage.

Acute Medicine: A Practical Guide to the Management of Medical Emergencies, Fifth Edition. Edited by David Springings and John B. Chambers.
© 2018 John Wiley & Sons Ltd. Published 2018 by John Wiley & Sons Ltd.

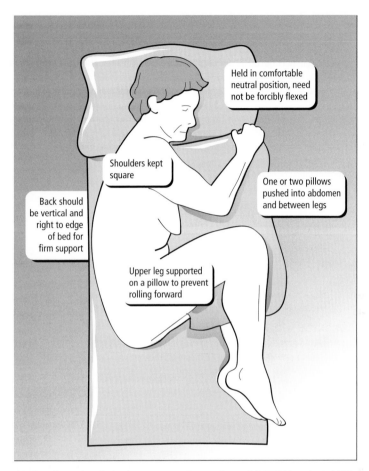

Figure 123.1 Positioning the patient for lumbar puncture. Source: Patten J (1977) *Neurological Differential Diagnosis*. London: Harold Starke, p. 262.

11 Cap the top of the manometer with your finger, disconnect it from the needle and put the CSF in the glucose tube. Collect three samples (about 2 mL each) in the plain sterile bottles.

12 In patients with suspected multiple sclerosis, a fourth sample should be collected, together with a paired serum sample for testing for oligoclonal bands in the immunology laboratory.

13 In suspected idiopathic intracranial hypertension, if the CSF opening pressure is markedly elevated, that is >30 cm, then removal of 20–30 mL CSF may result in temporary improvement of symptoms and help protect optic nerve function.

14 Remove the needle and place a small dressing over the puncture site.

Final points

15 Clear up and dispose of sharps safely. Ensure that the CSF samples are sent promptly to the microbiology laboratory (for red/white cell count, Gram stain, and other tests as indicated: Ziehl-Neelsen stain if suspected tuberculous meningitis, India ink preparation if suspected cryptococcal meningitis; polymerase chain reaction testing for viral DNA if suspected viral meningitis/encephalitis) and biochemistry laboratory (for protein and glucose concentrations, and spectrophotometry of bilirubin if suspected subarachnoid haemorrhage).

Table 123.1 Lumbar puncture: indications, contraindications and potential complications.

Indications

Suspected meningitis. **If you suspect bacterial meningitis take blood cultures and start antibiotic therapy immediately, before lumbar puncture** (Chapter 68).

Suspected encephalitis. **If you suspect viral encephalitis start aciclovir immediately, before lumbar puncture** (Chapter 69).

Suspected subarachnoid haemorrhage. **Wait 12 h from onset of headache before performing lumbar puncture** (Chapter 67).

Suspected idiopathic intracranial hypertension. **Other causes of raised CSF pressure must be excluded first** (Chapter 72).

Suspected Guillain-Barré syndrome (Chapter 71).

Suspected new acute presentation of multiple sclerosis.

Contraindications*

Reduced level of consciousness

Papilloedema

Focal neurological signs

Recent seizure

Bleeding disorder (including platelet count $<50 \times 10^9/l$, INR >1.5, receiving oral anticoagulant or anticoagulant-dose heparin)

Local skin infection

Anatomical abnormality, for example myelomeningocoele

Complications

Post-lumbar puncture headache (reportedly less frequent with atraumatic needle)

Cerebral herniation (can occur in setting of internal CSF pressure gradient)

Nerve root injury causing radicular pain or sensory disturbance

Bleeding causing spinal cord injury

Meningitis due to introduction of infection

* Lumbar puncture may be performed in patients with relative contraindications, but only after obtaining expert advice from a neurologist or neurosurgeon. Normal neuroimaging does not always exclude an internal CSF pressure gradient.

16 Write a note of the procedure in the patient's record, documenting: indications/lumbar interspace used/ needle size/opening pressure/appearance of CSF/samples sent/any complications.

Troubleshooting

You hit bone

Withdraw the needle. Recheck the patient's position and the bony landmarks. Try again, taking particular care to keep the needle parallel to the ground. If this fails, modify the angle of the needle in the sagittal plane.

Table 123.2 Lumbar puncture: equipment needed.

Sterile gloves and surgical mask

Sterile drapes (×2)

Sterile gauze swabs

Antiseptic solution for skin preparation (e.g. chlorhexidine in alcohol)

Small wound dressing

5 mL syringe, 25 G and 21 G needles, 1% lidocaine

Spinal needle (20 or 22 G)

Manometer and three-way tap

Three numbered plain sterile containers (in patients with suspected multiple sclerosis, a fourth sample should be collected, together with a paired serum sample, for testing for oligoclonal bands in the immunology laboratory)

Fluoride tube for glucose (to be sent with blood glucose sample taken before lumbar puncture)

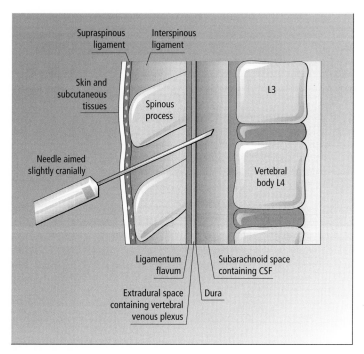

Figure 123.2 Anatomy of lumbar puncture.

If you are still unsuccessful, try another space or ask a colleague for assistance.

Consider placing patient in sitting position: seated on edge of bed, with back arched by leaning over a table or cushion. Accurate pressure measurement cannot be made in this position.

If the patient complains of shooting pains radiating into the legs (indicating that the needle is touching a lateral nerve root) withdraw and reposition the needle less laterally.

You obtain heavily blood-stained fluid

The possibilities are subarachnoid haemorrhage, traumatic tap or puncture of the venous plexus. If the fluid appears to be venous blood (slow ooze), try again in another space, after flushing the needle.

Deteriorating conscious level after lumbar puncture

Seek urgent advice from a neurologist or neurosurgeon. Give mannitol 20% 100–200 mL (0.5 g/kg) IV over 10 min. Check plasma osmolality: further mannitol may be given until plasma osmolality is 320 mosmol/kg.

Arrange transfer to the intensive therapy unit in case intubation and ventilation are needed. If intubated, hyperventilate to an arterial $PaCO_2$ of 4.0 kPa (30 mmHg).

Prolonged post-lumbar puncture headache

Low-pressure headache as a complication of lumbar puncture nearly always resolves spontaneously. Caffeine supplementation has been reported to help. Severe headache lasting longer than two weeks may be treated by an epidural blood patch (placed by an anaesthetist at the level of the original lumbar puncture).

Interpretation of CSF formula

See Tables 123.3 and 123.4.

Table 123.3 Cerebrospinal fluid (CSF): normal values and correction for traumatic tap.

Opening pressure:	7–18 cm CSF
Cell count:	0–5/mm^3, all lymphocytes
Protein concentration:	0.15–0.45 g/L (15–45 mg/dl)
Glucose concentration:	2.8–4.2 mmol/L
CSF: blood glucose ratio	>50%
Correction of cell count and protein concentration in traumatic tap: for every 1000 RBC/mm^3, subtract 1 WBC/mm^3 and 0.015 g/L (1.5 mg/dl) protein	

RBC, red blood cells; WBC, white blood cells.
From Normal reference values. *N Engl J Med* 1986, 314, 39–49. Gottlieb, A.J. *et al.* (1980) *The whole internist catalog.* Philadelphia: WB Saunders, 127–128.

Table 123.4 Cerebrospinal fluid (CSF) formulae in meningitis and encephalitis.

Element	Pyogenic meningitis	Viral meningitis	Tuberculous meningitis	Cryptococcal meningitis	Viral encephalitis
White cell count/mm^3	>1000	<500	<500	<150	<250
Predominant cell type	Polymorphs	Lymphocytes	Lymphocytes	Lymphocytes	Lymphocytes
Protein concentration (g/L)	>1.5	0.5–1.0	1.0–5.0	0.5–1.0	0.5–1.0
CSF: blood glucose	<50%	>50%	<50%	<50%	>50%

- The values given are typical, but many exceptions occur
- Red cells may be seen in the CSF in herpes encephalitis, reflecting cerebral necrosis
- Antibiotic therapy substantially changes the CSF formula in pyogenic bacterial meningitis, leading to a fall in cell count, increased proportion of lymphocytes and fall in protein level. However, the low CSF glucose level usually persists.

Subarachnoid haemorrhage

The definitive CSF test is identification by spectrophotometry of bilirubin (a breakdown product of haemoglobin). This is more accurate than visual analysis for xanthochromia or estimating the number of red blood cells in the first and third bottles collected. The lumbar puncture should be delayed for 12 h from the onset of the headache to allow for red blood cell breakdown. Evidence of subarachnoid haemorrhage may be present in CSF up to two weeks after the onset.

Guillain-Barré syndrome

CSF analysis is typically normal except for raised protein.

Multiple sclerosis

The CSF typically shows a raised white cell count (<50/mm^3) during acute presentation and positive oligoclonal bands (with no bands in serum sample).

Further reading

Doherty CM, Forbes RB. (2014) Diagnostic lumbar puncture. *Ulster Med J* 83, 93–102.
Wright BLC, Lai JTF, Sinclair AJ. (2012) Cerebrospinal fluid and lumbar puncture: a practical review. *J Neurol* 259, 1530–1545. DOI: 10.1007/s00415-012-6413-x

CHAPTER 124

Aspiration of the knee joint

KEHINDE SUNMBOYE

Indications, contraindications and potential complications are summarized in Table 124.1. If you are not familiar with joint aspiration, ask the help of a rheumatologist or orthopaedic surgeon.

Technique

1 Confirm the indications for joint aspiration. Explain the procedure to the patient and obtain consent. Verbal consent is sufficient.

2 The patient should lie down with the knee slightly flexed. The knee joint can be aspirated from the medial or lateral side. The needle should pass from a skin entry point 1 cm medial or lateral to the superior, middle or inferior third of the patella (see Figure 124.1). Points marked with X medially and laterally are the preferred entry sites due to the proximity to the suprapatellar pouch where effusions usually accumulate. Check the bony landmarks and mark the skin entry point with the tip of the needle cover.

3 Put on gloves. Prepare the skin with chlorhexidine or povidone-iodine. Anaesthetize the skin with 2 mL of lidocaine 1% using a 25 G (orange) needle. Then infiltrate a further 5 mL of lidocaine along the planned needle path.

Table 124.1 Aspiration of a knee joint: indications, contraindications and potential complications.

Indications
To confirm or exclude septic arthritis
To establish the diagnosis in acute mono- or polyarthritis
To relieve symptoms from a tense effusion by draining the joint

Contraindications
Cellulitis of overlying skin
Bleeding disorder (including platelet count $<50 \times 10^9$/L, INR >2 or receiving anticoagulant-dose heparin). Liaise with haematologist as indicated.

Potential complications
Introduction of infection: rarely occurs (<1/10,000) with appropriate sterile technique
Bleeding into the joint in patients with bleeding disorder
Cartilage injury

INR, international normalized ratio.

Acute Medicine: A Practical Guide to the Management of Medical Emergencies, Fifth Edition. Edited by David Sprigings and John B. Chambers.
© 2018 John Wiley & Sons Ltd. Published 2018 by John Wiley & Sons Ltd.

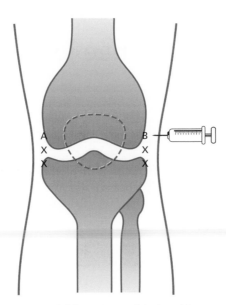

Figure 124.1 Points of needle entry (marked X) for aspiration of the knee joint.

4 Give the local anaesthetic time to work. Mount a 21 G (green) needle on a 20 mL syringe and then advance along the anaesthetized path, directing the needle perpendicularly behind the patella. Aspirate as you advance.

5 When you enter the effusion, hold the needle steady and aspirate to dryness (two syringes may be needed if the effusion is large). Remove the needle and place a small dressing over the puncture site. Send samples of the effusion for analysis: ethylene diaminetetra-acetic acid (EDTA) tube for white cell count; plain sterile container for Gram stain and culture; plain sterile container for microscopy for crystals.

6 Clear up and dispose of sharps safely. Write a note of the procedure in the patient's record: approach/appearance of synovial fluid/volume aspirated/samples sent. Ensure the samples are sent promptly for analysis.

Troubleshooting
Dry tap
- This may be due to misdiagnosis of effusion, or obesity with resulting difficulty in accurately identifying the bony landmarks.
- Try again from the lateral approach if the medial approach was used, and vice versa.
- If you still cannot obtain fluid, and septic arthritis needs to be excluded, use ultrasound to confirm the presence of the effusion and identify the appropriate puncture site and depth of needle insertion.

Interpreting the results

See Table 124.2.

Table 124.2 Findings on analysis of synovial fluid.

Classification of effusion	Features	White cell count	Causes
Normal synovial fluid	Clear colourless, viscus	<200/mm^3 <25% polymorphs	
Non-inflammatory	Cloudy, yellow, viscus	200–2000/mm^3 <25% polymorphs	Common: • Osteoarthritis • Trauma Uncommon: • Early or subsiding inflammation, Osteochrondritis dissecans • Neuropathic arthropathy, • Pigmented villonodular synovitis
Inflammatory	Cloudy, yellow, watery	2000–100,000/mm^3 >50% polymorphs	Common: • Rheumatoid arthritis • Crystal arthropathies • Psoriatic arthritis Uncommon: • Reiter syndrome • Ankylosing spondylitis • Arthritis associated with inflammatory bowel disease • Rheumatic fever • Systemic lupus erythematosus • Hypertrophic osteoarthropathy • Scleroderma
Septic	Purulent	>80,000/mm^3 >75% polymorphs	Common: • Bacterial • Mycobacterial Uncommon: • Fungal

Further reading

Roberts WN Jr. Joint aspiration or injection in adults: Technique and indications. UpToDate. Topic last updated February 2016. https://www.uptodate.com/contents/joint-aspiration-or-injection-in-adults-technique-and-indications?source=search_result&search=joint%20aspiration&selectedTitle=1~108.

CHAPTER 125

Insertion of a Sengstaken-Blakemore tube

Ben Warner and Mark Wilkinson

Indications, contraindications and potential complications of insertion of a Sengstaken-Blakemore tube are given in Table 125.1.

- Sengstaken-Blakemore tubes should only be inserted by those who are competent at placing them because of the risks of oesophageal perforation. They are usually inserted at the time of the endoscopy, if variceal bleeding cannot be controlled.
- See Table 125.2 for equipment needed for placement.

Technique

Preparation

1 If the patient has a reduced conscious level (grade 2 encephalopathy or more), endotracheal intubation should be done by an anaesthetist before insertion of the tube to prevent misplacement of the tube in the trachea or inhalation of blood.

2 If the patient has a normal conscious level, explain the procedure and obtain consent. Give supplemental oxygen via nasal cannulae, with monitoring of oxygen saturation by oximetry. Attach an ECG monitor. Sedation with midazolam can be given but only if an anaesthetist is available in case endotracheal intubation becomes necessary.

3 Put on apron, mask and gloves. Check the suction equipment works. Anaesthetize the patient's throat with lidocaine spray.

Placement of the tube

4 Ideally, the tube should be kept in the fridge beforehand so as to stiffen the tubing ready for easier insertion. Lubricate the end of the tube with KY jelly and pass it through the gap between your index and middle fingers placed on the tongue: this reduces the chance of the tube curling. Ask the patient to breathe quietly through his or her mouth throughout the procedure. Steadily advance the tube until it is inserted to the hilt. An assistant should aspirate blood from the mouth and from all lumens while you insert the tube.

5 If at any stage of the procedure the patient becomes dyspnoeic, withdraw the tube immediately and start again after endotracheal intubation.

6 Inflate the gastric balloon with the water/contrast mixture (310 mL). Insert a bung or clamp the tube. If there is resistance to inflation, deflate the balloon and check the position of the tube with X-ray screening. Pull the tube back gently until resistance is felt.

7 Never inflate the oesophageal balloon unless trained in the reasons to do so.

Acute Medicine: A Practical Guide to the Management of Medical Emergencies, Fifth Edition. Edited by David Springings and John B. Chambers.
© 2018 John Wiley & Sons Ltd. Published 2018 by John Wiley & Sons Ltd.

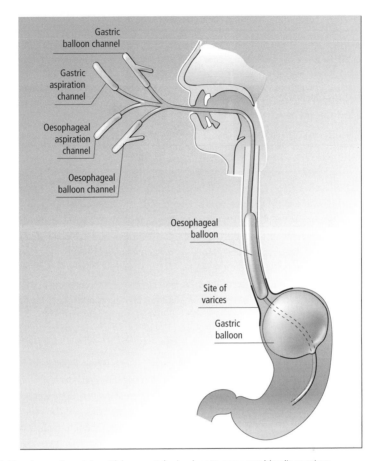

Figure 125.1 Four-lumen Sengstaken-Blakemore tube in place to compress bleeding varices.
Source: Thompson R (1985) *Lecture Notes on the Liver*. Oxford: Blackwell Scientific Publications. p. 37.

Table 125.1 Insertion of a Sengstaken-Blakemore tube: indications, contraindications and potential complications.

Indications
Failure to control variceal bleeding endoscopically (endoscopy is first-line management for patients with variceal bleeding. Senstaken-Blakemore tubes can be inserted at the same time as endoscopy under direct vision).

Contraindications
If the patient has a reduced conscious level (grade 2 encephalopathy or more), endotracheal intubation should be done by an anaesthetist before insertion of the tube to prevent misplacement of the tube in the trachea or inhalation of blood.

Potential complications
Inhalation of blood and secretions causing respiratory failure/pneumonia
Placement of tube in trachea causing respiratory failure
Oesophageal rupture due to inflation of gastric balloon in the oesophagus
Mucosal ulceration after placement of balloon

Table 125.2 Insertion of a Sengstaken-Blakemore tube: equipment needed.

Sengstaken-Blakemore tube (Figure 125.1). If this has only three lumens, tape a standard medium-bore nasogastric tube with the perforations just above the oesophageal balloon to allow aspiration of the oesophagus. The lumens of the tube are not always labelled; if not, label them now with tape.
Water (300 mL) for inflation of gastric balloon (with 10 mL of contrast medium (e.g. Gastrografin) added so you can see where it is); the balloon is less likely to deflate (with consequent displacement) if water is used rather than air (400 mL).
Bladder syringe for aspirating the oesophageal drainage tube.
Suction equipment.

8 Firm traction on the gastric balloon is usually sufficient to stop the bleeding since this occurs at the filling point of the varices in the lower few centimetres of the oesophagus.
9 Place a sponge pad (as used to support endotracheal tubes in ventilated patients) over the side of the patient's mouth to prevent the tube rubbing. Strap the tube to the cheek. Fixation with weights over the end of the bed is less effective, and may lead to displacement, especially in agitated patients. Mark the tube in relation to the teeth so that movement can be detected more easily.
10 Obtain a chest X-ray to check the position of the tube. Write a note of the procedure in the patient's record, documenting: monitoring/sedation if given/any complications/post-procedure chest X-ray findings/plan of management.

Aftercare
11 Continue terlipressin infusion and other supportive therapy (Chapter 77). If facilities for variceal injection/banding are available, the tube should be removed in the endoscopy suite immediately before this, which can be done as soon as the patient is haemodynamically stable (and usually within 12 h). If endoscopic therapy is not possible, discuss the case with the regional liver unit and arrange transfer if appropriate. Alternatively, start planning for oesophageal transection within 24 h if bleeding recurs when the balloon is deflated.
12 Do not leave the tube in for longer than 24 h because of the risk of mucosal ulceration. Changing the side of the attachment to the cheek every 2 h reduces the risk of skin ulceration, but should be done carefully because of the risk of displacement.

Further reading

Bajaj JS, Sanyal AJ. Methods to achieve hemostasis in patients with acute variceal hemorrhage UpToDate. Topic last updated November 2015. https://www.uptodate.com/contents/methods-to-achieve-hemostasis-in-patients-with-acute-variceal-hemorrhage?source=search_result&search=Sengstaken&selectedTitle=1~6.
Tripathi DJ, Stanley AJ, Hayes PC (2015) UK guidelines on the management of variceal haemorrhage in cirrhotic patients. *Gut* 0, 1–25. DOI: 10.1136/gutjnl-2015-309262.

Index

abbreviated mental test score, delirium 24, 26, 32
ABCDE protocol 2–8, 10–13, 16–22, 24–7, 36–9, 40–5,
    46–52, 68–71, 103–7, 114–15, 119–22, 289–91, 322,
    396–8, 413, 416, 419, 442, 534–6, 540, 615, 620–2
abcixamab 599
abdomen 7, 133–6, 138–43, 144–9, 150–4, 157–9, 205–6,
    211–14, 349, 352, 356, 462–6, 469–70, 481–6, 495–8,
    514–17, 518–20, 562–5, 587–8, 601–4, 610–11, 624,
    652–4, 655, 663–4
    see also ascites
abdominal aortic aneurysm 7, 9–11, 138–42
abdominal pain 7, 133–6, 138–43, 144–9, 150–4, 157–9,
    205–6, 211–14, 462–6, 469–70, 481–6, 495–8,
    514–17, 518–20, 562–5, 587–8, 610–11, 624, 652–3
    see also bowel obstructions; gastrointestinal system;
    pancreatitis; peritonitis; ruptured abdominal aortic
    aneurysm
    assessment 138–42, 144, 150–3, 157–9, 205–6, 211–12,
    214
    background 133, 138–43, 144–9, 150–4, 157–9, 205–6,
    211–14
    causes 138–42, 150–3, 157–9, 214
    examination 140–1
    management flowchart 134, 138
abdominal scans, ultrasound-guided approach 652, 653–4,
    655
abdominal tenderness/guarding 7, 25–6, 133–6, 138–42,
    144, 150–4, 157–9, 226, 227, 229, 462–6, 479
abdominal thrusts, upper airway obstruction 372–6
abnormal voice, breathlessness 68–72
abscesses 89–90, 100–2, 106–8, 210, 226, 227, 288, 333–8,
    392, 423, 426, 428, 433, 443–5, 506, 659–64
ACE-inhibitors 87, 115, 122, 155–7, 163–8, 179–82,
    255, 297, 314–16, 351–2, 503–7, 511–12, 627–31
acetylcysteine 238, 241, 242–5, 468, 554
acid-base disorders 4–8, 246–51, 495–8, 510–12, 514–17,
    518–20, 646–50, 674, 677–80
    see also acidosis; alkalosis; *individual disorders*
    background 246–51, 495–8, 510–12, 677–80
    causes 249–51
    classification 246, 247–8
    consequences 246, 249
    metabolic compensation 246

severity gradings 246, 248
acidity of arterial blood 246, 247
acidosis 4–8, 9–15, 72, 73–8, 103–8, 166–8, 213–14,
    230–1, 235–8, 239–40, 247–51, 384–9, 492–4,
    495–8, 511–12, 522–4, 573–6, 616–18, 646–50,
    677–80
    see also ketoacidosis; metabolic . . . ; respiratory . . . ;
    shock
acids 239, 241–5, 246–51
acitretin 549–54
acquired angioedema (AAE) 179–82
acromegaly 515–17, 522–4, 538–9
activated charcoal 234, 238–9, 241, 242–5, 599
activated partial thromboplastin time (APTT) 202–6, 360–5,
    471, 578–83, 586–8, 590–9
active bleeding, heart valve disease 331–2
Actrapid insulin 510–12
acute adrenal insufficiency 11–15, 22, 135–6, 525–9,
    574
    assessment 11–13, 22, 135, 525–9, 574
    causes 525, 526, 528–9
    definition 525
    drug therapy 528–9
    mortality rates 528
acute aortic syndromes 321–7
    see also aortic dissection
acute arrhythmias 4–8, 11–15, 61–6, 259–62, 264, 294–7,
    317–19, 366–70, 381, 397, 606–11, 617–18, 685,
    692–5
    see also arrhythmias
    assessments 4–7, 11–13, 14–15, 61–3, 259–61,
    685
    differential diagnosis 259, 261
acute arthritis 183–6, 191–3, 226, 227, 229, 232, 546,
    555–7, 709–11
    see also arthritis
    assessment 183–6, 191–3, 709–11
    causes 183–4, 186
    examination 185
    management flowchart 184
    sepsis 226, 227, 229, 232
acute cholangitis 28, 152–4, 478–80
acute circulatory collapse 525–9

Acute Medicine: A Practical Guide to the Management of Medical Emergencies, Fifth Edition. Edited by
David Sprigings and John B. Chambers.
© 2018 John Wiley & Sons Ltd. Published 2018 by John Wiley & Sons Ltd.

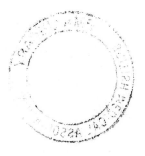